Nursing and COVID-19 II

Nursing and COVID-19 II

Nursing and COVID-19 II

Editors

Richard Gray
Sonia Udod

MDPI

Basel • Beijing • Wuhan • Barcelona • Belgrade • Novi Sad • Cluj • Manchester

Editors

Richard Gray
La Trobe University
Melbourne
Australia

Sonia Udod
University of Manitoba Winnipeg
Winnipeg
Canada

Editorial Office
MDPI
St. Alban-Anlage 66
4052 Basel, Switzerland

This is a reprint of articles from the Special Issue published online in the open access journal *International Journal of Environmental Research and Public Health* (ISSN 1660-4601) (available at: https://www.mdpi.com/journal/ijerph/special_issues/Nursing_Covid).

For citation purposes, cite each article independently as indicated on the article page online and as indicated below:

Lastname, A.A.; Lastname, B.B. Article Title. *Journal Name* **Year**, *Volume Number*, Page Range.

ISBN 978-3-0365-9194-0 (Hbk)
ISBN 978-3-0365-9195-7 (PDF)
doi.org/10.3390/books978-3-0365-9195-7

Contents

About the Editors

Richard Gray

Professor Richard Gray has been working at La Trobe University since 2017, becoming Theme Lead (Healthy Peoples Families and Communities) in 2021. He provides research leadership across La Trobe University, with an overall responsibility over the research theme of "Healthy People Families and Communities", facilitating research and industry opportunities in consultation and collaboration with Deans, Associate Deans, and Research Center Directors. Prof. Gray supports the Deputy Vice-Chancellor in the leadership and management of research at La Trobe University. He originally trained and worked as a Mental Health Nurse at the Maudsley Hospital in London before training in epidemiology and public health at the London School of Hygiene and Tropic Medicine. Subsequently, he has worked as a mental health services researcher focused on improving physical health outcomes for people experiencing mental ill-health, initially at the Institute of Psychiatry, King's College London, and later at the University of East Anglia and finally, La Trobe University. He is an Elsevier highly cited researcher, and his work has directly impacted the care and treatment of people experiencing mental ill-health in Australia and internationally. He is the Editor-in-Chief of Nursing Reports and is actively involved in the open science movement. He is a Fellow of the Royal Society of Public Health.

Sonia Udod

Dr. Sonia Udod has an active program of research in organizational leadership, the role of the nurse leader and nurse work environments. Her research focuses on nurse leader development, important for the creation of high-quality healthcare workplaces, leading to quality nurse, patient, and organizational outcomes. She is passionate about enhancing nurse leader capacity in the workplace and teaching students to be effective leaders. She has teaching expertise in leadership and management and advanced qualitative methods. She is committed to knowledge dissemination through peer-reviewed publications.

She has received numerous awards and scholarships, including the following: the Professional Nursing Award of Excellence in Research from the Association of Regulated Nurses of Manitoba, Top Researcher in Socio-Health, New Investigator Establishment Grant Award, Saskatchewan Health Research Foundation, Gail Donner Fellowship in Nursing, and Rosenstadt Doctoral Dissertation Award from the Faculty of Nursing, University of Toronto.

She has held several positions in service as Chair of the Leadership, Management and Policy Interest Group, Canadian Association Schools of Nursing, and International Director for the Association of Leadership Science in Nursing, and she is an inaugural member of the Leadership Institute in the Asper School of Business, University of Manitoba.

International Journal of
Environmental Research and Public Health

MDPI

Article

Longitudinal Study of the Mental Health, Resilience, and Post-Traumatic Stress of Senior Nursing Students to Nursing Graduates during the COVID-19 Pandemic

Ana Isabel Cobo-Cuenca [1], Beatriz Fernández-Fernández [2], Juan Manuel Carmona-Torres [1,*], Diana P. Pozuelo-Carrascosa [3], José Alberto Laredo-Aguilera [1], Benjamín Romero-Gómez [4], Sergio Rodríguez-Cañamero [5], Esperanza Barroso-Corroto [1] and Esmeralda Santacruz-Salas [1]

1 Facultad de Fisioterapia y Enfermería, Grupo IMCU, Departamento de Enfermería, Fisioterapia y Terapia Ocupacional, Universidad de Castilla-La Mancha, Campus de Fábrica de Armas, Av de Carlos III s/n, 45071 Toledo, Spain
2 Hospital General Nuestra Sra. Del Prado, Servicio de Salud de Castilla-La Mancha (SESCAM), Av. Extremadura KM 114, 45600 Talavera de la Reina, Spain
3 Facultad de Enfermería, Grupo IMCU, Universidad de Castilla-La Mancha, Santa Teresa Jornet s/n, 16071 Cuenca, Spain
4 Hospital El Tomillar de Sevilla, Servicio Andaluz de Salud (SAS), 41500 Alcalá de Guadaira, Spain
5 Clínica Hemodiálisis Avericum Toledo, Calle Alemania 141, 45005 Toledo, Spain
* Correspondence: juanmanuel.carmona@uclm.es

Abstract: This study analyzed changes in the psychological health of students who were in the final year of their nursing degree during the COVID-19 pandemic and later served as nursing professionals in hospitals. Methods: A prospective longitudinal study was conducted over two periods of time (the first in April 2020 and the second 6 months later, in December 2020) with 296 students for a T0 baseline (rate response 68.83%) and 92 students for a T1 post-test sample (response rate 31.08%). The data were electronically collected using the Hospital Anxiety and Depression Scale, the Life Satisfaction Questionnaire, the Resilience Scale, and a post-traumatic stress questionnaire. The mean age of the sample participants was 24.17 years (SD = 5.51), and 89.11% were female. During the pandemic, 14.11% of students showed scores that indicated depression, and 32.61% showed scores that indicated anxiety. In December 2020, 86.5% of the participants were working as nurses, and the percentages of those with anxiety (12%) and depression (4.3%) were significantly lower than in the first sample period. A total of 20.7% of the participants had post-traumatic stress. High scores for resilience were significantly associated with better quality of life and lower levels of anxiety, depression, and post-traumatic stress. Conclusions: Although the percentages of participants with anxiety and depression decreased, they still presented with mental health problems.

Keywords: COVID-19; anxiety; coping strategies; health; students; nursing

Citation: Cobo-Cuenca, A.I.; Fernández-Fernández, B.; Carmona-Torres, J.M.; Pozuelo-Carrascosa, D.P.; Laredo-Aguilera, J.A.; Romero-Gómez, B.; Rodríguez-Cañamero, S.; Barroso-Corroto, E.; Santacruz-Salas, E. Longitudinal Study of the Mental Health, Resilience, and Post-Traumatic Stress of Senior Nursing Students to Nursing Graduates during the COVID-19 Pandemic. *Int. J. Environ. Res. Public Health* **2022**, *19*, 13100. https://doi.org/10.3390/ijerph192013100

Academic Editors: Richard Gray and Sonia Udod

Received: 10 September 2022
Accepted: 9 October 2022
Published: 12 October 2022

1. Introduction

In December 2019, the first case of pneumonia originating from the SARS-CoV-2 virus was identified in the city of Wuhan, China. The virus was named according to its clinical similarity to the SARS virus that was identified in 2003 and determined to be responsible for the COVID-19 disease [1]. The virus's great capacity for infection and propagation led the World Health Organization to declare COVID-19 a pandemic on 11 March 2020 [2].

Due to this increase in the number of cases, on 14 March 2020, a state of alarm was decreed for the entire national territory of Spain, and the confinement of the population was mandated. The declaration of a state of alarm places all powers in the hands of the central government with the objective of mobilizing all available means to protect the state's health resources [3]. Despite all the measures that were adopted, the total number of diagnosed cases and deaths in the first weeks of the state of alarm was very high, as was the proportion of health personnel who were infected due to the lack of material resources, such as masks and personal protective equipment (PPE) [4,5]. In fact, at the end of May 2020, Spain (Madrid, Castile-La Mancha, and Castile-Leon) and Italy (Lombardy) were the regions with the highest excess mortality rates from COVID-19, both of which were approximately 30% [6]. A report issued by the National Institute of Statistics of Spain on 15 November 2021 showed that the COVID disease was the main cause of death in Spain in 2020, with its highest impact in the months of March and April (with 60,358 deaths and a deathrate of 127.5 per 100,000 inhabitants) [7]. Of the confirmed cases, 26% were health professionals, and Spain was the country with the highest number of health professionals infected by COVID-19 [8].

In terms of the impacts of COVID-19 on education, efforts to reduce the spread of COVID-19 through social isolation and mandatory social immobilization led to the closure of higher education institutions. University education was no longer provided via in-person classroom instruction; COVID-19 forced a change in the learning structure in university education and in the ways of teaching, with technologies playing a significant role [9]. At the University of Castilla-La Mancha (UCLM), the rector suspended in-person learning by enforcing the resolution of 11 March 2020, which adopted preventive measures and public health recommendations related to the university community as a result of issues surrounding the situation and evolution of COVID-19 [10]. At that time, the clinical practice of nursing students was interrupted. Due to the lack of health personnel and the overflow of patients in the health system, on 27 March 2020 [11], the Spanish government adopted measures to strengthen the health system. These measures included the authorization of students in their last year of nursing school to work at health centers as health assistants. Many of fourth-year students volunteered to provide health care in the absence of health personnel.

Public health emergencies can have many psychological effects on university students, including anxiety, fear, and worry [12]. A study of 52,730 people in China conducted during the initial phase of the pandemic found that 35% of the participants experienced psychological stress, with higher levels among those aged 18 to 30 years and, particularly, among women. Another study conducted in China revealed that 24.9% of university students suffered anxiety due to the COVID-19 outbreak [12]. The anxiety of university students as a result of COVID-19 may have been related to the effect of the virus on their studies, their use of social networks as their main means of information [13], and their fears of contagion [13], social distancing, and social alarmism [14], as well as anxiety surrounding their future job prospects [15]. These results indicate that the COVID-19 crisis could have had a significant psychological impact on university students. For nursing students, this impact would have been greater. In Spain, during the first wave, many nursing students had contact with COVID-19 patients during clinical practice, some contracted the disease, and many final-year students provided health care. Several studies explored the psychological and mental health impacts of the first wave of the COVID-19 epidemic on nursing students, showing an increase in fear, anxiety, depression, and sleep problems [16,17].

Similar data were found with healthcare professionals during the first pandemic period, with studies reporting a high incidence of anxiety, depression, and post-traumatic stress among participants [18–20]. The impact of COVID-19 was not equal among all healthcare professionals: gender (female), profession (nurse), and shift work increased the incidences of anxiety, depression, and post-traumatic stress. Despite this, resilience has also been considered a protective factor, which would be the person's ability to confront adversities and thereby reduce anxious, depressive, post-traumatic stress, and burnout symptoms [18–20].

After the first wave, longitudinal studies were conducted on the general population [21–23]. Luceño et al. (2021) [24] found that the levels of post-traumatic stress, anxiety, and depression of healthcare professionals was reduced with time, although there was not a full recovery.

However, to our knowledge, there are no known longitudinal studies that have evaluated mental health in students who were in their final year of study (fourth-year students in Spain) who have since graduated and are working as nurses.

Therefore, our starting hypothesis for this research was that university nursing students experienced a psychological impact from COVID-19 and may be suffering from anxiety/stress, which can last for several months.

The aims of this study were to analyze the psychological impacts of the COVID-19 pandemic on students who were in the last year of their nursing degree (and who provided health care during that period) and to assess their subsequent psychological health after they graduated from nursing school and began working as nurses in hospitals in Spain. The second objective was to determine the relationships between the different variables and mental health.

2. Materials and Methods

2.1. Design

This was a prospective longitudinal cohort study with 2 data collection periods (T0: from April to May 2020 and T1: December 2020) with students in the nursing program at the University of X. The Strengthening the Reporting of Observational Studies in Epidemiology (STROBE) guideline has been followed.

The inclusion criteria included:

- Enrolment in the fourth year of the nursing degree program at the University of X during the 2019/2020 academic year.

The exclusion criteria included:

- Students having abandoned their studies during the 2019/20 academic year.

To calculate the sample size, the prevalence of anxiety (24.9%) among university students in China was used [12]. The reference population was estimated to be 400 fourth year undergraduate students at the University of X [25].

The sample size was calculated with the GRANMO program (v 7.12 April 2012) to determine an estimate with respect to a reference (proportional). Accepting an alpha risk of 0.05 and a beta risk of 0.2 in a two tailed comparison, 45 subjects were required to detect a difference equal to or greater than 0.2 units. It was assumed that the proportion of the reference group was 24.9%. A loss-to-follow-up rate of 10% was estimated.

The questionnaire was sent in 2 stages to all fourth-year nursing students at the University of X. During the first stage (T0), in which all participants were still nursing students, 296 responses were received (the pretest response rate was 68.83%); for the follow-up survey, which was administered 6 months later, 92 responses were received (T0 baseline–T1 post-test response rate of 31.08% (N = 296 students who responded to the first survey) and T0–T1 test response rate of 22.5% (N = 400 enrolled students)).

2.2. Variables

- The independent variables were age, gender, smoking status (yes/no), number of cigarettes smoked, and previous pathologies.
- The dependent variables were:
    - anxiety and depression
    - satisfaction with life
    - resilience
    - post-traumatic stress

2.3. Instruments

- The Hospital Anxiety and Depression Scale [26], validated in Spanish by Herrera et al. [27], is a self-administered scale with 2 subscales, each of which includes 7 items (14 items in total). Scores of between 0 and 7 on each scale indicate no concerns regarding anxiety/depression, scores of between 8 and 10 indicate possible anxiety/depression, and scores of above 11 indicate probably anxiety/depression. The scale has an internal consistency by Cronbach's alpha of 0.90 for the full scale, 0.85 for the anxiety scale, and 0.84 for the depression scale.

- LISAT-8, the Spanish version of the LISAT-8 [28], is a self-administered questionnaire consisting of 8 items rated on a Likert scale. The items measure the respondent's satisfaction with 8 different aspects of life (life, sexual life, relationship with their partner, family life, relationship with friends and acquaintances, leisure, work situation, and financial situation). The final score is calculated by adding the scores of all the items (total possible scores range from 8 to 48). The scale comprises 3 dimensions: satisfaction with social life (items 1, 4, 5, and 6), satisfaction with emotional life (items 2 and 3) and satisfaction with work or financial life (items 7 and 8). The scale has a sensitivity of 81.7% (CI: 80.5–82.9) and a reliability of 79.2% (CI: 77.5–80.8) [19].
- The 10-item short version of the CD-RISC (2003) [29] proposed by Campbell and Stein (2003) [30], adapted to the university population by Notario et al. (2011) [31], was used. This is a self-administered questionnaire comprised of 10 items that uses a Likert scale for answers, with 5 response options ranging from 0 (never) to 4 (almost always). The final score of the questionnaire is the sum of the responses obtained for each item (range of 0–40). A higher score indicates a higher level of resilience. The Cronbach's alpha was 0.85 and the test-retest intraclass correlation coefficient was 0.71.
- The short version of the Davidson Trauma Scale (DTS) by Connor and Davidson (2000) [32], adapted to Spanish by Bobes et al. (2000) [33], is a questionnaire comprising 8 items answered using a 5-point Likert scale (0–4 points). It quantifies the frequency and severity of each symptom of post-traumatic stress disorder and the results in a total score of between 0 and 32 points. The cut-off scores proposed by the authors were as follows: 0–7, no post-traumatic stress disorder, and 12 or higher: post-traumatic stress disorder. The Cronbach's alpha was 0.83.

2.4. Procedure

An online questionnaire was developed. Five faculty members at the University of X were contacted and asked to pass the questionnaire link to their fourth-year students.

The questionnaire was distributed at 2 time points:

- First data collection period (T0): the HADS questionnaire was administered from April to May 2020 to determine the psychological state of nursing students during social isolation and confinement.
- Second data collection period (T1): All the students who completed the online questionnaire during phase 1 were invited to participate in the second phase of the study, which aimed to determine the evolution of the psychological impacts of COVID-19. This assessment was performed in December 2020. In this phase, all the participants now graduated nurses. The questionnaires used were HADS, LISAT 8, CD-RISC, and DTS.

2.5. Data Analysis

For the statistical analysis, SPSS version 22 (IBM Corp. Armonk, NY, USA), licensed by the University of Castilla-La Mancha, was used. Qualitative variables are reported as counts and percentages. Quantitative variables are expressed as the arithmetic means (m) and standard deviations (SD). An inferential analysis was performed to identify the relationships between the independent variables and the dependent variables, as follows:

- For qualitative variables: proportions of categorical variables were compared using χ^2 tests for contingency tables; for 2 × 2 tables, the χ^2 statistics with a Yates correction was used, and when the expected frequency was ≤5, Fisher's exact test was applied.
- For quantitative variables: first, the goodness of fit to a normal distribution was determined using the Shapiro–Wilk test, and then the homogeneity of the variances was determined using the Levene test. As the data did not follow a normal distribution, we used the appropriate nonparametric (Mann–Whitney U) test.

We used Spearman's correlation analysis (Rho) to explore the relationships between the different dependent variables (anxiety, depression, satisfaction with life, resilience and post-traumatic stress). In addition, to control the influence of gender, a partial correlation analysis was performed.

To identify the differences in anxiety and depression in the pre-test with those of the post-test, the Wilcoxon rank test was used.

All hypothesis comparisons were two-tailed. For all statistical tests, significant values were those with a p value of <0.05 at a confidence interval of 95%.

2.6. Ethical Considerations

The present study was approved by the Clinical Research Ethics Committee of the Health Area of X with the code 24/2020. The research respected the fundamental principles of the Declaration of Helsinki of the European Convention on Human Rights and Biomedicine. All participant data were treated confidentially in accordance with Organic Law 3/2018 of December 5 on the Protection of Personal Data and Guarantee of Digital Rights, maintaining strict confidentiality and preventing access to unauthorized third parties. All participants read the information sheet and gave their consent to participate in the study.

3. Results

During the first administration (T0), which took place during the confinement period, 296 students (response rate of 68.83%) aged between 21 and 54 years (m = 23.4; SD = 4.79) answered the questionnaires in full.

A total of 92 students participated in both data collection phases (T0 and T1). All were fourth-year students at the time of their inclusion in the study, and 86.5% were working as nurses during the second data collection period. A total of 89.1% were women and 10.9% were men; their ages were between 21 and 54 years (mean = 24.17, SD = 5.51). The majority (76.1%) had no previous pathology. A total of 5.4% were previously diagnosed with anxiety, 2.2% had a previous diagnosis of asthma, 2.2% had previous diagnoses of hypertension and dyslipidemia, and 1.1% had a previous diagnosis of hypothyroidism. With respect to tobacco, only 13 people smoked, and the number of cigarettes they smoked did not change (T0–T1).

Regarding the pre-test phase T0 (May 2020), 47.8% of the participants had provided health care assistance to the public health system in Spain due to the pandemic situation. Of these, 25.60% worked in a call center, 7.41% in intensive care units, and the rest in hospitalization units. With respect to shifts, 74.41% worked rotating shifts, and while doing so, 69.8% always had access to protective material against COVID-19 and only 3.5% underwent testing for COVID-19. During this phase (T0) (April–May 2020), 32.6% suffered from anxiety and 14.1% experienced depression.

Regarding coping with problems during the confinement period (April–May 2020), 51.1% of the respondents performed physical activity several times per week (21.1% were active every day), 35.6% talked to friends every day, 35.6% watched movies or TV shows to distract themselves every day, 34.4% tried to distract themselves with things they liked to avoid thinking about anything several times per week, 22.2% were angrier than usual several times week, 27.8% were more sad than usual several times per week, and 18.9% cried several times per week.

Regarding coping strategies and anxiety and depression during T0, talking with friends every day was associated with less depression ($\chi^2 = 9.80$, $p = 0.020$), and engaging in physical activity every day or several times per week was associated with less depression ($\chi^2 = 10.69$, $p = 0.03$). Being angrier than usual several times per week was related to more anxiety ($\chi^2 = 26.88$, $p < 0.001$) and crying more than usual several times per week was related to anxiety ($\chi^2 = 26.56$, $p < 0.001$).

During the T1 phase (December 2020), 86.5% of the participants were working as nurses. A total of 20.7% of the participants had post-traumatic stress, while 55.1% considered their quality of life to be high. Finally, the respondents had a mean resilience score of 27.03 (SD ± 8.27). Their responses to the different scales are shown in Table 1.

Table 1. Responses to the different scales during the post-test phase (December 2020) (by analyzed total responses and by gender).

	Men *n* (%)	Women *n* (%)	Total *n* (%)	*p*
Post-traumatic Stress				
No	6 (60%)	64 (81.7%)	73 (79.3%)	0.12 (1)
Yes	4 (40%)	15 (18.3%)	19 (20.7%)	
Anxiety				
No	9 (90%)	72 (87.8%)	81 (88%)	0.658 (1)
Yes	1 (10%)	10 (12.2%)	11 (12%)	
Depression				
No	8 (80%)	80 (97.6%)	88 (95.7%)	0.057 (1)
Yes	2 (20%)	2 (2.4%)	4 (4.3%)	
Overall LISAT				
Low	1 (10%)	1 (1.3%)	2 (2.2%)	0.164 (1)
Medium	5 (50%)	33 (41.8%)	38 (42.7%)	
High	4 (40%)	45 (57%)	49 (55.1%)	
Social LISAT				
Low	1 (10%)	0	1 (1.1%)	0.011 *(1)
Medium	5 (50%)	29 (36.7%)	34 (38.2%)	
High	4 (40%)	50 (63.3%)	54 (60.7%)	
Sexual LISAT				
Low	3 (42.9%)	23 (33.8%)	26 (34.7%)	0.89 (1)
Medium	3 (42.9%)	33 (48.5%)	36 (48%)	
High	1 (14.3%)	12 (17.6%)	13 (17.3%)	
Financial LISAT				
Low	4 (40%)	20 (25.6%)	24 (27.3%)	0.626 (1)
Medium	5 (50%)	47 (60.3%)	52 (59.1%)	
High	1 (10%)	11 (14.1%)	12 (13.6%)	
Resilience	26.3 (± 7.54)	27.12 (± 8.39)	27.03 (± 8.27)	0.656 (2)

* $p < 0.05$; LISAT, satisfaction with life; (1) significant value of χ^2 test; (2) significant value of Mann–Whitney U test; anxiety > 11; depression > 11; post-traumatic stress > 12; overall LISAT (good (36–48), medium (21–35), and low (20–8)); social LISAT (good (18–24), medium (11–17), low (4–109)); sexual and financial LISATs (good (10–12), medium (4–9), and low (4–8)).

Table 2 presents the differences in anxiety and depression between the two study phases. There were significant differences because the percentages of anxiety and depression decreased during the post-test phase.

Table 3 shows the correlations among the scores on the different scales during T1. Anxiety was positively associated with depression and post-traumatic stress. Depression was positively associated with post-traumatic stress. However, depression was negatively associated with resilience and the LISAT-8 scores. The LISAT-8 scores were positively associated with resilience and negatively associated with post-traumatic stress. When we conducted the sex-adjusted partial correlation, the results were similar, except for depression, which was not significantly associated with resilience and the LISAT-8 scores.

Table 2. T0–T1 mean anxiety and depression scores.

	Pre-Test (May 2020)	Post-Test (December 2020)	p
	n (SD)	n (SD)	
Anxiety	8.36 (± 4.11)	6.83 (± 3.53)	< 0.001 [(1)]
Depression	5.77 (± 3.52)	4.24 (± 3.36)	< 0.001 [(1)]
	n (%)	n (%)	
Anxiety			
No anxiety (<7)	41 (44.6%)	54 (58.7%)	< 0.001 [(2)]
Possible anxiety (8–11)	21 (22.8%)	27 (29.3%)	
Anxiety (>11)	30 (32.6%)	11 (12%)	
Depression			
No depression (<7)	61 (63.3%)	76 (82.6%)	< 0.001 [(2)]
Possible depression (7–11)	18 (19.6%)	12 (13%)	
Depression (>11)	13 (14.1%)	4 (4.3%)	

SD, standard deviation; [(1)] significant value of paired Wilcoxon test; [(2)] significant value of χ^2 test.

Table 3. Correlations between anxiety, depression, and post-traumatic stress and satisfaction with life.

	Simple Correlation					Partial Correlation				
	Anxiety	Depression	LISAT Total	Resilience	Post-Traumatic Stress	Anxiety	Depression	LISAT Total	Resilience	Post-Traumatic Stress
Anxiety	-	0.647 **	−0.159	−0.250	0.457 **	-	0.650 **	0.023	−0.097	0.440 *
Depression		-	−0.314 *	−0.288 *	0.546 **		-	−0.073	−0.126	0.508 *
Overall LISAT			-	0.664 **	−0.409 **			-	0.805 **	−0.264 *
Resilience				-	−0.333 *				-	−0.269 *
Post-traumatic stress					-					-

Data are presented in the correlation coefficient Rho. * $p < 0.05$; ** $p < 0.001$. Abbreviations: LISAT: life satisfaction. Adjusted for sex.

4. Discussion

The aim of this study was to analyze the psychological health of students who were in the last year of their nursing degree during the COVID-19 pandemic and their subsequent psychological health after they graduated from nursing school and began working as nurses in hospitals in Spain.

Many studies have evaluated the impact of the COVID-19 pandemic on the mental health of the general population, health personnel, and nursing students [25–27]. However, to our knowledge, this impact has not been longitudinally evaluated in nursing students who were providing health care assistance during the first wave of COVID-19 (March–May 2020) and again 6 months later, when they had graduated and were working as nurses (December 2020).

During the first wave of the pandemic, most university students had to stop attending classes in person. However, in Spain, students in their last year of nursing school had the opportunity to develop health care skills due to the collapse of the health system [11], which created the need for them to serve as front-line health workers in April and May without having finished their studies. This first wave of the pandemic was characterized by a very high mortality rate and little knowledge of the disease [7,8]. In our study, we observed that during the first wave, 47.8% of the participants provided health care assistance to the public health system in Spain prior to the completion of their studies.

In the first wave in Spain, during the confinement period, more than half of the students had symptoms of anxiety, and one-third of the total sample scored above the cut-off point for a diagnosis of anxiety disorder. Additionally, one-third of the participants scored high on the depression scale and 14% met the criteria for depressive disorder. The levels of both anxiety and depression were not related to age, whether the participants had provided health care assistance to the public, work locations, or work shifts. This increase in anxiety and depression during confinement coincided with other studies of nursing students, such as those by Patelarou et al. (2021) [16] and Romero et al. [17], and with other studies of health professionals [18,20]. In other studies [18], anxiety and depression were related to age, with the youngest participants having the highest scores. In our study, this was not the case, possibly because the students in our study were of similar ages and had not previously worked in the health system; they only had experience in clinical practice. They may also have had less fear of being infected [34] or of the repercussions of the disease, which caused higher mortality in older people [7,8].

Another fact that is not consistent with some previous studies [18,20,24,35] is the absence of a significant relationship between gender, anxiety, and depression, which is atypical and could be due to the presence of mental health problems prior to confinement, although none of the participants indicated that they had any diagnosed mental health pathology prior to the pandemic. Another possible explanation is that, as other studies have identified [20,24,35,36], women experience work overload in addition to the responsibility of caring for their children and homes, which increases their anxiety [35–37]. However, this did not occur in our sample because none of the students had family burdens, such as caring for children.

In our sample, we observed a high incidence of anxiety and depression during confinement. Six months later, the participants reported more normalized levels of anxiety and depression. This is consistent with population studies [21–23] and studies of Italian university students [38] and Spanish health professionals [24]. However, the longitudinal study [22] that included the general Spanish population showed that although depression levels had decreased, they did not return to pre-pandemic levels.

Resilience is the ability to face adversities and recover from them. Different studies have identified resilience as a protective factor against the development of post-traumatic stress disorders [39], mental health problems [40], and burnout [41]. Bonanno (2004) [39] found that in emergency situations, people make use of their internal resources to maintain their mental health. Resilience is related to less anxiety and depression, less psychological distress, and increased well-being [18,20,39]. In our study, people who scored high in resilience had a higher quality of life score and a lower prevalence of depression and post-traumatic stress disorders. Resilience can help people cope with adverse situations and is a great resource for mitigating anxiety symptoms and improving well-being [34].

Other studies [22,24,28] have found differences in resilience according to age and gender, with males presenting higher resilience scores. In our study, we did not find such differences. Resilience can be reinforced by experience and education; in fact, a study of nursing students in Israel [34] showed that students in advanced courses showed more resilience, possibly because their experience with clinical practice in real-life settings improved their ability to mitigate stress.

Previous studies have shown that rotating shifts are related to a high risk of post-traumatic stress, depression, and anxiety [18,41]. In our study, variables such as having worked in units with COVID patients, on rotating shifts, and with low levels of experience did not show any relationship with any psychological variable. However, the professionals in our sample had only worked as nurses for 6 months, which may explain the lack of significant relationships between these factors.

To our knowledge, this is the first longitudinal study conducted in Spain that evaluates the evolution of the mental health of nursing students over two periods: from the students' last semester of study to 6 months later, after they had graduated and were working as nurses during the pandemic.

This study is not exempt from limitations—data collection took place online, the response rate was low, and it is possible that the people who responded were those who had less anxiety and more resilience. Because the study was conducted online, we cannot determine the real response rate since we do not know how many members of the population the survey reached. The data are self-reported, and resilience, post-traumatic stress, and satisfaction with life were not measured at T0. The study design did not allow for causality to be established among the different variables. Nonetheless, this study highlights that the mental health of fourth-year nursing students was altered during the confinement period of the pandemic, although anxiety and depression decreased 6 months later, when the participants had graduated and were working as nurses. Universities and health services must make plans to provide mental health services to protect and help health professionals. It would be interesting to continue studying the evolution of the mental health of these professionals, as it has been 2 years since the pandemic began and there have since been more than six waves of the pandemic, each characterized by high mortality and workload and signs of mental fatigue, depression, etc.

Relevance to Clinical Practice

This study highlights the importance of resilience in protecting against problems with anxiety, depression, and post-traumatic stress disorders and improving quality of life. More than two years have passed since the onset of the COVID-19 pandemic and healthcare professionals have suffered the most from the negative impacts on their psychological health. However, few health policies have been implemented to reduce this problem. Therefore, work conditions should be improved and strategic lines of mental health support should be established by universities and health services to prevent mental pathologies. Teaching strategies that increase resilience can help health professionals cope with future pandemic waves or emergency situations.

5. Conclusions

The COVID-19 pandemic has had a negative impact on the mental health of nursing students in Spain. This study shows the evolution of anxiety and depression levels of nursing students from the first period of confinement to 6 months later. During the period of confinement in the first wave of the pandemic, students scored high on the anxiety and depression scales. After 6 months, their anxiety and depression levels had decreased.

Resilience is related to a better quality of life and less anxiety and depression, and it may be a protective factor for mental health. Unlike other studies, no relationship was found with gender, age, and work shifts, which was observed in health professionals with more work experience. Universities and, subsequently, health services should increase interventions to improve and promote training in mental health and resilience.

Author Contributions: Conceptualization, A.I.C.-C. and J.M.C.-T.; methodology, A.I.C.-C. and J.M.C.-T.; software, J.A.L.-A.; validation, all authors; formal analysis, J.M.C.-T.; investigation, all authros; data curation, A.I.C.-C. and J.M.C.-T.; writing—original draft preparation, A.I.C.-C. and J.M.C.-T.; writing—review and editing, all authors; visualization, all authors; supervision, A.I.C.-C. and J.M.C.-T.; project administration, A.I.C.-C. and J.M.C.-T.; funding acquisition, A.I.C.-C. and J.M.C.-T. All authors have read and agreed to the published version of the manuscript.

Funding: This research was funded by the FEDER-UCLM, grant number UCLM 2021.

Institutional Review Board Statement: The study was conducted in accordance with the Declaration of Helsinki and approved by the Ethics Committee of the Health Area of X (protocol code 24/2020).

Informed Consent Statement: Informed consent was obtained from all subjects involved in the study.

Data Availability Statement: The data that support the findings of this study are available from the corresponding author, upon reasonable request.

Conflicts of Interest: The authors declare no conflict of interest.

References

1. Guan, W.J.; Ni, Z.Y.; Hu, Y.; Liang, W.H.; Qu, C.Q.; He, J.X.; Liu, L.; Shan, H.; Lei, C.L.; Hui, D.S.C.; et al. Clinical Characteristics of coronavirus disease 2019 in China. *N. Engl. J. Med.* **2020**, *382*, 1708–1720. [CrossRef]
2. World Health Organization (WHO). Opening Address by the Director-General of WHO at the Press Conference on COVID-19 Held on 11 March 2020. Available online: https://www.who.int/es/dg/speeches/detail/who-director-general-s-opening-remarks-at-the-media-briefing-on-covid-19---11-march-2020 (accessed on 29 April 2020).

3. Gobierno de España. Real Decreto 463/2020, de 14 de Marzo, por el que se Declara el Estado de Alarma para la Gestión de la Situacion de Crisis Sanitaria Ocasionada por el COVID-19. 2020. Available online: https://www.boe.es/eli/es/rd/2020/03/14/463 (accessed on 28 June 2020).
4. Arango, C. Lessons Learned From the Coronavirus Health Crisis in Madrid, Spain: How COVID-19 Has Changed Our Lives in the Last 2 Weeks. *Biol. Psychiatry* **2020**, *88*, e33. [CrossRef] [PubMed]
5. Raurell-Torreda, M.; Martinez-Estalella, G.; Frade-Mera, M.J.; Carrasco Rodriguez-Rey, L.F.; Romero de San Pio, E. Reflections arising from the COVID-19 pandemic. *Enferm. Intensiv.* **2020**, *31*, 90–93. [CrossRef] [PubMed]
6. Konstantinoudis, G.; Cameletti, M.; Gómez-Rubio, V.; Gómez, I.L.; Pirani, M.; Baio, G.; Larrauri, A.; Riou, J.; Egger, M.; Vineis, P.; et al. Regional excess mortality during the 2020 COVID-19 pandemic in five European countries. *Nat. Commun.* **2022**, *13*, 482. [CrossRef]
7. Instituto Nacional de Estadistica. Defunciones Según la Causa de Muerte Año 2020. 2021. Available online: https://www.ine.es/dyngs/INEbase/es/operacion.htm?c=Estadistica_C&cid=1254736176780&menu=ultiDatos&idp=1254735573175 (accessed on 10 November 2021).
8. Redacción Médica. Coronavirus: El 26% de los Contagios en España Son Sanitarios. 2020. Available online: https://www.redaccionmedica.com/secciones/sanidad-hoy/coronavirus-espana-casi-tiene-3-veces-mas-sanitarios-infectados-que-italia-6826 (accessed on 29 April 2020).
9. Torrecillas Bautista, C. El Reto de la Docencia Online Para las Universidades Públicas Españolas ante la Pandemia del COVID-19 ICEI Papers COVID-19. 2020. Available online: https://www.ucm.es/icei/file/iceipapercovid16 (accessed on 10 November 2021).
10. Rectorado de la Universidad de Castilla-La Mancha. Resolución del Rector de la Universidad de Castilla-La Mancha, de 11 de Marzo, por la que se Adoptan Medidas Preventivas y Recomendaciones de Salud Pública Relativas a la Comunidad Universitaria Como Consecuencia de la Situación, Evolución y Perspectivas del Coronavirus (COVID-19). 2020. Available online: https://bellasartes.uclm.es/wp-content/uploads/2020/03/Resoluci%C3%B3n-11-de-marzo-rector-medidas-preventivas-firmada.pdf (accessed on 1 May 2020).
11. Gobierno de España. Orden SND/299/2020, de 27 de Marzo, por la que se Modifica la Orden SND/232/2020, de 15 de Marzo, por la que se Adoptan Medidas en Materia de Recursos Humanos y Medios para la Gestion de la Situacion de Crisis Sanitaria Ocasionada por el COVID-19. 2020. Available online: https://www.boe.es/eli/es/rd/2020/03/4174 (accessed on 28 June 2020).
12. Gao, J.; Zheng, P.; Jia, Y.; Chen, H.; Mao, Y.; Chen, S.; Wang, Y.; Fu, H.; Dai, J. Mental health problems and social media exposure during COVID-19 outbreak. *PLoS ONE* **2020**, *15*, e0231924. [CrossRef]
13. Qiu, J.; Shen, B.; Zhao, M.; Wang, Z.; Xie, B.; Xu, Y. A nationwide survey of psychological distress among Chinese people in the COVID-19 epidemic: Implications and policy recommendations. *Gen. Psychiatry* **2020**, *33*, e100213. [CrossRef]
14. Venkatesh, A.; Edirappuli, S. Social distancing in COVID-19: What are the mental health implications? *BMJ* **2020**, *369*, m1379. [CrossRef] [PubMed]
15. Wang, C.; Pan, R.; Wan, X.; Tan, Y.; Xu, L.; Ho, C.S.; Ho, R.C. Immediate Psychological Responses and Associated Factors during the Initial Stage of the 2019 Coronavirus Disease (COVID-19) Epidemic among the General Population in China. *Int. J. Environ. Res. Public Health* **2020**, *17*, 1729. [CrossRef] [PubMed]
16. Patelarou, A.; Mechili, E.A.; Galanis, P.; Zografakis-Sfakianakis, M.; Konstantinidis, T.; Saliaj, A.; Bucaj, J.; Alushi, E.; Carmona-Torres, J.M.; Cobo-Cuenca, A.I.; et al. Nursing students, mental health status during COVID-19 quarantine: Evidence from three European countries. *J. Ment. Health* **2021**, *30*, 164–169. [CrossRef]
17. Romero-Blanco, C.; Rodríguez-Almagro, J.; Onieva-Zafra, M.D.; Parra-Fernández, M.L.; Prado-Laguna, M.D.C.; Hernández-Martínez, A. Sleep Pattern Changes in Nursing Students during the COVID-19 Lockdown. *Int. J. Environ. Res. Public Health* **2020**, *17*, 5222. [CrossRef] [PubMed]
18. Luceño-Moreno, L.; Talavera-Velasco, B.; García-Albuerne, Y.; Martín-García, J. Symptoms of Posttraumatic Stress, Anxiety, Depression, Levels of Resilience and Burnout in Spanish Health Personnel during the COVID-19 Pandemic. *Int. J. Environ. Res. Public Health* **2020**, *17*, 5514. [CrossRef] [PubMed]
19. Pappa, S.; Ntella, V.; Giannakas, T.; Giannakoulis, V.G.; Papoutsi, E.; Katsaounou, P. Prevalence of depression, anxiety, and insomnia among healthcare workers during the COVID-19 pandemic: A systematic review and meta-analysis. *Brain Behav. Immun.* **2020**, *88*, 901–907, Erratum in: *Brain Behav Immun.* **2021**, *92*, 247. [CrossRef] [PubMed]
20. Peñacoba, C.; Velasco, L.; Catalá, P.; Gil-Almagro, F.; García-Hedrera, F.J.; Carmona-Monge, F.J. Resilience and anxiety among intensive care unit professionals during the COVID-19 pandemic. *Nurs. Crit. Care* **2021**, *26*, 501–509. [CrossRef] [PubMed]
21. Wan, Z.; Lian, M.; Ma, H.; Cai, Z.; Xianyu, Y. Factors associated with burnout among Chinese nurses during COVID-19 epidemic: A cross-sectional study. *BMC Nurs.* **2022**, *21*, 51. [CrossRef] [PubMed]
22. González-Sanguino, C.; Ausín, B.; Castellanos, M.; Saiz, J.; Muñoz, M. Mental health consequences of the COVID-19 outbreak in Spain. A longitudinal study of the alarm situation and return to the new normality. *Prog. Neuro-Psychopharmacol. Biol. Psychiatry* **2020**, *107*, 110219. [CrossRef] [PubMed]
23. Hyland, P.; Shevlin, M.; Murphy, J.; McBride, O.; Fox, R.; Bondjers, K.; Karatzias, T.; Bentall, R.P.; Martinez, A.; Vallières, F. A longitudinal assessment of depression and anxiety in the Republic of Ireland before and during the COVID-19 pandemic. *Psychiatry Res.* **2021**, *300*, 113905. [CrossRef]

24. Luceño-Moreno, L.; Talavera-Velasco, B.; Vázquez-Estévez, D.; Martín-García, J. Mental Health, Burnout and Resilience in Healthcare Professionals after the First Wave of COVID-19 Pandemic in Spain: A Longitudinal Study. *J. Occup. Environ. Med.* **2021**, *64*, e114–e123. [CrossRef]
25. Universidad de Castilla-La Mancha. Portal de Transparencia: Estadísticas de Estudiantes. Available online: https://www.uclm.es/misiones/lauclm/institucional/transparencia/estadisticaestudiantes (accessed on 5 May 2020).
26. Zigmond, A.S.; Snaith, R.P. The hospital anxiety and depression scale. *Acta Psychiatr. Scand.* **1983**, *67*, 361–370. [CrossRef] [PubMed]
27. Herrero, M.J.; Blanch, J.; Peri, J.M.; De Pablo, J.; Pintor, L.; Bulbena, A. A validation study of the hospital anxiety and depression scale (HADS) in a Spanish population. *Gen. Hosp. Psychiat.* **2003**, *25*, 277–283. [CrossRef]
28. Moncada, I.; Micheltorena, C.F.; Martínez-Sánchez, E.M.; Gutiérrez, J.R. Evaluation of the Psychometric Properties of the Life Satisfaction Checklist as a Screening Tool for Erectile Dysfunction. *J. Sex. Med.* **2008**, *5*, 83–91. [CrossRef]
29. Connor, K.M.; Davidson, J.R.T. Development of a new resilience scale: The Connor-Davidson Resilience Scale (CD-RISC). *Depress. Anxiety* **2003**, *18*, 76–82. [CrossRef] [PubMed]
30. Campbell-Sills, L.; Stein, M.B. Psychometric analysis and refinement of the connor–davidson resilience scale (CD-RISC): Validation of a 10-item measure of resilience. *J. Trauma. Stress Off. Publ. Int. Soc. Trauma. Stress Stud.* **2007**, *20*, 1019–1028. [CrossRef] [PubMed]
31. Notario-Pacheco, B.; Solera-Martínez, M.; Serrano-Parra, M.D.; Bartolomé-Gutiérrez, R.; García-Campayo, J.; Martínez-Vizcaíno, V. Reliability and validity of the Spanish version of the 10-item Connor-Davidson Resilience Scale (10-item CD-RISC) in young adults. *Health Qual. Life Outcomes* **2011**, *9*, 63. [CrossRef] [PubMed]
32. Connor, K.M.; Davidson, J.R. Further psychometric assessment of the TOP-8: A brief interview-based measure of PTSD. *Depress. Anxiety* **2000**, *9*, 135–137. [CrossRef]
33. Bobes, J.; Calcedo-Barba, A.; García, M.; Francois, M.; Rico-Villademoros, F.; González, M.P.; Bousoño, M. Evaluación de las propiedades psicométricas de la versión española de cinco cuestionarios para la evaluación del trastorno de estrés postraumático. *Actas Esp. Psiquiatr.* **2000**, *28*, 207–218.
34. Drach-Zahavy, A.; Goldblatt, H.; Admi, H.; Blau, A.; Ohana, I.; Itzhaki, M. A multi-level examination of nursing students' resilience in the face of the COVID-19 outbreak: A cross-sectional design. *J. Adv. Nurs.* **2022**, *78*, 109–120. [CrossRef]
35. Manzo, L.K.C.; Minello, A. Mothers, childcare duties, and remote working under COVID-19 lockdown in Italy: Cultivating communities of care. *Dialog- Hum. Geogr.* **2020**, *10*, 120–123. [CrossRef]
36. Salk, R.H.; Hyde, J.S.; Abramson, L.Y. Gender differences in depression in representative national samples: Meta-analyses of diagnoses and symptoms. *Psychol. Bull.* **2017**, *143*, 783–822. [CrossRef]
37. Ausín, B.; González-Sanguino, C.; Castellanos, M.; Muñoz, M. Gender-related differences in the psychological impact of confinement as a consequence of COVID-19 in Spain. *J. Gend. Stud.* **2020**, *30*, 29–38. [CrossRef]
38. Meda, N.; Pardini, S.; Slongo, I.; Bodini, L.; Zordan, M.A.; Rigobello, P.; Visioli, F.; Novara, C. Students' mental health problems before, during, and after COVID-19 lockdown in Italy. *J. Psychiatr. Res.* **2021**, *134*, 69–77. [CrossRef]
39. Bonanno, G.A. Loss, trauma, and human resilience: Have we underestimated the human capacity to thrive after extremely aversive events? *Am. Psychol.* **2004**, *59*, 20. [CrossRef] [PubMed]
40. Perlman, D.; Patterson, C.; Moxham, L.; Taylor, E.K.; Brighton, R.; Sumskis, S.; Heffernan, T. Understanding the influence of resilience for people with a lived experience of mental illness: A self-determination theory perspective. *J. Community Psychol.* **2017**, *45*, 1026–1032. [CrossRef]
41. Luceño-Moreno, L.; Talavera-Velasco, B.; Martín-García, J. Predictors of burnout in female nurses during the COVID-19 pandemic. *Int. J. Nurs. Pract.* **2022**, *28*, e13084. [CrossRef] [PubMed]

International Journal of
Environmental Research and Public Health

MDPI

Article

Protective Factors against Morally Injurious Memories from the COVID-19 Pandemic on Nurses' Occupational Wellbeing: A Cross-Sectional Experimental Study

Mihaela Alexandra Gherman *, Laura Arhiri, Andrei Corneliu Holman and Camelia Soponaru

Faculty of Psychology and Education Sciences, Alexandru Ioan Cuza University, Str. Toma Cozma 3, 700554 Iasi, Romania
* Correspondence: alexandra.gherman@uaic.ro

Abstract: The COVID-19 pandemic was a fertile ground for nurses' exposure to self- and other-Potentially Morally Injurious Events (PMIEs). Our study explored the effects of nurses' memories of self- and other-PMIEs on occupational wellbeing and turnover intentions. Using an experimental design on a convenience sample of 634 Romanian nurses, we tested a conceptual model with PLS-SEM, finding adequate explanatory and predictive power. Memories of self- and other-PMIEs were uniquely associated with work engagement, burnout, and turnover intentions, compared to a control group. These relationships were mediated by the three basic psychological needs. Relatedness was more thwarted for memories of other-PMIEs, while competence and autonomy were more thwarted for memories of self-PMIEs. Perceived supervisor support weakened the indirect effect between type of PMIE and turnover intentions, through autonomy satisfaction, but not through burnout. Self-disclosure weakened the indirect effect between type of PMIE and turnover intentions, through autonomy satisfaction, and both burnout and work engagement. Our findings emphasize the need for different strategies in addressing the negative long-term effects of nurses' exposure to self- and other-PMIEs, according to the basic psychological need satisfaction and type of wellbeing indicator.

Keywords: potentially morally injurious event (PMIE); turnover intentions; COVID-19 pandemic; basic psychological need satisfaction; nurses; burnout; episodic memories; self-determination theory; self-disclosure; perceived autonomy support

Citation: Gherman, M.A.; Arhiri, L.; Holman, A.C.; Soponaru, C. Protective Factors against Morally Injurious Memories from the COVID-19 Pandemic on Nurses' Occupational Wellbeing: A Cross-Sectional Experimental Study. *Int. J. Environ. Res. Public Health* **2022**, *19*, 11817. https://doi.org/10.3390/ijerph191811817

Academic Editors: Richard Gray and Sonia Udod

Received: 31 July 2022
Accepted: 14 September 2022
Published: 19 September 2022

1. Introduction

The fourth wave of the COVID-19 pandemic had a dramatic impact in Romania, with unprecedentedly high infection rates, registering the second highest per capita COVID-19 death rate in the world in October 2021 [1]. With one of the most underdeveloped healthcare systems in the European Union regarding infrastructure, sufficient staffing, and financing [2], the Romanian healthcare system quickly became overwhelmed [3,4]. Mirroring the global trend, nurses' exposure to PMIEs spiked during this pandemic in Romania, with severe consequences on their wellbeing and psychological health, including—but not restricted to—moral injury [5–9].

Potentially Morally Injurious Events (PMIEs) are events which imply "perpetrating, failing to prevent, bearing witness to, or learning about acts that transgress deeply held moral beliefs and expectations" [10] (p. 697). Self-PMIEs are moral transgressions enacted under perceived external coercion, while other-PMIEs are moral transgressions to which the person assists without speaking/acting out, despite feeling as if they should. Exposure to PMIEs was associated with poorer COVID-19 psycho-social functional improvement over time in healthcare providers, especially for self-perpetrated PMIEs [11]. One potential explanation for this trend is the negative impact of the repeated recall of autobiographical episodic memories of these events. Thus, studies found that nurses' episodic memories of PMIEs can have a unique negative association with their burnout, work motivation, work satisfaction, and adaptive performance several months after the event, mediated by autonomy thwarting [12]. Memories of self-PMIEs had stronger associations with burnout and turnover intentions compared to memories of other-PMIEs (i.e., enacted vs. witnessed PMIEs), mediated by the thwarting of all three basic psychological needs [13]. However, it remains unclear whether both memories of self-PMIEs and other-PMIEs would be associated with more burnout and turnover intentions when compared to a control group. This would be important to ascertain because it would contribute to our currently limited understanding of the distinctive harmful outcomes of exposure to self- and other-PMIEs [5,14–16]. Thus, our first aim was to experimentally investigate these differential associations with nurses' occupational wellbeing and turnover intentions, mediated by the thwarting of all three basic psychological needs [17].

To date, protective factors against the negative effects of autobiographical episodic memories on psychological health and wellbeing have not been investigated, to the best of our knowledge. Previous findings suggest that nurses' memories of PMIEs from the COVID-19 pandemic may not have yet been integrated in their autobiographical knowledge, an integration which might dramatically affect their work identities, behavior, and psychological health, with potential consequences on the healthcare organizational system [13]. Thus, departing from the mediating factors proposed, we set out to explore two potential moderators for the impact of memories of self- and other-PMIEs on burnout, turnover intentions, and work engagement. Perceived supervisor support and self-disclosure were assessed as moderators for autonomy and, respectively, relatedness thwarting.

1.1. Episodic Memories of PMIEs

Although correlated, self-PMIEs and other-PMIEs are distinct concepts, affecting psychological health differently [5,15,16]. However, this differential impact is still controversial. Thus, one study found that both were associated with increased depressive symptomatology in healthcare workers, but only self-PMIEs were associated with increased anxiety, PTSD, burnout, and disengagement [5]. Another study indicated that both types of PMIE could be associated with higher burnout, higher depressive symptoms, and worse quality of life in healthcare workers during the COVID-19 pandemic [14].

According to Self-Determination Theory (SDT), the three basic psychological needs are autonomy (i.e., the need to feel volitional and authentic in actions), competence (i.e., the need to feel effective and efficacious), and relatedness (i.e., the need to feel mutual connectedness and caring) [17]. In a previous study we conducted, our findings suggested that nurses' work-related, autobiographical episodic memories of PMIEs during the COVID-19 pandemic had unique associations with increased burnout and, respectively, decreased work motivation, work satisfaction, and adaptive performance compared to their memories of severe moral transgressions (SMTs) [12]. In this study, we used SMTs as a control group, because they are similar to PMIEs in perceived moral severity, but different in terms of perceived external coercion. Thus, one of the defining characteristics of PMIEs is that they are moral transgressions perpetrated/witnessed against the person's will (e.g., a nurse who prioritizes a younger patient over an older patient, based on directives according to which age is an indicator of odds of survival, and against their moral and professional ethical code, which would lead them to prioritize according to how critical the patient's condition was) [5–12]. In contrast, SMTs are more similar to medical errors, in that the outcome of the transgression is very harmful (i.e., high in moral severity) [18–20], but the transgression is enacted in the absence of perceived external pressures (i.e., a nurse who chooses to come to work even if they are aware of being infected with the new coronavirus and spreads the disease to their patients) [20]. The differential associations of PMIEs and SMTs with the outcomes specified above were mediated by the extent to which nurses' autonomy was thwarted in the two memories. Memories of PMIEs were associated with higher autonomy thwarting than memories of SMTs, which, in turn, was associated with more negative psychological health outcomes. However, we did not distinguish between self- and other-PMIEs in this study, treating PMIEs as a singular construct. We also did not explore the mediational role of the other two basic psychological needs (i.e., competence and autonomy) in the differences between PMIEs and SMTs in burnout. We address both these aspects in the current study.

In a different study, we compared nurses' memories of self-PMIEs to their memories of other-PMIEs during the COVID-19 pandemic and found that the former had a stronger association with increased burnout and turnover intentions, mediated by all three basic psychological needs [13]. Thus, memories of self-PMIEs were more autonomy- and competence-thwarting than memories of other-PMIEs, a difference which we attributed to the omission bias [19]. When people enact a moral violation, they judge it as more harmful and blameworthy than when they allow it to happen without interfering. Hence, when forced to perpetrate an immoral act, it is likely that nurses perceived they had less autonomy than when forced to passively witness one, to justify their immoral behavior to themselves [20]. With moral values being central to their professional identities [21], their competence was also more threatened during self-PMIEs, which constituted a more direct threat to their identity compared to other-PMIEs [20,22]. In contrast, relatedness was more thwarted in memories of other-PMIEs compared to self-PMIEs, because they represent acts of organizational betrayal, put in motion by their peers or superiors [5,15,16]. Other-PMIEs were shown to be perceived as signs of disrespect towards nurses and exclusion from medical decision making [23–25], while self-PMIEs represent more distal acts of betrayal [15,16]. However, in this research, we did not use a control group in our design, nor did we explore differences in work engagement. Investigating work engagement alongside burnout is important because, although they do not form a single construct, work engagement contributes to our understanding of occupational wellbeing by adding the dimension of studying the characteristics of normal and satisfactory activity to the more pathology-oriented dimensions of burnout [26,27].

To our knowledge, so far, there are no studies which compare nurses' memories of self-PMIEs and other-PMIEs from the COVID-19 pandemic to SMTs (i.e., a control group) in terms of associations with occupational wellbeing, comprising work engagement, and burnout, and, respectively, turnover intentions. Given the mixed findings on the effects of exposure to self- and other-PMIEs [5,13–16], it could be that the impact of memories of other-PMIEs is either not different or smaller than the impact of SMTs, since the latter can be need-thwarting as well, especially in terms of competence. On the other hand, this impact could be greater, because they could be more autonomy-thwarting than memories of SMTs [12,13], since they constitute passive moral transgressions perpetrated under environmental constraint [15,16]. These perceived environmental constraints represent morally laden limitations imposed on nurses by peers/supervisors/legislators during the pandemic, which could lead to more intense feelings of being disconnected from others and uncared for by them [15,16], which could, in turn, translate into more relatedness thwarting for memories of other-PMIEs compared to SMTs. The differential need thwarting of these types of events has direct implications for the types of interventions necessary for addressing the deficits in occupational wellbeing and turnover intentions associated with the two types of memories [10,16], as well as for prevention and reparatory efforts, which may focus on improving certain protective factors, such as perceived supervisor support and self-disclosure.

1.2. Perceived Supervisor Support

Perceived supervisor support is an organizational factor shown to influence nurses' work satisfaction, job performance, and turnover intentions [28–31]. When nurses believe their supervisors value their contributions and care about their wellbeing [28], they experience more autonomy and job satisfaction, have lower turnover intentions, and provide better patient care [30,32]. Then, higher perceived supervisor support could decrease the impact of memory-related autonomy thwarting on wellbeing and turnover intentions. Knowing that their supervisor is fair and generally supportive of their autonomy could help them restructure their PMIE memories upon repeated recall as caused by exceptional circumstances uncharacteristic for their workplace [33].

1.3. Self-Disclosure

Self-disclosure is the process through which people allow themselves to be known by others [34], helping them cope with traumatic events [35,36], and operating as a protective factor against suicidal behavior [37]. By boosting social support and belongingness, it also protected war veterans against suicidal ideation after exposure to PMIE [38]. As such, nurses with higher levels of self-disclosure share their PMIE-related experiences, increasing their sense of belonging and social support, which could mitigate the negative influence of relatedness thwarting on their wellbeing and turnover intentions.

1.4. Occupational Wellbeing and Turnover Intentions during the COVID-19 Pandemic

Nurses' wellbeing and turnover intentions were dramatically impacted by the COVID-19 pandemic, with consequences on patient care and their health [39,40]. Exposure to PMIEs and subsequent moral injury have been associated with decreased wellbeing and increased turnover intentions in healthcare providers and other populations, especially since the beginning of the COVID-19 pandemic [16,41–43]. With severe negative consequences at the individual and the organizational levels, more in-depth investigation in this area is necessary [39,41,44].

Two central work-related wellbeing indicators are work engagement and burnout [45]. Work engagement is an emotional and cognitive state manifested in vigor, dedication, and absorption [46]. While nurses' pandemic-related stress and worries about their own health led to lower work engagement [47], concerns about the wellbeing of patients predicted higher work engagement [48,49]. Consequently, since being exposed to a PMIE leads to feelings of guilt and shame, adversely affecting the self-concept, we can expect that concerns about oneself are stronger than for SMTs, especially due to the high autonomy thwarting in memories of PMIEs [12]. Thus, after perpetrating an SMT, morally upward counterfactuals help restore the person's morally good self-concept [12], guiding their future actions in that direction [22]. This emphasizes reparatory actions toward the harmed patients, which should lead to higher work engagement. In contrast, memories of PMIEs are not followed by morally upward counterfactuals to the same extent due to higher autonomy thwarting, which blocks mental simulations of alternative future courses of action [12,22]. As such, it is likely that work engagement is lower in this case, since the focus of the concerns would be the person rather than the patients.

Burnout is a syndrome characterized by the constant experiencing of work-related stress, expressed through exhaustion, cynicism, negative work attitudes, and low professional efficacy [50]. Having soared among nurses during this pandemic, it was predicted by nurses' memories of self- and other-PMIEs, through basic psychological need thwarting [12,13,51], which alone can have a negative effect on burnout for up to two years after the event [52]. Turnover intentions were found to be the strongest predictor for turnover behavior, designating a conscious and deliberate willfulness to leave the workplace [53]. They represent "the last in a sequence of withdrawal cognitions, a set to which thinking of quitting and intent to search for alternative employment also belong" [54] (p. 262). Already higher in nursing [44], they spiked during the COVID-19 pandemic [55], being associated with memories of self-and other-PMIEs in this population [13].

Previous research suggested that burnout and work engagement may be antecedents of nurses' turnover intentions [56,57]. Burnout mediated the relationship between perceived organizational justice and respect, work values, fairness, appropriate recognition and compensation, and, respectively, turnover intentions [58]. These workplace characteristics were previously linked to low relatedness satisfaction (i.e., low respect and fairness), low autonomy satisfaction (i.e., low perceived organizational justice), and low competence satisfaction (i.e., low recognition and compensation) [17]. As such, burnout might mediate the relationships between need satisfaction and turnover intentions in our model [58]. Low autonomy was associated with a decreased work engagement in nurses, as they found their jobs less meaningful and felt less responsible for their work, which was associated with higher turnover intentions [56]. Work engagement also mediated the relationship between ethical leadership and decision authority, associated with lower competence and relatedness satisfaction [58], and, respectively, turnover intentions [56]: the more nurses felt connected to and respected by their leaders, and the more their merits were acknowledged fairly, the lower their turnover intentions [57]. As such, work engagement might mediate the relationships between need satisfaction and turnover intentions in our model [54–58].

1.5. Present Study

In our study, our first goal is to investigate whether other- and self-PMIEs may differently influence nurses' occupational wellbeing and turnover intentions compared to SMTs, according to the thwarting of nurses' basic psychological needs associated to each type of memory (Figure 1). As such, we hypothesized:

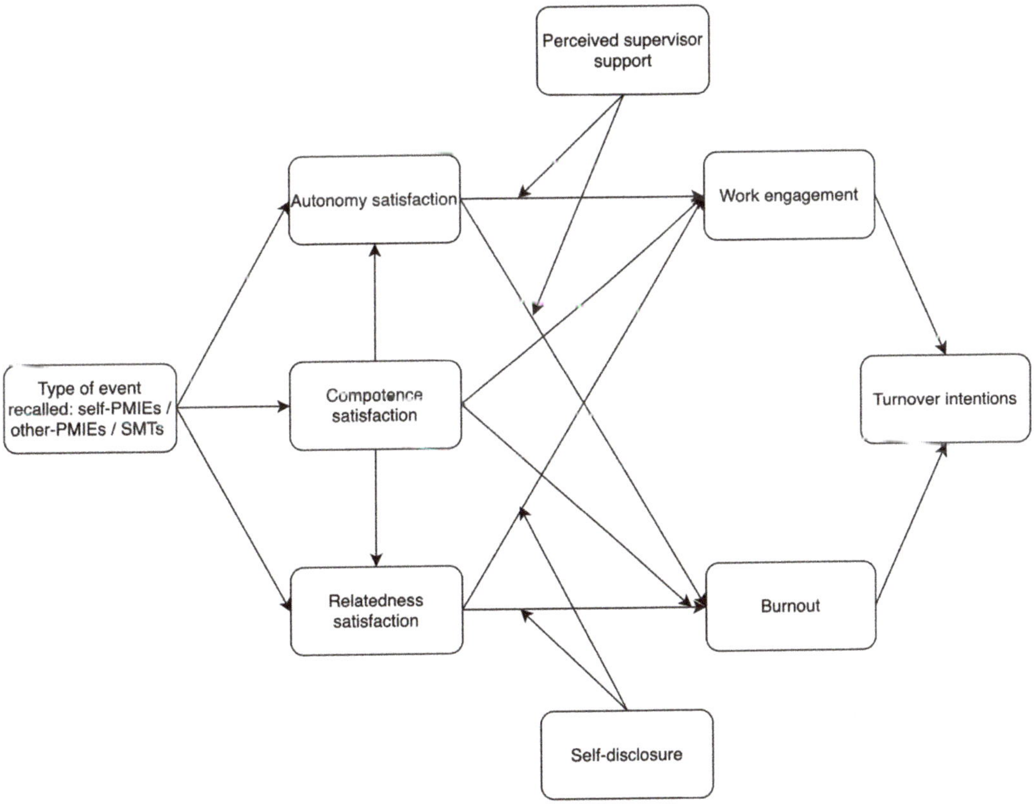

Figure 1. Conceptual model.

H1: *Autonomy will be more thwarted in memories of self-PMIEs than in memories of other-PMIEs and in memories of SMTs.*

H2: *Autonomy will be more thwarted in memories of other-PMIEs than in memories of SMTs.*

H3: *Competence will be more thwarted in memories of self-PMIEs and, respectively, in memories of SMTs compared to memories of other-PMIEs.*

H4: *Relatedness will be more thwarted in memories of other-PMIEs than in memories of self-PMIEs and in memories of SMTs.*

H5: *Relatedness will be more thwarted in memories of self-PMIEs than in memories of SMTs.*

H6: *Memories of self-PMIEs will be associated with lower work engagement, higher burnout, and more turnover intentions compared to memories of SMTs and other-PMIEs.*

H7: *Memories of other-PMIEs will be associated with lower work engagement, higher burnout, and more turnover intentions compared to memories of SMTs.*

H8: *Autonomy, competence, and relatedness thwarting will mediate the differences in burnout, turnover intentions, and work engagement between memories of self-PMIEs, other-PMIEs, and SMTs.*

Our second aim was to investigate whether self-disclosure and perceived autonomy support may operate as protective factors against the influence of basic psychological need thwarting on nurses' occupational wellbeing and turnover intentions. Thus, we hypothesized:

H9: *Nurses with higher levels of perceived autonomy support would experience lower burnout and turnover intentions, and, respectively, higher work engagement, when their memories are highly autonomy-thwarting, compared to nurses with lower levels of perceived autonomy support.*

H10: *Nurses with higher levels of self-disclosure would experience lower burnout and turnover intentions, and, respectively, higher work engagement, when their memories are highly relatedness-thwarting, compared to nurses with lower levels of perceived autonomy support.*

H11: *Burnout and work engagement will mediate the relationships between the types of events recalled, competence, relatedness, and autonomy satisfaction, and, respectively, turnover intentions.*

2. Materials and Methods

The manuscript complies with STROBE reporting guidelines for observational research [59].

2.1. Participants

A convenience sample of 634 Romanian nurses working in hospitals selected through snowballing techniques participated in our study, conducted in February 2022. We collected our data after the fourth wave of the COVID-19 pandemic hit Romania, with a devastating effect on the healthcare system. Infection rates soared to over 20,000 daily new cases, while mortality peaked at 500 deaths per day, in a country with 19 million inhabitants [60]. Given the unpreparedness of the medical system to handle this critical situation and relying on findings from previous waves in Romania [6], we anticipated that nurses in many specialties could have been exposed to PMIEs and attempted to include multiple specialties in our sample to boost representativeness.

First, we invited 608 nurses to participate to our research via e-mail and/or phone, and to extend the invitation to peers who met the inclusion criterion: having worked as a nurse in a hospital for more than six months during the COVID-19 pandemic. We obtained their contact information during previous data collection stages for other studies, when participants agreed to be contacted again for this purpose. A total of 524 of them agreed to participate, and another 241 nurses responded to the invitation extended by their peers, per our request. We randomized the 765 in the three experimental conditions and sent them links to Google Forms. Overall, 52 participants withdrew from the study, and 15 were eliminated because they failed the attention check. Another 64 participants from the self- and other-PMIE conditions were eliminated because their recalled events did not constitute PMIEs, according to their scores on the Moral Injury Events Scale. Hence, our final sample comprised 634 nurses, with 235 in the control group (37.06%), 214 in the other-PMIE condition (33.75%), and 185 in the self-PMIE condition (29.19%), from varied specialties (Table 1).

Table 1. Participants' characteristics.

	Experimental Condition						Total (*N* = 634)	
	Other-PMIE (*N* = 214)		Self-PMIE (*N* = 185)		SMT (*N* = 235)			
Specialty								
Dentistry	0	0%	1	0.54%	0	0%	1	0.15%
Emergency	23	10.75%	12	6.49%	20	8.51%	55	8.67%
Gastroenterology	6	2.8%	3	1.62%	8	3.4%	17	2.68%
Hematology	6	2.8%	7	3.78%	6	2.55%	19	3%
Intensive Care Units	20	9.35%	7	3.78%	16	6.81%	43	6.78%
Infectious Diseases	9	4.21%	8	4.32%	23	9.79%	40	6.31%
Internal Medicine	11	5.14%	11	5.95%	14	5.96%	36	5.68%
Chronic Internal Medicine	10	4.67%	13	7.03%	6	2.55%	29	4.57%
Neurology	16	7.48%	17	9.19%	20	8.51%	53	8.36%
Obstetrics Gynecology	7	3.27%	5	2.7%	12	5.11%	24	3.79%
Oncology	25	11.68%	26	14.05%	29	12.34%	80	12.62%
Palliation	24	11.21%	25	13.51%	34	14.47%	83	13.09%
Pneumology	12	5.61%	15	8.11%	10	4.26%	37	5.84%
Psychiatry	21	9.81%	10	5.41%	12	5.11%	43	6.78%
Radiology	2	0.94%	2	1.09%	2	0.85%	6	0.95%
Surgery	22	10.28%	23	12.43%	23	9.78%	68	10.73%
Age								
$M \pm SD$	38.8 ± 8.75		37.3 ± 9.72		39.2 ± 8.49		38.5 ± 8.97	
Range	21–57		22–57		21–55		21–57	
Sex								
Female	191	89.25%	154	83.24%	193	82.13%	538	84.86%
Male	23	10.74%	31	16.76%	42	17.87%	96	15.14%
Education								
Post-secondary studies	186	86.92%	166	89.73%	218	92.76%	570	89.90%
Bachelor's degree	20	9.35%	9	4.86%	12	5.11%	41	6.50%
Master's degree	8	3.74%	10	5.41%	5	2.13%	23	3.60%
Work experience (years)								
$M \pm SD$	13.6 ± 8.77		13 ± 10.4		13.9 ± 8.29		13.5 ± 9.11	
Range	1–36		1–38		1–35		1–38	

We proceeded in accordance with the ethical rules stipulated in the Declaration of Helsinki. We were granted approval by the ethics committee of our faculty. All participants were legally adults and consented to take part in our study. They were told that their participation was voluntary, and that dropout was possible at any stage. They were informed about anonymity and confidentiality of the information they provided. Due to the delicate nature of the information requested from them, we let them know that none of their data would be shared publicly or seen by any other third party, except for the first two authors. We decided to guarantee this aspect to our participants because they were reluctant to disclose the data needed for this study. In order to avoid social desirability in their responses, we offered them these guarantees. The information we gathered in this study remained securely stored for analyses only. Participants were rewarded for their willingness to take part in the study with five money prizes, each amounting to 100 RON, awarded to them based on a draw.

2.2. Procedure and Instruments

The study was self-paced. After reading and providing their informed consent, participants completed a series of socio-demographic items (i.e., age, sex, education, work experience, current specialty). Then, they filled in the measures of perceived supervisor support and self-disclosure.

Perceived Supervisor Support was measured with the six-item version of the Work Climate Questionnaire (WCQ) [61]. The final score ($\alpha = 0.933$) was the sum of the individual scores, with answers provided on a seven-point Likert-type scale, from 1—"Strongly Disagree" to 7—"Strongly Agree" (e.g., "I feel that my manager provides me choices and options.").

Self-Disclosure was measured with the 12-item Distress Disclosure Index (DDI; e.g., "When something unpleasant happens to me, I often look for someone to talk to.") [62]. Answers were given on a five-point Likert-type scale, from 1—"Strongly disagree" to 5—"Strongly agree". Alpha was 0.966.

Then, participants recalled episodic memories of self- and other-PMIEs and of SMTs, according to the experimental condition in which they had been randomly placed, after reading definitions and examples of the three constructs (see Appendix A for a detailed account of the experimental procedure). The nine-item Moral Injury Events Scale (MIES) modified to assess PMIEs among healthcare workers during the COVID-19 pandemic was filled in next [11]. (e.g., "I acted in a way that violated my own moral code or values in this instance."). The scale was tested and used on Romanian healthcare staff [6]. Responses were provided from 1—"Strongly Agree" to 6—"Strongly Disagree". To evaluate if memories constituted PMIEs, final scores were dichotomized, with answers of "Moderately Agree" to "Strongly Agree" on any of the nine items coded as exposure to a PMIE [11], eliminating participants not recounting PMIEs from the study.

Participants were also asked to morally judge the events recalled from 1—"Slightly Morally Wrong" to 7—"Very Morally Wrong" ("How morally wrong was your behavior in this instance?") [22]. To check the manipulation of recalling SMTs and, respectively, PMIEs, we asked participants to rate the extent to which they perceived themselves as moral victims and transgressors in those circumstances in two items, with answers ranging from 1—"Not at All" to 7—"Very Much" [11]. To check the manipulation of recalling other-PMIEs and, respectively, self-PMIEs, we added an item to evaluate the degree to which participants perceived themselves as witnesses during the events on a scale ranging from 1—"Not at All" to 7—"Very Much".

The level of need satisfaction experienced during their memories was self-rated, since previous research revealed a significant association between participants' and independent judges' ratings [63]. Each need was assessed through two items on a seven-point Likert scale, ranging from −3 (Strongly disagree) to +3 (Strongly agree), with 0—Do not agree nor disagree or not applicable: autonomy (e.g., "I felt free to do things and to think how I wanted"), competence (e.g., "I felt capable and skillful."), and relatedness (e.g., "I felt connected to one or more people") [63–69]. Individual scores for each need were averaged, with higher scores reflecting higher need satisfaction. Scores above zero indicated a need-satisfying memory, and scores under zero, a need-thwarting memory. The scale was used in previous research e.g., [12,13,52,63–69]. The reliability for the three scales was evaluated: Cronbach's alpha for Autonomy = 0.922; Cronbach's alpha for Competence = 0.862; and Cronbach's alpha for Relatedness = 0.910.

Then, participants filled in the scales for burnout, turnover intentions, and work engagement. *Burnout* was measured with the Maslach Burnout Inventory, validated on the Romanian population [70]. The total score ($\alpha = 0.962$) was the sum of the scores on the three dimensions evaluated: *emotional exhaustion* (EE; nine items; $\alpha = 0.985$), *depersonalization* (DP; five items; $\alpha = 0.977$), and *personal accomplishment* (PA; eight items; $\alpha = 0.986$). Answers were given on a seven-point Likert-type scale, from 0—"Never" to 6—"Everyday".

Nurses' turnover intentions were evaluated with the three-item scale from the Michigan Organizational Assessment Questionnaire [71] (e.g., "I will probably look for a new job in the next year."). Answers were given on a seven-point Likert-type scale, from 1—"Strongly disagree" to 7—"Strongly agree". Alpha was 0.943.

Work engagement was measured with a shortened, nine-item version of the original Utrecht Work Engagement scale (UWES-9) [46]. The total score ($\alpha = 0.898$) was the sum of the scores on the three dimensions evaluated: *vigor* (three items: e.g., "At work, I feel that I am bursting with energy."; $\alpha = 0.954$), *absorption* (three items: e.g., "I am immersed in my work."; $\alpha = 0.959$), and *dedication* (three items: e.g., "I am enthusiastic about my job.";

$\alpha = 0.957$). Answers were given on a seven-point Likert-type scale, from 1—"Never" to 7—"Daily".

We employed the attention check used by Stanley et al. [22]: "Do you feel that you paid attention, avoided distractions, and took the survey seriously?" Participants were informed that their answers would not influence their participation in the prize draw. Responses ranged from: 1—"No, I was distracted"; 2—"No, I had trouble paying attention"; 3—"No, I did not take this study seriously"; 4—"No, something else effected my participation negatively"; 5—"Yes". We eliminated from our data analysis participants who responded 1, 2, 3, or 4.

3. Results

3.1. Data Analysis Strategy

First, we verified the validity of our experimental manipulations and participant randomization in the three experimental conditions with one-way and mixed repeated measures ANOVAs, and with chi-square tests of association. Second, socio-demographic differences in outcomes of interest were assessed with Welch's independent sample t-tests and one-way ANOVAs, due to violations of the assumption of equal variances and unequal sample sizes (Table A2). For this purpose, we stratified "age" and "work experience". Correlations between outcomes of interest were also computed. These data analyses were conducted in Jamovi 2 (The jamovi group, Sydney, Australia).

Second, we proceeded to assess our hypotheses, graphically depicted in the conceptual model presented in Figure 1. Since the type of event recalled was a categorical variable with three levels, we dummy-coded it and ran the analysis twice. According to our hypotheses, we first assessed differences between recalling other-PMIEs and recalling SMTs, and, respectively, between recalling self-PMIEs and recalling SMTs (i.e., SMTs were coded with 0, and self-PMIEs and other-PMIEs with 1). The second time we ran the model, we assessed differences between other-PMIEs and self-PMIEs and, respectively, SMTs and self-PMIEs (i.e., SMTs and other-PMIEs were coded with 1, while self-PMIEs with 0). Aside from these exogenous variables, our model included another two exogenous variables, respectively, the two moderators—self disclosure and perceived supervisor support. Autonomy, competence, and relatedness satisfaction were included as mediators of the relationships between the type of event recalled and work engagement, turnover intentions, and burnout. In turn, the mediating role of work engagement and burnout on the relationship between need satisfaction and turnover intentions was also evaluated. Finally, our model tested whether self-disclosure moderated the effects of relatedness on work engagement, burnout, and turnover intentions, and, respectively, whether perceived supervisor support moderated the effects of autonomy on those three outcomes. We controlled for age and education level.

Work engagement and burnout are three-dimensional constructs. Treating multi-dimensional psychological constructs as reflective–reflective has been a contested practice, with newer perspectives suggesting that they should be considered reflective–formative second-order constructs [72]. Construct dimensions (i.e., first-order constructs) are considered reflective because their indicators (i.e., the items on the scales) can be removed or changed. By the same logic, if the second-order constructs were reflective–reflective, their dimensions could be removed or changed. However, this is not the case, because second-order constructs such as burnout and work engagement are formed by their dimensions; in line with previous research, we treated them as type II second-order reflective–formative constructs [73–75].

Given our reflective–formative constructs, average sample size, and non-normally distributed data for our endogenous constructs (work engagement: $W = 0.99$, $p < 0.001$; burnout: $W = 0.98$, $p < 0.001$; turnover intentions: $W = 0.99$, $p < 0.001$; autonomy: $W = 0.97$, $p < 0.001$; competence: $W = 0.96$, $p < 0.001$; relatedness: $W = 0.98$, $p < 0.001$), we assessed our model with partial least squares structural equation modelling (PLS-SEM), according to the recommendations of Becker et al. [76], Ringle et al. [77,78] and Hair et al. [79–81], and in line with previous research [73–75]. The minimum sample size needed for PLS-SEM does not depend on how complex the model is, but rather on the probability that the ratio of a path coefficient and its standard error is higher compared to the critical value of a test statistic for a given significance level [82]. Using the inverse square root method, and assuming a common power level of 80% and significance levels of 5%, the minimum sample size for our model would be 619, for minimum path coefficients of 0.05 to 0.1. The analyses were run in SmartPLS 4.0 [78]. Significance was assessed following a non-parametric bias-corrected and accelerated bootstrapping procedure with 10,000 subsamples [79–81].

First, we assessed our measurement model and examined factor loadings (>0.5), internal consistency (Cronbach's Alpha > 0.7), composite reliability (rhoA and rhoC values > 0.7), convergent validity (AVE > 0.5), and discriminant validity (Fornell and Larcker criterion, HTMT, and cross-loadings) [79–81,83–86]. Our higher constructs were validated with the disjoint two-stage approach, an alternative to the repeated indicators approach, which was problematic for higher-order constructs [79–81,84,86]. First, we modelled our reflective lower-order constructs with their respective indicators, and all the relationships among them, except for moderations. Next, we modelled work engagement and burnout as formative constructs based on the latent scores obtained in the previous step for their respective dimensions, and we assessed multicollinearity with VIF values (<5) and outer weights and loadings based on significance ($p < 0.001$).

Second, we tested our hypotheses by evaluating our structural model with the PROCESS module in SmartPLS [87]. Similar to the PROCESS macro for SPSS, the PROCESS module in SmartPLS can be used for path analyses, as it estimates a set of equations with observed variables [88]. However, in SmartPLS, the indicators of a construct are automatically equally weighted [80]. We assessed direct, indirect, and moderating relationships, followed by conditional mediations, according to our hypotheses. Significance was assessed following a non-parametric bias-corrected and accelerated bootstrapping procedure with 10,000 subsamples [80].

The model's predictive power was assessed with PLSpredict, a procedure used for out-of-sample prediction [89], which estimates the model on a training sample and assesses its predictive power on a holdout sample [90]. The root-mean-square error (RMSE) is usually employed to evaluate the degree of prediction error (i.e., differences between actual and predicted values). RMSE values are compared to naïve linear regression model benchmarks: if all PLS-SEM indicators have lower RMSE values compared to LM, then the model has high predictive power; if most PLS-SEM indicators have lower RMSE values compared to LM, then the model has medium predictive power; and if few PLS-SEM indicators have lower RMSE values compared to LM, then the model has low predictive power [90]. R^2 and f^2 coefficients (i.e., assessing the changes in R^2 when any one predictor is excluded from the model) were examined to assess the explanatory power of our model, and Q^2 was examined for predictive relevance.

3.2. Manipulation and Randomization Checks

To check our experimental manipulations, we ran a one-way and, respectively, a mixed repeated measures ANOVA to assess differences between the three experimental groups according to the perceived moral severity of the recalled PMIE, and, respectively, according to the perceived role in the event (i.e., witness, moral victim, moral perpetrator). Results showed no differences according to moral severity, as well as significant differences in terms of the three roles, supporting the validity of the experimental manipulation (Appendix B, Table A1).

To check participant randomization in the three experimental groups, we ran four one-way ANOVAs to assess differences in age, work experience, perceived supervisor support, and self-disclosure, and, respectively, two chi-square tests of association to assess differences in sex and in education levels. Results showed no significant differences for any of the participants' characteristics (Appendix B, Table A1).

3.3. Participants' Characteristics and Differences between Them according to Outcome Variables

Participants with less work experience (i.e., less than or equal to 10 years) had significantly lower *self-disclosure* than participants with more work experience (i.e., between 11 to 38 years). Similarly, younger participants (i.e., 21–30 years old) had lower self-disclosure compared to participants aged 41–57 years old ($t(631) = -2.82$, $p = 0.014$, $d = -0.29$) (Table A2).

Participants with less work experience (i.e., less than or equal to 10 years) experienced significantly less *work engagement* than participants with more work experience (i.e., between 11 to 36 years). Similarly, younger participants (i.e., 21–30 years old) experienced less work engagement compared to participants aged 31–40 years old ($t(631) = -3.94$, $p < 0.001$, $d = -0.42$) and compared to participants aged 41–57 years old ($t(631) = -4.42$, $p < 0.001$, $d = -0.46$). Participants with post-secondary studies experienced more work engagement than both participants with bachelor's degrees ($t(631) = 2.52$, $p = 0.032$, $d = 0.54$), who experienced more work engagement than participants with master's degrees ($t(631) = 3$, $p = 0.008$, $d = 0.78$) (Table A2).

Participants with less work experience reported more burnout than participants with more work experience. This trend was mirrored by the effects of participants' age, with those aged 21 to 30 reporting more burnout than those aged 31 to 40 ($t(631) = 2.57$, $p = 0.028$, $d = 0.27$) and more than those aged 41 to 57 ($t(631) = 4.17$, $p < 0.001$, $d = 0.43$). We also looked at differences according to the three dimensions of burnout (EE, DP, PA) and found the same pattern of results for EE, with slight differences for PA and DP (Table A2).

Turnover intentions were stronger for the youngest participants (i.e., 21–30 years) than for their older counterparts (compared to 31–40 years: $t(631) = 2.52$, $p = 0.032$, $d = 0.27$; compared to 41–57 years: ($t(631) = 2.39$, $p = 0.046$, $d = 0.25$). Participants with bachelor's studies had lower turnover intentions than participants with master's degrees ($t(631) = -2.47$, $p = 0.037$, $d = -0.64$) (Table A2).

3.4. Correlational Analyses

Pearson's correlations were computed to assess the associations between nurses' well-being and turnover intentions, and, respectively, their self-disclosure, perceived supervisor support, and basic psychological need satisfaction in the recalled memories (Table A3). The higher the burnout, the higher the turnover intentions and, respectively, the lower their work engagement, perceived supervisor support, self-disclosure, and need satisfaction. The higher their work engagement, the lower their turnover intentions, and respectively, the higher their perceived supervisor support, autonomy, and relatedness satisfaction. The higher their turnover intentions, the lower their perceived supervisor support, self-disclosure, and need satisfaction. High perceived supervisor support was associated with high self-disclosure and competence satisfaction. Higher self-disclosure was associated with higher competence and autonomy satisfaction.

3.5. Measurement Model

In the first stage of the disjoint approach, we assessed the factor loadings, validity, and reliability of the model with lower-order constructs only. All factor loadings exceeded 0.5, so we kept all items (Table A4, Appendix D). Internal consistency reliability was satisfactory, with Cronbach's alpha and rhoA values exceeding 0.7 (Table A4, Appendix D). Convergent validity was also satisfactory, with AVE values exceeding 0.50 (Table A4, Appendix D). Discriminant validity was established, according to the Fornell and Larcker [83] criterion (the square roots of AVE for all constructs were greater than their correlations with the other latent constructs—Table A5, Appendix D) and HTMT values (all values below 0.85—Table A5, Appendix D). Cross-loading analyses also showed that all indicators correlated more strongly with their own constructs compared to other constructs in the model.

In the second stage of the disjoint approach, we validated our two higher-order reflective formative constructs: burnout and work engagement. We checked the VIF values of the reflective–formative constructs, and they were below 5. Outer weights were significant, and outer loadings were above 0.5 (Table A6, Appendix D), according to the results of a 10,000-resample bootstrapping analysis.

3.6. Structural Model

To test our hypotheses, we ran two 10,000-sample bootstrapping analyses on unstandardized data, and we found that all R^2 coefficients were larger than 0.10, which indicates that our proposed paths explained the variance of the endogenous constructs adequately [91], with contributions ranging from moderate to substantial [92] (Table A7, Appendix D). The f^2 coefficients, indicative of effect sizes, ranged from high (0.438 for differences between the self-PMIE group and the control group in predicting autonomy) to negligeable (0.011 for differences between the self-PMIE group and the control group in predicting turnover intentions), in line with the complexity of the model [92] (Table A7, Appendix D). The Q^2 values for our endogenous constructs were larger than 0, suggesting predictive relevance. The predictive power of the model was medium, with most PLS-SEM indicators having lower RMSE values compared to LM benchmarks, and with Q^2 values for the indicators of our constructs above 0 (Table A8, Appendix D).

To test our first four hypotheses, we examined the paths from the type of event recalled to each of the three basic psychological needs (Table 2). Autonomy satisfaction was lower in memories of other-PMIEs ($M = -0.75$, $SD = 1.09$) compared to memories of SMTs ($M = 0.24$, $SD = 1.16$), and lower in memories of self-PMIEs ($M = -1.59$, $SD = 1.08$) than in memories of SMTs and other-PMIEs, confirming H1 and H2. Competence satisfaction was higher in memories of other-PMIEs ($M = -0.75$, $SD = 1.06$) compared to memories of SMTs ($M = -1.5$, $SD = 1$) and compared to memories of self-PMIEs ($M = -1.49$, $SD = 0.9$), confirming H3. Relatedness satisfaction was lower in memories of other-PMIEs ($M = -1.35$, $SD = 1.16$) compared to memories of SMTs ($M = 0.19$, $SD = 1.19$) and compared to memories of self-PMIEs ($M = -0.67$, $SD = 1.1$), but lower in memories of self-PMIEs than in memories of SMTs, confirming H4 and H5.

Table 2. Structural Model. Direct Relationships Testing H1–H4.

Paths	Path Coefficients	SE	T	95% CI	
				LL	UL
H1: S/SMT → A	−1.823	0.11	16.64	−1.999	−1.639
H1: O/S → A	0.836	0.109	7.669	0.658	1.016
H2: O/SMT → A	−0.986	0.106	9.306	−1.158	−0.811
H3: O/S → C	0.742	0.098	7.541	0.578	0.901
H3: O/SMT → C	0.744	0.087	8.544	0.601	0.883
H4: O/SMT → R	−1.536	0.111	13.875	−1.718	−1.355
H4: O/S → R	−0.677	0.113	5.997	−0.866	−0.493
H4: S/SMT → R	−0.858	0.112	7.682	−1.04	−0.671

Note: S/SMT = self-PMIEs compared to SMTs, O/S = other-PMIEs compared to self-PMIEs, O/SMT = other-PMIEs compared to SMTs, A = autonomy satisfaction, C = competence satisfaction, R = relatedness satisfaction.

3.6.1. Basic Psychological needs, Work Engagement, and Burnout Were Mediators between Type of Event Recalled and Turnover Intentions

We found significant indirect effects of type of event recalled on turnover intentions through the degree to which relatedness, autonomy, and competence were satisfied, work engagement, and burnout, confirming H8 and H11 (Table 3).

Table 3. Mediation Analysis Results—H8.

Relationships	Total Effects					Direct Effects					Indirect Effects				
	Path Coeff.	SE	T	95%CI		Path Coeff.	SE	T	95%CI		Path Coeff.	SE	T	95%CI	
				LL	UL				LL	UL				LL	UL
H6 and H8: S/SMT → R → UWES → TI											0.083	0.03	2.733	0.044	0.149
H6 and H8: S/SMT → R → BRN → TI	1.563	0.252	6.211	1.162	1.994	−0.065	0.141	0.461	−0.292	0.172	0.038	0.019	1.985	0.015	0.08
H6 and H8: S/SMT → A → UWES → TI											0.168	0.058	2.877	0.089	0.286
H6 and H8: S/SMT → A → BRN → TI											0.043	0.032	1.33	0.003	0.11
H7 and H8: O/SMT → R → UWES → TI											0.149	0.05	2.964	0.081	0.251
H7 and H8: O/SMT → R → BRN → TI											0.067	0.032	2.074	0.027	0.138
H7 and H8: O/SMT → A → UWES → TI	1.203	0.210	5.721	0.866	1.561	−0.11	0.107	1.029	−0.283	0.067	0.091	0.033	2.75	0.048	0.159
H7 and H8: O/SMT → A → BRN → TI											0.023	0.018	1.313	0.002	0.061
H7 and H8: O/SMT → C → BRN → TI											−0.008	0.005	1.515	−0.019	−0.002
H7 and H8: O/SMT → C → UWES → TI											−0.012	0.007	1.655	−0.027	−0.003
H6 and H8: O/S → A → BRN → TI											−0.02	0.015	1.308	−0.363	−0.047
H6 and H8: O/S → A → UWES → TI											−0.077	0.028	2.744	−0.149	−0.044
H6 and H8: O/S → C → BRN → TI	−0.36	0.142	2.530	−0.588	−0.120	−0.045	0.107	0.42	−0.222	0.130	−0.008	0.005	1.523	0.008	0.036
H6 and H8: O/S → C → UWES → TI											−0.012	0.007	1.661	−0.025	0.012
H6 and H8: O/S → R → BRN → TI											0.03	0.015	1.991	−0.35	0.003
H6 and H8: O/S → R → UWES → TI											0.066	0.024	2.777	−0.019	−0.002

Note: S/SMT = self-PMIEs compared to SMTs, O/S = other-PMIEs compared to self-PMIEs, O/SMT = other-PMIEs compared to SMTs, A = autonomy satisfaction, C = competence satisfaction, R = relatedness satisfaction, BRN = burnout, UWES = work engagement, DDI = self-disclosure, TI = turnover intentions.

Thus, the differences in turnover intentions between memories of self-PMIEs (M = 14.9, SD = 3.19) and the control group (M = 12, SD = 3.32) could be explained by differences in autonomy and relatedness satisfaction, which were both associated with decreased work engagement for self-PMIEs (M = 23.4, SD = 6.7) compared to the control group (M = 36.4, SD = 7.87) and increased burnout for self-PMIEs (M = 88.1, SD = 22.6) compared to the control group (M = 55.3, SD = 17.6). The total effect of the differences in turnover intentions between memories of self-PMIEs and the control group was significant, but the direct effect was insignificant, suggesting full mediation.

The differences in turnover intentions between memories of other-PMIEs M = 13.2, SD = 3.49) and the control group (M = 12, SD = 3.32) could also be explained by differences in autonomy, relatedness, and competence satisfaction, which were all associated with decreased work engagement for other-PMIEs (M = 30.8, SD = 5.48) compared to the control group (M = 36.4, SD = 7.87), as well as increased burnout for other-PMIEs (M = 72.4, SD = 14.8) compared to the control group (M = 55.3, SD = 17.6). The total effect the differences in turnover intentions between memories of other-PMIEs and the control group was significant, but the direct effect was insignificant, suggesting full mediation.

The differences in turnover intentions between memories of other-PMIEs and self-PMIEs could be explained by differences in autonomy, which were associated with decreased work engagement and increased burnout for self-PMIEs compared to other-PMIEs. They were also explained by differences in competence, associated with increased burnout for self-PMIEs compared to other-PMIEs. However, differences in competence did not have a significant effect on work engagement which could explain the differences in turnover intentions, higher for self PMIEs than for SMTs. Concerning differences in relatedness between self- and other-PMIEs, they accounted for differences in work engagement (higher for other-PMIEs), which explained differences in turnover intentions (higher for self-PMIEs). However, differences in relatedness did not account for differences in burnout, explaining differences in turnover intentions for these two types of events recalled. As such, the mediation was partial. For the other mediations in the model, see Table A9 (Appendix D).

3.6.2. Moderation Analyses

To test H9, we assessed the moderating role of perceived supervisor support on the relationships between autonomy satisfaction and burnout, autonomy satisfaction and work engagement, and, respectively, autonomy satisfaction and turnover intentions in our model. To test H10, we assessed the moderating role of self-disclosure on the relationships between relatedness satisfaction and burnout, relatedness satisfaction and work engagement, and, respectively, autonomy satisfaction and turnover intentions in our model. We were interested in assessing the rates of change in the indirect effects between the types of events recalled and turnover intentions at lower and higher levels of the two moderators (Table 4; for direct and interaction effects, see Table A10, Appendix D; for conditional direct effects and other conditional indirect effects in our model, please see Table A11 and, respectively, Table A12 in Appendix D).

To do this, we computed indices of moderated mediation [93].

The index value of perceived supervisor support for the moderated mediation effect between other-PMIEs compared to the control group and turnover intentions, through autonomy satisfaction and burnout, was not statistically significant ($\omega = -0.003$, $SE = 0.004$, $T = -0.68$, 95% CI = $[-0.011, 0.003]$). This suggests that, at higher levels of perceived supervisor support, the indirect effect of self-PMIEs compared to the control group was not statistically significantly lower compared to the indirect effect at low perceived supervisor support (Figure 2).

Table 4. Conditional Moderation Analyses.

Paths	Path Coefficient	SE	T	95%CI	
				LL	UL
O/SMT → A → BRN → TI conditional on PSS at −1 SD	0.016	0.008	1.912	0.005	0.033
O/SMT → A → BRN → TI conditional on PSS at Mean	0.013	0.006	1.984	0.005	0.027
O/SMT → A → BRN → TI conditional on PSS at +1 SD	0.01	0.007	1.345	0.001	0.026
O/SMT → A → UWES → TI conditional on PSS at −1 SD	0.043	0.014	3.022	0.024	0.073
O/SMT → A → UWES → TI conditional on PSS at Mean	0.024	0.009	2.595	0.012	0.044
O/SMT → A → UWES → TI conditional on PSS at +1 SD	0.005	0.01	0.532	−0.011	0.023
O/SMT → R → BRN → TI conditional on DDI at −1 SD	0.033	0.014	2.313	0.015	0.062
O/SMT → R → BRN → TI conditional on DDI at Mean	0.018	0.01	1.774	0.006	0.041
O/SMT → R → BRN → TI conditional on DDI at +1 SD	0.004	0.013	0.292	−0.015	0.028
O/SMT → R → UWES → TI conditional on DDI at −1 SD	0.062	0.02	3.136	0.035	0.102
O/SMT → R → UWES → TI conditional on DDI at Mean	0.025	0.013	1.864	0.006	0.051
O/SMT → R → UWES → TI conditional on DDI at +1 SD	−0.012	0.02	0.613	−0.048	0.017
S/SMT → A → BRN → TI conditional on PSS at −1 SD	0.029	0.015	1.94	0.01	0.06
S/SMT → A → BRN → TI conditional on PSS at Mean	0.024	0.012	2.006	0.009	0.049
S/SMT → A → BRN → TI conditional on PSS at +1 SD	0.018	0.014	1.352	0.002	0.048
S/SMT → A → UWES → TI conditional on PSS at −1 SD	0.08	0.025	3.15	0.045	0.13
S/SMT → A → UWES → TI conditional on PSS at Mean	0.045	0.017	2.641	0.022	0.08
S/SMT → A → UWES → TI conditional on PSS at +1 SD	0.01	0.019	0.532	−0.02	0.042
S/SMT → R → BRN → TI conditional on DDI at −1 SD	0.018	0.008	2.212	0.008	0.036
S/SMT → R → BRN → TI conditional on DDI at Mean	0.01	0.006	1.737	0.003	0.023
S/SMT → R → BRN → TI conditional on DDI at +1 SD	0.002	0.007	0.291	−0.008	0.016
S/SMT → R → UWES → TI conditional on DDI at −1 SD	0.035	0.012	2.899	0.019	0.06
S/SMT → R → UWES → TI conditional on DDI at Mean	0.014	0.008	1.827	0.004	0.029
S/SMT → R → UWES → TI conditional on DDI at +1 SD	−0.007	0.011	0.605	−0.027	0.009
O/S → A → BRN → TI conditional on PSS at −1 SD	−0.013	0.007	1.871	−0.029	−0.004
O/S → A → BRN → TI conditional on PSS at Mean	−0.011	0.006	1.922	−0.023	−0.004
O/S → A → BRN → TI conditional on PSS at +1 SD	−0.008	0.006	1.319	−0.023	−0.001
O/S → A → UWES → TI conditional on PSS at −1 SD	−0.036	0.012	2.946	−0.063	−0.02
O/S → A → UWES → TI conditional on PSS at Mean	−0.021	0.008	2.481	−0.038	−0.01
O/S → A → UWES → TI conditional on PSS at +1 SD	−0.005	0.009	0.525	−0.02	0.009
O/S → R → BRN → TI conditional on DDI at −1 SD	0.015	0.007	2.181	0.006	0.029
O/S → R → BRN → TI conditional on DDI at Mean	0.008	0.005	1.686	0.003	0.019
O/S → R → BRN → TI conditional on DDI at +1 SD	0.002	0.006	0.287	−0.006	0.013
O/S → R → UWES → TI conditional on DDI at −1 SD	0.027	0.01	2.879	0.015	0.048
O/S → R → UWES → TI conditional on DDI at Mean	0.011	0.006	1.765	0.003	0.024
O/S → R → UWES → TI conditional on DDI at +1 SD	−0.005	0.009	0.607	−0.021	0.007

Note: S/SMT = self-PMIEs compared to SMTs, O/S = other-PMIEs compared to self-PMIEs, O/SMT = other-PMIEs compared to SMTs, A = autonomy satisfaction, C = competence satisfaction, R = relatedness satisfaction, BRN = burnout, UWES = work engagement, DDI = self-disclosure, TI = turnover intentions.

The index value of perceived supervisor support for the moderated mediation effect between other-PMIEs compared to the control group and turnover intentions, through autonomy satisfaction and work engagement, was significant (ω = −0.019, *SE* = 0.008, T = −2.29, 95% CI = [−0.033, −0.007]). This suggests that, at higher levels of perceived supervisor support, the indirect effect of self-PMIEs compared to the control group was lower compared to the indirect effect at low perceived supervisor support. With an increase in perceived supervisor support, differences between other-PMIEs and the control group in turnover intentions were reduced (Figure 3).

The index value of self-disclosure for the moderated mediation effect between other-PMIEs compared to the control group and turnover intentions, through relatedness satisfaction and burnout, was significant (ω = 0.028, *SE* = 0.02, T = 1.87, 95% CI = [0.04, 0.05]). This suggests that, at higher levels of self-disclosure, the indirect effect of self-PMIEs compared to the control group was lower compared to the indirect effect at low self-disclosure. With an increase in self-disclosure, differences between other-PMIEs and the control group in turnover intentions were reduced (Figure 4).

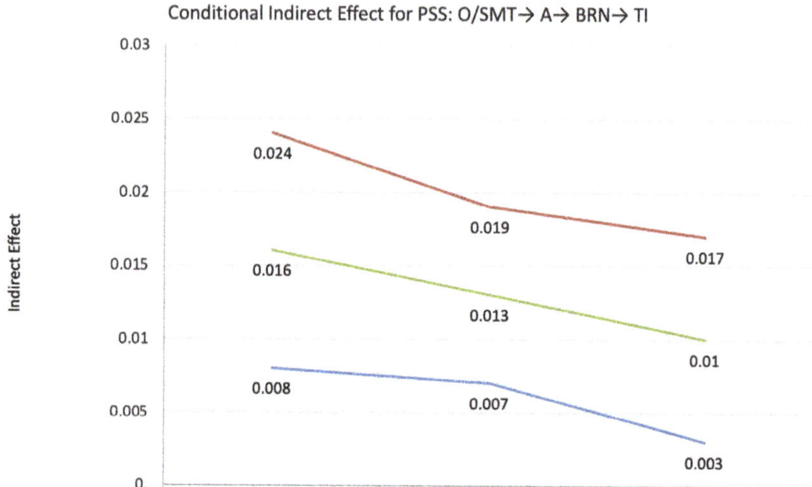

	-5.958	0	5.958
Indirect Effect (IE)	0.016	0.013	0.01
Lower Bound	0.008	0.007	0.003
Upper Bound	0.024	0.019	0.017

Figure 2. Conditional indirect effects of the difference between other-PMIEs compared to the control group on turnover intentions at low, average and high levels of perceived supervisor support, through autonomy satisfaction and burnout.

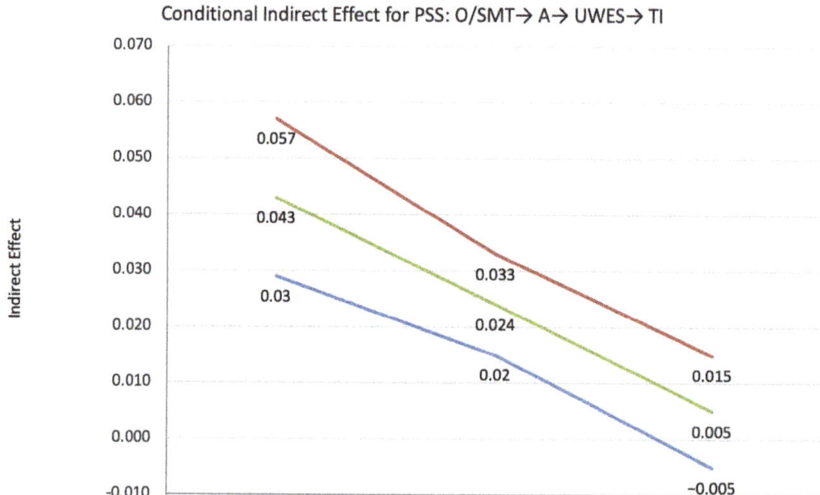

	-5.598	0	5.958
Indirect Effect (IE)	0.043	0.024	0.005
Lower Bound	0.029	0.015	-0.005
Upper Bound	0.057	0.033	0.015

Figure 3. Conditional indirect effects of the difference between other-PMIEs compared to the control group on turnover intentions at low, average and high levels of perceived supervisor support, through autonomy satisfaction and work engagement.

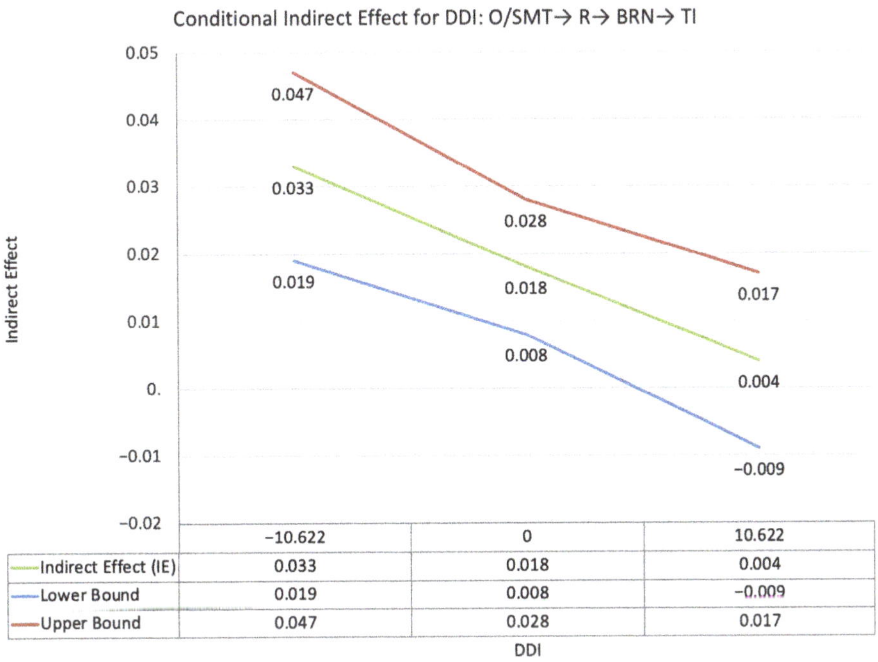

Figure 4. Conditional indirect effects of the difference between other-PMIEs compared to the control group on turnover intentions at low, average and high levels of self-disclosure, through relatedness satisfaction and burnout.

The index value of self-disclosure for the moderated mediation effect between other-PMIEs compared to the control group and turnover intentions, through relatedness satisfaction and work engagement, was significant (ω = −0.018, *SE* = 0.007, T = −2.43, 95% CI = [−0.03, −0.007]). This suggests that, at higher levels of self-disclosure, the indirect effect of self-PMIEs compared to the control group was lower compared to the indirect effect at low self-disclosure. With an increase in self-disclosure, differences between other-PMIEs and the control group in turnover intentions were reduced (Figure 5).

The index value of perceived supervisor support for the moderated mediation effect between self-PMIEs compared to the control group and turnover intentions, through autonomy satisfaction and burnout, was not statistically significant (ω = 0.006, *SE* = 0.008, T = 0.69, 95% CI = [−0.006, 0.02]). This suggests that, although at higher levels of perceived supervisor support, the indirect effect of self-PMIEs compared to the control group is slightly lower compared to the indirect effect at low perceived supervisor support, this difference does not reach statistical significance (Figure 6).

The index value of perceived supervisor support for the moderated mediation effect between self-PMIEs compared to the control group and turnover intentions, through autonomy satisfaction and work engagement, was significant (ω = 0.035, *SE* = 0.015, T = 2.38, 95% CI = [0.013, 0.06]). This suggests that, at higher levels of perceived supervisor support, the indirect effect of self-PMIEs compared to the control group was lower compared to the indirect effect at low perceived supervisor support. With an increase in perceived supervisor support, differences between self-PMIEs and the control group in turnover intentions were reduced (Figure 7).

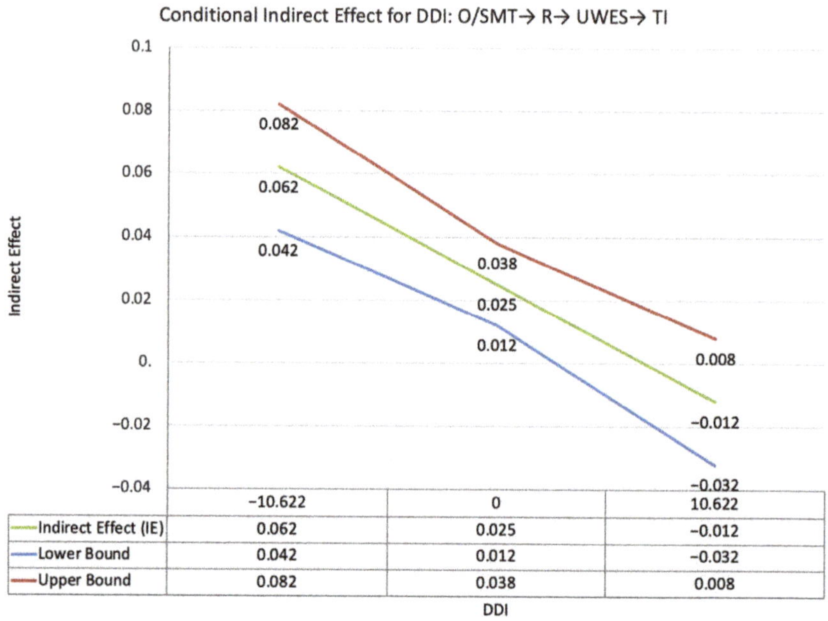

Figure 5. Conditional indirect effects of the difference between other-PMIEs compared to the control group on turnover intentions at low, average and high levels of self-disclosure, through relatedness satisfaction and work engagement.

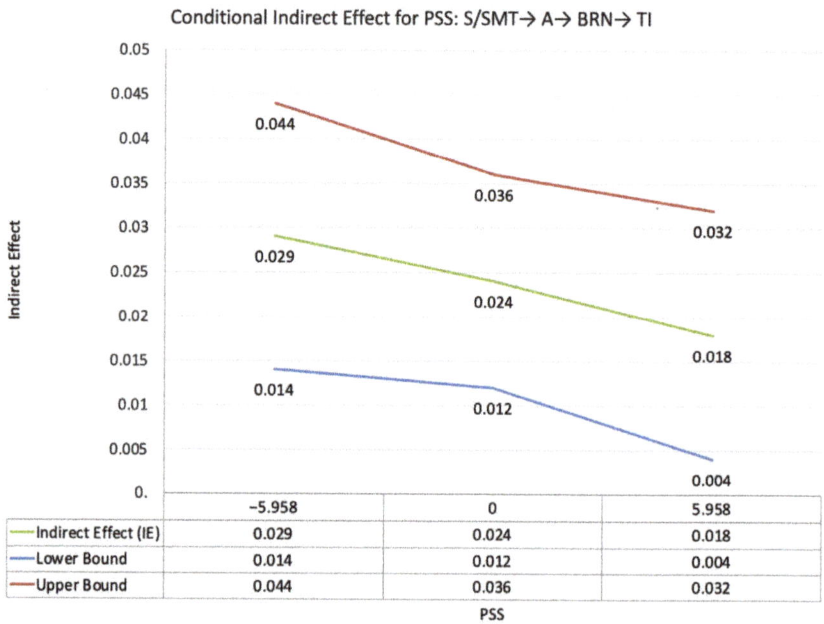

Figure 6. Conditional indirect effects of the difference between self-PMIEs compared to the control group on turnover intentions at low, average and high levels of perceived supervisor support, through autonomy satisfaction and burnout.

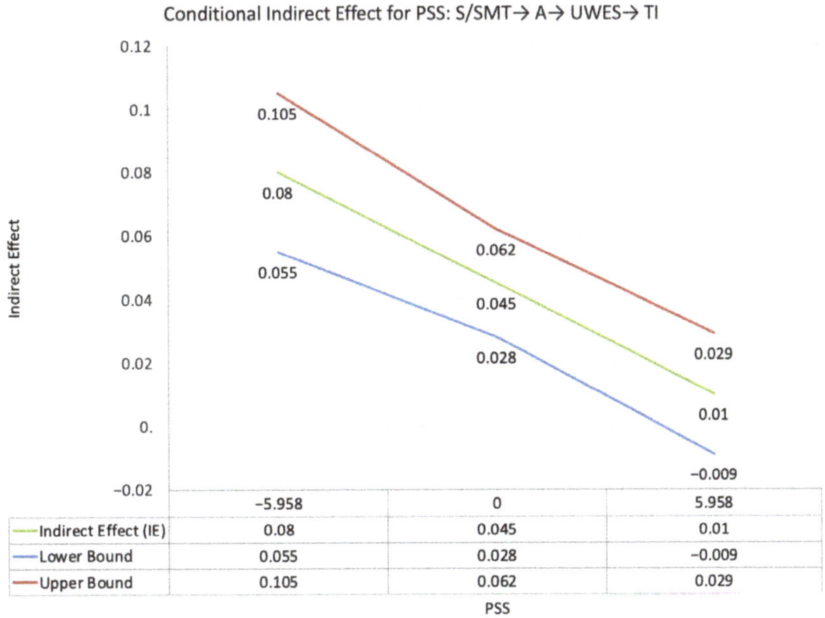

	-5.958	0	5.958
Indirect Effect (IE)	0.08	0.045	0.01
Lower Bound	0.055	0.028	−0.009
Upper Bound	0.105	0.062	0.029

Figure 7. Conditional indirect effects of the difference between self-PMIEs compared to the control group on turnover intentions at low, average and high levels of perceived supervisor support, through autonomy satisfaction and work engagement.

The index value of self-disclosure for the moderated mediation effect between self-PMIEs compared to the control group and turnover intentions, through relatedness satisfaction and burnout, was significant (ω = 0.009, SE = 0.006, T = 1.58, 95% CI = [0.001, 0.019]). This suggests that, at higher levels of self-disclosure, the indirect effect of self-PMIEs compared to the control group was lower compared to the indirect effect at low self-disclosure. With an increase in self-disclosure, differences between self-PMIEs and the control group in turnover intentions were reduced (Figure 8).

The index value of self-disclosure for the moderated mediation effect between self-PMIEs compared to the control group and turnover intentions, through relatedness satisfaction and work engagement, was significant (ω = 0.023, SE = 0.01, T = 2.39, 95% CI = [0.009, 0.004]). This suggests that, at higher levels of self-disclosure, the indirect effect of self-PMIEs compared to the control group was lower compared to the indirect effect at low self-disclosure. With an increase in self-disclosure, differences between self-PMIEs and the control group in turnover intentions were reduced (Figure 9).

The index value of perceived supervisor support for the moderated mediation effect between self-PMIEs compared to other-PMIEs and turnover intentions, through autonomy satisfaction and burnout, was not statistically significant (ω = 0.003, SE = 0.004, T = 0.686, 95% CI = [−0.003, 0.009]). This suggests that, at higher levels of perceived supervisor support, the indirect effect of self-PMIEs compared other-PMIEs was not significantly lower compared to the indirect effect at low perceived supervisor support (Figure 10).

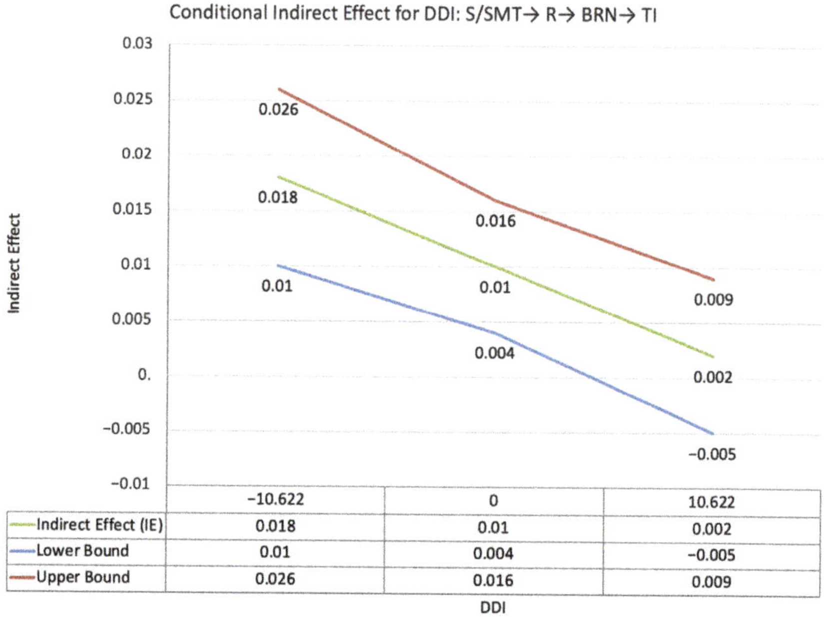

Figure 8. Conditional indirect effects of the difference between self-PMIEs compared to the control group on turnover intentions at low, average and high levels of self-disclosure, through relatedness satisfaction and burnout.

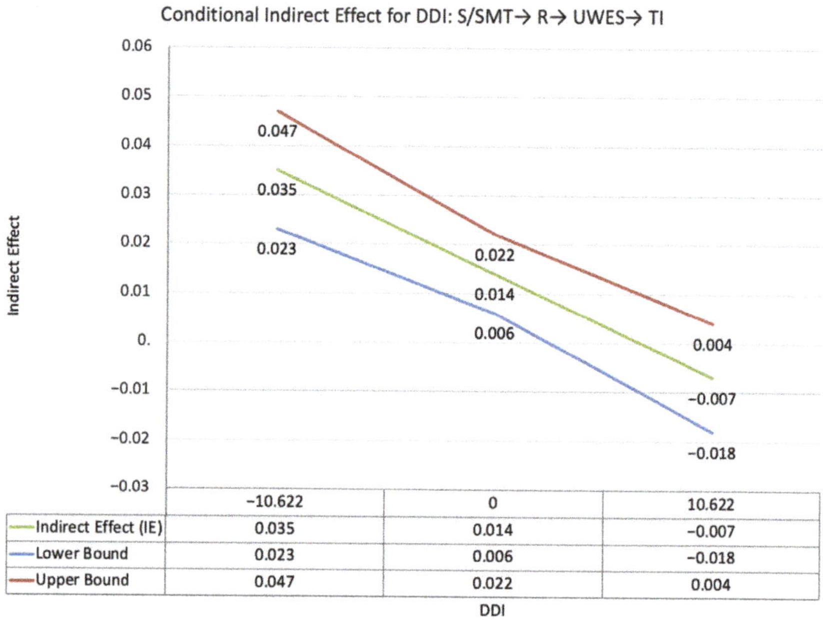

Figure 9. Conditional indirect effects of the difference between self-PMIEs compared to the control group on turnover intentions at low, average and high levels of self-disclosure, through relatedness satisfaction and work engagement.

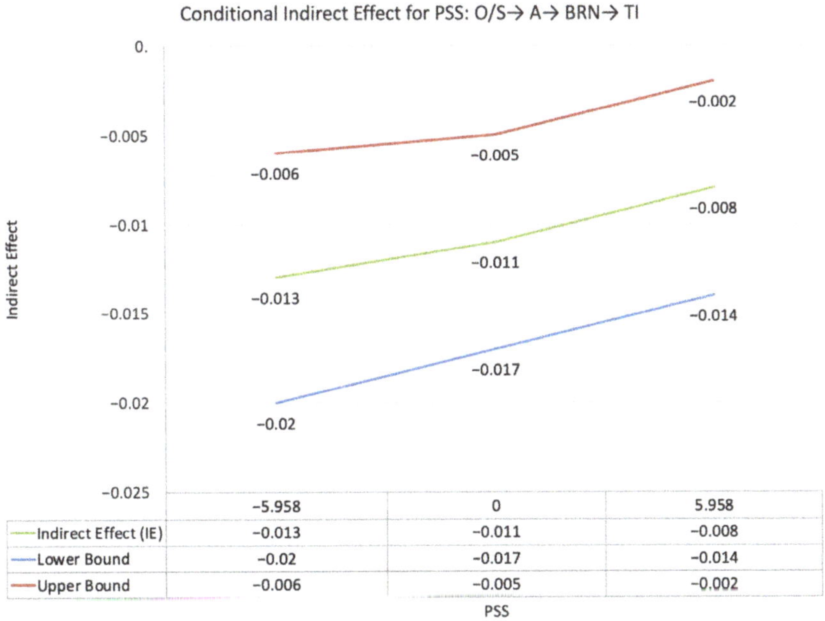

Figure 10. Conditional indirect effects of the difference between self-PMIEs compared to other-PMIEs on turnover intentions at low, average and high levels of perceived supervisor support, through autonomy satisfaction and burnout.

The index value of perceived supervisor support for the moderated mediation effect between self-PMIEs compared to other-PMIEs and turnover intentions, through autonomy satisfaction and work engagement, was significant (ω = 0.016, *SE* = 0.007, T = 2.31, 95% CI = [0.006, 0.028]). This suggests that, at higher levels of perceived supervisor support, the indirect effect of self-PMIEs compared to other-PMIEs was lower compared to the indirect effect at low perceived supervisor support. With an increase in perceived supervisor support, differences between self-PMIEs and other-PMIEs in turnover intentions were reduced (Figure 11).

The index value of self-disclosure for the moderated mediation effect between self-PMIEs compared to other-PMIEs and turnover intentions, through relatedness satisfaction and burnout, was significant (ω = −0.024, *SE* = 0.013, T = −1.83, 95% CI = [−0.47, −0.004]). This suggests that, at higher levels of self-disclosure, the indirect effect of self-PMIEs compared to other-PMIEs was lower compared to the indirect effect at low self-disclosure. With an increase in self-disclosure, differences between self-PMIEs and other-PMIEs in turnover intentions were reduced (Figure 12).

The index value of self-disclosure for the moderated mediation effect between self-PMIEs compared to other-PMIEs and turnover intentions, through relatedness satisfaction and work engagement, was significant (ω = −0.018, *SE* = 0.007, T = −2.43, 95% CI = [−0.03, −0.007]). This suggests that, at higher levels of self-disclosure, the indirect effect of self-PMIEs compared to other-PMIEs was lower compared to the indirect effect at low self-disclosure. With an increase in self-disclosure, differences between self-PMIEs and other-PMIEs in turnover intentions were reduced (Figure 13).

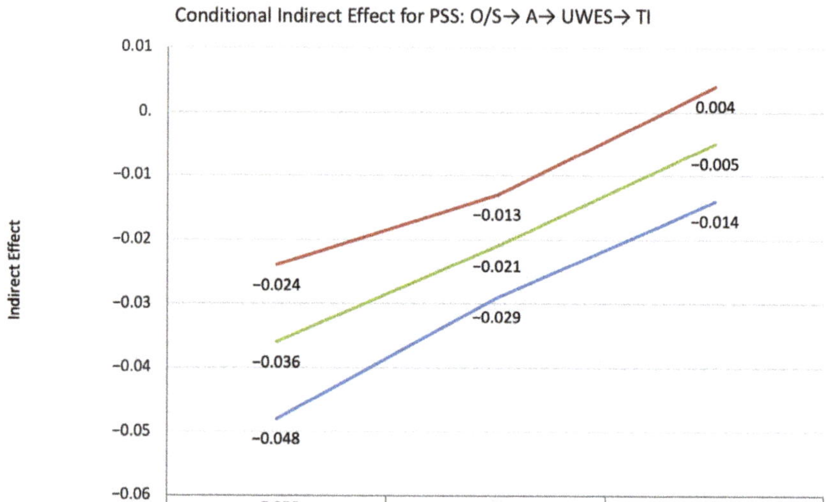

	−5.958	0	5.958
Indirect Effect (IE)	−0.036	−0.021	−0.005
Lower Bound	−0.048	−0.029	−0.014
Upper Bound	−0.024	−0.013	0.004

PSS

Figure 11. Conditional indirect effects of the difference between self-PMIEs compared to other-PMIEs on turnover intentions at low, average and high levels of perceived supervisor support, through autonomy satisfaction and work engagement.

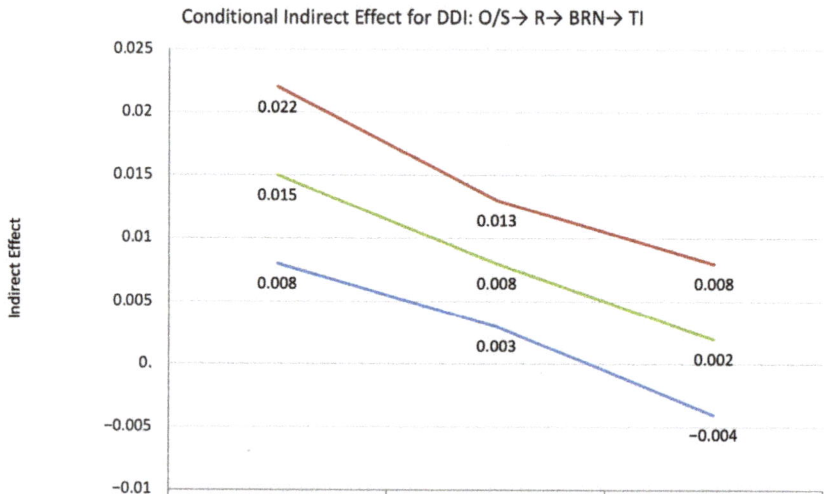

	−10.622	0	10.622
Indirect Effect (IE)	0.015	0.008	0.002
Lower Bound	0.008	0.003	−0.004
Upper Bound	0.022	0.013	0.008

DDI

Figure 12. Conditional indirect effects of the difference between self-PMIEs compared to other-PMIEs on turnover intentions at low, average and high levels of self-disclosure, through relatedness satisfaction and burnout.

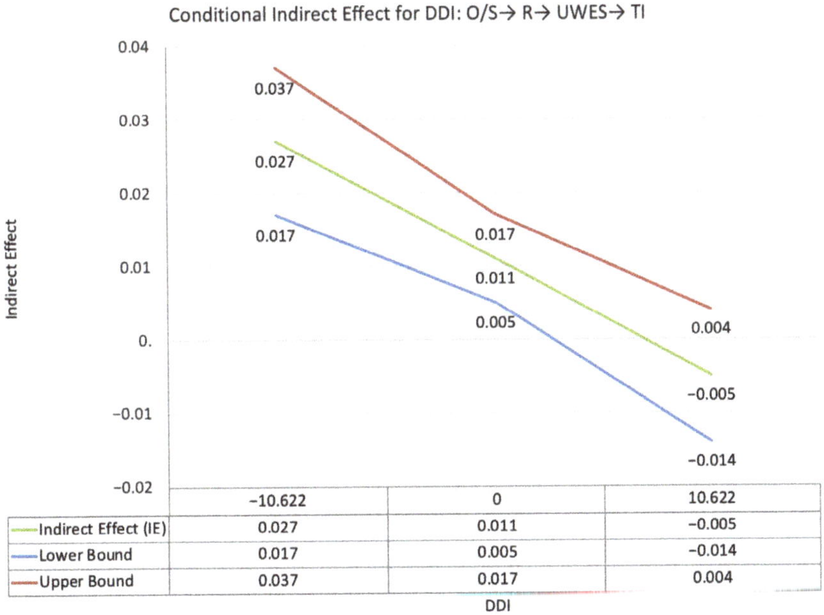

Figure 13. Conditional indirect effects of the difference between self-PMIEs compared to other-PMIEs on at low, average and high levels of self-disclosure, through relatedness satisfaction and work engagement.

4. Discussion

The Romanian healthcare system was the most affected one in Europe during the fourth wave of the COVID-19 pandemic, in terms of the disproportion between resources of all types (e.g., medical supplies, understaffing, insufficient time for patient care) and number of patients requiring medical attention [1–4]. Previous research showed that this constituted a fertile ground for PMIEs [5–16]. This study aimed to investigate the differential effects of Romanian nurses' episodic memories of self- and other-PMIEs during the fourth wave of the COVID-19 pandemic compared to a control group on their occupational wellbeing and turnover intentions, according to basic psychological need thwarting, as well as two potential protective factors for these relationships: perceived supervisor support and self-disclosure. Building on previous studies comparing memories of self-PMIEs to other-PMIEs [13] and memories of undifferentiated PMIEs to memories of SMTs [12], we designed an experiment to better isolate the potential outcomes of nurses' exposure to self-PMIEs from exposure to other-PMIEs, in line with past recommendations [5,13–16]. Our results partially supported our initial hypotheses. The differences in turnover intentions between nurses who recalled memories of self- and other-PMIEs, compared to each other and to the control group, were associated with significant differences in autonomy, competence, and relatedness, which, in turn, were associated with differences in burnout and work engagement. Higher levels of self-disclosure operated as a protective factor for burnout and work engagement, by weakening the strength of their association with relatedness satisfaction and with turnover intentions. Higher perceived supervisor support also helped weaken the association between autonomy satisfaction and work engagement, but it did not have the same effect on burnout in our sample.

The COVID-19 pandemic constituted an unprecedented crisis for healthcare systems all around the world, dramatically impacting patientcare and the psycho-social health and functioning of healthcare professionals. As frontline workers, nurses were among the most affected social categories, especially in terms of exposure to PMIEs [5–11]. This occurred because of the sudden ethical shift brought about by the pandemic: from nursing ethics, which include values from the patient-centered model of care, rooted in deontological ethics, to the public-health-centered approach, rooted in consequentialist ethics, adopted out of necessity during the pandemic [94–96]. As such, the transition from morally valuing the life of each patient to maximizing the number of lives saved led to ethical conflicts, amounting to PMIEs in many instances [5–11]. Aside from moral injury, exposure to PMIEs may have long-term consequences on a multitude of (occupational) health indicators, many of which remain uninvestigated and unaddressed by specific interventions [11,15,16]. Of these, the impact of the autobiographical episodic memories of self- and other-PMIEs should be of immediate concern, given that research suggests they might not have been integrated in autobiographical knowledge yet [13].

Autobiographical knowledge refers to semantic information about the self-concept, informing us about who we are and how we should act. Episodic memories of events which are in stark contrast with what we already know about ourselves are difficult to integrate into autobiographical knowledge, but they can guide behavior and shape attitudes prior to integration as well [64]. For nurses, integrating memories of PMIEs would change their self-concept and work identities, expanding the moral boundaries encompassing their schemas about patientcare and their roles in it [13]. If they internalize such "lessons" from the pandemic, according to which they and their peers are capable of, for instance, prioritizing resources according to arbitrary (and sometimes, discriminatory) criteria e.g., age; [95,96], acts that were once inconceivable outside of crisis situations become possible in more ordinary times. This could result in a catastrophic setback from the model of patient-centered care in nursing.

Aside from organizational and systemic consequences, nurses integrating such morally dissonant identity elements would lead to dehumanization, dissociation mechanisms, and a wide array of pathological outcomes [15,16], which could also contribute to decreasing the quality of patientcare. Thus, as our findings show, both memories of self- and other-PMIEs were associated with significant decreases in work engagement and, respectively, increases in burnout and turnover intentions, compared to a control group, outcomes which contribute to poorer job performance [97,98]. To prevent and treat these consequences of nurses' exposure to self- and other-PMIEs, we first have to better distinguish the unique effects of each on occupational wellbeing and turnover intentions, and to identify the mechanisms through which the memories of these events negatively affect these outcomes. This would expand our search for potential paths of intervention, from reconstructing memories to addressing the basic psychological need thwarting through which they might impair nurses' occupational wellbeing and turnover intentions.

Nurses' memories of self-PMIEs were associated with lower work engagement, higher burnout, and more turnover intentions compared to both memories of other-PMIEs and memories of SMTs. Furthermore, memories of other-PMIEs were also associated with a similar decrease in nurses' occupational wellbeing and, respectively, increase in turnover intentions compared to SMTs. These results support previous findings which showed that self-PMIEs have more negative effects on psychological health and functioning compared to other-PMIEs [5,13,15,16], in contrast to research showing similar effects for these two types of PMIEs [14].

However, these events thwarted basic psychological needs differently. While autonomy satisfaction was lower in memories of both self- and other-PMIEs compared to the control group, it was most thwarted for memories of self-PMIEs, which significantly mediated the associations with burnout, work engagement, and turnover intentions. Competence satisfaction, on the other hand, was highest in memories of other-PMIEs and lowest in memories of self-PMIEs and SMTs. Finally, relatedness satisfaction was lowest in memories of other-PMIEs compared to memories of SMTs and memories of self-PMIEs, but lower for self-PMIEs than for SMTs. This implies that autonomy thwarting could be the main mechanism through which exposure to self-PMIEs may affect long-term psychosocial functioning and health in nurses, while relatedness thwarting could play this role for exposure to other-PMIEs. Finally, nurses feeling ineffective and inefficacious following exposure to self-PMIEs is comparable to the deficits in competence satisfaction occurring after they committed an SMT at their workplace. From an intervention standpoint, this result would indicate that strategies such as the ones used for overcoming medical errors could be efficient in addressing competence thwarting following exposure to self-PMIEs.

Nurses' experience of medical errors is arguably more complex compared to other healthcare providers due to their increased contact with patients, which often puts them in problematic situations after a medical error occurs [99]. Results of a systematic review suggest that disclosing medical errors to patients and family members enabled nurses to feel relief and closure, helping them to emotionally reconcile the event by taking the morally responsible action [100]. Organizational formal support and informal support from colleagues helped them restore personal integrity and implement constructive changes [101]. Future studies should investigate whether these two strategies could help restore nurses' sense of competence following self-PMIEs, although disclosing such events as medical errors to patients would mean taking full responsibility for them, which could be problematic, because of the autonomy thwarting associated with self-PMIEs. Considering that they perpetrated those events under perceived external coercion, future studies should test disclosure to patients as a joint endeavor of the medical staff to alleviate nurses' distress.

For the impact of the deficits in autonomy satisfaction associated with both memories of self- and other-PMIEs on our outcomes, we tested perceived supervisor support as a protective factor. Our results show that it operated as a protective factor against a decrease in work engagement for other-PMIEs, and against increases in turnover intentions for self- and other PMIEs, without contributing to lowering burnout. Having a higher general level of perceived supervisor support could have helped nurses understand that the autonomy thwarting experienced during the self- and other-PMIEs (and associated with their memories of them) are not representative for their workplace and relationship with their supervisors outside of the crisis created by the COVID-19 pandemic. As such, in line with previous research, higher perceived supervisor support lowered the impact of autonomy thwarting on their turnover intentions [30,32]. This implies that interventions focused on increasing perceived supervisor support could help prevent and, possibly, restore the increase in nurses' turnover intentions, attributable to exposure to self- and other-PMIEs during the COVID-19 pandemic. This also suggests that increasing perceived supervisor support could prevent the integration of these memories in nurses' autobiographical knowledge.

On the other hand, perceived supervisor support did not protect against autonomy thwarting for any of the three groups. One possible explanation could be that burnout is considered a more complex syndrome, which severely affects occupational health, with some arguing it should be included as a distinct mental disorder in the current diagnostic system [102]. In contrast, work engagement is a positive, affective-motivational state of fulfillment, characterized by vigor, dedication, and absorption [46], without pathological elements [103]. Higher levels of self-disclosure can have therapeutic properties, as people usually act on their tendency to share their emotional experiences with others, whereas perceived supervisor support is more descriptive of work relationships. This might explain why higher self-disclosure was a significant moderator in our model for burnout, but not for perceived supervisor support.

Unlike perceived supervisor support, which is a result of previous experiences, to a certain extent, self-disclosure is a process of communication in which one naturally engages intentionally, with the purpose of sharing information about themselves and meaningful life events [34]. Previous studies suggest that self-disclosure leads to decreased loneliness [104,105], aiding people to perceive their contexts as empathic, helpful, and affirmative [106]. Thus, in opposition to perceived supervisor support, which describes a previous mode of relating, self-disclosure could have helped nurses experience social support *after* being exposed to PMIEs, and thus exert a reparatory influence. Our results on self-disclosure are in line with past research, which showed that recovery from moral injury was associated with seeking out social support [107] and reconnection activities [108]. This could also occur because sharing one's experience could help them find redemptive meaning in these traumatic events, an ability essential for healing and moving past a PMIE [107–109]. In contrast, perceived lack of support following PMIEs led to sustained psychological distress and to the reinforcement of veterans' sense of moral injury [110,111].

The stronger influence of self-disclosure for self-PMIEs can also be explained by past findings. Since self-PMIE exposure was associated with intense shame and guilt [15,16], disclosing personal information could open new perspectives about the self and the PMIE, fostering the construction of more affirmative narratives of the events [36]. Thus, self-disclosing emotions and information about a PMIE could help adaptive coping by moving from distrust and betrayal to bonding, trust, and empowerment [111].

Our research is not without limitations. Our research was cross-sectional, and we cannot derive any definitive conclusions regarding causality. Future studies should test our results longitudinally. Our sample was not representative of the population of Romanian nurses, although we aimed to collect data from nurses from various specialties. Furthermore, future studies should also explore the content of nurses' memories of self- and other-PMIEs from the COVID-19 pandemic thematically. Although it would have enriched our research to have participants permit us to employ their data for this purpose, they did not agree, due to its delicate nature. Future studies should aim to achieve this purpose. Finally, we conducted three separate studies in 2022 (including the present study) in which we explored associations between Romanian nurses' autobiographical episodic memories from the COVID-19 pandemic and several occupational health outcomes. For all three, we employed snowballing sampling. We first contacted participants who took part in previous studies on different topics and invited them to: (a) participate in the current study; and (b) to contact other potential participants from their personal networks who met the eligibility criteria. Since we extended this invitation for all three studies, we may have had people who took part in all three of them, which might have led to their becoming familiar with the purpose of our studies, since they were debriefed after each one. It should also be noted that their personal contacts may have shared socio-demographic characteristics with them, since they were more likely to contact friends/colleagues of similar age and background. This might have decreased the heterogeneity of our samples, but also the external validity of our findings. Future studies should test our results in different geo-cultural settings and on representative samples of nurses.

5. Conclusions

Our study experimentally assessed the differential associations between nurses' autobiographical episodic memories of self- and other-PMIEs from the COVID-19 pandemic and burnout, work engagement, and turnover intentions, compared to a control group. We also explored whether differences in the three basic psychological needs (i.e., autonomy, competence, and relatedness) mediated this differential impact. In addition, we tested two potential protective factors: perceived supervisor support for autonomy satisfaction and self-disclosure for relatedness satisfaction. To the best of our knowledge, this is the first study which focuses on exploring these potential avenues for prevention and reparations following nurses' exposure to self- and other-PMIEs during the COVID-19 pandemic. Our results suggest that both self- and other-PMIEs have unique associations with work engagement, burnout, and turnover intentions though different basic psychological need thwarting. As such, relatedness was more thwarted for memories of other-PMIEs, whereas competence and autonomy were more thwarted in memories of self-PMIEs. High perceived supervisor support can constitute a protective factor against the increase in turnover intentions associated to both types of PMIE memories, rendering the associations between autonomy thwarting and turnover intentions insignificant. It can also constitute a protective factor against the decrease in work engagement associated with memories of other-PMIEs, in a similar fashion. High self-disclosure can constitute a protective factor against the decrease in work engagement and, respectively, the increase in burnout, rendering the associations between relatedness thwarting and these two outcomes insignificant or less significant. All in all, our findings suggest that different strategies for moral repair should be employed to address the deleterious effects of the exposure of nurses to self- and other-PMIEs, highlighting the relevance of the nature of the outcome as well.

Author Contributions: Authors had equal contributions to this research. Conceptualization, M.A.G., L.A., A.C.H. and C.S.; methodology, M.A.G., L.A., A.C.H. and C.S.; investigation, M.A.G., L.A., A.C.H. and C.S.; data curation, M.A.G., L.A., A.C.H. and C.S.; writing—original draft preparation, M.A.G., L.A., A.C.H. and C.S.; writing—review and editing, M.A.G., L.A., A.C.H. and C.S. All authors have read and agreed to the published version of the manuscript.

Funding: This work was supported by a grant of the Romanian Ministry of Education and Research, CNCS—UEFISCDI, project number PN-III-P1-1.1-PD-2019-0982, within PNCDI III. The sponsor did not have any involvement in study design, collection, analysis and interpretation of data, writing of the report or decision to submit the article for publication. Authors are also thankful to the Romanian Ministry of Research, Innovation and Digitization, within Program 1—Development of the national RD system, Subprogram 1.2—Institutional Performance—RDI excellence funding projects, Contract no.11PFE/30.12.2021, for financial support.

Institutional Review Board Statement: The study was conducted in accordance with the Declaration of Helsinki and approved by the Ethics Committee of the Faculty of Psychology and Education Sciences, Alexandru Ioan Cuza University, Iasi, Romania (protocol numbers are not issued by this Ethics Committee; the date of approval was 27 November 2020).

Informed Consent Statement: Informed consent was obtained from all subjects involved in the study.

Data Availability Statement: The data presented in this study are available on request from the corresponding author. The data are not publicly available due to ethical constraints created by the sensitive topic investigated, which precludes us from sharing the content of the memories of moral transgressions recalled by participants, as well as information based on which participants could be identified.

Conflicts of Interest: The authors declare no conflict of interest. The funders had no role in the design of the study; in the collection, analyses, or interpretation of data; in the writing of the manuscript, or in the decision to publish the results.

Appendix A

Experimental Procedure

First, all participants read definitions and examples for the roles of "moral victims" and "moral transgressors". Moral transgressors were defined as "individuals whose intentions and actions bring about harmful events" and moral victims as "individuals who experience feelings and emotions brought about by the moral transgressor's actions" [9]. They were told that the same person can be a moral transgressor or a moral victim at different times or at the same time. The examples of moral transgressors and victims were the ones used by Gherman et al. [12], fitted for the nurses' work environment and depicting severe moral transgressions (i.e., having had harmful effects for patients) [20,22]. The example for the role of moral transgressor was:

> *"Laura is a nurse at a hospital in Romania. One morning during the 4th wave of the COVID-19 pandemic, she woke up feeling sick, and tested herself for COVID-19 at home with three rapid tests. Although all three tests were positive, she went to work anyway, because she had the opportunity to work an extra shift and make more money. Patients and colleagues contracted the infection from her and several of them are still in the ICU, with reserved prognoses. Laura felt terribly guilty and ashamed about the consequences of her action".*

The example for the role of moral victim was:

> *"Laura is a nurse at a hospital in Romania. During the 4th wave of the COVID-19 pandemic, she unknowingly cared for a patient who was infected with COVID-19. The patient knew about the infection, but lied about it, taking advantage of the fact that patients were not tested prior to being committed. Laura, along with several other*

patients and colleagues, contracted COVID-19 from the patient, and she is now in the ICU, with a reserved prognosis. Laura felt betrayed and angered about the consequences of the patient's action".

Next, all participants read definitions and examples for self-PMIEs, other-PMIEs, and SMTs. All examples depicted severe moral transgressions, with severity operationalized as the magnitude of the harmful effects on patients [18] and were devised according to Brüggemann et al. [18] and Gherman et al. [12].

Self-PMIEs were defined as: "events or action during which you felt as both a moral victim and a moral transgressor, when you did something that you felt was morally wrong not because you wanted to, but because you felt as if you did not have a choice" [9].

The example for self-PMIEs was: "Laura is a nurse at a hospital in Romania. During the 4th wave of the COVID-19 pandemic, the beds in the ICU were all occupied, and she had to care for several patients with COVID-19 in the ER. Four patients were rapidly deteriorating, all of them badly needing access to ventilators. None were available, and Laura had to decide to start manual ventilation on one of them. The physicians on call were not answering, and patients' oxygen saturations were dropping quickly. In the spur of the moment, she started the procedure on the youngest patient, a 12-year-old child. Until other nurses could join her, the oldest patient of the four died. Laura felt incredibly guilty for not having saved his life".

Other-PMIEs were defined as: "events or action during which you felt as both a moral victim and a moral transgressor, when you witnessed something that you felt was morally wrong and failed to act or speak out not because you wanted to, but because you felt as if you did not have a choice" [9].

The example for others-PMIEs was: "Laura is a nurse at a hospital in Romania. During the 4th wave of the COVID-19 pandemic, the beds in the ICU were all occupied, and she had to care for several patients with COVID-19 in the ER. Four patients were rapidly deteriorating, all of them badly needing access to ventilators. None were available, and the physician on call had to decide to start manual ventilation on two of them. He told Laura to start the procedure on the youngest patient, a 12-year-old child, while he proceeded to do the same on a 26-year-old female. Until other medical staff could join them, the oldest patient of the four died. Laura felt incredibly guilty for not having saved his life, since, in her opinion, his condition was the most critical of the four, but felt that she could not have disobeyed the doctor's order".

SMTs were defined as: "events or action during which you felt as a moral transgressor, when you did something that you felt was morally wrong in the absence of any external pressures to do so" [9,12].

The example for SMTs was the same as the one for the role of moral transgressor, previously used by Gherman et al. [12]: "Laura is a nurse at a hospital in Romania. One morning during the 4th wave of the COVID-19 pandemic, she woke up feeling sick, and tested herself for COVID-19 at home with three rapid tests. Although all three tests were positive, she went to work anyway, because she had the opportunity to work an extra shift and make more money. Patients and colleagues contracted the infection from her and several of them are still in the ICU, with reserved prognoses. Laura felt terribly guilty and ashamed about the consequences of her action".

All examples depicted work-related incidents to prepare participants for the recall tasks.

Next, participants in the self-PMIE condition received the following instruction, adapted from previous research [12,13,52,63–69]: "Please describe a personal memory of a specific event related to your work during the COVID-19 pandemic which you consider a self-PMIE, as defined and exemplified above. Select a memory significant to you which is at least six-months-old, and which often comes to your mind. This memory should be of the most morally wrong thing you have done during the pandemic with harmful consequences on a patient, under environmental constraints. Describe in a general fashion what happened, where it happened, who you were with (if anyone), and how you and other people reacted. Please remember we are not interested in the identities of anybody involved, so feel free to use phrases such as 'a colleague', 'a boss', 'a patient', and other generic denominators. What is important to us is for you to remember specific details, not for us to know them. Describe your role and what have been the consequences of your reaction or of your actions during this event. Please provide enough details so that we can fully understand what happened, as if you were telling a story to someone. We would also like to assure you that the content of your memories will not be shared with anybody outside of the two first authors and it will not be used in our analyses".

Participants in the other-PMIE condition received the same instruction, with the first two sentences modified as such: "Please describe a personal memory of a specific event related to your work during the COVID-19 pandemic which you consider an other-PMIE, as defined and exemplified above. Select a memory significant to you which is at least six-months-old, and which often comes to your mind. This memory should be of the most morally wrong thing you have witnessed during the pandemic with harmful consequences on a patient, against which you wanted to speak out or take action, but you felt you could not".

Finally, participants in the SMT condition also received the same instruction, with the first two sentences modified as such: "Please describe a personal memory of a specific event related to your work during the COVID-19 pandemic which you consider a severe moral transgression, as defined and exemplified above. Select a memory significant to you which is at least six-months-old, and which often comes to your mind. This memory should be of the most morally wrong thing you have done during the pandemic with harmful consequences on a patient, without any external pressure to do so".

Appendix B

Manipulation Checks Results

To check for differences in perceived moral severity of the events recalled across the three experimental conditions, we conducted a one-way ANOVA, which showed no significant differences between the three groups: $F_{(6, 631)} = 0.08$, $p = 0.923$, $\eta^2 = 0$ (Table A1)

To assess differences between the three experimental groups according to the perceived role in the event (i.e., witness, moral victim, moral perpetrator), we ran a mixed repeated measures ANOVA, with the experimental group as the between-subjects factor, and the perceived role as the within-subjects factor. Mauchly's test of sphericity showed the violation of the assumption of sphericity, $\chi^2_{(2)} = 0.906$, $p < 0.001$, so we used a Greenhouse–Geisser correction for within-subjects effects. The results of the three-way mixed ANOVA showed significant main effects for type of role ($F_{(1.83, 1153.54)} = 418$, $p < 0.001$, $\eta_p^2 = 0.399$), experimental condition ($F_{(2, 631)} = 465$, $p < 0.001$, $\eta_p^2 = 0.596$), and the interaction between them ($F_{(3.66, 1153.54)} = 587$, $p < 0.001$, $\eta_p^2 = 0.651$). Post-hoc tests with Tukey corrections showed that, for the witness role, there were no significant differences between the SMT ($M = 1.96$, $SD = 0.83$) and the self-PMIE ($M = 2.16$, $SD = 1.01$) groups ($t_{(631)} = 2.18$, $p = 0.417$), and people recalling other-PMIEs ($M = 5.91$, $SD = 0.99$) perceived themselves as moral transgression witnesses significantly more than the ones recalling self-PMIEs ($t_{(631)} = 41.27$, $p < 0.001$) and SMTs ($t_{(631)} = -41.58$, $p < 0.001$). For the perpetrator role, there were no significant differences between the SMT ($M = 5.85$, $SD = 1$) and the self-PMIE ($M = 5.85$, $SD = 1.15$) groups ($t_{(631)} = 0.02$, $p = 1$), and people recalling other-PMIEs ($M = 4.08$, $SD = 2.01$) perceived themselves as moral transgressors significantly less than the ones recalling self-PMIEs ($t_{(631)} = -11.99$, $p < 0.001$) and SMTs ($t_{(631)} = 12.76$, $p < 0.001$). For the victim role, there were no significant differences between the other-PMIE ($M = 5.87$, $SD = 1.1$) and the self-PMIE ($M = 5.83$, $SD = 1.07$) groups ($t_{(631)} = 0.39$, $p = 1$), and people recalling SMTs ($M = 2.11$, $SD = 1.03$) perceived themselves as moral victims significantly less than the ones recalling self-PMIEs ($t_{(631)} = -35.4$, $p < 0.001$) and other-PMIEs ($t_{(631)} = -37.24$, $p < 0.001$). People recalling SMTs felt less like moral witnesses than moral perpetrators ($t_{(631)} = -31.86$, $p < 0.001$), and more like moral perpetrators than moral victims ($t_{(631)} = 31.05$, $p < 0.001$), with no significant differences between the roles of moral witness and moral victim ($t_{(631)} = 0.55$, $p = 1$). People recalling other-PMIEs felt more like moral witnesses than moral perpetrators ($t_{(631)} = 15.06, p < 0.001$), and less like moral perpetrators than moral victims ($t_{(631)} = -14.14, p < 0.001$), with no significant differences between the roles of moral witness and moral victim ($t_{(631)} = 0.44, p = 1$). People recalling self-PMIEs felt less like moral witnesses than moral perpetrators ($t_{(631)} = -29.82, p < 0.001$), and less like moral witnesses than moral victims ($t_{(631)} = -37.33, p < 0.001$), with no significant differences between the roles of moral perpetrator and moral victim ($t_{(631)} = 0.16, p = 1$).

Table A1. Differences between the three experimental groups according to perceived moral severity, age, work experience, perceived supervisor support, self-disclosure, sex, education.

	Self-PMIE	Other-PMIE	SMT				
	$M \pm SD$	$M \pm SD$	$M \pm SD$	F	df	p	η^2
Moral severity	6.06 ± 0.8	6.07 ± 0.82	6.04 ± 0.76	0.08	2, 631	0.923	0
Age	39.2 ± 8.49	38.8 ± 8.75	37.3 ± 9.72	2.66	2, 631	0.07	0.008
Work experience	13.9 ± 8.29	13.6 ± 8.78	13 ± 10.4	0.43	2, 631	0.65	0.001
PSS	21.1 ± 5.37	21.4 ± 5.28	20.9 ± 7.28	0.31	2, 631	0.735	0.001
Self-Disclosure	35.3 ± 10.7	35.2 ± 10.3	36.1 ± 11	0.39	2, 632	0.674	0.001
	Observed frequencies			χ^2	df	p	n
Sex (Male/Female)	31/154	23/191	42/193	4.95	2	0.084	634
Education (PS/B/M)	166/9/10	186/20/8	218/12/5	7.65	4	0.105	634

Note: SMT = severe moral transgressions; self-PMIEs = potentially morally injurious events perpetrated by the self; other-PMIEs = potentially morally injurious events witnessed by the self; PS = Post-secondary Studies; B = Bachelor's Degree; M = Master's Degree; PSS = perceived supervisor support.

Appendix C

Table A2. Socio-demographic differences in perceived supervisor support, self-disclosure, work engagement, emotional exhaustion, depersonalization, personal accomplishment, burnout, and turnover intentions.

Characteristics	N	$M \pm SD$	t/F	Cohen's d/η^2	Post-Hoc Tests [a]
		Perceived Supervisor Support			
Sex			$t(632) = -0.23, p = 0.818$	−0.03	
Male	96	21 ± 6.53			
Female	538	21.2 ± 5.86			
Work experience (years)			$t(632) = -1.95, p = 0.052$	−0.16	-
0.5–10	298	20.6 ± 6.1			
11–38	336	21.6 ± 5.8			
Age (years)			$F(2, 631) = 1.19, p = 0.304$	0	
21–30	144	20.5 ± 6.27			
31–40	232	21.1 ± 5.86			
41–57	158	21.5 ± 5.86			
Education			$F(2, 631) = 2.18, p = 0.113$	0.01	-
PS	570	21 ± 5.95			
B	41	23 ± 5.89			
M	23	20.8 ± 6.01			
		Self-Disclosure			
Sex			$t(632) = -0.34, p = 0.732$	−0.04	
Male	96	35.1 ± 10.89			
Female	538	35.5 ± 10.58			
Work experience (years)			$t(632) = -3.26, p = 0.001$	−0.26	-
0.5–10	298	34 ± 10.61			
11–38	336	36.8 ± 10.49			
Age (years)			$F(2, 631) = 4.48, p = 0.012$	0.01	21–30 < 41–57 *
21–30	144	33.8 ± 10.8			
31–40	232	34.9 ± 10			
41–57	158	36.9 ± 10.9			
Education			$F(2, 631) = 1.07, p = 0.345$	0	-
PS	570	35.6 ± 10.7			
B	41	34.9 ± 11.5			
M	23	32.4 ± 6.79			
		Work Engagement			

Table A2. *Cont.*

Characteristics	N	$M \pm SD$	t/F	Cohen's d/η^2	Post-Hoc Tests [a]
Sex			$t(632) = -0.43, p = 0.670$	−0.05	
Male	96	30.4 ± 9.6			
Female	538	30.8 ± 8.41			
Work experience (years)			$t(632) = -3.75, p < 0.001$	−0.3	-
0.5–10	298	29.4 ± 8.53			
11–38	336	31.9 ± 8.48			
Age (years)			$F(2, 631) = 10.9, p < 0.001$	0.03	21–30 < 31–40 ***, 21–30 < 41–57 ***
21–30	144	27.9 ± 8.49			
31–40	232	31.4 ± 8.12			
41–57	158	31.7 ± 8.74			
Education			$F(2, 631) = 4.54, p = 0.011$	0.01	PS > M *, B > M **
PS	570	30.8 ± 8.71			
B	41	32.9 ± 7.69			
M	23	26.2 ± 5.08			
		Emotional Exhaustion			
Sex			$t(632) = 0.14, p = 0.889$	0.02	-
Male	96	29 ± 12.11			
Female	538	28.9 ± 11.52			
Work experience (years)			$t(632) = 2.66, p = 0.008$	0.21	-
0.5–10	298	30.2 ± 11.64			
11–38	336	27.7 ± 11.46			
Age (years)			$F(2, 631) = 8.63, p < 0.001$	0.03	21–30 > 31–40 *, 21–30 > 41–57 ***
21–30	144	32 ± 11.2			
31–40	232	29 ± 11.5			
41–57	158	27.1 ± 11.6			
Education			$F(2, 631) = 1.5, p = 0.223$	0.01	-
PS	570	28.6 ± 11.8			
B	41	30.3 ± 9.14			
M	23	32.4 ± 9.1			
		Depersonalization			
Sex			[b] $t(120) = -0.2, p = 0.845$	−0.02	-
Male	96	15.4 ± 7.45			
Female	538	15.6 ± 6.21			
Work experience (years)			$t(632) = 2.89, p = 0.004$	0.23	-
0.5–10	298	16.4 ± 6.43			
11–38	336	14.9 ± 6.32			
Age (years)			$F(2, 631) = 1.63, p = 0.197$	0.05	
21–30	144	16.4 ± 6.54			
31–40	232	15.4 ± 6.36			
41–57	158	15.3 ± 6.36			
Education			$F(2, 631) = 3.86, p = 0.022$	0.01	PS < B *, PS < M *
PS	570	15.5 ± 6.41			
B	41	15.1 ± 5.88			
M	23	19.2 ± 6.34			
		Personal Accomplishment			
Sex			$t(632) = 0.28, p = 0.779$	0.03	-
Male	96	26.5 ± 11.6			
Female	538	26.1 ± 10.78			
Work experience (years)			$t(632) = 3.39, p < 0.001$	0.27	-
0.5–10	298	27.7 ± 10.79			
11–38	336	24.8 ± 10.82			
Age (years)			$F(2, 631) = 5.21, p = 0.006$	0.02	21–30 > 41–57 **
21–30	144	28.4 ± 11.3			
31–40	232	26.3 ± 10.3			
41–57	158	24.8 ± 11			
Education			$F(2, 631) = 1.45, p = 0.236$	0.01	-
PS	570	26 ± 11.1			
B	41	26.7 ± 9.79			
M	23	29.9 ± 8.19			
		Burnout			

Table A2. *Cont.*

Characteristics	N	$M \pm SD$	t/F	Cohen's d/η^2	Post-Hoc Tests [a]
Sex			$t(632) = 0.14, p = 0.886$	0.02	-
Male	96	70.9 ± 24.21			
Female	538	70.6 ± 22.45			
Work experience (years)			$t(632) = 3.82, p < 0.001$	0.3	-
0.5–10	298	74.3 ± 22.93			
11–38	336	67.4 ± 22.04			
Age (years)			$F(2, 631) = 8.7, p < 0.001$	0.03	21–30 > 31–40 *, 21–30 > 41–57 ***
21–30	144	76.8 ± 23.5			
31–40	232	70.7 ± 21.7			
41–57	158	67.1 ± 22.4			
Education			$F(2, 631) = 2.87, p = 0.057$	0.01	-
PS	570	70.1 ± 23			
B	41	72 ± 19.9			
M	23	81.5 ± 16.5			
			Turnover Intentions		
Sex			$t(632) = 1.3, p = 0.194$	0.14	-
Male	96	13.7 ± 3.55			
Female	538	13.2 ± 3.53			
Work experience (years)			$t(632) = 1.43, p = 0.152$	0.11	-
0.5–10	298	13.5 ± 3.49			
11–38	336	13.1 ± 3.56			
Age (years)			$F(2, 631) = 3.7, p = 0.025$	0.01	21–30 > 31–40 *, 21–30 > 41–57 *
21–30	144	14 ± 3.47			
31–40	232	13 ± 3.28			
41–57	158	13.1 ± 3.74			
Education			$F(2, 631) = 3.64, p = 0.027$	0.01	B < M *
PS	570	13.3 ± 3.55			
B	41	12 ± 3.32			
M	23	14.3 ± 2.91			

Note: [a] Only significant post-hoc tests are summarily presented, [b] Levene's test was significant ($p < 0.05$), suggesting a violation of the assumption of equal variances. Therefore, Welch's t-test was reported. *** $p < 0.001$, ** $p < 0.01$, * $p < 0.05$. PS = Post-Secondary Studies; B = Bachelor's Degree; M = Master's Degree.

Table A3. Correlations between basic psychological need satisfaction in autobiographical memories, self-disclosure, perceived supervisor support, wellbeing, and turnover intentions. Skewness and kurtosis.

		Skewness	Kurtosis	1		2		3		4		5		6		7	
1	**Burnout**	−0.03	−0.84	—													
2	**Work engagement**	0.03	−0.72	−0.61	***	—											
3	**Turnover intentions**	−0.09	−0.23	0.44	***	−0.45	***	—									
4	**Perceived supervisor support**	0.33	−0.04	−0.15	***	0.11	**	−0.51	***	—							
5	**Self-disclosure**	0.11	−0.56	−0.46	***	0.06		−0.13	**	0.11	**	—					
6	**Autonomy**	0.12	−0.57	−0.42	***	0.41	***	−0.3	***	−0.02		0.08	*	—			
7	**Competence**	0.29	−0.41	−0.11	**	0.07		−0.09	*	0.16	***	0.17	***	−0.01		—	
8	**Relatedness**	0.11	−0.46	−0.25	***	0.24	***	−0.2	***	0.06		−0.01		0.22	***	−0.18	***

Note: * $p < 0.05$, ** $p < 0.01$, *** $p < 0.001$.

Appendix D

Table A4. Stage 1—Outer loadings, Reliability, Convergent Validity.

LOCs	Items	Outer Loadings	Alpha	rho_A	rho_C	AVE
A	A1	0.966	0.924	0.927	0.963	0.929
	A2	0.961				
C	C1	0.935	0.862	0.864	0.936	0.879
	C2	0.94				
R	R1	0.958	0.911	0.911	0.957	0.918
	R2	0.958				
Vigor	UWE1	0.957	0.958	0.965	0.972	0.921
	UWE2	0.962				
	UWE3	0.96				
Absorption	UWE4	0.96	0.96	0.964	0.974	0.926
	UWE5	0.965				
	UWE6	0.962				
Dedication	UWE7	0.962	0.957	0.957	0.972	0.921
	UWE8	0.958				
	UWE9	0.959				
EE	EE1	0.911	0.985	0.985	0.987	0.894
	EE2	0.952				
	EE3	0.953				
	EE4	0.95				
	EE5	0.948				
	EE6	0.949				
	EE7	0.945				
	EE8	0.951				
	EE9	0.953				
DP	DP1	0.959	0.978	0.979	0.982	0.918
	DP2	0.956				
	DP3	0.96				
	DP4	0.955				
	DP5	0.959				
PA	PA1	0.954	0.984	0.984	0.987	0.913
	PA2	0.954				
	PA3	0.956				
	PA4	0.959				
	PA5	0.958				
	PA6	0.956				
	PA7	0.952				
PSS	PSS1	0.856	0.933	0.939	0.947	0.75
	PSS2	0.861				
	PSS3	0.867				
	PSS4	0.87				
	PSS5	0.876				
	PSS6	0.866				
DDI	S1	0.856	0.966	0.967	0.97	0.73
	S2	0.828				
	S3	0.842				
	S4	0.852				
	S5	0.862				
	S6	0.839				
	S7	0.874				
	S8	0.861				
	S9	0.852				
	S10	0.857				
	S11	0.86				
	S12	0.867				
TI	TI1	0.949	0.944	0.944	0.964	0.899
	TI2	0.945				
	TI3	0.95				

Note. TI = Turnover Intentions, A = Autonomy satisfaction, C = Competence satisfaction, R = Relatedness satisfaction, DDI = Self-disclosure, PSS = Perceived Supervisor Support, PA = Personal Accomplishment, DP = Depersonalization, EE = Emotional Exhaustion.

Table A5. Stage 1—Discriminant Validity according to HTMT Values and the Fornell–Larcker Criterion.

		1	2	3	4	5	6	7	8	9	10	11	12
1	A	***0.964***	0.32	0.016	0.357	0.334	0.38	0.319	0.034	0.238	0.088	0.318	0.364
2	Absorption	0.302	***0.962***	0.077	0.346	0.434	0.417	0.359	0.126	0.16	0.073	0.365	0.401
3	C	−0.007	0.071	***0.938***	0.112	0.067	0.063	0.113	0.175	0.205	0.181	0.097	0.038
4	DP	−0.34	−0.337	−0.102	***0.958***	0.352	0.431	0.387	0.119	0.177	0.243	0.316	0.365
5	Dedication	0.314	0.417	0.06	−0.341	***0.96***	0.405	0.376	0.06	0.203	0.041	0.353	0.421
6	EE	−0.364	−0.407	−0.058	0.424	−0.394	***0.946***	0.429	0.103	0.193	0.418	0.366	0.399
7	PA	−0.304	−0.35	−0.104	0.381	−0.365	0.424	***0.955***	0.144	0.24	0.387	0.371	0.38
8	PAS	−0.016	0.122	0.154	−0.115	0.058	−0.101	−0.139	***0.866***	0.067	0.12	0.543	0.087
9	R	0.218	0.15	−0.182	−0.167	0.189	−0.183	−0.227	0.064	***0.958***	0.024	0.211	0.223
10	SD	0.084	0.072	0.166	−0.238	0.04	−0.409	−0.379	0.114	−0.006	***0.854***	0.133	0.028
11	TI	−0.298	−0.349	−0.087	0.304	−0.336	0.353	0.358	−0.51	−0.196	−0.127	***0.948***	0.395
12	Vigor	0.344	0.387	0.035	−0.355	0.405	−0.391	−0.371	0.083	0.209	0.019	−0.377	***0.96***

Note. Diagonal and bolded, italicized are the square roots of the AVE. Below the diagonal elements are correlations between constructs' values. Above the diagonal elements are the HTMT values. TI = Turnover Intentions, A = Autonomy satisfaction, C = Competence satisfaction, R = Relatedness satisfaction, DDI = Self-disclosure, PSS = Perceived Supervisor Support, PA = Personal Accomplishment, DP = Depersonalization, EE = Emotional Exhaustion.

Table A6. Stage 2—Higher Order Constructs Validation: Multicollinearity Analysis, Outer Weights, and Outer Loadings.

HOCs	LOCs	Items	VIF	Outer Weights		Outer Loadings	
	A	A1	3.793	0.54	***	0.967	***
		A2	3.793	0.497	***	0.961	***
	C	C1	2.352	0.515	***	0.933	***
		C2	2.352	0.552	***	0.942	***
	R	R1	3.32	0.523	***	0.958	***
		R2	3.32	0.521	***	0.958	***
UWES	Vigor	-	1.285	0.507	***	0.816	***
	Absorption	-	1.3	0.388	***	0.747	***
	Dedication	-	1.322	0.391	***	0.758	***
BRN	EE	-	1.352	0.509	***	0.831	***
	DP	-	1.297	0.276	***	0.676	***
	PA	-	1.297	0.485	***	0.806	***
	PSS	PSS1	2.834	0.162	***	0.855	***
		PSS2	2.61	0.232	***	0.864	***
		PSS3	2.942	0.173	***	0.866	***
		PSS4	2.826	0.211	***	0.869	***
		PSS5	3.008	0.189	***	0.874	***
		PSS6	2.834	0.188	***	0.865	***
	DDI	S1	3.204	0.096	***	0.856	***
		S2	2.842	0.079	***	0.828	***
		S3	3.018	0.09	***	0.842	***
		S4	3.116	0.1	***	0.852	***
		S5	3.297	0.102	***	0.862	***
		S6	2.893	0.096	***	0.839	***
		S7	3.553	0.105	***	0.874	***
		S8	3.299	0.098	***	0.861	***
		S9	3.096	0.1	***	0.852	***
		S10	3.216	0.101	***	0.857	***
		S11	3.23	0.106	***	0.86	***
		S12	3.452	0.096	***	0.867	***
	TI	TI1	4.494	0.36	***	0.949	***
		TI2	4.343	0.351	***	0.945	***
		TI3	4.768	0.344	***	0.95	***

Note. HOC = Higher-Order Constructs, LOC = Lower-Order Constructs, BRN = Burnout, UWES = Work Engagement, TI = Turnover Intentions, A = Autonomy satisfaction, C = Competence satisfaction, R = Relatedness satisfaction, DDI = Self-disclosure, PSS = Perceived Supervisor Support, PA = Personal Accomplishment, DP = Depersonalization, EE = Emotional Exhaustion. *** $p < 0.001$.

Table A7. Explanatory and Predictive Power of the Model.

Predictors	Outcomes	R2	f2	Q2
O/S	TI	0.467	0.011	0.945
SMT/S			0.011	
O/SMT			0.012	
A			0.033	
C			0.011	
R			0.014	
BRN			0.03	
UWES			0.07	
PSS × A			0.012	
DDI × R			0.011	
PSS			0.383	
DDI			0.011	
O/S	BRN	0.586	0.146	0.568
SMT/S			0.45	
O/SMT			0.125	
A			0.023	
C			0.018	
R			0.026	
PSS × A			0.014	
DDI × R			0.015	
PSS			0.027	
DDI			0.414	
O/S	UWES	0.43	0.168	0.383
SMT/S			0.352	
O/SMT			0.083	
A			0.038	
C			0.033	
R			0.04	
PSS × A			0.041	
DDI × R			0.029	
PSS			0.039	
DDI			0.031	
O/S	A	0.308	0.088	0.433
O/SMT			0.139	
SMT/S			0.438	
O/S	C	0.112	0.088	0.629
O/SMT			0.126	
SMT/S			0	
O/S	R	0.24	0.054	0.356
O/SMT			0.313	
SMT/S			0.09	

Note. O/S = other-PMIEs compared to self-PMIEs, O/SMT = other-PMIEs compared to SMTs, SMT/S = SMTs compared to self-PMIEs, BRN = Burnout, UWES = Work Engagement, TI = Turnover Intentions, A = Autonomy satisfaction, C = Competence satisfaction, R = Relatedness satisfaction, DDI = Self-disclosure, PSS = Perceived Supervisor Support, PA = Personal Accomplishment, DP = Depersonalization, EE = Emotional Exhaustion.

Table A8. Predictive Power of the Model.

Endogenous Constructs	Indicators	Q^2 Predict	PLS-SEM_RMSE	LM_RMSE
A	A1	0.32	1.099	1.105
	A2	0.247	1.254	1.265
C	C1	0.085	1.092	1.073
	C2	0.107	1.044	1.041
R	R1	0.217	1.248	1.27
	R2	0.215	1.201	1.219
UWES	Vigor	0.252	0.866	0.888
	Absorption	0.216	0.887	0.903
	Dedication	0.23	0.879	0.906
BRN	EE	0.405	0.772	0.787
	DP	0.254	0.865	0.881
	PA	0.363	0.799	0.805
TI	TI1	0.15	1.081	0.973
	TI2	0.144	1.212	1.093
	TI3	0.14	1.153	1.053

Note. BRN = Burnout, UWES = Work Engagement, TI = Turnover Intentions, A = Autonomy satisfaction, C = Competence satisfaction, R = Relatedness satisfaction, DDI = Self-disclosure, PSS = Perceived Supervisor Support, PA = Personal Accomplishment, DP = Depersonalization, EE = Emotional Exhaustion.

Table A9. Mediation Analyses—Other Results.

Paths	Total Indirect Effects					Direct Effects					Indirect Effects				
	Path Coeff	SE	T	95%CI		Path Coeff	SE	T	95%CI		Path Coeff	SE	T	95%CI	
				LL	UL				LL	UL				LL	UL
A → BRN → TI											−0.02	0.018	1.339	−0.06	−0
A → UWES → TI	−0.12	0.037	3.124	−0.18	−0.06	−0.235	0.113	2.084	−0.42	−0.05	−0.09	0.032	2.845	−0.16	−0.05
C → BRN → TI											−0.01	0.007	1.569	−0.02	−0
C → UWES → TI	−0.03	0.012	2.153	−0.05	−0.01	0.02	0.036	0.556	−0.04	0.078	−0.02	0.009	1.706	−0.04	−0
O/SMT → A → BRN											0.093	0.059	1.586	0.002	0.195
O/SMT → C → BRN											−0.03	0.016	1.902	−0.06	−0.01
O/SMT → R → BRN	0.332	0.11	3.009	0.155	0.524	0.494	0.054	9.092	0.401	0.579	0.27	0.092	2.92	0.122	0.426
O/SMT → A → TI											0.232	0.118	1.974	0.051	0.438
O/SMT → BRN → TI											0.123	0.043	2.833	0.056	0.199
O/SMT → C → TI											0.015	0.027	0.552	−0.03	0.059
O/SMT → R → TI											0.383	0.144	2.654	0.155	0.629
O/SMT → UWES → TI	1.203	0.21	5.721	0.866	1.561	−0.11	0.107	1.029	−0.28	0.067	0.139	0.038	3.672	0.085	0.211
O/SMT → A → UWES											−0.32	0.088	3.615	−0.48	−0.19
O/SMT → C → UWES											0.042	0.024	1.783	0.007	0.084
O/SMT → R → UWES	−0.8	0.155	5.13	−1.05	−0.55	−0.487	0.087	5.57	−0.63	−0.34	−0.52	0.125	4.148	−0.73	−0.32
PSS → BRN → TI											−0.01	0.007	1.838	−0.03	−0
PSS → UWES → TI	−0.02	0.014	1.335	−0.05	0.002	−0.522	0.054	9.706	−0.61	−0.43	−0.01	0.011	0.544	−0.03	0.012
PSS x A → BRN → TI											0.003	0.004	0.666	−0	0.012
PSS x A → UWES → TI	0.022	0.01	2.301	0.008	0.039	0.03	0.03	0.981	−0.02	0.081	0.019	0.008	2.364	0.008	0.036
R → BRN → TI											−0.04	0.021	2.115	−0.09	−0.02
R → UWES → TI	−0.14	0.038	3.695	−0.21	−0.09	−0.25	0.091	2.729	−0.4	−0.1	−0.1	0.032	3.028	−0.16	−0.05
DDI → BRN → TI											−0.09	0.029	2.934	−0.14	−0.04
DDI → UWES → TI	−0.08	0.034	2.435	−0.14	−0.03	0.061	0.056	1.095	−0.03	0.154	0.003	0.013	0.196	−0.02	0.025
DDI x R → BRN → TI											0.011	0.006	1.659	0.003	0.025
DDI x R → UWES → TI	0.038	0.013	2.871	0.018	0.062	0.07	0.031	2.255	0.019	0.121	0.027	0.01	2.622	0.013	0.048
S/SMT → A → BRN											0.172	0.107	1.611	−0	0.35
S/SMT → R → BRN	0.323	0.122	2.651	0.13	0.53	0.993	0.071	14.03	0.869	1.101	0.151	0.056	2.702	0.069	0.255
S/SMT → A → UWES											−0.59	0.151	3.885	−0.84	−0.35
S/SMT → R → UWES	−0.88	0.17	5.148	−1.17	−0.61	−1.19	0.098	12.18	−1.35	−1.03	−0.29	0.081	3.599	−0.44	−0.17
S/SMT → A → TI											0.429	0.208	2.066	0.091	0.776
S/SMT → BRN → TI											0.247	0.086	2.884	0.11	0.39
S/SMT → R → TI											0.214	0.085	2.524	0.088	0.369
S/SMT → UWES → TI	1.563	0.252	6.211	1.162	1.994	−0.065	0.141	0.461	−0.29	0.172	0.341	0.075	4.547	0.225	0.473
O/S → A → BRN											−0.08	0.05	1.577	−0.17	−0
O/S → C → BRN											−0.03	0.016	1.909	−0.06	−0.01
O/S → R → BRN	−0.49	0.084	5.81	−0.62	−0.34	−0.499	0.059	8.426	−0.59	−0.4	0.119	0.044	2.734	0.056	0.199
O/S → A → UWES											0.269	0.075	3.571	0.158	0.407
O/S → C → UWES											0.042	0.023	1.798	0.007	0.083
O/S → R → UWES	0.785	0.116	6.771	0.589	0.969	0.704	0.074	9.517	0.578	0.823	−0.23	0.062	3.697	−0.34	−0.14
O/S → A → TI											−0.2	0.095	2.062	−0.36	−0.05
O/S → BRN → TI											−0.12	0.046	2.731	−0.2	−0.06
O/S → C → TI											0.015	0.027	0.55	−0.03	0.06
O/S → R → TI											0.169	0.069	2.467	0.069	0.299
O/S → UWES → TI	−0.4	0.147	2.752	−0.64	−0.16	−0.045	0.107	0.42	−0.22	0.13	−0.2	0.046	4.344	−0.29	−0.13

Note: S/SMT = self-PMIEs compared to SMTs, O/S = other-PMIEs compared to self-PMIEs, O/SMT = other-PMIEs compared to SMTs, A = autonomy satisfaction, C = competence satisfaction, R = relatedness satisfaction, BRN = burnout, UWES = work engagement, DDI = self-disclosure, TI = turnover intentions.

Table A10. Moderation Analyses—Direct and Interaction Effects.

Relationship	Path Coefficients	SE	T	95%CI	
				LL	UL
S/SMT → BRN	0.993	0.071	14.029	0.869	1.101
S/SMT → UWES	−1.19	0.098	12.182	−1.349	−1.026
S/SMT → TI	−0.065	0.141	0.461	−0.292	0.172
O/SMT → BRN	0.494	0.054	9.092	0.401	0.579
O/SMT → UWES	−0.487	0.087	5.57	−0.627	−0.339
O/SMT → TI	−0.11	0.107	1.029	−0.283	0.067
O/S → BRN	−0.499	0.059	8.426	−0.592	−0.399
O/S → UWES	0.704	0.074	9.517	0.578	0.823
O/S → TI	−0.045	0.107	0.420	−0.222	0.130
A → BRN	−0.095	0.058	1.622	−0.191	0.002
A → UWES	0.322	0.083	3.863	0.186	0.459
A → TI	−0.235	0.113	2.084	−0.422	−0.049
C → BRN	−0.042	0.021	1.998	−0.076	−0.007
C → UWES	0.056	0.031	1.849	0.007	0.107
C → TI	0.02	0.036	0.556	−0.041	0.078
R → BRN	−0.176	0.058	3.027	−0.27	−0.079
R → UWES	0.339	0.079	4.312	0.211	0.468
R → TI	−0.25	0.091	2.729	−0.401	−0.1
BRN → TI	0.249	0.081	3.066	0.114	0.379
UWES → TI	−0.286	0.059	4.887	−0.383	−0.191
PSS → BRN	−0.053	0.027	1.968	−0.1	−0.01
PSS → UWES	0.021	0.038	0.544	−0.042	0.084
PSS → TI	−0.522	0.054	9.706	−0.609	−0.431
DDI → BRN	−0.347	0.035	9.841	−0.407	−0.291
DDI → UWES	−0.009	0.045	0.199	−0.083	0.066
DDI → TI	0.061	0.056	1.095	−0.028	0.154
PSS × A → BRN	0.012	0.016	0.731	−0.015	0.039
PSS × A → UWES	−0.067	0.023	2.977	−0.105	−0.03
PSS × A → TI	0.03	0.03	0.981	−0.02	0.081
DDI × R → BRN	0.043	0.021	2.039	0.007	0.078
DDI × R → UWES	−0.095	0.029	3.343	−0.142	−0.048
DDI × R → TI	0.07	0.031	2.255	0.019	0.121

Note: S/SMT = self-PMIEs compared to SMTs, O/S = other-PMIEs compared to self-PMIEs, O/SMT = other-PMIEs compared to SMTs, A = autonomy satisfaction, C = competence satisfaction, R = relatedness satisfaction, BRN = burnout, UWES = work engagement, DDI = self-disclosure, TI = turnover intentions.

Table A11. Moderation Analyses—Conditional Direct Effects.

Paths	Path Coefficient	SE	T	95%CI	
				LL	UL
A → BRN conditional on PSS at −1 SD	−0.064	0.023	2.797	−0.102	−0.026
A → BRN conditional on PSS at Mean	−0.052	0.018	2.851	−0.083	−0.023
A → BRN conditional on PSS at +1 SD	−0.041	0.026	1.564	−0.084	0.001
A → TI conditional on PSS at −1 SD	−0.16	0.045	3.525	−0.236	−0.086
A → TI conditional on PSS at Mean	−0.13	0.033	3.93	−0.185	−0.076
A → TI conditional on PSS at +1 SD	−0.101	0.044	2.271	−0.172	−0.027
A → UWES conditional on PSS at −1 SD	0.152	0.035	4.339	0.094	0.209
A → UWES conditional on PSS at Mean	0.086	0.028	3.105	0.041	0.131
A → UWES conditional on PSS at +1 SD	0.019	0.036	0.537	−0.04	0.078
R → BRN conditional on DDI at −1 SD	−0.086	0.021	4.12	−0.121	−0.052
R → BRN conditional on DDI at Mean	−0.048	0.019	2.52	−0.08	−0.017
R → BRN conditional on DDI at +1 SD	−0.01	0.032	0.316	−0.063	0.042
R → TI conditional on DDI at −1 SD	−0.104	0.037	2.844	−0.165	−0.046
R → TI conditional on DDI at Mean	−0.042	0.03	1.391	−0.091	0.007
R → TI conditional on DDI at +1 SD	0.02	0.045	0.458	−0.053	0.093
R → UWES conditional on DDI at −1 SD	0.141	0.03	4.772	0.093	0.191
R → UWES conditional on DDI at Mean	0.057	0.027	2.082	0.011	0.101
R → UWES conditional on DDI at +1 SD	−0.027	0.044	0.628	−0.099	0.045

Note: S/SMT = self-PMIEs compared to SMTs, O/S = other-PMIEs compared to self-PMIEs, O/SMT = other-PMIEs compared to SMTs, A = autonomy satisfaction, C = competence satisfaction, R = relatedness satisfaction, BRN = burnout, UWES = work engagement, DDI = self-disclosure, TI = turnover intentions.

Table A12. Moderation Analyses—Other Conditional Indirect Effects.

Paths	Path Coefficient	SE	T	95%CI	
				LL	UL
A → BRN → TI conditional on PSS at −1 SD	−0.016	0.008	1.968	−0.033	−0.005
A → BRN → TI conditional on PSS at Mean	−0.013	0.006	2.041	−0.026	−0.005
A → BRN → TI conditional on PSS at +1 SD	−0.01	0.007	1.367	−0.026	−0.001
A → UWES → TI conditional on PSS at −1 SD	−0.044	0.014	3.164	−0.071	−0.025
A → UWES → TI conditional on PSS at Mean	−0.025	0.009	2.7	−0.043	−0.012
A → UWES → TI conditional on PSS at +1 SD	−0.006	0.01	0.535	−0.023	0.011
O/SMT → A → BRN conditional on PSS at −1 SD	0.063	0.024	2.675	0.027	0.105
O/SMT → A → BRN conditional on PSS at Mean	0.052	0.019	2.737	0.024	0.086
O/SMT → A → BRN conditional on PSS at +1 SD	0.04	0.026	1.542	0	0.086
O/SMT → A → TI conditional on PSS at −1 SD	0.158	0.05	3.175	0.083	0.247
O/SMT → A → TI conditional on PSS at Mean	0.128	0.036	3.563	0.074	0.194
O/SMT → A → TI conditional on PSS at +1 SD	0.099	0.045	2.228	0.029	0.176
O/SMT → A → UWES conditional on PSS at −1 SD	−0.15	0.038	3.971	−0.217	−0.093
O/SMT → A → UWES conditional on PSS at Mean	−0.085	0.029	2.94	−0.136	−0.041
O/SMT → A → UWES conditional on PSS at +1 SD	−0.019	0.036	0.534	−0.079	0.038
O/SMT → R → BRN conditional on DDI at −1 SD	0.133	0.034	3.852	0.078	0.191
O/SMT → R → BRN conditional on DDI at Mean	0.074	0.03	2.448	0.026	0.125
O/SMT → R → BRN conditional on DDI at +1 SD	0.015	0.049	0.315	−0.064	0.097
O/SMT → R → TI conditional on DDI at −1 SD	0.16	0.058	2.766	0.071	0.258
O/SMT → R → TI conditional on DDI at Mean	0.064	0.046	1.379	−0.009	0.144
O/SMT → R → TI conditional on DDI at +1 SD	−0.031	0.069	0.456	−0.145	0.082
O/SMT → R → UWES conditional on DDI at −1 SD	−0.217	0.048	4.559	−0.299	−0.142
O/SMT → R → UWES conditional on DDI at Mean	−0.087	0.042	2.063	−0.158	−0.019
O/SMT → R → UWES conditional on DDI at +1 SD	0.042	0.067	0.626	−0.069	0.153
R → BRN → TI conditional on DDI at −1 SD	−0.022	0.009	2.375	−0.04	−0.009
R → BRN → TI conditional on DDI at Mean	−0.012	0.007	1.806	−0.026	−0.004
R → BRN → TI conditional on DDI at +1 SD	−0.002	0.009	0.292	−0.018	0.01
R → UWES → TI conditional on DDI at −1 SD	−0.04	0.013	3.208	−0.065	−0.023
R → UWES → TI conditional on DDI at Mean	−0.016	0.009	1.879	−0.033	−0.004
R → UWES → TI conditional on DDI at +1 SD	0.008	0.013	0.615	−0.011	0.031
S/SMT → A → BRN conditional on PSS at −1 SD	0.117	0.043	2.748	0.047	0.188
S/SMT → A → BRN conditional on PSS at Mean	0.096	0.034	2.799	0.042	0.155
S/SMT → A → BRN conditional on PSS at +1 SD	0.074	0.048	1.555	−0.002	0.155
S/SMT → A → TI conditional on PSS at −1 SD	0.291	0.085	3.412	0.156	0.438
S/SMT → A → TI conditional on PSS at Mean	0.237	0.064	3.736	0.138	0.348
S/SMT → A → TI conditional on PSS at +1 SD	0.183	0.083	2.217	0.051	0.322
S/SMT → A → UWES conditional on PSS at −1 SD	−0.278	0.066	4.239	−0.387	−0.172
S/SMT → A → UWES conditional on PSS at Mean	−0.157	0.052	2.998	−0.244	−0.073
S/SMT → A → UWES conditional on PSS at +1 SD	−0.035	0.066	0.533	−0.146	0.07
S/SMT → R → BRN conditional on DDI at −1 SD	0.074	0.022	3.443	0.042	0.113
S/SMT → R → BRN conditional on DDI at Mean	0.041	0.018	2.346	0.015	0.073
S/SMT → R → BRN conditional on DDI at +1 SD	0.009	0.027	0.314	−0.036	0.055
S/SMT → R → TI conditional on DDI at −1 SD	0.089	0.034	2.617	0.04	0.152
S/SMT → R → TI conditional on DDI at Mean	0.036	0.026	1.351	−0.004	0.083
S/SMT → R → TI conditional on DDI at +1 SD	−0.018	0.039	0.452	−0.083	0.045
S/SMT → R → UWES conditional on DDI at −1 SD	−0.121	0.031	3.934	−0.178	−0.076
S/SMT → R → UWES conditional on DDI at Mean	−0.049	0.024	2.014	−0.091	−0.011
S/SMT → R → UWES conditional on DDI at +1 SD	0.024	0.038	0.619	−0.037	0.088

Note: S/SMT = self-PMIEs compared to SMTs, O/S = other-PMIEs compared to self-PMIEs, O/SMT = other-PMIEs compared to SMTs, A = autonomy satisfaction, C = competence satisfaction, R = relatedness satisfaction, BRN = burnout, UWES = work engagement, DDI = self-disclosure, TI = turnover intentions.

References

1. Euronews with AP. COVID-19: Romania in Eye of Storm with Record Infections and Deaths. 19 October 2021. Available online: https://www.euronews.com/2021/10/19/romania-in-eye-of-covid-storm-with-death-rate-among-world-s-highest (accessed on 31 May 2022).
2. Popescu, M.; Stefan, O.M.; Stefan, M.; Valeanu, L.; Tomescu, D. ICU-Associated Costs during the Fourth Wave of the COVID-19 Pandemic in a Tertiary Hospital in a Low-Vaccinated Eastern European Country. *Int. J. Environ. Res. Public Health* **2022**, *19*, 1781. [CrossRef] [PubMed]
3. Reuters. Romania's COVID-19 Deaths Hit Record as Intensive Care Beds Run out. 19 October 2021. Available online: https://www.reuters.com/world/europe/romania-reports-record-number-deaths-covid-19-infections-2021-10-19/ (accessed on 31 May 2022).

4. Furlong, A. Romania Suspends Surgeries, Asks EU for Help as It Battles Coronavirus Wave. 5 October 2021. Available online: https://www.politico.eu/article/romania-surgeries-eu-coronavirus-help/ (accessed on 31 May 2022).
5. Dale, L.P.; Cuffe, S.P.; Sambuco, N.; Guastello, A.D.; Leon, K.G.; Nunez, L.V.; Bhullar, A.; Allen, B.R.; Mathews, C.A. Morally Distressing Experiences, Moral Injury, and Burnout in Florida Healthcare Providers during the COVID-19 Pandemic. *Int. J. Environ. Res. Public Health* **2021**, *18*, 12319. [CrossRef] [PubMed]
6. Maftei, A.; Holman, A.C. The prevalence of exposure to potentially morally injurious events among physicians during the COVID-19 pandemic. *Eur. J. Psychotraumatol.* **2021**, *12*, 1898791. [CrossRef] [PubMed]
7. Riedel, P.-L.; Kreh, A.; Kulcar, V.; Lieber, A.; Juen, B. A Scoping Review of Moral Stressors, Moral Distress and Moral Injury in Healthcare Workers during COVID-19. *Int. J. Environ. Res. Public Health* **2022**, *19*, 1666. [CrossRef]
8. Rushton, C.H.; Thomas, T.A.; Antonsdottir, I.M.; Nelson, K.E.; Boyce, D.; Vioral, A.; Swavely, D.; Ley, C.D.; Hanson, G.C. Moral Injury and Moral Resilience in Health Care Workers during COVID-19 Pandemic. *J. Palliat. Med.* **2021**, *25*, 712–719. [CrossRef]
9. Williamson, V.; Murphy, D.; Greenberg, N. COVID-19 and experiences of moral injury in front-line key workers. *Occup. Med.* **2020**, *70*, 317–319. [CrossRef]
10. Litz, B.T.; Stein, N.; Delaney, E.; Lebowitz, L.; Nash, W.P.; Silva, C.; Maguen, S. Moral injury and moral repair in war veterans: A preliminary model and intervention strategy. *Clin. Psychol. Rev.* **2009**, *29*, 695–706. [CrossRef]
11. Borges, L.M.; Holliday, R.; Barnes, S.M.; Bahraini, N.H.; Kinney, A.; Forster, J.E.; Brenner, L.A. A longitudinal analysis of the role of potentially morally injurious events on COVID-19-related psychosocial functioning among healthcare providers. *PLoS ONE* **2021**, *16*, e0260033. [CrossRef]
12. Gherman, M.A.; Arhiri, L.; Holman, A.C.; Soponaru, C. The Moral Impact of the COVID-19 Pandemic on Nurses' Burnout, Work Satisfaction and Adaptive Work Performance: The Role of Autobiographical Memories of Potentially Morally Injurious Events and Basic Psychological Needs. *Int. J. Environ. Res. Public Health* **2022**, *19*, 7645. [CrossRef]
13. Gherman, M.A.; Arhiri, L.; Holman, A.C.; Soponaru, C. Injurious Memories from the COVID-19 Frontline: The Role of Autobiographical Episodic Memories of Self- and Other-Potentially Morally Injurious Events on Romanian Nurses' Burnout, Turnover Intentions and Basic Need Satisfaction. *Int. J. Environ. Res. Public Health* **2022**, *19*, 9604. [CrossRef]
14. Nieuwsma, J.A.; O'Brien, E.C.; Xu, H.; Smigelsky, M.A.; VISN 6 MIRECC Workgroup; HERO Research Program; Meador, K.G. Patterns of Potential Moral Injury in Post-9/11 Combat Veterans and COVID-19 Healthcare Workers. *J. Gen. Intern. Med.* **2022**, *37*, 2033–2040. [CrossRef]
15. Griffin, B.J.; Purcell, N.; Burkman, K.; Litz, B.T.; Bryan, C.J.; Schmitz, M.; Villerme, C.; Walsh, J.; Maguen, S. Moral injury: An Integrative Review. *J. Trauma. Stress* **2019**, *23*, 350–362. [CrossRef]
16. Michaud, K.; Suurd Ralph, C.; Connick-Keefer, S.J.A. Operational stressors, psychological distress, and turnover intentions: The impact of potentially morally injurious experiences. *Mil. Psychol.* **2021**, *33*, 250–263. [CrossRef]
17. Ryan, R.M.; Deci, E.L. *Self-Determination Theory: Basic Psychological Needs in Motivation, Development, and Wellness*; The Guilford Press: New York, NY, USA, 2017. [CrossRef]
18. Brüggemann, A.J.; Wijma, B.; Swahnberg, K. Abuse in health care: A concept analysis. *Scand. J. Caring Sci.* **2012**, *26*, 123–132. [CrossRef]
19. Yeung, S.K.; Yay, T.; Feldman, G. Action and Inaction in Moral Judgments and Decisions: Meta-Analysis of Omission Bias Omission-Commission Asymmetries. *Pers. Soc. Psychol. Bull.* **2021**, *48*, 1461672211042315. [CrossRef]
20. Helion, C.; Helzer, E.G.; Kim, S.; Pizarro, D.A. Asymmetric memory for harming versus being harmed. *J. Exp. Psychol. Gen.* **2020**, *149*, 889–900. [CrossRef]
21. McHan, K.; Johnston-Taylor, E.; Piscopo, B.; Abate, E.; Dehom, S. Nursing values and moral identity in baccalaureate nursing students. *J. Prof. Nurs.* **2022**, *39*, 171–176. [CrossRef]
22. Stanley, M.L.; Cabeza, R.; Smallman, R.; De Brigard, F. Memory and Counterfactual Simulations for Past Wrongdoings Foster Moral Learning and Improvement. *Cogn. Sci.* **2021**, *45*, e13007. [CrossRef]
23. Fruet, I.M.A.; Dalmolin, G.D.L.; Barlem, E.L.D.; Silva, R.M.d.; Andolhe, R. Aplicabilidade da Moral Distress Scale adaptada no cenário da enfermagem em hemato-oncologia. *Rev. Gaucha Enferm.* **2018**, *38*, e63060. [CrossRef]
24. Soleimani, M.A.; Sharif, S.P.; Yaghoobzadeh, A.; Panarello, B. Psychometric evaluation of the Moral Distress Scale-Revised among Iranian Nurses. *Nurs. Ethics* **2019**, *26*, 1226–1242. [CrossRef]
25. Abdolmaleki, M.; Lakdizaji, S.; Ghahramanian, A.; Allahbakhshian, A.; Behshid, M. Relationship between autonomy and moral distress in emergency nurses. *Indian J. Med. Ethics* **2019**, *4*, 20–25. [CrossRef]
26. Özkan, A.H. The effect of burnout and its dimensions on turnover intention among nurses: A meta-analytic review. *J. Nurs. Manag.* **2022**, *30*, 660–669. [CrossRef]
27. Leiter, M.P.; Maslach, C. Nurse turnover: The mediating role of burnout. *J. Nurs. Manag.* **2009**, *17*, 331–339. [CrossRef]
28. Chen, Z.; Sun, H.; Lam, W.; Hu, Q.; Huo, Y.; Zhong, J.A. Chinese hotel employees in the smiling masks: Roles of job satisfaction, burnout, and supervisory support in relationships between emotional labor and performance. *Int. J. Hum. Resour.* **2012**, *23*, 826–845. [CrossRef]
29. St-Pierre, I.; Holmes, D. The relationship between organizational justice and workplace aggression. *J. Adv. Nurs.* **2010**, *66*, 1169–1182. [CrossRef]

30. Gillet, N.; Fouquereau, E.; Bonnaud-Antignac, A.; Mokounkolo, R.; Colombat, P. The mediating role of organizational justice in the relationship between transformational leadership and nurses' quality of work life: A cross-sectional questionnaire survey. *Int. J. Nurs. Stud.* **2013**, *50*, 1359–1367. [CrossRef]
31. Caesens, G.; Stinglhamber, F.; Luypaert, G. The impact of work engagement and workaholism on well-being: The role of work-related social support. *Career Dev. Int.* **2014**, *19*, 813–835. [CrossRef]
32. Gillet, N.; Fouquereau, E.; Coillot, H.; Cougot, B.; Moret, L.; Dupont, S.; Bonnetain, F.; Colombat, P. The effects of work factors on nurses' job satisfaction, quality of care and turnover intentions in oncology. *J. Adv. Nurs.* **2018**, *74*, 1208–1219. [CrossRef]
33. Nelson, D.L.; Canas, J.; Bajo, M.-T. The effects of natural category size on memory for episodic encodings. *Mem. Cognit.* **1987**, *15*, 133–140. [CrossRef] [PubMed]
34. Jourard, S.M. *Self-Disclosure: An Experimental Analysis of the Transparent Self*; Wiley-Interscience: Hoboken, NJ, USA, 1971; ISBN 978-0471451501.
35. Smyth, J.M.; Pennebaker, J.W.; Arigo, D. What Are the HEALTH Effects of Disclosure? In *Handbook of Health Psychology*; Baum, A., Revenson, T.A., Singer, J., Eds.; Psychology Press: London, UK, 2012; pp. 175–191. ISBN 978-0805864618.
36. Levi-Belz, Y.; Lev-Ari, L. "Let's talk about it": The moderating role of self-disclosure on complicated grief over time among suicide survivors. *Int. J. Environ. Health Res.* **2019**, *16*, 3740. [CrossRef] [PubMed]
37. Gvion, Y.; Levi-Belz, Y. Serious suicide attempts: Systematic review of psychological risk factors. *Front. Psychiatry* **2018**, *9*, 56. [CrossRef] [PubMed]
38. Levi-Belz, Y.; Shemesh, S.; Zerach, G. Moral injury and suicide ideation among combat veterans: The moderating role of self-disclosure. *Crisis* **2022**. advance online publication. [CrossRef] [PubMed]
39. Falatah, R. The Impact of the Coronavirus Disease (COVID-19) Pandemic on Nurses' Turnover Intention: An Integrative Review. *Nurs. Rep.* **2021**, *11*, 787–810. [CrossRef] [PubMed]
40. Couper, K.; Murrells, T.; Sanders, J.; Anderson, J.E.; Blake, H.; Kelly, D.; Kent, B.; Maben, J.; Rafferty, A.M.; Taylor, R.M.; et al. The impact of COVID-19 on the wellbeing of the UK nursing and midwifery workforce during the first pandemic wave: A longitudinal survey study. *Int. J. Nurs. Stud.* **2022**, *127*, 104155. [CrossRef]
41. Irshad, M.; Khattak, S.A.; Hassan, M.M.; Majeed, M.; Bashir, S. Withdrawn: How perceived threat of COVID-19 causes turnover intention among Pakistani nurses: A moderation and mediation analysis. *Int. J. Ment. Health Nurs.* **2020**, *30*, 350. [CrossRef]
42. Lake, E.T.; Narva, A.M.; Holland, S.; Smith, J.G.; Cramer, E.; Rosenbaum, K.E.F.; French, R.; Clark, R.R.S.; Rogowski, J.A. Hospital nurses' moral distress and mental health during COVID-19. *J. Adv. Nurs.* **2022**, *78*, 799–809. [CrossRef]
43. Saragih, I.D.; Tonapa, S.I.; Saragih, I.S.; Advani, S.; Batubara, S.O.; Suarilah, I.; Lin, C.J. Global prevalence of mental health problems among healthcare workers during the COVID-19 pandemic: A systematic review and meta-analysis. *Int. J. Nurs. Stud.* **2021**, *121*, 104002. [CrossRef]
44. Kim, Y.-J.; Lee, S.-Y.; Cho, J.-H. A Study on the Job Retention Intention of Nurses Based on Social Support in the COVID-19 Situation. *Sustainability* **2020**, *12*, 7276. [CrossRef]
45. Santos, A.; Chambel, M.J.; Castanheira, F. Wellbeing among hospital nurses: A cross-sectional study of the contributions of relational job characteristics. *Int. J. Nurs. Stud.* **2020**, *105*, 103438. [CrossRef]
46. Schaufeli, W.B.; Salanova, M.; González-Romá, V.; Bakker, A.B. The measurement of engagement and burnout: A two sample confirmatory factor analytic approach. *J. Happiness Stud.* **2002**, *3*, 71–92. [CrossRef]
47. Demerouti, E.; Bakker, A.B.; Nachreiner, F.; Schaufeli, W.B. The job demands-resources model of burnout. *J. Appl. Psychol.* **2001**, *86*, 499–512. [CrossRef]
48. Wildgruber, D.; Frey, J.; Seer, M.; Pinther, K.; Koob, C.; Reuschenbach, B. Arbeitsengagement und Belastungserleben von Health Professionals in Zeiten der Corona-Pandemie—Eine Querschnittstudie. *Pflege* **2020**, *33*, 299–307. [CrossRef]
49. Zhang, M.; Zhang, P.; Liu, Y.; Wang, H.; Hu, K.; Du, M. Influence of perceived stress and workload on work engagement in front-line nurses during COVID-19 pandemic. *J. Clin. Nurs.* **2021**, *30*, 1584–1595. [CrossRef]
50. Maslach, C.; Jackson, S.E.; Leiter, M.P. *MBI: Maslach Burnout Inventory*; Consulting Psychologists Press: Palo Alto, CA, USA, 1996.
51. Norman, S.B.; Feingold, J.H.; Kaye-Kauderer, H.; Kaplan, C.A.; Hurtado, A.; Kachadourian, L.; Feder, A.; Murrough, J.W.; Charnie, D.; Southwick, S.M.; et al. Moral distress in frontline healthcare workers in the initial epicenter of the COVID-19 pandemic in the United States: Relationship to PTSD symptoms, burnout, and psychosocial functioning. *Depress. Anxiety* **2021**, *38*, 1007–1017. [CrossRef]
52. Philippe, F.L.; Lopes, M.; Houlfort, N.; Fernet, C. Work-related episodic memories can increase or decrease motivation and psychological health at work. *Work Stress* **2019**, *33*, 366–384. [CrossRef]
53. Griffeth, R.W.; Hom, P.W.; Gaertner, S. A meta-analysis of antecedents and correlates of employee turnover: Update, moderator tests, and research implications for the next millennium. *J. Manag.* **2000**, *26*, 463–488. [CrossRef]
54. Tett, R.P.; Meyer, J.P. Job satisfaction, organizational commitment, turnover intention, and turnover: Path analyses based on meta-analytic findings. *Pers. Psychol.* **1993**, *46*, 259–293. [CrossRef]
55. Nikkhah-Farkhani, Z.; Piotrowski, A. Nurses' turnover intention—A comparative study between Iran and Poland. *Med. Pract.* **2020**, *71*, 413–420. [CrossRef]
56. Gabel Shemueli, R.; Dolan, S.L.; Suárez Ceretti, A.; Nunez del Prado, P. Burnout and engagement as mediators in the relationship between work characteristics and turnover intentions across two Ibero-American nations. *Stress Health* **2016**, *32*, 597–606. [CrossRef]

57. McKenna, J.; Jeske, D. Ethical leadership and decision authority effects on nurses' engagement, exhaustion, and turnover intention. *J. Adv. Nurs.* **2021**, *77*, 198–206. [CrossRef]
58. Wan, Q.; Li, Z.; Zhou, W.; Shang, S. Effects of work environment and job characteristics on the turnover intention of experienced nurses: The mediating role of work engagement. *J. Adv. Nurs.* **2018**, *74*, 1332–1341. [CrossRef]
59. von Elm, E.; Altman, D.; Egger, M.; Pocock, S.J.; Gøtzsche, P.C.; Vandenbroucke, J.P. STROBE Initiative.The Strengthening the Reporting of Observational Studies in Epidemiology (STROBE) statement: Guidelines for reporting observational studies. *J. Clin. Epidemiol.* **2008**, *61*, 344–349. [CrossRef]
60. Dascalu, S.; Geambasu, O.; Raiu, V.C.; Azoicai, D.; Popovici, D.E.; Apetrei, C. COVID-19 in Romania: What Went Wrong? *Front. Public Health* **2021**, *9*, 813941. [CrossRef]
61. Baard, P.P.; Deci, E.L.; Ryan, R.M. Intrinsic need satisfaction: A motivational basis of performance and well-being in two work settings. *J. Appl. Soc. Psychol.* **2004**, *34*, 2045–2068. [CrossRef]
62. Kahn, J.H.; Hessling, R.M. Measuring the tendency to conceal versus disclose psychological distress. *J. Soc. Clin. Psychol.* **2001**, *20*, 41–65. [CrossRef]
63. Philippe, F.L.; Koestner, R.; Beaulieu-Pelletier, G.; Lecours, S. The role of need satisfaction as a distinct and basic psychological component of autobiographical memories: A look at well-being. *J. Pers.* **2011**, *79*, 905–938. [CrossRef]
64. Philippe, F.L. Episodic memories as proxy or independent representations: A theoretical review and an empirical test of distinct episodic memories on work outcomes. *New Ideas Psychol.* **2022**, *64*, 100913. [CrossRef]
65. Milyavskaya, M.; Philippe, F.L.; Koestner, R. Psychological need satisfaction across levels of experience: Their organization and contribution to general well-being. *J. Res. Pers.* **2013**, *47*, 41–51. [CrossRef]
66. Philippe, F.L.; Bernard-Desrosiers, L. The odyssey of episodic memories: Identifying the paths and processes through which they contribute to well-being. *J. Pers.* **2017**, *85*, 518–529. [CrossRef]
67. Philippe, F.L.; Koestner, R.; Beaulieu-Pelletier, G.; Lecours, S.; Lekes, N. The role of episodic memories in current and future well-being. *Pers. Soc. Psychol. Bull.* **2012**, *38*, 505–519. [CrossRef]
68. Philippe, F.L.; Koestner, R.; Lecours, S.; Beaulieu-Pelletier, G.; Bois, K. The role of autobiographical memory networks in the experience of negative emotions: How our remembered past elicits our current feelings. *Emotion* **2011**, *11*, 1279–1290. [CrossRef] [PubMed]
69. Philippe, F.L.; Koestner, R.; Lekes, N. On the directive function of episodic memories in people's lives: A look at romantic relationships. *J. Pers. Soc. Psychol.* **2013**, *104*, 164–179. [CrossRef] [PubMed]
70. Bria, M.; Spânu, F.; Băban, A.; Dumitrașcu, D.L. Maslach burnout inventory–general survey: Factorial validity and invariance among Romanian healthcare professionals. *Burn. Res.* **2014**, *1*, 103–111. [CrossRef]
71. Cammann, C.; Fichman, M.; Jenkins, D.; Klesh, J. *The Michigan Organizational Assessment Questionnaire*; University of Michigan: Ann Arbor, MI, USA, 1979; unpublished manuscript.
72. Lee, N.; Cadogan, J.W. Problems with formative and higher- order reflective variables. *J. Bus. Res.* **2013**, *66*, 242–247. [CrossRef]
73. Gisilanbe Vetbuje, B.; Farmanesh, P.; Sousan, A. Relationship between perceived threat of COVID-19 and burnout among frontline nurses: A mediation analysis. *Brain Behav.* **2022**, *12*, e2601. [CrossRef]
74. Roșca, A.C.; Mateizer, A.; Dan, C.-I.; Demerouti, E. Job Demands and Exhaustion in Firefighters: The Moderating Role of Work Meaning. A Cross-Sectional Study. *Int. J. Environ. Res. Public Health* **2021**, *18*, 9819. [CrossRef]
75. Vîrgă, D.; Pattusamy, M.; Kumar, D.P. How psychological capital is related to academic performance, burnout, and boredom? The mediating role of study engagement. *Curr. Psychol.* **2020**. [CrossRef]
76. Becker, J.-M.; Klein, K.; Wetzels, M. Hierarchical latent var- iable models in PLS-SEM: Guidelines for using reflective-formative type models. *Long Range Plann.* **2012**, *45*, 359–394. [CrossRef]
77. Ringle, C.M.; Sarstedt, M.; Straub, D.W. Editor's comments: A critical look at the use of PLS-SEM in "MIS quarterly". *MIS Q.* **2012**, *36*, iii–xiv. [CrossRef]
78. Ringle, C.M.; Wende, S.; Becker, J.-M. SmartPLS 4. 2022. Boenningstedt: SmartPLS. Available online: https://www.smartpls.com (accessed on 1 August 2022).
79. Hair, J.F.; Risher, J.J.; Sarstedt, M.; Ringle, C.M. When to Use and How to Report the Results of PLS-SEM. *Eur. Bus. Rev.* **2019**, *31*, 2–24. [CrossRef]
80. Hair, J.F.; Hult, G.T.M.; Ringle, C.M.; Sarstedt, M. *A Primer on Partial Least Squares Structural Equation Modeling (PLS-SEM)*, 3rd ed.; Sage: Thousand Oaks, CA, USA, 2022; ISBN 978-1544396408.
81. Hair, J.F.; Hult, G.T.M.; Ringle, C.M.; Sarstedt, M.; Danks, N.P.; Ray, S. *Partial Least Squares Structural Equation Modeling (PLS-SEM) Using R: A Workbook*; Springer Nature: Cham, Switzerland, 2021; ISBN 978-3-030-80518-0.
82. Kock, N.; Hadaya, P. Minimum sample size estimation in PLS-SEM: The inverse square root and gamma-exponential methods. *Inf. Syst. J.* **2018**, *28*, 227–261. [CrossRef]
83. Fornell, C.; Larcker, D.F. Evaluating structural equation models with unobservable variables and measurement error. *J. Mark. Res.* **1981**, *18*, 39–50. [CrossRef]
84. Henseler, J.; Ringle, C.; Sarstedt, M. A new criterion for assessing discriminant validity in variance-based structural equation modeling. *J. Acad. Mark. Sci.* **2015**, *43*, 115–135. [CrossRef]
85. Agarwal, R.; Karahanna, E. Time flies when you're having fun: Cognitive absorption and beliefs about information technology usage. *MIS Q.* **2000**, *24*, 665–694. [CrossRef]

86. Wetzels, M.; Odekerken-Schröder, G.; Van Oppen, C. Using PLS path modeling for assessing hierarchical construct models: Guidelines and empirical illustration. *MIS Q.* **2009**, *33*, 177–195. [CrossRef]
87. Sarstedt, M.; Hair, J.F.; Nitzl, C.; Ringle, C.M.; Howard, M.C. Beyond a Tandem Analysis of SEM and PROCESS: Use of PLS-SEM for Mediation Analyses! *Int. J. Mark. Res.* **2020**, *62*, 288–299. [CrossRef]
88. Hayes, A.F. *Introduction to Mediation, Moderation, and Conditional Process Analysis: A Regression-Based Approach*, 3rd ed.; Guilford Press: New York, NY, USA, 2022; ISBN 978-1-462-54903-0.
89. Shmueli, G.; Ray, S.; Estrada, J.M.V.; Chatla, S.B. The elephant in the room: Predictive performance of PLS models. *J. Bus. Res.* **2016**, *69*, 4552–4564. [CrossRef]
90. Shmueli, G.; Sarstedt, M.; Hair, J.F.; Cheah, J.H.; Ting, H.; Vaithilingam, S.; Ringle, C.M. Predictive model assessment in PLS-SEM: Guidelines for using PLSpredict. *Eur. J. Mark.* **2019**, *53*, 2322–2347. [CrossRef]
91. Falk, R.F.; Miller, N.B. *A Primer for Soft Modeling*; University of Akron Press: Akron, OH, USA, 1992; ISBN 978-0-962-26284-5.
92. Cohen, J. *Statistical Power Analysis for the Behavioral Sciences*; Lawrence Erlbaum: Hillsdale, NJ, USA, 1988; ISBN 978-0-203-77158-7.
93. Hayes, A.F. An index and test of linear moderated mediation. *Multivar. Behav. Res.* **2015**, *50*, 1–22. [CrossRef]
94. Emanuel, E.J.; Persad, G.; Upshur, R.; Thome, B.; Parker, M.; Glickman, A.; Zhang, C.; Boyle, C.; Smith, M.; Phillips, J.P. Fair Allocation of Scarce Medical Resources in the Time of COVID-19. *N. Engl. J. Med.* **2020**, *382*, 2049–2055. [CrossRef]
95. Apriceno, M.; Lytle, A.; Monahan, C.; Macdonald, J.; Levy, S.R. Prioritizing health care and employment resources during COVID-19: Roles of benevolent and hostile ageism. *Gerontologist* **2021**, *61*, 98–102. [CrossRef]
96. Guidet, B.; Flaatten, H.; Leaver, S.K. Age is just a number: How should we triage old patients in the coronavirus disease 2019 pandemic? *Eur. J. Emerg. Med.* **2021**, *28*, 92–94. [CrossRef]
97. An, M.; Shin, E.S.; Choi, M.Y.; Lee, Y.; Hwang, Y.Y.; Kim, M. Positive Psychological Capital Mediates the Association between Burnout and Nursing Performance Outcomes among Hospital Nurses. *Int. J. Environ. Res. Public Health* **2020**, *17*, 5988. [CrossRef] [PubMed]
98. Keyko, K.; Cummings, G.G.; Yonge, O.; Wong, C.A. Work engagement in professional nursing practice: A systematic review. *Int. J. Nurs. Stud.* **2016**, *61*, 142–164. [CrossRef]
99. Institute of Medicine. *Keeping Patients Safe: Trans-Forming the Work Environment of Nurses*; National Academies Press: Washington, DC, USA, 2004. [CrossRef]
100. Lewis, E.J.; Baernholdt, M.; Hamric, A.B. Nurses' Experience of Medical Errors: An Integrative Literature Review. *J. Nurs. Care Qual.* **2013**, *28*, 153–161. [CrossRef]
101. Levi-Belz, Y.; Gvion, Y.; Horesh, N.; Fischel, T.; Treves, I.; Or, E.; Orit, S.R.; Weiser, M.; Shem, H.; Apter, D.; et al. Mental Pain, Communication Difficulties, and Medically Serious Suicide Attempts: A Case-Control Study. *Arch. Suicide Res.* **2014**, *18*, 74–87. [CrossRef]
102. Nadon, L.; De Beer, L.T.; Morin, A.J.S. Should Burnout Be Conceptualized as a Mental Disorder? *Behav. Sci.* **2022**, *12*, 82. [CrossRef]
103. Maslach, C.; Leiter, M.P. *The Truth About Burnout*; Jossey-Bass: San Francisco, CA, USA, 1997; ISBN 978-0-470-42356-1.
104. King, M. Working to Address the Loneliness Epidemic: Perspective-Taking, Presence, and Self-Disclosure. *Am. J. Health Promot.* **2018**, *32*, 1315–1317. [CrossRef]
105. Ferrajão, P.C.; Oliveira, R.A. The effects of combat exposure, abusive violence, and sense of coherence on PTSD and depression in Portuguese colonial war veterans. *Psychol. Trauma.* **2016**, *8*, 1–8. [CrossRef]
106. Gray, M.J.; Schorr, Y.; Nash, W.; Lebowitz, L.; Amidon, A.; Lansing, A.; Maglione, M.; Lang, A.J.; Litz, B.T. Adaptive disclosure: An open trial of a novel exposure-based intervention for service members with combat-related psychological stress injuries. *Behav. Ther.* **2012**, *43*, 407–415. [CrossRef]
107. Currier, J.M.; Holland, J.M.; Marlott, J. Moral injury, meaning making, and mental health in returning veterans. *J. Clin. Psychol.* **2015**, *71*, 229–240. [CrossRef] [PubMed]
108. Currier, J.M.; Holland, J.M.; Drescher, K.; Foy, D. Initial psychometric evaluation of the moral injury questionnaire—Military version. *Clin. Psychol. Psychother.* **2015**, *22*, 54–63. [CrossRef] [PubMed]
109. Ferrajão, P.C.; Aragão Oliveira, R. Portuguese war veterans: Moral injury and factors related to recovery from PTSD. *Qual. Health Res.* **2016**, *26*, 204–214. [CrossRef] [PubMed]
110. Scandlyn, J.; Hautzinger, S. 'Victim/volunteer': Heroes versus perpetrators and the weight of US service-members' pasts in Iraq and Afghanistan. *Int. J. Hum. Rights* **2015**, *19*, 555–571. [CrossRef]
111. Shay, J. *Combat and the Undoing of Character*; Scribner: New York, NY, USA, 1994; ISBN 978-0684813219.

International Journal of
Environmental Research and Public Health

MDPI

Article

Competencies of Nurse Managers as Predictors of Staff Nurses' Job Satisfaction and Turnover Intention

Pin-Pin Choi [1,*], Wai-Man Lee [1], Suet-Shan Wong [1] and Mei-Ha Tiu [2]

[1] School of Nursing and Health Studies, Hong Kong Metropolitan University, Hong Kong
[2] School of Nursing, St. Teresa's Hospital, Hong Kong
* Correspondence: sppchoi@hkmu.edu.hk; Tel.: +852-3970-8704

Abstract: Nurse managers have played an integral role in stabilizing the nursing work environment and workforce in the face of the COVID-19 pandemic, yet the competencies required for such a feat are largely unknown. This study was conducted during the pandemic to identify the specific domains of nurse manager competencies that associate with nurse outcomes. A cross-sectional survey was conducted on a convenience sample of 698 staff nurses to measure the perceived competence of their nurse managers and their job satisfaction and turnover intention levels. The overall perceived nurse manager competency level in our sample was 3.15 out of 5 (SD = 0.859). The findings indicated that 34.3% of nurses were dissatisfied with their current jobs, and 36.3% of nurses were considering leaving their current workplace. Regression analyses identified "Team Communication and Collaboration" ($\beta = 0.289$; $p = 0.002$), "Staff Advocacy and Development" ($\beta = 0.229$; $p = 0.019$), and "Quality Monitoring and Pursuance" ($\beta = 0.213$; $p = 0.031$) as significant predictors of staff nurses' job satisfaction and "Staff Advocacy and Development" ($\beta = -0.347$; $p < 0.000$) and "Team Communication and Collaboration" ($\beta = -0.243$; $p = 0.012$) as significant predictors of nurses' turnover intention. The findings of the study have implications for the future recruitment, training, and performance evaluation of nurse managers.

Keywords: management; professional roles; survey; workforce

Citation: Choi, P.-P.; Lee, W.-M.; Wong, S.-S.; Tiu, M.-H. Competencies of Nurse Managers as Predictors of Staff Nurses' Job Satisfaction and Turnover Intention. *Int. J. Environ. Res. Public Health* **2022**, *19*, 11461. https://doi.org/10.3390/ijerph191811461

Academic Editors: Richard Gray and Sonia Udod

Received: 10 August 2022
Accepted: 8 September 2022
Published: 12 September 2022

1. Introduction

1.1. Challenges in Modern Healthcare

Modern healthcare continues to face increasing challenges due to growing aging populations and the escalating demands of care recipients for quality care [1]. The boom in the medical sciences and technology has added to these challenges by contributing to new knowledge on disease management, leading to constant changes in healthcare policies and care delivery processes [1]. The outbreak of the coronavirus disease 2019 (COVID-19) has further intensified the complexity of the healthcare environment. Healthcare workers have developed psychological distress and burnout due to overwhelming patient loads, inadequate manpower and time off, and separation from family members during the pandemic [2]. The same applies to nurses, who make up the largest proportion of the healthcare workforce and provide round-the-clock care to patients. The pandemic has increased their job demands, leading to feelings of loss of control, burnout, and moral distress [3]. The International Council of Nurses (ICN) published a report entitled "The global nursing workforce and the COVID-19 pandemic" in January 2022 to raise an urgent appeal about the sustainability of the nursing workforce [4]. The nurse understaffing phenomenon is expected to persist for some years, and the ICN has prompted health service providers to develop effective strategies to mitigate the impact of the pandemic on the phenomenon [4].

1.2. The Pivotal Role of First-Line Nurse Managers

First-line nurse managers play a central role in confronting the challenges in healthcare as they are responsible for overseeing the operation of individual work units, and for providing direct supervision and work support to frontline nurses [1,5,6]. Their competencies, namely the specific attributes and behaviors crucial for effective performance, were extensively studied. Previous research on nurse manager competencies focused on examining their leadership styles and management practices, which have been cited as integral to staff satisfaction and retention [5,7–10]. Cummings and colleagues [7] conducted a systematic review and found a strong linkage between leadership and management behaviors and various nurse outcomes, including individual productivity and effectiveness, staff health and well-being, and staff satisfaction and retention. Many scholars further pinpointed a lack of attention paid by researchers, hospital administrators, and policy makers to the importance of unit-level management, and they have called for more systematic studies to examine the competencies required of nurse managers and the management skills and practices that determine nurse outcomes [5,11,12].

During the COVID-19 pandemic, there has been increasing scholarly interest in examining workforce issues in nursing. Researchers are cognizant of the exacerbating effect of the pandemic on nurse shortages and turnover. Most studies focused on the work-related outcomes and experiences of nurses, capturing their perceived stress, satisfaction, support, intent to stay/leave, and quality of care [13,14], as well as their lived experiences of caring for patients during the pandemic [15,16], through survey and qualitative approaches. There is also growing evidence confirming the relationship between the quality of the practice environment and nurse outcomes, with management support being one of the dimensions underlying the construct of the practice environment [17,18]. However, very few studies have examined the management behaviors that support nursing work during the pandemic. Researchers examined the associations between nurse outcomes and their practice environment, and noted that "dissatisfaction with management" is the top-ranked factor leading to the intention of nurses to leave their workplace [19]. They emphasized the role of nurse managers in rebuilding the nursing work environment and retaining nurses and stressed that there is an urgent need to further explore issues related to the competencies of nurse managers and nurse outcomes in light of the pandemic [19,20].

1.3. Background of This Study

This study was conducted during the COVID-19 pandemic and was developed based on a phenomenological study that delineated the perceptions of first-line nurse managers and staff nurses about what constitutes the managerial effectiveness of nurse managers [21]. The study generated a list of narrative descriptions that captured the competencies required of nurse managers and laid the foundation for this study. According to the extant literature, nurse manager competencies are closely associated with nurse outcomes [7,8]. This study set out to test this hypothesis and to shed light on the competencies of nurse managers as perceived by staff nurses and nurse satisfaction and turnover during the pandemic.

2. Aim

The aim of this study was to identify the specific domains of nurse manager competency that associate with nurse outcomes, namely the job satisfaction and turnover intention of staff nurses.

3. Methods

3.1. Design

A cross-sectional survey design using online questionnaires was employed in this study.

3.2. Sampling and Data Collection

Convenience and snowball sampling approaches were adopted. Potential respondents were invited to complete an electronic survey in a structured Google form, which was disseminated to the hospital administrators of both public and private hospitals in Hong Kong as well as through the research team's personal networks. Eligible respondents were those who were full-time staff nurses currently practicing in hospital settings in Hong Kong. The Google form contained an information sheet, and relevant questions to screen for eligibility of the respondents. Only one response per IP address was allowed. Nurse managers and administrators were excluded because they were not involved in direct patient care. Data collection was conducted from May to July 2022. The survey was distributed to 824 potential respondents, and the response rate was 84.7% ($N = 698$). Among them, 688 questionnaires were filled out completely and were used for the final analysis. The sample size of this study was estimated using G*Power v.3.1.9.4 (USA) for a multiple linear regression analysis, using a medium effect size of 0.15, an α error probability of 0.05, a power of 0.95, and five predictors. The sample size required was 138, and the sample size attained in this study was sufficient for statistical analyses.

Ethical approval was obtained from the institution with which the corresponding author was affiliated prior to the commencement of the study (Reference no: HE/RGC/2019-31). Respondents were provided with written information on the aim and process of the study, and on their right to confidentiality and to withdraw from the study. The survey was anonymous, so no personal identifying information was collected from the respondents. Informed consent regarding the voluntary participation of the respondents was indicated by the return of their questionnaires.

3.3. Measures

Data collection was performed using an instrument developed from a phenomenological study that involved individual interviews with both nurse managers and staff nurses to elicit their perspectives on the competencies required of nurse managers [21]. Nurse manager competencies refer to the attributes and behaviors essential for managerial competence [21]. A total of 63 descriptive expressions were generated from the verbatim transcripts, which were then content validated by four expert panels who were nurse managers and/or administrators with at least 15 years of experience in nursing leadership and management. Content validation involves examining whether an instrument is made up of an appropriate sample of items for measuring the construct under study [22]. All panel members consensually agreed that the items are appropriate for measuring the essential competencies of nurse managers. Minor modifications were made to two items to improve clarity, and no items were added or deleted from the instrument. The scale-level content validity index of the instrument was 0.94, which indicated a high level of relevance and clarity [22].

The instrument was named the *Nurse Manager Competency Scale*, and its psychometric properties were further evaluated by 970 staff nurses recruited from February to May 2022. The sample size was estimated based on a 1:10 item-to-response ratio [23], and sampling and data collection were conducted using the same approaches adopted in this study. Exploratory factor analysis (EFA) was adopted to examine the construct validity of the scale, which refers to the extent to which the instrument can represent a theoretical construct [24]. Principal axis factoring with varimax rotation was chosen as it allows for the existence of correlations among domains [25]. The Kaiser–Meyer–Olkin (KMO) test and Bartlett's test for sphericity were performed before the EFA. The number of factors extracted was conducted according to the Kaiser–Guttman rule, taking into consideration the following criteria: (1) eigenvalues of 1.0 or above; (2) scree plots; (3) items with salient factor loadings of $\geq$0.40; and (4) the meaning of the items [26]. The results yielded a five-factor structure that accounted for 58.3% of the total variance. Three items were removed as they were noted to be redundant and were with low factor loadings (<0.40). Internal consistency coefficients were computed using the Cronbach's alpha measure to indicate the degree to which the items measure the same trait [24]. The internal consistency coefficient of the overall scale was 0.96, reflecting that the instrument is reliable [27].

Three main variables were examined in this study, namely the nurse manager competencies, and job satisfaction and turnover intention of staff nurses. The resulting *Nurse Manager Competency Scale* adopted in this study was made up of 60 items that captured five domains of *nurse manager competencies*: (1) Staff Advocacy and Development [12 items], which measured the competencies in advocating for staff interests and developing staff potential; (2) Team Communication and Collaboration [15 items], which measured the competencies in building cohesive teams through fostering team communication and collaboration; (3) Change and Resource Management [10 items], which measured the competencies in facilitating and embracing changes and ensuring optimal resource allocation; (4) Quality Monitoring and Pursuance [11 items], which measured the competencies in safeguarding the quality of care and cultivating a quality culture in the work unit; and (5) Personal Mastery [12 items], which measured the competencies in knowing oneself, his or her own internal attributes, purpose and vision [21]. Respondents were asked to evaluate the competencies of their nurse managers by using a 5-point Likert scale, ranging from 1 (strongly disagree) to 5 (strongly agree). Average scores were computed for each subscale and the overall scale, with higher scores denoting a more positive perception towards the competencies of their nurse managers and vice versa. For nurse outcomes, in line with the extant literature, *job satisfaction* and *turnover intention* were measured using a single-item measure [28,29]. Respondents were asked to indicate their level of satisfaction with their current job, and their intention to leave their current workplace, by using a 5-point Likert scale, ranging from 1 (most dissatisfied/least intended to leave) to 5 (most satisfied/most intended to leave). For the job satisfaction measure, a higher score indicates a higher level of job satisfaction and vice versa, and it is postulated as positively related to the nurse manager competencies. For the turnover intention measure, a higher score indicates a higher level of intention to leave the current workplace, and vice versa, and it is postulated as negatively related to the nurse manager competencies. Demographic and work-related information, including gender, age, rank, years of work experience, and type of hospital and work setting were also collected.

Information regarding the instrument used in this study, and its psychometric properties (including the factor analysis results and Cronbach's alpha values of each domain) is presented in Table 1. The questionnaire was written in Chinese, and was translated into English for reporting purposes. Forward and backward translations were conducted by two research team members, and validation was carried out by a qualified language editor.

Table 1. Psychometric properties of the nurse manager competency scale.

Items	Factor Loading				
	Domain 1: Staff Advocacy and Development	**Domain 2: Team Communication and Collaboration**	**Domain 3: Change and Resource Management**	**Domain 4: Quality Monitoring and Pursuance**	**Domain 5: Personal Mastery**
1. Understands staff's unique needs	0.751				
2. Stands up and speaks for colleagues	0.724				
3. Offers prompt assistance to colleagues when needed	0.722				
4. Advocates for the interests of co-workers	0.702				
5. Develops staff potential	0.666				
6. Able to address the needs of staff	0.622				
7. Provides an accurate appraisal of staff performance	0.607				
8. Delegates work according to the individual's potential	0.589				
9. Provides advice to colleagues on their career development	0.521				
10. Offers learning opportunities to colleagues	0.483				

Table 1. *Cont.*

Items	Factor Loading				
	Domain 1: Staff Advocacy and Development	Domain 2: Team Communication and Collaboration	Domain 3: Change and Resource Management	Domain 4: Quality Monitoring and Pursuance	Domain 5: Personal Mastery
11. Offers promotion opportunities to colleagues	0.450				
12. Shares with others his/her own expertise	0.448				
13. Respects others' views		0.775			
14. Is willing to accept others' opinions		0.723			
15. Strives to listen to colleagues' voices		0.684			
16. Views issues from others' perspectives		0.676			
17. Establishes trusting relationships		0.655			
18. Collaborates effectively with colleagues		0.631			
19. Incorporates multiple perspectives when managing incidents at work		0.597			
20. Shows appreciation to others		0.571			
21. Provides communication platforms		0.540			
22. Mediates conflicts among colleagues		0.522			
23. Bridges communication between hospital administrators and frontline workers		0.507			
24. Cultivates team spirit		0.468			
25. Facilitates collaboration with other departments		0.462			
26. Maintains day-to-day communication with colleagues		0.442			
27. Leads the team effectively		0.421			
28. Is flexible enough to make changes			0.689		
29. Handles unexpected incidents efficiently			0.682		
30. Effectively responds to sudden increases in demand for resources			0.660		
31. Effectively responds to sudden increases in demand for manpower			0.649		
32. Is willing to adopt new technological innovations in healthcare			0.635		
33. Keeps abreast with changes in health technology			0.570		
34. Scrutinizes the use of resources during times of change			0.540		
35. Forecasts the resources needed during times of change			0.529		
36. Facilitates changes at work			0.464		
37. Transforms changes into opportunities for advancement			0.415		
38. Directs colleagues towards goal setting				0.665	
39. Incorporates professional values in goal setting				0.635	
40. Pursues quality of care				0.596	
41. Incorporates organizational values in goal setting				0.524	
42. Develops initiatives to promote quality of care				0.514	
43. Proactively identifies risks to safeguard quality of care				0.503	
44. Pursues advancements in nursing				0.499	
45. Monitors staff performance to ensure quality of care				0.487	

Table 1. *Cont.*

Items	Factor Loading				
	Domain 1: Staff Advocacy and Development	Domain 2: Team Communication and Collaboration	Domain 3: Change and Resource Management	Domain 4: Quality Monitoring and Pursuance	Domain 5: Personal Mastery
46. Cultivates a culture of quality				0.489	
47. Values evidence-based practices				0.446	
48. Direct the team towards achieving quality of care				0.429	
49. Manages his/her own emotions well					0.666
50. Is open-minded					0.662
51. Is caring					0.607
52. Is fair					0.589
53. Is genuine					0.566
54. Is positive					0.551
55. Is knowledgeable about generational diversity					0.503
56. Is organized					0.478
57. Is hard-working and efficient					0.442
58. Is decisive					0.420
59. Is passionate about work					0.404
60. Is clinically knowledgeable and proficient					0.412
No. of items	12	15	10	11	12
Eigen values	4.22	3.54	2.65	2.13	1.85
Explained variance (%)	19.30	14.78	10.64	8.55	5.03
Cumulative explained variance (%)	19.30	34.08	44.72	53.27	58.30
Cronbach's alpha values	0.960	0.948	0.924	0.902	0.898

3.4. Data Analysis

Data were analyzed using SPSS version 26.0 software (Armonk, NY, USA: IBM Corporation). Demographic and work-related data, the perceived nurse manager competencies, and nurse outcome variables (namely job satisfaction and turnover intention) were summarized using descriptive statistics such as frequencies, percentages, means, and standard deviations (SDs). Pearson correlation analyses were performed to examine the associations among all the study variables. Multiple linear regression analyses were conducted to examine the relationships between the five domains of nurse manager competency (predictor variables) and the job satisfaction and turnover intention of frontline nurses (outcome variables). For all the analyses, a p value of <0.05 was regarded as statistically significant.

4. Results

4.1. Demographic and Work-Related Characteristics of the Respondents

The 688 respondents recruited in this study were from 24 hospitals and 88 work units. Among them, the majority were female (83.6%, n = 575), and were registered nurses (61.3%; n = 422) working in public hospitals in Hong Kong (83.9%; n = 577). Around half of them worked in general medical and surgical settings (46.7%; n = 321), and approximately 60% of them (n = 416) had more than 10 years of work experience. Details of the demographic and work-related characteristics of the respondents are presented in Table 2.

Table 2. Demographic and work-related characteristics of the respondents (N = 688).

	n (%)
Gender	
Male	113 (16.4)
Female	575 (83.6)
Age	
25 or below	34 (4.9)
26–35	227 (33.0)
36–45	178 (25.9)
46–55	187 (27.2)
56 or above	62 (9.0)
Rank	
Enrolled Nurse	87 (12.6)
Registered Nurse	422 (61.3)
Advanced Practice Nurse	179 (26.0)
Type of hospital	
Public acute hospital	451 (65.6)
Public sub-acute hospital	126 (18.3)
Private hospital	111 (16.1)
Type of clinical setting	
Medical	207 (30.1)
Surgical	114 (16.6)
Obstetrics	41 (6.0)
Psychiatry	75 (10.9)
Accident and Emergency	39 (5.7)
Operating Theatre	68 (9.9)
Out-patient Clinic/Community Nursing Service	59 (8.6)
Others	85 (12.4)
Years of working as a nurse	
1 to 3 years	55 (8.0)
4 to 10 years	217 (31.5)
11 to 20 years	159 (23.1)
21 to 30 years	172 (25.0)
>30 years	85 (12.4)

4.2. The Level of Nurse Manager Competencies and Nurse Outcomes

Table 3 lists the items along with the respondents' mean ratings of the nurse manager competencies. The overall mean score on *nurse manager competencies* in our sample was 3.15 out of 5 (SD = 0.859). Among the five domains of nurse manager competencies, the respondents rated "Quality Monitoring and Pursuance" (mean = 3.20; SD = 0.811) the highest, followed by "Personal Mastery" (mean = 3.16; SD = 0.859), "Change and Resource Management" (mean = 3.15; SD = 0.816), "Staff Advocacy and Development" (mean = 3.06; SD = 0.918), and lastly "Team Communication and Collaboration" (mean = 3.05; SD = 0.890). Respondents gave comparatively higher ratings to a few items, including the competencies of nurse managers in "monitoring staff performance to ensure quality of care" (item 45) under the domain of "Quality Monitoring and Pursuance"; "being passionate about work" (item 59); "being clinically knowledgeable and proficient" (item 60) under the domain of "Personal Mastery"; and "responding effectively to sudden increases in resource demand" (item 30) under the domain of "Change and Resource Management". Respondents gave relatively lower ratings to a number of items, concerning the competencies of nurse managers in "*understanding staff's unique needs*" (item 1), and "*addressing the needs of staff*" (item 6) under the domain of "Staff Advocacy and Development", and "*viewing from others' perspectives*" (item 16), "establishing trusting relationships" (item 17), and *"providing communication platforms"* (item 21) under the domain of "Team Communication and Collaboration".

Table 3. The level of nurse manager competencies (N = 688).

Domains and Items of the Nurse Manager Competency Scale	Mean ± SD
Domain 1: Staff Advocacy and Development	
1. Understands staff's unique needs	2.74 ± 1.178
2. Stands up and speaks for colleagues	2.92 ± 1.148
3. Offers prompt assistance to colleagues when needed	3.16 ± 1.119
4. Advocates for the interests of co-workers	3.00 ± 1.143
5. Develops staff potential	3.03 ± 1.053
6. Able to address the needs of staff	2.90 ± 1.111
7. Provides an accurate appraisal of staff performance	3.08 ± 1.019
8. Delegates work according to the individual's potential	3.06 ± 1.102
9. Provides advice to colleagues on their career development	3.11 ± 1.027
10. Offers learning opportunities to colleagues	3.23 ± 1.035
11. Offers promotion opportunities to colleagues	3.15 ± 1.027
12. Shares with others his/her own expertise	3.30 ± 1.002
Domain 2: Team Communication and Collaboration	
13. Respects others' views	3.01 ± 1.113
14. Is willing to accept others' opinions	2.92 ± 1.110
15. Strives to listen to colleagues' voices	3.00 ± 1.091
16. Views issues from others' perspectives	2.89 ± 1.121
17. Establishes trusting relationships	2.87 ± 1.137
18. Collaborates effectively with colleagues	3.07 ± 1.075
19. Incorporates multiple perspectives when managing incidents at work	3.16 ± 1.065
20. Shows appreciation to others	3.19 ± 1.015
21. Provides communication platforms	2.88 ± 1.116
22. Mediates conflicts among colleagues	3.00 ± 1.033
23. Bridges communication between hospital administrators and frontline workers	3.07 ± 1.116
24. Cultivates team spirit	3.14 ± 1.114
25. Facilitates collaboration with other departments	3.28 ± 1.052
26. Maintains day-to-day communication with colleagues	3.00 ± 1.067
27. Leads the team effectively	3.11 ± 0.960
Domain 3: Change and Resource Management	
28. Is flexible enough to make changes	3.05 ± 1.058
29. Handles unexpected incidents efficiently	3.35 ± 1.085
30. Effectively responds to sudden increases in demand for resources	3.41 ± 1.021
31. Effectively responds to sudden increases in demand for manpower	3.00 ± 1.197
32. Is willing to adopt new technological innovations in healthcare	3.24 ± 0.940
33. Keeps abreast with changes in health technology	3.26 ± 0.966
34. Scrutinizes the use of resources during times of change	3.10 ± 1.004
35. Forecasts the resources needed during times of change	3.09 ± 0.922
36. Facilitates changes at work	3.01 ± 1.071
37. Transforms changes into opportunities for advancement	3.02 ± 1.059
Domain 4: Quality Monitoring and Pursuance	
38. Directs colleagues towards goal setting	3.35 ± 0.942
39. Incorporates professional values in goal setting	3.10 ± 0.987
40. Pursues quality of care	3.10 ± 1.070
41. Incorporates organizational values in goal setting	3.14 ± 0.961
42. Develops initiatives to promote quality of care	3.14 ± 1.028
43. Proactively identifies risks to safeguard quality of care	3.03 ± 1.107
44. Pursues advancements in nursing	3.21 ± 1.014

Table 3. *Cont.*

Domains and Items of the Nurse Manager Competency Scale	Mean ± SD
45. Monitors staff performance to ensure quality of care	3.44 ± 0.974
46. Cultivates a culture of quality	3.26 ± 0.960
47. Values evidence-based practices	3.17 ± 0.950
48. Direct the team towards achieving quality of care	3.13 ± 1.034
Domain 5: Personal Mastery	
49. Manages his/her own emotions well	3.15 ± 1.171
50. Is open-minded	2.90 ± 1.143
51. Is caring	3.02 ± 1.107
52. Is fair	2.88 ± 1.131
53. Is genuine	3.15 ± 1.089
54. Is positive	3.17 ± 1.076
55. Is knowledgeable about generational diversity	2.98 ± 0.997
56. Is organized	3.13 ± 1.063
57. Is hard-working and efficient	3.17 ± 1.099
58. Is decisive	3.12 ± 1.037
59. Is passionate about work	3.44 ± 0.996
60. Is clinically knowledgeable and proficient	3.49 ± 0.968

For nurse outcomes, the mean *job satisfaction* level was 2.85 out of 5 (SD = 0.875), and the mean *turnover intention* level was 3.16 out of 5 (SD = 0.817). Only one-fourth of respondents (25.0%; $n = 172$) rated themselves as satisfied with their current jobs; more than one-third of respondents were dissatisfied with their current jobs (34.3%, $n = 236$) and were considering leaving their current workplace (36.3%, $n = 250$).

4.3. Correlations between Nurse Manager Competencies and Nurse Outcomes

Significant positive associations were noted between job satisfaction and the five domains of nurse manager competencies, and significant negative correlations were noted between turnover intention and the five domains of nurse manager competencies. The strength of the relationships detected was below 0.60, reflecting a moderate relationship between nurse manager competencies and nurse outcomes (Table 4).

Table 4. Associations between nurse manager competencies and nurse outcomes.

	Pearson's r *	
	Job Satisfaction	**Turnover Intention**
Nurse manager competencies	0.60	−0.58
Team Communication and Collaboration	0.59	−0.57
Staff Advocacy and Development	0.59	−0.58
Change and Resource Management	0.57	−0.52
Personal Mastery	0.58	−0.57
Quality Monitoring and Pursuance	0.56	−0.53

* All correlation were significant at $p < 0.001$.

4.4. Predictors of Nurse Outcomes

Multiple regression analyses were conducted to examine the associations between the five domains of nurse manager competencies and nurse outcomes. The five domains of nurse manager competencies were entered as predictor variables, and the job satisfaction and turnover intention measures were entered as the dependent variables. Correlation analyses revealed weak but significant correlations (r ranging from 0.108 to 0.200) between the nurse manager competencies and the demographic and work-related variables (such as age and years of work experience). The regression models were controlled for these personal and work-related variables. The presence of multicollinearity was excluded by examining the correlations among the predictor variables ($r < 0.60$), tolerance (ranging from 0.130 to 0.216), the variance inflation factor (ranging from 4.63 to 9.74), and the condition index (ranging from 1.00 to 8.53).

The overall regression was statistically significant in predicting the job satisfaction ($R^2 = 0.41$, $F = 159.82$, $p < 0.000$) and turnover intention ($R^2 = 0.34$, $F = 176.32$, $p < 0.000$) of nurses. Regression analyses identified "Team Communication and Collaboration", "Staff Advocacy and Development", and "Quality Monitoring and Pursuance" as significant predictors of nurses' job satisfaction and "Staff Advocacy and Development" and "Team Communication and Collaboration" as significant predictors of nurses' turnover intention (Table 5).

Table 5. Predictors of staff nurses' job satisfaction and turnover intention.

Predictor Variables	Job Satisfaction				Turnover Intention			
	B	β	t	*p*	B	β	t	*p*
Team Communication and Collaboration	0.284	0.289	3.035	0.002	−0.223	−0.243	−2.511	0.012
Staff Advocacy and Development	0.227	0.229	2.345	0.019	−0.309	−0.347	−3.581	0.000
Change and Resource Management	0.116	0.108	1.352	0.177	−0.036	−0.036	−0.424	0.672
Personal Mastery	0.142	0.140	1.264	0.207	−0.106	−0.111	−0.946	0.344
Quality Monitoring and Pursuance	0.203	0.213	2.164	0.031	−0.027	−0.027	−0.327	0.744

5. Discussion

The aim of this study was to examine the associations between nurse manager competencies and nurse outcomes. The findings were consistent with those of previous studies, upholding the role of nurse managers in stabilizing the nursing workforce in the face of the COVID-19 pandemic [12,30]. The findings supplemented the extant literature by providing empirical support for the specific domains of nurse manager competencies that predict the job satisfaction and turnover intention of staff nurses.

5.1. Discussion of the Findings

Regarding nurse outcomes, the findings of this study revealed that one-third of respondents were considering leaving their current workplace; the figure was comparable to or slightly better than those of previous studies, which reported that about 40 to 50 per cent of staff nurses intended to leave their current workplace in Taiwan and the United States [19,20,31]. This can be attributed to two factors. The first is that Hong Kong nurses had previously experienced a similar epidemic situation, which was the outbreak of the severe acute respiratory syndrome (SARS) in 2003; local nurses were more prepared for crises and might not have found the COVID-19 pandemic as distressing as nurses in other countries [32]. The second is that local nurses were noted to have gained a strong sense of professionalism from the public recognition that they received, which could have helped to retain them in the workplace [33].

Staff nurses in this study reported a more positive perception towards three domains of nurse manager competency, including "Change and Resource Management", "Personal Mastery", and "Quality Monitoring and Pursuance". "Change and Resource Management" and "Personal Mastery" were not identified as significant factors predicting the job satisfaction and turnover intention of staff nurses in this study. Past relevant studies conceptualized these areas of nurse manager competency as "Staffing and Resource Adequacy" and "Nurse Manager Ability", and conflicting findings were noted regarding their predictive effects on nurse outcomes [34,35]. Previous research conceptualized "Quality Monitoring and Pursuance" as "Nursing Foundations for Quality of Care" and "Patient Safety Culture", and similarly, no conclusive findings were yielded regarding their predictive effectives on nurse outcomes [28,36]. Further studies are required to examine the associations between these specific domains of nurse manager competency and nurse outcomes. The pandemic turned hospitals into battlefields, with nurse managers heavily engaged in effecting changes and directing staff to work according to standards to ensure quality of care [6]. During the period of crisis, intertwined challenges related to resource allocation and change and quality management arose [37]. Many of these challenges were exacerbated by the pandemic situation; for instance, the lack of hospital beds, manpower, and materials, such as personal protective equipment [38]. These challenges called for changes such as the development of new systems and protocols of care, and new ways of working, which were mostly coordinated by nurse managers [38]. Their role in sustaining the quality of care was rated the most important in past studies, involving personal mastery such as their abilities to handle contingencies and projecting a sense of confidence, calm, control, and security during crises [39–41].

Among the five domains of nurse manager competency, staff nurses reported a more negative perception towards "Staff Advocacy and Development" and "Team Communication and Collaboration". Past relevant studies described these areas of nurse manager competency as "Nurse Participation in Hospital Affairs" and "Collegial Relationships", respectively. Consistent with previous studies, this study identified these domains of nurse manager competency as the key predictors of nurse outcomes [28,35]. In previous research, nurse managers rated their advocacy skills lowest among their other skills, and many nurse managers indicated that they had not been prepared and trained to advocate for co-workers in the workplace [42,43]. They faced difficulties in advocating for professional autonomy or, more specifically, the inclusion of frontline nurses in decision-making processes [42,43]. Scholars have highlighted the need to uphold professional autonomy at work, as nurses with a poorer sense of professional autonomy tended to be more dissatisfied with their job and to experience burnout [44,45]. Regarding team effectiveness, findings of previous research indicated that communication and collaboration could directly impact nurse outcomes, and these were compromised due to the lack of time and increased workload resulting from the pandemic situation [6,46]. Elements underlying this area of competency were referred to in previous studies as "human skills", consisting of communication and relationship management skills [40], and as "directive functions", concerning the ability of nurse managers to effectively communicate and work with teams, be open to suggestions, and respect nurses.

5.2. Implications for Policy, Practice, and Education

The findings of this study have implications for the development of competency assessment tools or performance appraisal tools as well as for the designing of competency-based academic and training programs for nurse managers. The *Nurse Manager Competency Scale* captured the areas of competency crucial for managerial success. With further validation, it could be adopted as a tool to assess the competencies of nurse managers against standards of performance [47]. Regarding the training of nurse managers, previous studies have indicated that a one-off education program failed to improve the competencies of nurse managers [37], and many scholars have stressed the importance of providing systematic and continuous training to nurse managers [41,48]. The findings of this study can serve as a basis for designing these training programmes. Because the study was conducted during the COVID-19 pandemic, it has also taken into account the competencies that nurse managers should learn in order to manage crises or health catastrophes such as pandemics [39]. The efforts made by previous researchers to develop training and orientation programs based on nurse manager competencies have proven to be effective in facilitating the role transition of novice nurse managers and in bringing them success [37]. The findings of this study lay a foundation for the development of succession planning programs to identify the right person with the essential competency levels, and to facilitate the role transition of staff nurses to first-line nurse managers. There is also a need to conduct regular educational need assessments, as the competencies required for success may change with time [41,48].

With committed efforts, our future nurse leaders will be better prepared for the challenges ahead, which will ultimately lead to improved staff and organizational outcomes.

Among the various domains of nurse manager competencies, "Team Communication and Collaboration" and "Staff Advocacy and Development" were identified as the key predictors of nurse outcomes. To ensure team effectiveness, the initial effort should be to understand the views and needs of staff nurses, and to develop a clear and transparent chain of command and an open, two-way system of communication with them [6,38]. During periods of crisis and rapid changes, other than face-to-face interactions, nurse leaders may adopt digital platforms such as webinars and virtual meetings to share information and to network and exchange ideas with others during the pandemic [38,49]. Regarding the role of nurse managers in advocating for the interest of staff nurses, it should be noted that staff advocacy cannot be achieved without understanding matters of concern to nurses. Regular, short surveys can be adopted to facilitate nurses to voice their needs and concerns, and these types of advocacy strategies have been largely neglected in management training for nurse managers [38,42,43].

5.3. Limitations and Future Research

This study helped to fill the existing gap in the literature on the "critical success factors of nurse managers" (p. 5), which has been regarded by researchers as a growing global priority [12]. However, this study has a few limitations. While the study was cross-sectional and descriptive in nature, the influence of other political and economic factors that might have influenced the variables (e.g., nurse outcomes) under study were not examined. Future researchers can consider adopting longitudinal studies to further examine the causal relationships among multiple variables that have a bearing on nurse outcomes. In addition, the study was subjective in nature, as the measurement was based on the perceptions of staff nurses. Future studies can consider incorporating the use of more objective measures such as actual nurse turnover. The *Nurse Manager Competency Scale* adopted in this study comprised 60 items and was relatively lengthy, and the findings derived from the study were therefore subjected to acquiescence response bias [24]. Lastly, this study was conducted in a single region, and adopted non-random sampling approaches. This led to uncertainty regarding the representativeness of the findings and their applicability to the global context. Future researchers can replicate the study by adopting a more sophisticated sampling approach that allows for unit-level analyses so as to improve the generalizability of the study. The research team faced practical constraints in recruiting nurse managers to the study; further research can therefore be conducted to compare the nurse managers' perceptions of their own competencies with those evaluated by staff nurses so as to identify the gap in existing management practices.

6. Conclusions

The COVID-19 pandemic has brought about many challenges to contemporary healthcare, leading to rapid changes in the provision of care, and to a sense of uncertainly and insecurity among the workforce. Nurse managers play a pivotal role in ensuring both quality of care and workforce stability. This study adds knowledge to the specific domains of competencies that nurse managers require in order to ensure positive nurse outcomes and has implications for what they can put into practice to attain the goal of organizational and workforce stability.

Author Contributions: P.-P.C. was responsible for the acquisition of funding, conceptualization, methodology, data collection and analysis, and writing of the manuscript; S.-S.W., W.-M.L. and M.-H.T. were responsible for conceptualization, methodology, data collection and analysis, and for reviewing and editing the manuscript. All authors have read and agreed to the published version of the manuscript.

Funding: The work described in this paper was supported by a research donation to Hong Kong Metropolitan University (Project Reference No.: 2019/1004).

Institutional Review Board Statement: The study was conducted in accordance with the Declaration of Helsinki and approved by the Ethics Committee of the Hong Kong Metropolitan University (ethical approval code: HE-RGC2019/31) on 22 May 2019.

Informed Consent Statement: Informed consent was indicated by the return of the questionnaires.

Data Availability Statement: The data that support the findings of this study are available from the corresponding author upon reasonable request.

Acknowledgments: We would like to thank Sarah Tang, Bella Lau, and Reina Tsui for their contribution to data collection, data entry, and the translation of the instrument. We would also like to thank the respondents for sharing with us their perspectives on the study issue.

Conflicts of Interest: The authors declare no conflict of interest. The funders had no role in the design of the study; in the collection, analyses, or interpretation of the data; in the writing of the manuscript; or in the decision to publish the results.

References

1. Ann-Hughes, K.; Carryer, J.; Jones, M.; HlthMgt, S.G.G. Attributes of an effective nurse manager in New Zealand: An analysis of nurse manager perceptions. *Nurs. Prax. N. Z.* **2018**, *34*, 27–37. [CrossRef]
2. Phougeishangbam, P.D.; Mayanglambam, P. Impact of COVID 19 on health care personnel. *Indian J. Public Health Res. Dev.* **2020**, *11*, 79–83.
3. Tolksdorf, K.H.; Tischler, U.; Heinrichs, K. Correlates of turnover intention among nursing staff in the COVID-19 pandemic: A systematic review. *BMC Nurs.* **2022**, *21*, 174. [CrossRef]
4. Buchan, J.; Catton, H.; Shaffer, F. Sustain and Retain in 2022 and Beyond. *Int. Counc. Nurses* **2022**, *71*, 1–71.
5. Roche, M.R.; Duffield, C.M.; Dimitrelis, S.; Frew, B. Leadership skills for nursing unit managers to decrease intention to leave. *Nurs. Res. Rev.* **2015**, *5*, 57–64.
6. Galleryzki, A.R.; Hariyati, R.T.S. Overview of Nurses' Perceptions of the Headroom Management Function in Hospitals during the COVID-19 Pandemic. *J. Glob. Res. Public Health* **2021**, *6*, 136–142.
7. Cummings, G.G.; Tate, K.; Lee, S.; Wong, C.A.; Paananen, T.; Micaroni, S.P.; Chatterjee, G.E. Leadership styles and outcome patterns for the nursing workforce and work environment: A systematic review. *Int. J. Nurs. Stud.* **2018**, *85*, 19–60. [CrossRef]
8. Labrague, L.J.; Nwafor, C.E.; Tsaras, K. Influence of toxic and transformational leadership practices on nurses' job satisfaction, job stress, absenteeism and turnover intention: A cross-sectional study. *J. Nurs. Manag.* **2020**, *28*, 1104–1113. [CrossRef]
9. Abualrub, R.F.; Alghamdi, M.G. The impact of leadership styles on nurses' satisfaction and intention to stay among Saudi nurses. *J. Nurs. Manag.* **2012**, *20*, 668–678. [CrossRef]
10. Suliman, M.; Aljezawi, M.; Almansi, S.; Musa, A.; Alazam, M.; Ta'an, W.F. Effect of nurse managers' leadership styles on predicted nurse turnover. *Nurs Manag.* **2020**, *29*, 20–25. [CrossRef]
11. Kantanen, K.; Kaunonen, M.; Helminen, M.; Suominen, T. The development and pilot of an instrument for measuring nurse managers' leadership and management competencies. *J. Res. Nurs.* **2015**, *20*, 667–677. [CrossRef]
12. Warshawsky, N.E.; Cramer, E.; Grandfield, E.M.; Schlotzhauer, A.E. The influence of nurse manager competency on practice environment, missed nursing care, and patient care quality: A cross-sectional study of nurse managers in US hospitals. *J. Nurs. Manag.* 2022; *Online ahead of print*. [CrossRef] [PubMed]
13. Lavoie-Tremblay, M.; Gélinas, C.; Aubé, T.; Tchouaket, E.; Tremblay, D.; Gagnon, M.P.; Côté, J. Influence of caring for COVID-19 patients on nurse's turnover, work satisfaction and quality of care. *J. Nurs. Manag.* **2022**, *30*, 33–43. [CrossRef] [PubMed]
14. Sanner-Stiehr, E.; Garcia, A.; Polivka, B.; Dunton, N.; Williams, J.A.; Walpitage, D.L.; Hui, C.; Spreckelmeyer, K.; Yang, F. Support from work and intent to stay among nurses during COVID-19: An academic-practice collaboration. *Nurse Lead.* 2022; *Online ahead of print*.
15. Cadge, W.; Lewis, M.; Bandini, J.; Shostak, S.; Donahue, V.; Trachtenberg, S.; Grone, K.; Kacmarek, R.; Lux, L.; Matthews, C.; et al. Intensive care unit nurses living through COVID-19: A qualitative study. *J. Nurs. Manag.* **2021**, *29*, 1965–1973. [CrossRef]
16. Nelson, H.; Murdoch, N.H.; Norman, K. The Role of Uncertainty in the Experiences of Nurses During the Covid-19 Pandemic: A Phenomenological Study. *Can. J. Nurs. Res.* **2021**, *53*, 124–133. [CrossRef]
17. Al Sabei, S.D.; Al-Rawajfah, O.; AbuAlRub, R.; Labrague, L.J.; Burney, I.A. Nurses' job burnout and its association with work environment, empowerment and psychological stress during COVID-19 pandemic. *Int. J. Nurs. Pract.* **2022**, e13077. [CrossRef]
18. Gurková, E.; Mikšová, Z.; Šáteková, L. Missed nursing care in hospital environments during the COVID-19 pandemic. *Int. Nurs. Rev.* **2022**, *69*, 175–184. [CrossRef]
19. Taylor-Clark, T.M.; Swiger, P.A.; Anusiewicz, C.V.; Loan, L.A.; Olds, D.M.; Breckenridge-Sproat, S.T.; Raju, D.; Patrician, P.A. Identifying Potentially Preventable Reasons Nurses Intend to Leave a Job. *J. Nurs. Adm.* **2022**, *52*, 73–80. [CrossRef]
20. Raso, R.; Fitzpatrick, J.J.; Masick, K. Perceptions of US nurses and nurse leaders on authentic nurse leadership, healthy work environment, intent to leave and nurse well-being during a second pandemic year: A cross sectional study. *J. Nurs. Manag.* 2022; *Online ahead of print*. [CrossRef]

21. Choi, P.-P.; Wong, S.-S.; Lee, W.-M.; Tiu, M.-H. Multi-Generational Perspectives on the Competencies Required of First-Line Nurse Managers. *Int. J. Environ. Res. Public Health* **2022**, *19*, 10560. [CrossRef]
22. Shi, J.; Mo, X.; Sun, Z. Content validity index in scale development. *J. Cent. South Univ. (Med. Sci.)* **2012**, *37*, 152–155.
23. Streiner, D.L.; Norman, G.R.; Cairney, J. *Health Measurement Scales: A Practical Guide to Their Development and Use*, 5th ed.; Oxford University Press: Oxford, UK, 2015.
24. Polit, D.F.; Beck, C.T. *Essentials of Nursing Research: Appraising Evidence for Nursing Practice*, 10th ed.; Wolters Kluwer: Philadelphia, PA, USA, 2022.
25. Fabrigar, L.R.; Wegener, D.T.; MacCallum, R.C.; Strahan, E.J. Evaluating the use of exploratory factor analysis in psychological research. *Psychol. Methods.* **1999**, *4*, 272. [CrossRef]
26. Nunnally, J.C.; Bernstein, I.H. *Psychometric Theory*, 3rd ed.; McGraw-Hill: New York, NY, USA, 1994.
27. DeVellis, R.F. *Scale Development: Theory and Applications*, 4th ed.; Sage Publications: Thousand Oaks, CA, USA, 2016.
28. Nantsupawat, A.; Kunaviktikul, W.; Nantsupawat, R.; Wichaikhum, O.A.; Thienthong, H.; Poghosyan, L. Effects of nurse work environment on job dissatisfaction, burnout, intention to leave. *Int. Nurs. Rev.* **2017**, *64*, 91–98. [CrossRef] [PubMed]
29. Wanous, J.; Reichers, A.; Hudy, M. Overall job satisfaction: How good are single item measure? *J. Appl. Psychol.* **1997**, *82*, 247–252. [CrossRef] [PubMed]
30. Aydogdu, A.L.F. Nurse managers on front line against new coronavirus. *Management* **2020**, *8*, 21–24.
31. Chen, H.M.; Liu, C.C.; Yang, S.Y.; Wang, Y.R.; Hsieh, P.L. Factors Related to Care Competence, Workplace Stress, and Intention to Stay among Novice Nurses during the Coronavirus Disease (COVID-19) Pandemic. *Int. J. Environ. Res. Public Health* **2021**, *18*, 2122. [CrossRef]
32. Hung, L.S. The SARS epidemic in Hong Kong: What lessons have we learned. *J. R. Soc. Med.* **2003**, *96*, 374–378. [CrossRef]
33. Choi, S.P.P.; Cheung, K.; Pang, S.M.C. Attributes of nursing work environment as predictors of registered nurses' job satisfac-tion and intention to leave. *J. Nurs. Manag.* **2013**, *21*, 429–439. [CrossRef]
34. Cho, H.; Han, K.; Ryu, E. Unit work environment, psychological empowerment and support for patient activation among nurses. *J. Nurs. Manag.* **2021**, *29*, 1623–1630. [CrossRef]
35. Lee, S.E.; MacPhee, M.; Dahinten, V.S. Factors related to perioperative nurses' job satisfaction and intention to leave. *Jpn. J. Nurs. Sci.* **2020**, *17*, e12263. [CrossRef]
36. Kim, K.-J.; Yoo, M.S.; Seo, E.J. Exploring the Influence of Nursing Work Environment and Patient Safety Culture on Missed Nursing Care in Korea. *Asian Nurs. Res.* **2018**, *12*, 121–126. [CrossRef] [PubMed]
37. Kim, S.; Lim, J.-Y. Development and Evaluation of the "High-Up" Program for Enhancing the Nursing-Management Competency of Mid-Career Hospital Nurses: A Quasi-Experimental Study. *Int. J. Environ. Res. Public Health* **2022**, *19*, 4392. [CrossRef] [PubMed]
38. Rodriguez, K.M.A.; Cura, J.D.; Aringo, R.B., Jr. Fostering a culture of nursing excellence during the COVID-19 crisis. *Nurs. Manag.* **2022**, *53*, 18–27. [CrossRef] [PubMed]
39. Vázquez-Calatayud, M.; Regaira-Martínez, E.; Rumeu-Casares, C.; Paloma-Mora, B.; Esain, A.; Oroviogoicoechea, C. Experiences of frontline nurse managers during the COVID-19: A qualitative study. *J. Nurs. Manag.* **2022**, *30*, 79–89. [CrossRef]
40. Liou, Y.F.; Liaw, J.J.; Chang, Y.C.; Kao, J.H.; Feng, R.C. Psychometric properties and development of the competency inventory for Taiwanese nurse managers across all levels. *J. Nurs. Manag.* **2021**, *29*, 2092–2101. [CrossRef]
41. Shomura, M.; Okabe, H.; Tejima, Y.; Yaguchi, N.; Iwamoto, S.; Sakurai, D. Nurse managers' self-evaluations of their man-agement competencies and factors associated with their ability to develop staff. *J. Nurs. Educ. Pract.* **2019**, *9*, 99–107. [CrossRef]
42. MacLellan, L.; Levett-Jones, T.; Higgins, I. The enemy within: Power and politics in the transition to nurse practitioner. *Nurs. Open* **2017**, *2*, 1–7. [CrossRef]
43. Paarima, Y.; Ofei, A.M.A.; Kwashie, A.A. Managerial Competencies of Nurse Managers in Ghana. *Afr. J. Nurs. Midwifery* **2020**, *22*, 1–20. [CrossRef]
44. Putra, K.R.; Sutadi, H.; Setyowati, S.; Hariyati, R.T.S. The impact of nurse manager caring behaviors and work environment on burnout syndrome among nurses. *Kontakt* **2021**, *23*, 90–96. [CrossRef]
45. Dettmers, J.; Bredehöft, F. The Ambivalence of Job Autonomy and the Role of Job Design Demands. *Scand. J. Work Organ. Psychol.* **2020**, *5*, 8. [CrossRef]
46. Fowler, K.R.; Robbins, L.K.; Lucero, A. Nurse manager communication and outcomes for nursing: An integrative review. *J. Nurs. Manag.* **2021**, *29*, 1486–1495. [CrossRef] [PubMed]
47. Gonczi, A.; Hager, P.; Athanasou, J. *The Development of Competency-Based Assessment Strategies for the Professions*; Australian Government Publishing Service: Canberra, Australia, 1993.
48. Flatekval, A.M.; Corbo, S.A. Nurse manager self-reported competency levels. *Nurs. Manag.* **2019**, *50*, 28–33. [CrossRef] [PubMed]
49. Daradkeh, L.F.; Villar, R.C.; Nashwan, A.J. The perception of nursing leaders towards communication and relationship man-agement competencies while using digital platforms during COVID-19 pandemic in Qatar. *J. Nurs. Manag.* **2021**, 1–8. [CrossRef]

International Journal of
Environmental Research and Public Health

MDPI

Article

Working Conditions and Wellbeing among Prison Nurses during the COVID-19 Pandemic in Comparison to Community Nurses

Megan Guardiano [1], Paul Boy [1], Grigoriy Shapirshteyn [2], Lisa Dobrozdravic [2], Liwei Chen [3], Haiou Yang [4], Wendie Robbins [1,5] and Jian Li [1,5,*]

1 School of Nursing, University of California Los Angeles, Los Angeles, CA 90095, USA
2 Quality Management Support Unit, Avenal State Prison, Avenal, CA 93204, USA
3 Department of Epidemiology, Fielding School of Public Health, University of California Los Angeles, Los Angeles, CA 90095, USA
4 Center for Occupational and Environmental Health, University of California Irvine, Irvine, CA 92617, USA
5 Department of Environmental Health Sciences, Fielding School of Public Health, University of California Los Angeles, Los Angeles, CA 90095, USA
* Correspondence: jianli2019@ucla.edu

Abstract: The psychological health and work challenges of nurses working in prisons during the COVID-19 pandemic are understudied. We evaluated the work and wellbeing characteristics of a California prison nurse group, with a comparison to those of a community nurse group. From May to November 2020, an online survey measured psychosocial and organizational work factors, sleep habits, psychological characteristics, COVID-19 impacts, and pre-pandemic recall among 62 prison nurses and 47 community nurses. Prison nurses had significantly longer work hours (54.73 ± 14.52, $p < 0.0001$), higher pandemic-related work demands, and less sleep hours (5.36 ± 1.30, $p < 0.0001$) than community nurses. Community nurses had significantly higher pandemic-related fear levels (work infection: $p = 0.0115$, general: $p = 0.0025$) and lower perceived personal protective equipment (PPE) supply ($p = 0.0103$). Between pre-pandemic and pandemic periods, both groups had significantly increased night shift assignments and decreased sleep hours, but the prison group had increased work hours. Although not statistically significant, both groups had high occupational stress and prevalence of post-traumatic stress symptoms. Our results indicate that prison nurses experienced work and wellbeing challenges during the pandemic. Future research and practice ought to address nurses' workload, PPE, and psychological resources in correctional facilities and healthcare organizations.

Keywords: correctional nurses; occupational health; work conditions; mental health; prison; nurses; COVID-19

Citation: Guardiano, M.; Boy, P.; Shapirshteyn, G.; Dobrozdravic, L.; Chen, L.; Yang, H.; Robbins, W.; Li, J. Working Conditions and Wellbeing among Prison Nurses during the COVID-19 Pandemic in Comparison to Community Nurses. *Int. J. Environ. Res. Public Health* **2022**, *19*, 10955. https://doi.org/10.3390/ijerph191710955

Academic Editor: Paul B. Tchounwou

Received: 27 July 2022
Accepted: 30 August 2022
Published: 2 September 2022

1. Introduction

At the onset of the COVID-19 pandemic in 2020, an estimated 27,743 registered nurses (RNs) were actively working at United States (U.S.) correctional facilities, which include state prisons, as their primary employment, accounting for 0.8% of the U.S. RN population [1,2]. Throughout the pandemic, the National Institute for Occupational Safety and Health [3] and the National Academy of Medicine [4] have advocated for the occupational mental health and wellbeing of healthcare workers. The National Commission on Correctional Health Care, aligned with the Nurse Code of Ethics, supports correctional nurse health to optimize care for incarcerated individuals [5].

The job demands–resources (JD-R) theory provides a framework to demonstrate how the occupational environment and conditions may influence wellbeing among nurses working in prison settings. Initially, the occupational theory of JD-R related the concepts of elevated job demands and insufficient job resources with lower motivation and the outcome of burnout among workers [6]. The JD-R theory has been developed to broadly involve multiple [7] and various job demands, job resources, and worker health outcomes [8], applicable to any occupation [6]. Among nurses, evidence suggests that high psychological and physical job demands are related to the intention to quit nursing, emphasizing the relevance of the JD-R theory to this population [9]. Additional significant findings from research applications of the JD-R theory in the COVID-19 pandemic context indicate a negative association between the perception of work organization support and post-traumatic stress disorder symptoms in a sample of U.S. nurses working in COVID-19 hospital units [10]. As an extension of the JD-R theory to our study of prison nurses, the domain of job demands includes efforts, work hours, and the types of shift assignment and patient care. The job resources domain encompasses PPE supply and work-related rewards. The wellbeing outcome measures are the psychological characteristics of anxiety, depression, and post-traumatic stress symptoms. Thus, research applying this JD-R theory to correctional nurses working during the COVID-19 pandemic will further characterize the job demands, resources, and outcomes unique to this population and compounded by the pandemic.

Prior to the COVID-19 pandemic, published reviews related to nurses and other health professionals working in correctional facilities identified occupational stressors including security prioritization, conflicts, fear, job demands [11], burnout, stress [12], and secondary trauma [13]. Within North America, older U.S. studies have demonstrated moderate [14] and high [15] work-related mean stress levels among correctional nurses. Other North American pre-pandemic studies of correctional worker mental health in Canada have included nurses, but within healthcare worker subgroups [16,17].

A recent study of U.S. correctional workers during the COVID-19 pandemic found that correctional healthcare workers reporting any degree of depression, anxiety, burnout, and post-traumatic stress symptoms ranged from 37% to 50% [18]. However, this study was concentrated on correctional facilities located in eastern U.S. states [18]. To the best of our knowledge, there are no available scientific reports focused solely on prison nurses and their working conditions and wellbeing during the COVID-19 pandemic.

The prevalence of COVID-19 cases in U.S. correctional facilities has been significantly higher than that of the general population. Based on the facilities' available reports, which vary in data quality, there were 42,107 COVID-19 cases among incarcerated individuals in U.S. federal and state prisons, a rate that was five-and-a-half-fold greater than that of the U.S. population, between March and June 2020 [19,20]. There were 13,781 documented or reported COVID-19 cases specifically in California correctional institutions, a rate that was on average over eight-and-a-half-fold greater than that of the aggregated Californian population between September and November 2020 [21].

Research on healthcare workers and nurses working through the COVID-19 pandemic has demonstrated elevated levels of occupational and psychological concerns. Studies conducted in Europe and Asia have identified elevated levels of occupational stress [22,23], insomnia, workload, anxiety, and depression [22]. Additionally, effort and over-commitment have been associated with anxiety and depression [24]. Literature reviews and meta-analyses of international healthcare workers have reinforced these individual study findings, with pooled prevalence rates ranging from 43% to 56.5% for stress, 40% to 44% for sleep issues [25–27], and 18.75% to 48% for post-traumatic stress [26–28].

Qualitative and quantitative research on U.S. nurses during the COVID-19 pandemic have recognized occupational challenges regarding patient care, increased workload, and inadequate personal protective equipment (PPE), as well as psychological outcomes including post-traumatic stress, depression, and anxiety [29–32]. However, these studies heavily focus on hospital settings, and are mostly concentrated in the U.S. Northeast, South, and Midwest [29,30]. A December 2020 national survey that provided state-specific data reported that the majority of California nurses felt exhausted, overwhelmed, and anxious, with 52% expressing neutrality or disagreement with the statement that their workplace valued employee safety and health [33]. Yet, there was minimal representation of correctional nurses in California [33]. In California correctional settings, the Legislative Analyst's Office 2019 report acknowledged the California Department of Corrections and Rehabilitation's (CDCR) use of mandatory overtime for nursing staff, despite previous state agreement to decrease this practice [34].

The underrepresentation of correctional nurses in California and the combined challenges intrinsic to the correctional work setting and to the COVID-19 pandemic warrant further investigation. To the best of our knowledge, this is the first study in the western U.S. region to exclusively target prison nurses and their working conditions and wellbeing in the context of the COVID-19 pandemic, and compared to a non-correctional worker group. This study aims to evaluate a group of California prison nurses and compare their work characteristics and wellbeing outcomes with those of a community nurse group.

2. Materials and Methods

2.1. Design

This cross-sectional study with convenience sampling utilized a one-time online survey to compare the occupational and wellbeing characteristics of nurse participants working in a prison (prison group) to those working in other clinical settings (community group).

2.2. Setting and Sample

Recruitment for the community group occurred through nursing organization websites during an approximate 1.5-month survey window between late May and early July 2020. Most of the community nurse participants were in California. The prison nurse group was subsequently enrolled through collaboration with healthcare administrators at a California state prison. The survey window for the prison nurse group was about two months, from early September to late November 2020. For both groups, eligible nurses had to have current paid employment in a healthcare setting since the start of the COVID-19 pandemic.

Informed consent was obtained from participants at the initiation of the online survey. Each participant received a USD 10 gift card incentive. This study was reviewed and approved by the University of California, Los Angeles Institutional Review Board (IRB#20-000804 and IRB#20-001440), and followed the Declaration of Helsinki guidelines, as well as the Strengthening the Reporting of Observational Studies in Epidemiology (STROBE) reporting guideline.

2.3. Measures

The "Survey of Nurses Work and Wellbeing during the COVID-19 Outbreak" was administered online to both groups of participants. The survey included validated instruments, Likert-type scales, visual analog scales, and numeric and free text responses to measure the working conditions and wellbeing of nurses before and during the pandemic (current context). Specifically, the survey focused on 3 domains of assessments on working conditions: psychosocial characteristics, organizational work characteristics, and the COVID-19 working characteristics. The survey also focused on 3 domains of assessments on psychological wellbeing, including sleep characteristics, psychological characteristics, and post-traumatic stress disorder. Pre-pandemic recall and current reports were requested for the variables of weekly work and sleep hours and night shift assignment. All other variables were one-time measurements.

2.3.1. Psychosocial and Organizational Work Characteristics

The Effort–Reward Imbalance (ERI) scale was used to measure psychosocial factors at work, consisting of 10 items, 3 for effort, and 7 for reward [35–37]. The effort score ranges from 3 to 12 and the reward score ranges from 7 to 28, with high scores corresponding with high magnitudes of effort and reward [35–37]. The E–R ratio score ranges between 0.25 and 4.00, with scores above one suggesting high work stress [35–37]. The Cronbach's alpha coefficients were 0.80 for the effort subscale, and 0.78 for the reward subscale. The ERI measure has been widely used among nurses in Europe [38], as well as healthcare workers, including nurses in the United States [39]. During the COVID-19 pandemic, several studies used the ERI for measuring work stress in frontline healthcare workers [22–24,40].

The organizational work characteristics included work years, as well as pre-pandemic and current (at the time of survey) measurements of weekly average work hours and frequency of night shift assignment.

2.3.2. COVID-19 Characteristics

The COVID-19 working characteristics included perceptions of general pandemic-related fear, fear of infection, adequacy of PPE supply, magnitude of COVID-19 patient contact, requests or history of work department redeployment, and history of COVID-19 symptoms, testing, and diagnosis.

2.3.3. Sleep Characteristics

Pre-pandemic and current weekly averages of sleep hours were collected. To measure insomnia levels, three items about sleep within the last month were obtained from the National Health and Nutritional Examination Survey [41]. Scores range between 0 and 12, with higher numbers associated with higher degrees of insomnia [41]. This insomnia measure had a Cronbach's alpha of 0.83.

2.3.4. Psychological Characteristics

The Patient Health Questionnaire-4 (PHQ-4) measured depression and anxiety. The PHQ-4 features two two-item subscales to measure depression and anxiety symptoms over the past month [42]. Each subscale's score ranges from 0 to 6, with higher numbers relating to higher levels of depression and anxiety [42]. For both conditions, scores of 3 and above represent positive cases of depression and anxiety [42]. Both subscales were reliable, with a Cronbach's alpha of 0.82 for depression and 0.9 for anxiety. Previous studies utilized this brief instrument during the COVID-19 pandemic among a hospital nurse sample in Romania [43], and a hospital nurse and nurse assistant sample in the United States [29].

Post-Traumatic Stress Disorder (PTSD) symptoms over the past month were measured with a six-item screening instrument [44]. Scores range from 6 to 30, with elevated scores reflecting elevated PTSD symptoms [44]. A score of 14 or above indicates PTSD [44]. The Cronbach's alpha for this scale was 0.88. This instrument has been used in a United Kingdom healthcare worker sample during the COVID-19 pandemic [45].

2.4. Statistical Analyses

Participants with partial responses were included using pairwise deletion, with the omission of non-responses per variable rather than the implementation of missing value replacements. Data were analyzed with Mann–Whitney U and *t*-tests for continuous data, and Fisher's exact and Chi-Square tests for categorical data. The Shapiro–Wilk test checked for normal distributions. Wilcoxon signed-rank and McNemar's tests compared pre-pandemic and current data. Means, standard deviations, and ranges were calculated. Calculations and analyses were conducted using SAS 9.4 (SAS Institute Inc., Cary, NC, USA).

3. Results

Among the 114 participants that originally submitted the survey, 5 participant entries were removed due to lack of consent or nonresponse on all items, resulting in a total sample of 109 with at least partial responses. Of this total sample, 79.82% completed the entire survey, with similar completion rates between the prison (79.03% of 62) and community (80.85% of 47) groups. The analysis incorporated the remaining participants' partial responses.

Table 1 shows the demographic characteristics of the study participants, with no significant differences between the two groups for gender, race, marital status, and age. The majority of participants in both groups were female, married or partnered, with a mean age within the 40-year age range. The largest racial subgroup was non-Hispanic White for both groups.

Table 1. Sociodemographic data.

Variables	Prison (n = 62)		Community (n = 47)		p-Value
	n [a]	%	n [a]	%	
Gender					
Female	45	93.75	36	85.71	
Male	3	6.25	5	11.90	0.36 [b]
Transgender	0	0	1	2.38	
Race					
Non-Hispanic White	18	35.29	16	38.10	
Non-Hispanic Black	3	5.88	4	9.52	
Non-Hispanic Asian	10	19.61	13	30.95	0.41 [b]
Hispanic or Latino	16	31.37	7	16.67	
Other	4	7.84	2	4.76	
Marital Status					
Single	15	30.00	13	31.71	
Married or Partnered	28	56.00	24	58.54	0.83 [c]
Separated or Divorced or Widowed	7	14.00	4	9.76	
Age in Years (mean ± SD)	44.29 ± 9.44		41.29 ± 12.78		0.12 [d]

[a] Sample sizes vary per variable due to missing data. [b] Fisher's exact. [c] Chi-Square. [d] Mann–Whitney U.

Table 2 indicates the organizational characteristics before and during the pandemic. Both prison and community nurses had mean work years of about 15 years, with a minimum of 2 years, without significant differences. The pre-pandemic and current weekly mean hours of work were significantly higher for prison nurses compared to community nurses. For prison nurses, work hours significantly increased during the pandemic. Although there were no significant differences in night shift assignment between the groups before the pandemic and currently, the amount of prison nurses working any night shifts significantly increased after the start of the pandemic. There were no significant differences in psychosocial work stress experiences in terms of effort-reward imbalance between the groups, but stress levels in both groups were relatively high (E-R ratio > 1.0).

Table 3 reports working conditions during COVID-19. Prison nurses reported significantly more direct COVID-19 patient contact, and had more requests to work, or had worked, in other departments. However, significantly more prison nurses perceived adequate PPE supply and had COVID-19 testing compared to community nurses. Significantly more community nurses expressed fear of contracting COVID-19 at work, and had a higher level of general fear towards the COVID-19 outbreak.

Table 4 focuses on the psychological wellbeing of the study participants. The prison nurses' mean daily sleep hours were significantly lower than those of community nurses before the pandemic and currently. Sleep hours significantly decreased for both groups compared to before the pandemic. Mean scores for total insomnia and the sleep-related items indicating "trouble falling asleep" and "waking up at night" were elevated in the prison group compared to the community group, but these differences were not statistically significant. Both groups did not significantly differ in their mean PTSD scores, but both mean scores were above the cutoff score of 14. The percentage of nurses with a PTSD score equal to or above 14 was 49.02% in the prison group and 69.05% in the community group. Although depression and anxiety mean scores were more elevated in the community group, they did not significantly differ from those of the prison group. For both groups, the depression and anxiety mean scores were below the cutoff, and the prevalence of depression and anxiety cases was low.

Table 2. Psychosocial and organizational work characteristics.

Variables	Prison		Community		*p*-Value
	Mean ± SD				
Effort–Reward Imbalance					
E–R Ratio	1.32 ± 0.44		1.28 ± 0.58		0.46 [a]
Effort Score	9.62 ± 1.69		9.40 ± 2.06		0.65 [a]
Reward Score	17.95 ± 3.82		18.73 ± 3.76		0.27 [a]
Work Years (mean ± SD, range)	15.93 ± 10.52, 2–42		15.32 ± 12.49, 2–45		0.34 [a]
Pre-Pandemic Work Hours (weekly mean)	41.51 ± 8.21		33.51 ± 13.95		<0.0001 [a]
Pandemic Work Hours (weekly mean)	54.73 ± 14.52		33.51 ± 15.27		<0.0001 [a]
Pre-Pandemic vs. Pandemic Work Hours (*p*-values)	<0.0001 [b]		0.48 [b]		
Pre-Pandemic Night Shift	*n* [c]	%	*n* [c]	%	
No	44	78.57	38	82.61	0.61 [d]
Yes	12	21.43	8	17.39	
Pandemic Night Shift					
No	33	57.89	35	76.09	
Yes	24	42.11	11	23.91	0.0526 [d]
Pre-Pandemic vs. Pandemic Night Shift (*p*-values)	0.0017 [e]		<0.0001 [e]		

[a] Mann–Whitney U. [b] Wilcoxon signed rank. [c] Sample sizes vary per variable due to missing data. [d] Chi-Square. [e] McNemar's Test.

Table 3. COVID-19 characteristics.

Variables	Prison		Community		*p*-Value
	n [a]	%	*n* [a]	%	
COVID-19 Patient Contact					
Direct patient contact	53	91.38	24	52.17	
No direct patient contact but work with other HCW(s) who have direct patient(s)	5	8.62	12	26.09	<0.0001 [b]
No direct patient contact but shared common spaces with other worker(s) and/or patient(s)	0	0	4	8.70	
No contact	0	0	6	13.04	
PPE Supply					
Adequate	46	77.97	25	54.35	0.0103 [c]
Inadequate	13	22.03	21	45.65	
Volunteered or Asked to Work in Other Department					
Yes	54	87.10	19	40.43	<0.0001 [c]
No	8	12.90	28	59.57	
Fear of Work Infection					
Strongly Agree	18	31.03	21	44.68	
Agree	19	32.76	22	46.81	0.0115 [b]
Disagree	14	24.14	3	6.38	
Strongly Disagree	7	12.07	1	2.13	
Fear of Outbreak (0–100, mean ± SD)	51.80 ± 28.65		67.85 ± 22.96		0.0025 [d]
COVID-19 Symptoms	*n* [a]	%	*n* [a]	%	
Yes	22	40.00	16	39.02	0.92 [c]
No	33	60.00	25	60.98	
COVID-19 Testing					
Yes	55	100.00	20	46.51	<0.0001 [c]
No	0	0	23	53.49	
COVID-19 Diagnosis					
Yes	7	12.73	3	6.98	
No	48	87.27	40	93.02	0.51 [b]

HCWs = healthcare workers. [a] Sample sizes vary per variable due to missing data. [b] Fisher's exact. [c] Chi-Square. [d] Mann–Whitney U.

Table 4. Sleep and psychological characteristics.

Variables	Prison		Community		*p*-Value
	Mean ± SD				
Pre-Pandemic Sleep (mean daily hours)	6.60 ± 1.10		7.20 ± 1.13		0.0156 [a]
Pandemic Sleep (mean daily hours)	5.36 ± 1.30		6.65 ± 1.51		<0.0001 [a]
Pre-Pandemic vs. Pandemic Sleep (*p*-values)	<0.0001 [b]		0.0099 [b]		
Insomnia Score	6.20 ± 2.98		5.68 ± 3.45		0.44 [a]
Trouble falling asleep	3.29 ± 1.08		2.98 ± 1.27		0.16 [a]
Waking up at night	3.09 ± 1.14		2.86 ± 1.30		0.31 [a]
Waking up too early	2.82 ± 1.25		2.84 ± 1.38		0.97 [a]
PTSD					
Mean Score	14.57 ± 5.95		15.88 ± 5.42		0.17 [a]
Score ≥ 14 (n [c], %)	25	49.02	29	69.05	0.0514 [d]
Depression					
Mean Score	1.24 ± 1.48		1.76 ± 1.51		0.06 [a]
Score ≥ 3 (n [c], %)	8	16.00	9	21.95	0.47 [d]
Anxiety					
Mean Score	1.50 ± 1.61		2.02 ± 2.02		0.28 [a]
Score ≥ 3 (n [c], %)	9	18.75	11	26.83	0.36 [d]

[a] Mann–Whitney U. [b] Wilcoxon signed rank. [c] Sample sizes vary per variable due to missing data. [d] Chi-Square.

4. Discussion

Significant findings from this study provide insight into prison nurses' intensified challenges, including longer work hours, less sleep hours, more COVID-19 patient care demand, higher perceived PPE supply, and lower pandemic-related fear levels compared to community nurses. Although not statistically different, the occupational stress and mental distress results of prison nurses and community nurses are concerning, and reflect the pandemic context.

The weekly work hours of the prison nurse study participants contrasted with those of the U.S. nurse population. Among the estimated U.S. population, 58.7% of nurses worked 32 to 40 h weekly between February and June 2020 [1]. While the community group's mean pre-pandemic and current weekly hours were within this range, those of the prison group exceeded the national population estimate. Additionally, this finding of long working hours among the prison nurse study participants may be related to the previously mentioned issue of mandated overtime among some California state institutions [34]. The World Health Organization and International Labor Organization have confirmed that long working hours of 55 or more weekly hours are an occupational risk factor for cardiovascular disease [46].

Our study's findings on sleep hours and related issues align with a pre-pandemic Washington state prison study, in which the majority of correctional staff and healthcare workers had less than five hours of sleep, 53% had zero to two hours of sleep between work shifts, and 40.7% to 47.2% of participants reported over thrice-weekly trouble falling asleep and nightly waking [47]. In contrast, among East U.S. correctional healthcare workers during the pandemic, 81.57% did not have sleep disturbances, indicated by normal score ranges, but their mean sleep disturbance scores were significantly higher compared to correctional officer mean scores [18].

The prison nurse study participants experienced higher pandemic-related work demand, schedule, and environment adjustments through increased COVID-19 patient care, increased night shift assignments, and increased department redeployment requests. The elevated California correctional facility COVID-19 case rate [21] may have contributed to these occupational changes. Furthermore, a 2022 report from the National Commission on Correctional Health Care featured the ongoing issue of understaffing among certified correctional health professionals throughout the two years of the pandemic [48]. COVID-19 patient contact, shift assignment, and department redeployment work changes were similarly identified as challenges in the pandemic experience of U.S. hospital nurses [32]. COVID-19 patient care has been associated with increased risk of infection, anxiety, and emotional distress among nurses working in hospitals and other clinical settings [49–51].

The perception of adequate PPE supply may have been related to the lower degrees of COVID-19 general and work infection fears, despite significantly increased COVID-19 patient care among prison nurses. In contrast, among community nurses, there was a higher proportion that perceived inadequate PPE supply, elevated COVID-19-related fears, and a lower proportion of COVID-19 patient care. The perception of adequate PPE availability has been previously associated with a reduced probability of COVID-19 infection among U.S. healthcare workers across multiple clinical settings [49].

The history of the CDCR's mandatory overtime practice [34] and our prison nurse study participants' long working hours and COVID-19-related work changes exemplify the influence of occupational policy on nurses' health and wellbeing, as well as highlight implications for organizational interventions. A scoping review of nurses' coping during COVID-19 emphasized the importance of work hour and schedule flexibility and occupational safety via PPE and training [52], encompassing organizational responsibilities.

Considering our findings of elevated work hours and COVID-19 patient care, lowered sleep hours, and sleep quality issues, our sample of prison nurses may be at risk of high fatigue. There have been associations of increased work hours and COVID-19 patient care with increased fatigue among hospital nurses working through the pandemic [29].

Although other nurse- and work-related stress instruments have been used within this population before the pandemic [14,15], the ERI instrument has not been previously applied to correctional nurses to measure occupational stress. The similar mean E–R ratio scores among the prison and community nurses corroborate previous ERI results from other nurse and healthcare worker populations working through the pandemic. Italian hospital healthcare workers had a mean E–R ratio over 1 [22], and three-fourths of nurses working in Greek hospitals scored E–R ratios over 1, demonstrating occupational stress in the context of the COVID-19 pandemic [23]. In contrast, pre-pandemic studies among correctional officers in China and general nurses in Europe indicated a mean E–R ratio score under 1 [38,53]. With respect to the findings of our study, it is suggested that the current pandemic circumstances may contribute to increased occupational stress in all types of nurses.

Addressing the high levels of occupational stress suggested by both nurse groups may imply feasible approaches with symptom reduction interventions. The published reviews of individual-based nurse intervention studies have identified evidence of mindfulness interventions as being helpful in the reduction of work stress and burnout [54], as well as the prominent use of technological mediums to promote intervention accessibility [55]. Therefore, potential interventions to reduce stress among nurses working in prisons and within the community may involve mindfulness techniques administered through a digital format.

Regarding psychological measures, the high prevalence of PTSD symptoms in our study contrasts with the findings of previous studies on correctional healthcare workers. Pre-pandemic Canadian studies that categorized nurses within a minority subgroup of correctional wellness workers found a lower prevalence of positive PTSD screens, at 16.7% and 17.2%, which suggests the pandemic's effect on correctional healthcare worker post-traumatic stress symptoms [16,17]. Considering the COVID-19 pandemic, our study's psychological findings differ from those of a recent East U.S. correctional worker study. Almost half of our prison nurse group had positive PTSD screens, while in the latter study, 43.27% of correctional healthcare workers had normal PTSD scores and 20.29% had moderate and severe scores [18]. Both our prison group and the East U.S. healthcare worker subgroup had a low prevalence of depression and anxiety screens [18]. The prevalence contrasts among these studies may be due to differences in instrumentation, timing, and setting. Although the scope of our study may not provide causal inferences, our prison group's higher prevalence of PTSD may be related to our single-site focus and a previous finding among hospital nurses of significantly elevated PTSD scores associated with COVID-19 patient care [29].

This study had the following limitations, including its relatively small sample size. Our findings from one California prison may not be generalizable to all California prisons, nor the whole correctional nurse population. Although most of the nurses in the community group were from California and worked in hospital settings, the heterogeneity of this group may present a nonequivalent comparison to the single-site prison nurse group due to potential differences in the work settings. The extended and nonoverlapping survey windows of the two groups also present the possibility of different historical effects affecting each group. The self-report nature of the survey and the retrospective items referring to before the pandemic may have introduced recall bias. Regarding the possible generalizability between our study participants and the correctional and general U.S. nurse populations, the demographics of our study participants reflect those of the 2020 U.S. nurse population estimates, with a female and White majority [1]. However, the sample and population estimate distributions underrepresent male nurses and nurses of other ethnicities, warranting future research to investigate the occupational experiences and needs of these minority groups.

The study's strengths include its timing within the first year of the COVID-19 pandemic, which provides data of the pandemic's initial impact on the prison and community healthcare settings. Despite limitations from the study design decision to retroactively add the prison nurse group, this addition contributes to the representation of the correctional nurse population. Likewise, the allowance of one- to two-month survey windows and the use of short-form versions of validated instruments were intended to accommodate participants' time and stress while working during this phase of the COVID-19 pandemic. The comparative study design between a specialized nurse group and a general nurse group, rather than a different occupation, highlights the needs and circumstances of prison nurses. The participants in both study groups were experienced nurses, with a minimum of 2 years and a mean of about 15 years of work, which avoids potential confounding from newer nurses transitioning into the practice. This study addresses the geographical and nursing specialty knowledge gaps by providing data on Californian prison nurses. Although the prison nurse group sample size was small, our study may be considered a pilot study, contributing knowledge related to the COVID-19 pandemic in the context of the need for data on the correctional nursing workforce [2].

5. Conclusions

Our group of prison nurse participants significantly differed from the community nurses, with longer work hours, fewer sleep hours, higher COVID-19 patient care, higher perceptions of adequate PPE supply, and lower pandemic-related fear levels. Occupational stress and mental distress impacted both groups of nurses. Our findings suggest the need for and importance of future research and practice to improve correctional nurse occupational wellbeing, and consequently, the care and wellbeing of incarcerated individuals. Although our study was limited to a relatively small sample at a single prison, our findings may be considered preliminary for future studies involving multiple correctional facilities.

Addressing excessive working hours and sleep deficiencies among correctional nurses may involve the revision of institution policies regarding mandatory overtime, staffing, and more equitable distributions of workload. Additional organizational support in both correctional and healthcare settings may include sufficient PPE supply and accessible interventions and resources to manage mental distress among nurses in the workplace.

Author Contributions: Conceptualization, W.R. and J.L.; data curation, M.G., W.R. and J.L.; formal analysis, M.G.; investigation, P.B., G.S., L.D., W.R. and J.L.; methodology, L.C., H.Y., W.R. and J.L.; project administration, W.R. and J.L. supervision, W.R. and J.L.; visualization, M.G.; writing—original draft preparation, M.G., W.R. and J.L.; writing—review and editing, M.G., P.B., G.S., L.D., L.C., H.Y.,

W.R. and J.L. Note, W.R. and J.L. made equal contributions to this piece of research work. All authors have read and agreed to the published version of the manuscript.

Funding: M.G. was partially supported by the National Institute for Occupational Safety and Health (NIOSH) Occupational and Environmental Health Nursing Program of the Southern California Education and Research Center (SCERC), Grant Agreement Number T42 OH008412 from the Centers for Disease Control and Prevention (CDC). Its contents are solely the responsibility of the authors and do not necessarily represent the official view of the U.S. CDC.

Institutional Review Board Statement: The study was conducted according to the guidelines of the Declaration of Helsinki and approved by the Institutional Review Board of the University of California, Los Angeles (protocol code 20-000804 and 20-001440).

Informed Consent Statement: Informed consent was obtained from all subjects involved in the study.

Data Availability Statement: The data presented in this study are available on request from the corresponding author. The data are not publicly available due to privacy reasons.

Acknowledgments: We thank all nurse participants for their daily work and their contributions to this study.

Conflicts of Interest: The authors declare no conflict of interest.

References

1. Smiley, R.A.; Ruttinger, C.; Oliveira, C.M.; Hudson, L.R.; Allgeyer, R.; Reneau, K.A.; Silvestre, J.H.; Alexander, M. The 2020 National Nursing Workforce Survey. *J. Nurs. Regul.* **2021**, *12*, S1–S96. [CrossRef]
2. Shelton, D.; Maruca, A.T.; Wright, R. Nursing in the American justice system. *Arch. Psychiatr. Nurs.* **2020**, *34*, 304–309. [CrossRef] [PubMed]
3. National Institute for Occupational Safety and Health. Healthcare Workers: Work Stress & Mental Health. Available online: https://www.cdc.gov/niosh/topics/healthcare/workstress.html (accessed on 1 May 2022).
4. National Academy of Medicine. Action Collaborative on Clinician Well-Being and Resilience. Available online: https://nam.edu/initiatives/clinician-resilience-and-well-being/ (accessed on 1 May 2022).
5. Roscoe, L. Ethical Issues, Moral Courage and Moral Resiliency in Correctional Nursing. Available online: https://www.ncchc.org/correctional-nursing-practice-what-you-need-to-know/ethical-issues-moral-courage-and-moral-resiliency-in-correctional-nursing/ (accessed on 18 July 2022).
6. Demerouti, E.; Bakker, A.B.; Nachreiner, F.; Schaufeli, W.B. The job demands-resources model of burnout. *J. Appl. Psychol.* **2001**, *86*, 499–512. [CrossRef] [PubMed]
7. Bakker, A.B.; Demerouti, E.; Verbeke, W. Using the job demands-resources model to predict burnout and performance. *Hum. Resour. Manag.* **2004**, *43*, 83–104. [CrossRef]
8. Schaufeli, W.B.; Taris, T.W. *A Critical Review of the Job Demands-Resources Model: Implications for Improving Work and Health*; Springer: Dordrecht, The Netherlands, 2014; pp. 43–68. [CrossRef]
9. Van Der Heijden, B.; Brown Mahoney, C.; Xu, Y. Impact of job demands and resources on nurses' burnout and occupational turnover intention towards an age-moderated mediation model for the nursing profession. *Int. J. Environ. Res. Public Health* **2019**, *16*, 2011. [CrossRef]
10. Cockerham, M.; Beier, M.E.; Branson, S.; Boss, L. Nurse adaptability and post-traumatic stress disorder symptoms during the COVID-19 pandemic: The effects of family and perceived organizational support. *Front. Psychol.* **2021**, *12*, 749763. [CrossRef]
11. Keller, E.; Boch, S.; Hittle, B.M. Unsafe and unsettling: An integrative review on correctional nursing work environments and stressors. *J. Forensic Nurs.* **2022**, *online ahead of print*. [CrossRef]
12. Simon, L.; Beckmann, D.; Stone, M.; Williams, R.; Cohen, M.; Tobey, M. Clinician experiences of care provision in the correctional setting: A scoping review. *J. Correct. Health Care* **2020**, *26*, 301–314. [CrossRef]
13. Wright, R.M. The relationship among secondary trauma, self-efficacy, and correctional nurses. *J. Correct. Health Care* **2020**, *26*, 207–214. [CrossRef]
14. Flanagan, N.A. Testing the relationship between job stress and satisfaction in correctional nurses. *Nurs. Res.* **2006**, *55*, 316–327. [CrossRef]
15. El Ghaziri, M.; Dugan, A.G.; Zhang, Y.; Gore, R.; Castro, M.E. Sex and gender role differences in occupational exposures and work outcomes among registered nurses in correctional settings. *Ann. Work Expo. Health* **2019**, *63*, 568–582. [CrossRef] [PubMed]
16. Fusco, N.; Ricciardelli, R.; Jamshidi, L.; Carleton, R.N.; Barnim, N.; Hilton, Z.; Groll, D. When our work hits home: Trauma and mental disorders in correctional officers and other correctional workers. *Front. Psychiatry* **2021**, *11*, 10. [CrossRef] [PubMed]
17. Carleton, R.N.; Ricciardelli, R.; Taillieu, T.; Mitchell, M.M.; Andres, E.; Afifi, T.O. Provincial correctional service workers: The prevalence of mental disorders. *Int. J. Environ. Res. Public Health* **2020**, *17*, 2203. [CrossRef] [PubMed]
18. Burhanullah, M.H.; Rollings-Mazza, P.; Galecki, J.; Van Wert, M.; Weber, T.; Malik, M. Mental health of staff at correctional facilities in the United States during the COVID-19 pandemic. *Front. Psychiatry* **2022**, *12*, 767385. [CrossRef] [PubMed]

19. Saloner, B.; Parish, K.; Ward, J.A.; Dilaura, G.; Dolovich, S. COVID-19 cases and deaths in federal and state prisons. *JAMA* **2020**, *324*, 602. [CrossRef] [PubMed]
20. DeWolf, L.; Rajeshwar, P.; Tyagi, E. Missing the Mark: Data Reporting and Quality Scorecard. Available online: https://uclacovidbehindbars.org/blog/scorecard (accessed on 17 July 2022).
21. California Department of Corrections and Rehabilitation. CDCR Patients: COVID-19 Cases and Outcomes. Available online: https://www.cdcr.ca.gov/covid19/population-status-tracking/ (accessed on 22 May 2022).
22. Magnavita, N.; Soave, P.M.; Antonelli, M. Prolonged stress causes depression in frontline workers facing the COVID-19 pandemic—A repeated cross-sectional study in a COVID-19 hub-hospital in central Italy. *Int. J. Environ. Res. Public Health* **2021**, *18*, 7316. [CrossRef]
23. Tzenetidis, V.; Papathanasiou, I.; Tzenetidis, N.; Nikolentzos, A.; Sarafis, P.; Malliarou, M. Effort reward imbalance and insomnia among Greek healthcare personnel during the outbreak of COVID-19. *Mater. Sociomed* **2021**, *33*, 124–130. [CrossRef]
24. Zhang, J.; Wang, Y.; Xu, J.; You, H.; Li, Y.; Liang, Y.; Li, S.; Ma, L.; Lau, J.T.-F.; Hao, Y.; et al. Prevalence of mental health problems and associated factors among front-line public health workers during the COVID-19 pandemic in China: An effort–reward imbalance model-informed study. *BMC Psychol.* **2021**, *9*, 55. [CrossRef]
25. Al Maqbali, M.; Al Sinani, M.; Al-Lenjawi, B. Prevalence of stress, depression, anxiety and sleep disturbance among nurses during the COVID-19 pandemic: A systematic review and meta-analysis. *J. Psychosom. Res.* **2021**, *141*, 110343. [CrossRef]
26. Dragioti, E.; Tsartsalis, D.; Mentis, M.; Mantzoukas, S.; Gouva, M. Impact of the COVID-19 pandemic on the mental health of hospital staff: An umbrella review of 44 meta-analyses. *Int. J. Nurs. Stud.* **2022**, *131*, 104272. [CrossRef]
27. Marvaldi, M.; Mallet, J.; Dubertret, C.; Moro, M.R.; Guessoum, S.B. Anxiety, depression, trauma-related, and sleep disorders among healthcare workers during the COVID-19 pandemic: A systematic review and meta-analysis. *Neurosci. Biobehav. Rev.* **2021**, *126*, 252–264. [CrossRef] [PubMed]
28. Saragih, I.D.; Tonapa, S.; Saragih, I.S.; Advani, S.; Batubara, S.O.; Suarilah, I.; Lin, C.J. Global prevalence of mental health problems among healthcare workers during the Covid-19 pandemic: A systematic review and meta-analysis. *Int. J. Nurs. Stud.* **2021**, *121*, 104002. [CrossRef] [PubMed]
29. Sagherian, K.; Steege, L.M.; Cobb, S.J.; Cho, H. Insomnia, fatigue and psychosocial well-being during COVID-19 pandemic: A cross-sectional survey of hospital nursing staff in the United States. *J. Clin. Nurs.* **2020**, *Online ahead of print*. [CrossRef] [PubMed]
30. Mensinger, J.L.; Brom, H.; Havens, D.S.; Costello, A.; D'Annunzio, C.; Durning, J.D.; Bradley, P.K.; Copel, L.; Maldonado, L.; Smeltzer, S.; et al. Psychological responses of hospital-based nurses working during the COVID-19 pandemic in the United States: A cross-sectional study. *Appl. Nurs. Res.* **2022**, *63*, 151517. [CrossRef] [PubMed]
31. Shechter, A.; Diaz, F.; Moise, N.; Anstey, D.E.; Ye, S.; Agarwal, S.; Birk, J.L.; Brodie, D.; Cannone, D.E.; Chang, B.; et al. Psychological distress, coping behaviors, and preferences for support among New York healthcare workers during the COVID-19 pandemic. *Gen. Hosp. Psychiatry* **2020**, *66*, 1–8. [CrossRef]
32. Kelley, M.M.; Zadvinskis, I.M.; Miller, P.S.; Monturo, C.; Norful, A.A.; O'Mathuna, D.; Roberts, H.; Smith, J.; Tucker, S.; Zellefrow, C.; et al. United States nurses' experiences during the COVID-19 pandemic: A grounded theory. *J. Clin. Nurs.* **2022**, *31*, 2167–2180. [CrossRef]
33. American Nurses Foundation. Pulse on the Nation's Nurses COVID-19 Survey Series: Mental Health and Wellness Survey 2. December 2020. Available online: https://www.nursingworld.org/practice-policy/work-environment/health-safety/disaster-preparedness/coronavirus/what-you-need-to-know/mental-health-and-wellness-survey-2/ (accessed on 21 July 2022).
34. MOU Analysis. MOU Fiscal Analysis: Bargaining Units 1, 3, 4, 11, 14, 15, 17, 20, and 21 (SEIU Local 1000). Available online: https://lao.ca.gov/Publications/Report/4094 (accessed on 20 August 2022).
35. Li, J.; Leineweber, C.; Nyberg, A.; Siegrist, J. Cost, gain, and health: Theoretical clarification and psychometric validation of a work stress model with data from two national studies. *J. Occup. Environ. Med.* **2019**, *61*, 898–904. [CrossRef]
36. Siegrist, J.; Wege, N.; Puhlhofer, F.; Wahrendorf, M. A short generic measure of work stress in the era of globalization: Effort-reward imbalance. *Int. Arch. Occup. Environ. Health* **2009**, *82*, 1005–1013. [CrossRef]
37. Chin, D.L.; Kyung, M.; Li, J.; Phelps, S.; Hong, O. The short form effort-reward imbalance: Measure of occupational stress for firefighters. *Am. J. Ind. Med.* **2022**, *65*, 492–499. [CrossRef]
38. Li, J.; Galatsch, M.; Siegrist, J.; Müller, B.H.; Hasselhorn, H.M. Reward frustration at work and intention to leave the nursing profession—Prospective results from the European longitudinal NEXT study. *Int. J. Nurs. Stud.* **2011**, *48*, 628–635. [CrossRef]
39. Gillen, M.; Yen, I.H.; Trupin, L.; Swig, L.; Rugulies, R.; Mullen, K.; Font, A.; Burian, D.; Ryan, G.; Janowitz, I.; et al. The association of socioeconomic status and psychosocial and physical workplace factors with musculoskeletal injury in hospital workers. *Am. J. Ind. Med.* **2007**, *50*, 245–260. [CrossRef] [PubMed]
40. Schug, C.; Geiser, F.; Hiebel, N.; Beschoner, P.; Jerg-Bretzke, L.; Albus, C.; Weidner, K.; Morawa, E.; Erim, Y. Sick leave and intention to quit the job among nursing staff in German hospitals during the COVID-19 pandemic. *Int. J. Environ. Res. Public Health* **2022**, *19*, 1947. [CrossRef] [PubMed]
41. Chakravorty, S.; Siu, H.Y.K.; Lalley-Chareczko, L.; Brown, G.K.; Findley, J.C.; Perlis, M.L.; Grandner, M.A. Sleep duration and insomnia symptoms as risk factors for suicidal ideation in a nationally representative sample. *Prim. Care Companion CNS Disord.* **2015**, *17*, 10.4088/PCC.13m01551. [CrossRef] [PubMed]
42. Kroenke, K.; Spitzer, R.L.; Williams, J.B.; Lowe, B. An ultra-brief screening scale for anxiety and depression: The PHQ-4. *Psychosomatics* **2009**, *50*, 613–621. [CrossRef] [PubMed]

43. Petrișor, C.; Breazu, C.; Doroftei, M.; Mărieș, I.; Popescu, C. Association of moral distress with anxiety, depression, and an intention to leave among nurses working in intensive care units during the COVID-19 pandemic. *Healthcare* **2021**, *9*, 1377. [CrossRef] [PubMed]
44. Lang, A.J.; Stein, M.B. An abbreviated PTSD checklist for use as a screening instrument in primary care. *Behav. Res. Ther.* **2005**, *43*, 585–594. [CrossRef]
45. Lamb, D.; Gnanapragasam, S.; Greenberg, N.; Bhundia, R.; Carr, E.; Hotopf, M.; Razavi, R.; Raine, R.; Cross, S.; Dewar, A.; et al. Psychosocial impact of the COVID-19 pandemic on 4378 UK healthcare workers and ancillary staff: Initial baseline data from a cohort study collected during the first wave of the pandemic. *Occup. Environ. Med.* **2021**, *78*, 801–808. [CrossRef]
46. Pega, F.; Nafradi, B.; Momen, N.C.; Ujita, Y.; Streicher, K.N.; Pruss-Ustun, A.M.; Descatha, A.; Driscoll, T.; Fischer, F.M.; Godderis, L.; et al. Global, regional, and national burdens of ischemic heart disease and stroke attributable to exposure to long working hours for 194 countries, 2000–2016: A systematic analysis from the WHO/ILO Joint Estimates of the Work-related Burden of Disease and Injury. *Environ. Int.* **2021**, *154*. [CrossRef]
47. James, L.; Todak, N.; Best, S. The negative impact of prison work on sleep health. *Am. J. Ind. Med.* **2017**, *60*, 449–456. [CrossRef] [PubMed]
48. National Commission on Correctional Health Care. Pandemic Taking a Toll on Correctional Health Care Staff. Available online: https://www.ncchc.org/pandemic-taking-a-toll-on-correctional-health-care-staff/ (accessed on 20 August 2022).
49. Firew, T.; Sano, E.D.; Lee, J.W.; Flores, S.; Lang, K.; Salman, K.; Greene, M.C.; Chang, B.P. Protecting the front line: A cross-sectional survey analysis of the occupational factors contributing to healthcare workers' infection and psychological distress during the COVID-19 pandemic in the USA. *BMJ Open* **2020**, *10*, e042752. [CrossRef] [PubMed]
50. Burstyn, I.; Holt, K. A cross-sectional survey of the workplace factors contributing to symptoms of anxiety and depression among nurses and physicians during the first wave of COVID-19 pandemic in two US healthcare systems. *Ann. Work. Expo. Health* **2021**, *66*, 312–333. [CrossRef] [PubMed]
51. Da Rosa, P.; Brown, R.; Pravecek, B.; Carotta, C.; Garcia, A.S.; Carson, P.; Callies, D.; Vukovich, M. Factors associated with nurses emotional distress during the COVID-19 pandemic. *Appl. Nurs. Res.* **2021**, *62*, 151502. [CrossRef] [PubMed]
52. Rahman, A. A scoping review of COVID-19-related stress coping resources among nurses. *Int. J. Nurs. Sci.* **2022**, *9*, 259–267. [CrossRef]
53. Hu, S.; Wang, J.N.; Liu, L.; Wu, H.; Yang, X.; Wang, Y.; Wang, L. The association between work-related characteristic and job burnout among Chinese correctional officers: A cross-sectional survey. *Public Health* **2015**, *129*, 1172–1178. [CrossRef]
54. Wexler, T.M.; Schellinger, J. Mindfulness-based stress reduction for nurses: An integrative review. *J. Holist. Nurs.* **2022**. *online ahead of print*. [CrossRef] [PubMed]
55. Velana, M.; Rinkenauer, G. Individual-level interventions for decreasing job-related stress and enhancing coping strategies among nurses: A systematic review. *Front. Psychol.* **2021**, *12*, 708696. [CrossRef] [PubMed]

International Journal of
Environmental Research and Public Health

MDPI

Article

Psychometric Properties of the WHO-5 Well-Being Index among Nurses during the COVID-19 Pandemic: A Cross-Sectional Study in Three Countries

Mariela Loreto Lara-Cabrera [1,2,*], Moisés Betancort [3], Amparo Muñoz-Rubilar [4], Natalia Rodríguez-Novo [5], Ottar Bjerkeset [6] and Carlos De las Cuevas [7,8]

1 Department of Mental Health, Faculty of Medicine and Health Sciences, Norwegian University of Science and Technology (NTNU), 7091 Trondheim, Norway
2 Nidelv Community Mental Health Centre, Division of Psychiatry, St Olavs Hospital Trondheim University Hospital, 7006 Trondheim, Norway
3 Department of Clinical Psychology, Psychobiology and Methodology, Universidad de La Laguna, 38200 San Cristóbal de La Laguna, Spain
4 Faculty of Health Sciences, Universidad Central de Chile, Santiago 8370178, Chile
5 Departament of Nursing, Universidad de La Laguna, 38200 San Cristóbal de La Laguna, Spain
6 Faculty of Nursing and Health Sciences, Nord University, Levanger Campus, 8026 Levanger, Norway
7 Department of Internal Medicine, Dermatology and Psychiatry, Universidad de La Laguna, 38200 San Cristóbal de La Laguna, Spain
8 Instituto Universitario de Neurociencia (IUNE), Universidad de La Laguna, 38200 San Cristobal de La Laguna, Spain
* Correspondence: mariela.lara@ntnu.no

Citation: Lara-Cabrera, M.L.; Betancort, M.; Muñoz-Rubilar, A.; Rodríguez-Novo, N.; Bjerkeset, O.; De las Cuevas, C. Psychometric Properties of the WHO-5 Well-Being Index among Nurses during the COVID-19 Pandemic: A Cross-Sectional Study in Three Countries. *Int. J. Environ. Res. Public Health* **2022**, *19*, 10106. https://doi.org/10.3390/ijerph191610106

Academic Editors: Richard Gray and Sonia Udod

Received: 22 July 2022
Accepted: 9 August 2022
Published: 16 August 2022

Abstract: Nurses' well-being has been increasingly recognised due to the ongoing pandemic. However, no validation scales measuring nurses' well-being currently exist. Thus, we aimed to validate the WHO-5 Well-Being Index (WHO-5) in a sample of nurses. A cross-sectional multinational study was conducted, and a total of 678 nurses who worked during the COVID-19 pandemic in Spain (36.9%), Chile (40.0%) and Norway (23.1%) participated in this study. The nurses completed the WHO-5, the Patient Health Questionnaire-2 (PHQ-2), the Generalized Anxiety Disorder-2 (GAD-2) and three questions about the quality of life (QoL). The WHO-5 demonstrated good reliability and validity in the three countries. Cronbach's alphas ranged from 0.81 to 0.90. High correlations were found between the WHO-5 and the psychological well-being dimension of QoL, and negative correlations between the WHO-5 and PHQ-2. The unidimensional scale structure was confirmed in all the countries, explaining more than 68% of the variance. The item response theory likelihood ratio model did not show discernible differences in the WHO-5 across the countries. To conclude, the WHO-5 is a psychometrically sound scale for measuring nurses' well-being during a pandemic. The scale showed strong construct validity for cross-cultural comparisons; however, more research is required with larger sample sizes.

Keywords: COVID-19; cross-cultural; item response theory; measurement invariance; mental health; nursing staff; pandemics; public health; validation; WHO-5 Well-Being Index

1. Introduction

Psychological well-being is a relative rather than an absolute concept [1]. Thus, one's satisfaction or happiness is influenced by a blend of objective reality and one's subjective reactions to it. This is affected by how well a person functions and how much their aspirations differ from their current situation [1,2]. As a part of the quality of life (QoL) concept, well-being is measured via diverse self-rated scales, although no consensus exists on a gold standard [3,4]. However, in recent years, collecting self-rated well-being data has become valuable for understanding well-being among the general population [5], in research [6,7], in clinical settings [7] and for understanding healthcare worker-reported outcomes in the workplace [5,8].

Nursing professionals frequently face burdensome workloads and are exposed to severe emotional demands and high perceived stress levels [9]. This is further complicated by the likelihood of understaffing and working during stressful events, such as a global pandemic. Furthermore, having to care for patients in an unsafe environment while exposed to personal risk can negatively affect nurses' physical health [10] and psychological well-being [10,11]. In addition to a potential reduction in work performance, these factors can be associated with anxiety and depression symptoms [12,13] with deterioration of psychological well-being [11,14]. Nurses' well-being is a significant determinant of a hospital's ability to provide patient care [9]. As significant concerns for nurses' well-being have been documented during the current global pandemic [5,11,15]; it is crucial to have a reliable self-reported scale that can adequately assess the well-being of nursing professionals. Thus, a critical nursing research goal is to capture and improve nurses' well-being worldwide, and the WHO-5 Well-Being Index (WHO-5) is potentially useful for measuring this [7].

The WHO-5 reflects positive affections, and this short scale captures subjective psychological well-being by measuring affective and hedonic dimensions of well-being [2,16]. This self-rated scale was developed to enable primary healthcare general practitioners to screen patients for signs of depression to reduce relapse of depression symptoms and suicide rates [17,18]. Since its development, the scale has been used to guide clinical practice worldwide [7]. As a generic self-rated well-being scale, previous research on its psychometric properties has focused primarily on students and patients in different settings, such as general practice, private clinics, and hospital settings [6,7]. In addition, it is increasingly used as a reliable measure to monitor depression [19], with excellent clinimetric cross-cultural sensitivity to detect depression [20]. Extensive research and translations into the languages of over 30 countries are among the advantages of the WHO-5, allowing the understanding of mental health from a well-being perspective. However, although previous work has reported adequate internal consistency and structural validity of the scale in several research fields [1,7], no cross-cultural validation scales measuring nurses' well-being currently exist.

When considering using a previously developed self-rated scale, examining validation and adaptation to specific context conditions of the population is recommended to ensure that the scale measures the originally intended construct [21]. Hence, researchers can determine the items' suitability to capture the construct in advance, increasing the certainty that the scale would provide reliable information. This would give the information required to justify using the scale if appropriate for the specific new population. Although the WHO-5 was first validated as a scale for psychological well-being among patients, other factors can affect the scale's psychometric properties. These factors could include cultural and socioeconomic background [22], and other factors that can highlight whether the hypothesised factor structure is the same across groups [21]. A recent validation study using item response theory (IRT) suggested that cross-cultural validation studies are needed for the WHO-5 [23]. This recommendation is consistent with recent studies suggesting that the cross-cultural validity of well-being scales remains an unexplored question [24]. These recommendations align with Boer et al. [25], suggesting that comparisons between countries may require assurance of measurement comparability before reliable conclusions can be drawn. However, despite previous use of the WHO-5 Well-Being Index in nursing studies [26], measurement invariance investigations of the WHO-5 have yet to be conducted among nurses. Furthermore, evidence-based psychometric evaluations in a pandemic context are relatively scarce.

The present study aimed to investigate the validity of the WHO-5 Well-Being Index among clinical nurses working in health services in Spain, Chile and Norway. This was performed by examining the internal consistency and conducting factor and IRT analyses, including assessing measurement invariance and differential item functioning (DIF) across countries and comparing the results obtained. Several a priori research hypotheses were tested to investigate the internal structure of the WHO-5. First, it was hypothesised that the WHO-5 would have good internal consistency, with Cronbach's alpha coefficients exceeding 0.75. Second, as previous research has suggested that subjective well-being is part of the concept of perceived QoL [27], we also expected a priori that the WHO-5 would show high and strong correlations with questions about QoL. As validation studies in recent years have suggested that psychological problems affect subjective well-being [28,29], we also expected that core anxiety symptoms would have a negative association with the WHO-5 and that the WHO-5 would be negatively associated with core symptoms of depression. Finally, it was hypothesised that the WHO-5 would have adequate structural validity and a good fit in a one-factor solution based on prior studies [7].

2. Materials and Methods

This cross-sectional multinational study with nonprobability snowball sampling was conducted following the guidelines of Consensus-Based Standards for the Selection of Health Measurement Instruments [30]. An online survey was used to collect the data, and the STROBE reporting guideline was followed.

2.1. Sample/Participants

The recruitment of nurses followed three steps. First, schools' management, nurse educators and the teaching staff at three universities invited nurses working in non-emergency clinical settings, including university hospitals, non-teaching hospitals and public community local health settings. Second, the survey was posted on the web pages of the associations of nurses. Finally, nurses connected to the university campus and potential participants were kindly asked to invite other nurses by forwarding the information about the study to other networks and via social media. Data were obtained during June and July 2020. Nurses were recruited to participate in the online survey by sending a welcoming email containing a hyperlink to the survey to all the nurses registered in professional associations in the areas of study (Tenerife Island in Spain, Santiago in Chile and Mid and West Norway).

Inclusion criteria were direct care nursing staff, working in inpatient wards, and employed by the hospitals. In the survey, questions about current working position were included, that is, whether they were involved with clinical, academic or administrative work, or were working with nursing education at the university. Participants were included if they were nurses, actively providing direct patient care in their respective countries, and agreed to participate.

2.2. Data Collection

We asked the participants to anonymously provide their sociodemographic information, through self-reporting, as part of the different questionnaires in the online survey. All the items were set as voluntary. To ensure that participants did not answer repeatedly, the online survey was set to reject multiple responses from the same IP address. We designed the survey to avoid burden on the respondents, maximise data quality and maintain ethically sound research. In addition, the online survey was designed so it was easy for the nurses to navigate. It was planned a priori to calculate item response rates and to exclude participants omitting answers/missing (if 25% or fewer items were missing). However, all participants answered the WHO-5 completely without omissions.

Before carrying out the investigation, the survey was piloted by five nurses and two professors. They examined the content validity of the items, reviewed their relevance, and provided feedback to ensure language representation for ease of understanding.

2.3. Measures

2.3.1. WHO-5 Well-Being Index

The nurses self-reported their well-being during the past two weeks. The scale has five items depicting feeling cheerful (Item 1: 'I have felt cheerful and in good spirits'), feeling calm (Item 2: 'I have felt calm and relaxed'), feeling active (Item 3: 'I have felt active and vigorous'), feeling rested when waking up (Item 4: 'I woke up feeling fresh and rested') and feeling that one's life is filled with exciting things (Item 5: 'My daily life has been filled with things that interest me'). The response options ranged from 0 to 5, with 0 representing 'at no time' and 5 'all the time' [6,7]. In the present study, the WHO-5 Well-Being Index was calculated as the sum of the scores of the responses, ranging from 0 (the worst imaginable well-being) to 25 (the best imaginable well-being). We used the Spanish version of the WHO-5, and this version was validated and tested for clarity in a sample of outpatients in community mental health settings [31]. The Norwegian version we used was validated among adolescents [32].

2.3.2. Quality of Life

The nurses' self-reported QoL was assessed using the Multidimensional Quality of Life Index (MQLI). The MQLI is a self-administered questionnaire. The items evaluated their physical well-being, psychological/emotional well-being and overall QoL on a 10-point line [27,33]. Responses to these three questions were scored from 0 (representing 'poor') to 10 (indicating 'excellent') by placing a mark on the value representing their experiences. The reliability and validity of the MQLI were established in the original validation study (Cronbach's alpha 0.92) and in the Norwegian validation study (Cronbach's alpha 0.73) [27,33]; however, investigations about the validity and reliability of the MQLI-3 items have not been conducted among nurses.

2.3.3. Anxiety and Depression

The nurses' self-reported anxiety was assessed using the Generalized Anxiety Disorder 2 (GAD-2) scale during the past two weeks [34]. In the present study, the GAD-2 was used as a self- administered questionnaire, and nurses were asked to report the presence of each symptom during the last 14 days. The questionnaire assessed how often they have been nervous ('feeling nervous, anxious or on edge') and worried ('not being able to stop or control worrying'). The responses were provided on a Likert scale, from 0 (representing 'not at all') to 3 (representing 'nearly every day'). The construct validity of the PHQ-2 was established in the original validation study [34].

The nurses' self-reported depression was assessed using the Patient Health Questionnaire-2 (PHQ-2) scale during the past two weeks [35]. In the present study, the PHQ-2 was used as a self-administered questionnaire. The questionnaire asks how often a person has been bothered by feeling a lack of interest ('little interest or pleasure in doing things') and feeling sad ('feeling down, depressed, or hopeless'). Nurses were asked to report the presence of each symptom during the last 14 days. Responses are provided on a Likert scale between 0 and 3, where 0 represents 'not at all', 1 represents 'several days', 2 represents 'more than half the days', and 3 represents 'nearly every day'. The PHQ-2 is widely used and considered to be a reliable measure. The construct and criterion validity of the PHQ-2 were established in the original validation study [35].

2.4. Data Analysis

The data were analysed using IBM SPSS Statistics for Macintosh, Version 25.0 (IBM Corp., Armonk, NY, USA), and R library psych with ULLRToolbox. Values were described with means, standard deviations, frequencies and percentages. Each survey was examined for completeness, floor, and ceiling effects. Internal consistency was calculated using Cronbach's alpha, and factor analyses were performed using principal component and minimum rank analysis. Two studies were conducted to assess the WHO-5 Well-Being Index invariance through the three samples (countries). First, an analysis was generated from IRT to study the consistency of the scale in a situation of invariance. A DIF study was conducted to assess item stability across different samples and test a potential source of systematic measurement bias in item responses regarding culture. The likelihood ratio chi-square test, the Nagelkerke and McFadden's pseudo-R were computed as magnitude measures with a minimum cell count of six. The study of the differential behaviour of the item allowed us to study the invariance of the construct through different groups of participants [36].

Simultaneously, a study of the construct invariance was conducted through a confirmatory factor analysis in which configurational and metric invariance across groups were tested [37,38]. The IRT analysis was conducted following a logistic ordinal regression differential item functioning model under invariance criteria [39], using the country variable as a grouping variable. Three search criteria for items were used according to the country (Spain, Chile, and Norway): chi-square, R^2 and beta. None of the cases was flagged. Our aim was to verify the linear item invariance [40] comprising the construct according to the country variable. The proposed models were compared following Satorra and Bentler approach [41].

Sample size estimates were based on factor analysis, requiring at least 10 participants per variable to achieve replicable findings, following the guidelines of Consensus-Based Standards for the Selection of Health Measurement Instruments [30].

2.5. Ethical Approval

The Research Ethics Committee of the Canary Islands Health Service, Spain, first approved the study (CHUC_2020_33), and subsequently, we obtained approvals in Chile and Norway (27/2020 and 155172). All the participants provided informed consent before participation.

3. Results

Completed data were obtained from 678 nurses. Their mean age was 39.3 years (standard deviation (SD) = 12.1), ranging from 36 to 48 years, and most nurses were female (74.5% for Chile, 88.9% for Norway, and 80.8% for Spain). There were no missing values. None of the items have floor/ceiling effects. The mean scores for each of the measures used in this study are shown in Table 1.

Table 1. Means (M), standard deviation (SD, ±) and bivariate correlations of the study variables.

Variables	Spain (n = 250)	Chile (n = 271)	Norway (n = 157)
WHO-5 Total Score, mean, SD ***	12.4 ± 4.9	11.9 ± 5.3	16.0 ± 3.7
MQLI-physical well-being, mean, SD ***	6.5 ± 2.3	6.1 ± 2.4	6.5 ± 2.1
MQLI-emotional well-being, mean, SD ***	6.2 ± 2.5	5.8 ± 2.7	7.0 ± 1.9
MQLI-quality of life, mean, SD ***	6.9 ± 2.4	6.4 ± 2.5	7.6 ± 1.8
GAD-2, mean, SD ***	2.5 ± 1.7	2.9 ± 1.8	1.2 ± 1.1
PHQ-2, mean, SD ***	2.0 ± 1.7	2.2 ± 1.7	1.1 ± 1.0
Correlations MQLI-physical well-being and WHO-5	0.592 **	0.662 **	0.683 **
Correlations MQLI-emotional well-being and WHO-5	0.721 **	0.738 **	0.610 **
Correlations MQLI-quality of life and WHO-5	0.630 **	0.724 ***	0.584 **
Correlations GAD-2 and WHO-5	−0.650 **	−0.733 **	−0.390 **
Correlations PHQ-2 and WHO-5	−0.726 **	−0.698 **	−0.563 **

** $p < 0.01$. *** $p < 0.001$. GAD-2 = Generalized Anxiety Disorder-2; MQLI = Multidimensional Quality of Life Index; PHQ-2 = Patient Health Questionnaire-2; WHO-5 = WHO-5 Well-Being Index.

The mean WHO-5 score for the global sample was 13.0 (SD = 5.1), the median score was 13.0, and the skewness was −0.17 (SE = 0.94). In the samples in Chile, Norway, and Spain, the WHO-5 items registered high correlations with each other (Chile: from 0.56 to 0.75; Norway: from 0.31 to 0.51; Spain: from 0.59 to 0.75), indicating that they measured the same construct. Similarly, the WHO-5 items showed a high correlation with the total scale score (Chile: from 0.70 to 0.82, Norway: from 0.53 to 0.73; and Spain: from 0.64 to 0.78).

Table 1 also shows the results regarding the hypotheses and correlations. Strong correlations were expected based on the assumption that the WHO-5 Well-Being Index is part of the concept of perceived QoL, measured using the MQLI-3. These were supported by the WHO-5 Well-Being Index and physical well-being ($r = 0.662$ for Chile, $r = 0.683$ for Norway, and $r = 0.592$ for Spain), psychological/emotional well-being ($r = 0.738$ for Chile, $r = 0.610$ for Norway, and $r = 0.721$ for Spain), and overall QoL ($r = 0.724$ for Chile, $r = 0.584$ for Norway, and $r = 0.630$ for Spain).

Based on previous studies, we expected that the WHO-5 Well-Being Index is a valid measure in the context of mental health, and strong correlations were expected with core symptoms of anxiety (GAD-2) and depression (PHQ-2). Table 1 shows adequate negative correlations obtained with GAD-2 (r ranging from −0.39 to −0.77) and PHQ-2 (r ranging from −0.56 to −0.73).

The WHO-5 Well-Being Index showed high internal consistency in the three countries (Table 2, Chile-Cronbach's alpha = 0.903; Spain-Cronbach's alpha = 0.883; and Norway-Cronbach's alpha = 0.810). No item deletion improved Cronbach's alpha in any of the samples studied.

Table 2. Means (M), standard deviation (SD, ±), factor loading and Cronbach's alpha for the three samples.

WHO-5 Item	Spain (n = 250)		Chile (n = 271)		Norway (n = 154)	
	Mean ± SD	**Factor Loading**	**Mean ± SD**	**Factor Loading**	**Mean ± SD**	**Factor Loading**
WHO-Item 1: Feeling cheerful	2.7 ± 1.1	0.869	2.7 ± 1.1	0.853	3.7 ± 0.6	0.699
WHO-Item 2: Feeling calm	2.4 ± 1.1	0.867	2.2 ± 1.2	0.874	3.3 ± 0.9	0.725
WHO-Item 3: Feeling active	2.6 ± 1.2	0.843	2.4 ± 1.2	0.896	3.0 ± 1.1	0.730
WHO-Item 4: Feeling rested	2.2 ± 1.2	0.794	2.1 ± 1.3	0.832	2.6 ± 1.2	0.843
WHO-Item 5: Feeling that one's life is filled with interesting things	2.5 ± 1.3	0.768	2.5 ± 1.3	0.801	3.4 ± 0.9	0.792
Cronbach's alpha	0.883		0.903		0.810	

The unidimensionality of the WHO-5 Well-Being Index was confirmed through factor analysis using principal component analysis as an extraction method. A single-factor structure was demonstrated, explaining 72.5% in Chile (factor loadings between 0.80 and 0.90), 57.7% in Norway (factor loadings between 0.70 and 0.84) and 68.7% of the variance in Spain (factor loadings between 0.77 and 0.87).

Table 2 shows the factor loadings. The Kaiser–Meyer–Olkin measures of sampling adequacy were 0.859 for Chile, 0.793 for Norway and 0.846 for Spain, indicating sample adequacy. Bartlett's test of sphericity values were 672.275 (Spain), 859.431 (Chile) and 257.384 (Norway; df = 10, $p < 0.0001$), all of them indicating an underlying structure in the scale and that factor analyses were justified in the samples.

The comparison data of both models can be seen in Table 3. As shown in Figure 1, a broad overlap was found between the Spain and Chile distributions, although the Norway sample showed a higher mean well-being score than Spain and Chile samples. With this setting in two iterations, three items were identified (flagged) as potential sources of differences regarding country: Item 1 ('I have felt cheerful and in good spirits'), Item 3 ('I have felt active and vigorous') and Item 4 ('I woke up feeling fresh and rested'; see Figure 1).

Table 3. Comparison data between models.

Models	Df	AIC	BIC	Chi-Square	Chi-Square Diff	Df Diff
Model 1	15	8771.5	8907.9	82.918		
Model 2	23	8801.7	8800.3	128.376	53.445	8 ***

*** $p < 0.001$. AIC = Akaike Information Criteria; BIC = Bayes Information Criteria; Df diff = Degree of Freedom differential analysis.

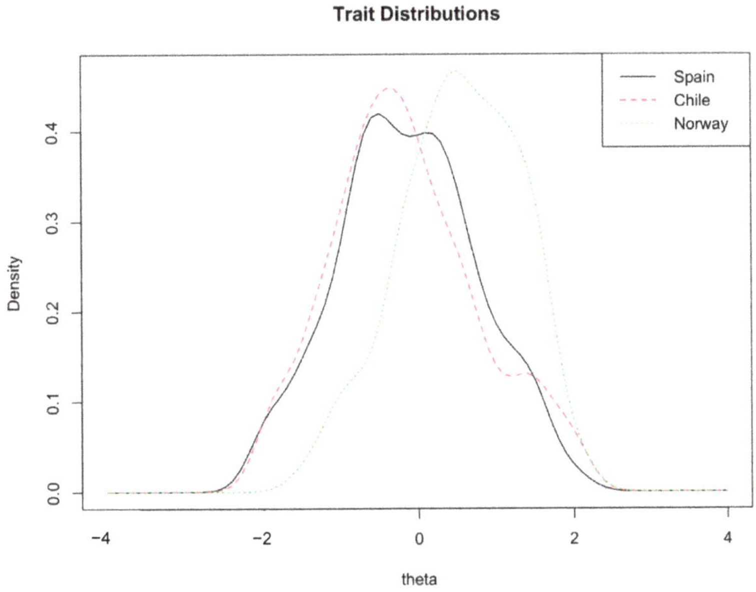

Figure 1. Graphic representation of the population latent trait distribution in the three countries.

Figure 2 shows the item true score function with a test for differential item functioning models (uniform vs. nonuniform) and item response function for Items 1, 3 and 4 with regression parameter values by country, indicating that the items with differential behaviour depending on the country were Items 1, 3 and 4. A differential effect was found in response to Item 1 depending on the type of country [$Pr(\chi^2_{12},2) < 0.001$]. The slope for the Norwegian sample was lower than that of the Spanish and Chilean samples (1.95 vs. 3.71 and 3.35). Data found in the item true score function showed that the responses of the Norwegian sample for this item were in a low–medium range of the trait compared to the Spanish and Chileans (Figure 2b). Item 3 showed a differential effect of the item [$Pr(\chi^2_{12},2) < 0.001$]. Differential behaviour was evident: the second graph of true item scores for Item 3 showed greater homogeneity between the three samples. Finally, Item 4, 'I have felt cheerful and in good spirits', also showed differential behaviour according to the country [$Pr(\chi^2_{12},2) < 0.001$]. Figure 2f shows the trait values according to the true response function, where the Norwegian sample showed higher trait values than the Spanish and Chilean samples.

The values of the differential-corrected and differential-uncorrected raw data per participant and group regarding the central 50% of the distribution showed an interquartile range between −0.04 and 0.02 with a median value of approximately 0.0. The differential behaviour of the scale according to the countries showed some spurious differences between the raw values and values according to the differential. The IRT differential item analysis showed a spurious bias response effect regarding Items 1, 3 and 4. We then considered whether some items exhibiting differential behaviour affected the internal validity of the scale structure according to the countries. Our aim was to verify the linear item invariance comprising the construct according to the country variable. The comparison of the configurational invariance, assuming the same measurement model per country, and the invariance in the beta regression coefficients (per country) were significant [$\chi 2$ diff(4) = 23, $p < 0.001$)]. A statistical significance was found, which reflected as a small effect size (w = 0.01). It was assumed that factorial weights differed by country. This spurious difference (located in the weights of Items 1, 3 and 4) was lower on average in the Norwegian sample (see Figure 2).

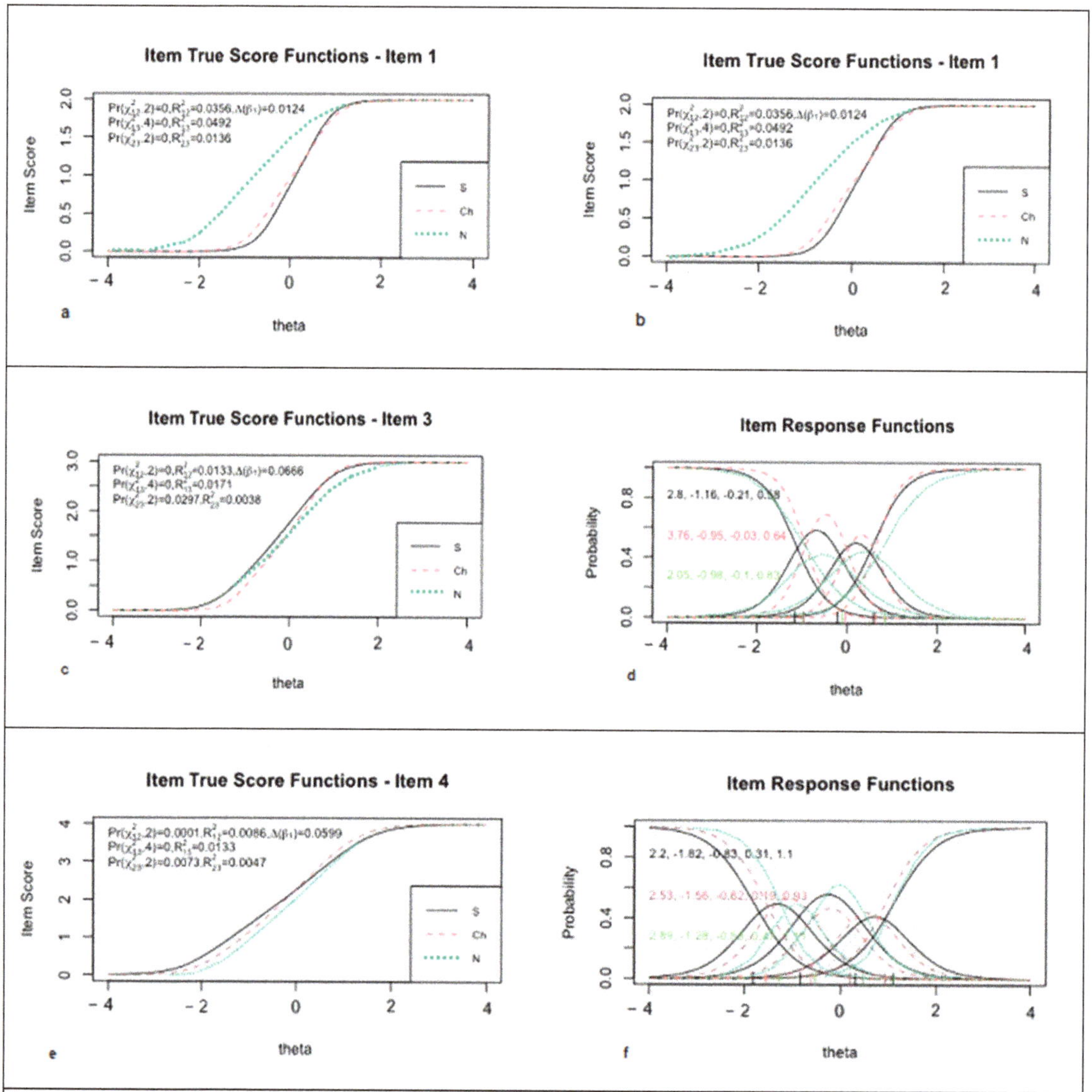

Items	Spain	Chile	Norway
WHO-Item 1: Feeling cheerful	0.83	0.82	0.66
WHO-Item 3: Feeling active	0.78	0.87	0.69
WHO-Item 4: Feeling rested	0.72	0.77	0.84

Figure 2. Item true score function with test for differential items functioning models (uniform vs. nonuniform) and item response function for Items 1 (**a**,**b**), 3 (**c**,**d**) and 4 (**e**,**f**) with regressions parameters values by country.

4. Discussion

This study aimed to investigate the validity of the WHO-5 Well-Being Index for nurses by examining internal consistency and conducting factor and IRT analyses. This was conducted to investigate the WHO-5's scale construct validity across three countries: Spain, Chile, and Norway.

Construct validity based on a priori hypothesis testing was supported. Contrary to previous studies showing low Cronbach's alpha [42], the WHO-5 Well-Being Index showed high internal consistency in the three countries, with Cronbach's alpha varying from 0.810 to 0.903 (Norway to Chile). These findings are within the range of Cronbach's alpha reported in validation studies among medical educators in Hong Kong [43], outpatients with epilepsy in Denmark [44], adults living with epilepsy and HIV in Kenya [45] and among Chinese university students [46].

Regarding hypotheses concerning well-being and QoL, our study revealed high correlation values between the WHO-5 Well-Being Index and the psychological/emotional well-being dimension of the MQLI and the overall QoL. These correlations are consistent with those Mundal et al. [27] reported in a previous validation study. Our results also indicated adequate negative correlations between well-being and anxiety, consistent with a previous study that found strong correlations between the WHO-5 Well-Being Index and anxiety [29]. Additionally, adequate negative correlations were found between well-being and depression, consistent with previous studies reporting that the WHO-5 correlated negatively with depression [28,47–52]. Together with the obtained internal consistency values, these findings support the construct validity of the well-being scale.

The unidimensionality of the WHO-5 was confirmed through factor analysis, with values from 57.7% (for the Norwegian sample) to 72.5% (for the Chilean sample). Our findings are consistent with prior research founding a one-factor structure [7,52], indicating that the WHO-5 can be used to measure the well-being of nurses in different countries for cross-cultural investigations. Notably, as IRT DIF analysis revealed, the WHO-5 performed differently for the well-being construct in the Norwegian sample than for the Spanish and Chilean ones. However, the differential patterns found were associated with negligible effect sizes below 0.13 [53]. Additionally, the Norwegian nurses had a greater probability of responding with high values on the scale than the Spanish and Chilean. This suggests that these items behave slightly differently depending on the country. Cultural differences are likely to have caused the differences in responses to the items. When measuring well-being in countries with different economic situations [22], for instance, developed countries such as Norway compared to other countries such as Chile, this difference in economic well-being could also be a source of bias.

It is noteworthy that differences between the samples could be explained by the impact of COVID-19, since Chile and Spain were hit much harder than Norway, specifically during the data collection period. As prior studies have suggested [54–56], factors such as self-perceived job insecurity, ethical dilemmas and stringency of government responses may affect well-being. Nevertheless, nurses in the Norwegian sample reported higher values when comparing the means between the three countries. These combined findings emphasize that nurses from Norway reported better well-being than those in Spain and Chile during the pandemic. These results appear consistent with studies reporting that the WHO-5 Well-Being Index can differentiate between populations [31,43,45]. However, further research, using several measurement points, is needed to investigate whether the nurses' mental well-being changes over time and whether the WHO-5 Well-Being Index can capture these changes.

Although it is unknown whether the pandemic might explain these differences or whether the differences might be explained by language differences in how nurses perceived their well-being, it is noteworthy that the overall mean of the WHO-5 was significantly lower for nurses from Chile and Spain, as this was higher compared to the WHO-5 means reported in a similar COVID-19 study in Vietnam [57]. Nurses in Chile and Spain had mean scores below 13, corresponding to depression. Our findings regarding the lack of well-being reported in all the countries have implications for government policies/policymakers, showing that they should focus on nurses' well-being. Additionally, nurses in the three countries reported variations in their well-being with a scale that also detects depression [7].

Our findings suggest that the COVID-19 pandemic influenced how nurses struggled with feeling 'calm and relaxed' and 'active and vigorous' and waking up 'feeling fresh and rested'. Such information will guide researchers seeking interventions to enhance well-being in different cultures.

Notably, nurses in Chile and Spain, countries hit hard by COVID-19, struggle more with mental health problems. This finding is in line with a prior study [58]. In countries where depression is associated with stigma [59], the WHO-5 Well-Being Index will be a better alternative to measure depression and lack of well-being. Thus, measuring nurses' well-being can guide hospital administrators in implementing strategies to protect nursing staff without time constraints and psychological burdens being viewed as a stigma. In addition, collecting such information in different countries can guide researchers in developing methods to improve nurses' well-being across countries and cultures.

Although the study's multi-country design, involving collecting data in three countries, and rigorous statistical analyses are strengths, the study has limitations. First, the nurses studied were convenience-sampled, using a non-probability snowball sampling approach, limiting the possibility to know the response rate of nurses who refused to participate in the study. Second, the sample is limited, as demographic differences existed between the countries. Finally, cultural differences may have caused the differences regarding Item 1, as our result suggested that this item could be understood differently in different countries. Nevertheless, while accepting this final limitation, it must be noted that when measuring well-being in countries with different economic situations, such as developed countries such as Norway as compared to countries such as Chile, this difference in economic well-being could be a source of bias. However, further studies are required due to the relatively limited sample size.

5. Conclusions

The WHO-5 Well-Being Index demonstrated its utility as a cross-cultural ultra-brief questionnaire for measuring subjective psychological well-being in Spanish, Chilean and Norwegian nurses. The scale showed high internal consistency in the three countries. Although the unidimensionality of the WHO-5 was confirmed through factor analysis, we found a non-invariance effect on the weights of items, and Item 1 appears somewhat less stable when comparing the Norwegian sample with the Spanish and Chilean samples. Although our findings support the scale's construct validity, allowing comparative analyses between countries, more research is required with larger sample sizes.

Author Contributions: Conceptualization, M.L.L.-C.; writing—original draft preparation, M.L.L.-C., A.M.-R. and C.D.l.C.; data collection, A.M.-R., O.B. and N.R.-N.; formal analysis, M.B. and C.D.l.C.; methodology, M.B. and C.D.l.C.; data curation, A.M.-R.; project administration and funding acquisition, M.L.L.-C.; writing—review and editing, A.M.-R., M.B., O.B., N.R.-N., C.D.l.C. and M.L.L.-C. All authors have read and agreed to the published version of the manuscript.

Funding: The corresponding author was funded by a post-doctoral grant while planning and conducting the study, grant number 90327500/2018, from the Central Norway Regional Health Authority.

Institutional Review Board Statement: The study was conducted in accordance with the Declaration of Helsinki. The Research Ethics Committee of the Canary Islands Health Service, Spain, first approved the study, and subsequently we obtained approvals in Chile and Norway (CHUC_2020_33, 155172 and 27/2020).

Informed Consent Statement: Informed consent was obtained from all subjects involved in the study.

Data Availability Statement: Due to the sensitive nature of the questions asked in this study, survey respondents were assured raw data would remain confidential and would not be shared. The data are not publicly available due to data protection regulations.

Acknowledgments: We are grateful to the nurses and organisations supporting this study.

Conflicts of Interest: The authors declare no conflict of interest.

rences

McDowell, I. Measures of self-perceived well-being. *J. Psychosom. Res.* **2010**, *69*, 69–79. [CrossRef] [PubMed]

Kusier, A.O.; Folker, A.P. The Well-Being Index WHO-5: Hedonistic foundation and practical limitations. *Med. Humanit.* **2019**, *30*, 30. [CrossRef] [PubMed]

3. Linton, M.J.; Dieppe, P.; Medina-Lara, A. Review of 99 self-report measures for assessing well-being in adults: Exploring dimensions of well-being and developments over time. *BMJ Open* **2016**, *6*, e010641. [CrossRef] [PubMed]
4. Lindert, J.; Bain, P.A.; Kubzansky, L.D.; Stein, C. Well-being measurement and the WHO health policy Health 2010: Systematic review of measurement scales. *Eur. J. Public Health* **2015**, *25*, 731–740. [CrossRef]
5. De Kock, J.H.; Latham, H.A.; Leslie, S.J.; Grindle, M.; Munoz, S.A.; Ellis, L.; Polson, R.; O'Malley, C.M. A rapid review of the impact of COVID-19 on the mental health of healthcare workers: Implications for supporting psychological well-being. *BMC Public Health* **2021**, *21*, 104. [CrossRef]
6. Lara-Cabrera, M.L.; Bjorkly, S.; De Las Cuevas, C.; Pedersen, S.A.; Mundal, I.P. Psychometric properties of the Five-item World Health Organization Well-being Index used in mental health services: Protocol for a systematic review. *J. Adv. Nurs.* **2020**, *76*, 2426–2433. [CrossRef]
7. Topp, C.W.; Ostergaard, S.D.; Sondergaard, S.; Bech, P. The WHO-5 Well-Being Index: A systematic review of the literature. *Psychother. Psychosom.* **2015**, *84*, 167–176. [CrossRef]
8. Blasco-Belled, A.; Tejada-Gallardo, C.; Fatsini-Prats, M.; Alsinet, C. Mental health among the general population and healthcare workers during the COVID-19 pandemic: A meta-analysis of well-being and psychological distress prevalence. *Curr. Psychol.* **2022**, 1–12. [CrossRef]
9. Hall, L.H.; Johnson, J.; Watt, I.; Tsipa, A.; O'Connor, D.B. Healthcare Staff Wellbeing, Burnout, and Patient Safety: A Systematic Review. *PLoS ONE* **2016**, *11*, e0159015. [CrossRef]
10. Fernandez, R.; Lord, H.; Halcomb, E.; Moxham, L.; Middleton, R.; Alananzeh, I.; Ellwood, L. Implications for COVID-19: A systematic review of nurses' experiences of working in acute care hospital settings during a respiratory pandemic. *Int. J. Nurs. Stud.* **2020**, *111*, 103637. [CrossRef]
11. Dragioti, E.; Tsartsalis, D.; Mentis, M.; Mantzoukas, S.; Gouva, M. Impact of the COVID-19 pandemic on the mental health of hospital staff: An umbrella review of 44 meta-analyses. *Int. J. Nurs. Stud.* **2022**, *131*, 104272. [CrossRef] [PubMed]
12. Zheng, R.; Zhou, Y.; Fu, Y.; Xiang, Q.; Cheng, F.; Chen, H.; Xu, H.; Fu, L.; Wu, X.; Feng, M.; et al. Prevalence and associated factors of depression and anxiety among nurses during the outbreak of COVID-19 in China: A cross-sectional study. *Int. J. Nurs. Stud.* **2021**, *114*, 103809. [CrossRef] [PubMed]
13. Slusarska, B.; Nowicki, G.J.; Niedorys-Karczmarczyk, B.; Chrzan-Rodak, A. Prevalence of Depression and Anxiety in Nurses during the First Eleven Months of the COVID-19 Pandemic: A Systematic Review and Meta-Analysis. *Int. J. Environ. Res. Public Health* **2022**, *19*, 1154. [CrossRef]
14. Huerta-Gonzalez, S.; Selva-Medrano, D.; Lopez-Espuela, F.; Caro-Alonso, P.A.; Novo, A.; Rodriguez-Martin, B. The Psychological Impact of COVID-19 on Front Line Nurses: A Synthesis of Qualitative Evidence. *Int. J. Environ. Res. Public Health* **2021**, *18*, 2975. [CrossRef]
15. Lara-Cabrera, M.L.; Betancort, M.; Muñoz-Rubilar, C.A.; Rodríguez Novo, N.; De las Cuevas, C. The Mediating Role of Resilience in the Relationship between Perceived Stress and Mental Health. *Int. J. Environ. Res. Public Health* **2021**, *18*, 9762. [CrossRef] [PubMed]
16. World Health Organization. Use of well-being measures in primary health care-the DepCare project health for all. *Target* **1998**, *12*, E60246.
17. Bech, P. *Clinical Psychometrics*; John Wiley & Sons: New York, NY, USA, 2012.
18. World Health Organization. *Wellbeing Measures in Primary Health care/The DepCare Project: Report on a WHO Meeting: Stockholm, Sweden, 12–13 February 1998*; World Health Organization Regional Office for Europe: Copenhagen, Denmark, 1998.
19. Newnham, E.A.; Hooke, G.R.; Page, A.C. Monitoring treatment response and outcomes using the World Health Organization's Wellbeing Index in psychiatric care. *J. Affect. Disord.* **2010**, *122*, 133–138. [CrossRef]
20. Carrozzino, D.; Christensen, K.S.; Patierno, C.; Woźniewicz, A.; Møller, S.B.; Arendt, I.-M.T.P.; Zhang, Y.; Yuan, Y.; Sasaki, N.; Nishi, D.; et al. Cross-cultural validity of the WHO-5 Well-Being Index and Euthymia Scale: A clinimetric analysis. *J. Affect. Disord.* **2022**, *311*, 276–283. [CrossRef]
21. Boateng, G.O.; Neilands, T.B.; Frongillo, E.A.; Melgar-Quinonez, H.R.; Young, S.L. Best Practices for Developing and Validating Scales for Health, Social, and Behavioral Research: A Primer. *Front. Public Health* **2018**, *6*, 149. [CrossRef]
22. Lomas, T. Positive cross-cultural psychology: Exploring similarity and difference in constructions and experiences of wellbeing. *Int. J. Wellbeing* **2015**, *5*, 60–77. [CrossRef]
23. Sischka, P.E.; Costa, A.P.; Steffgen, G.; Schmidt, A.F. The WHO-5 well-being index–validation based on item response theory and the analysis of measurement invariance across 35 countries. *J. Affect. Disord. Rep.* **2020**, *1*, 100020. [CrossRef]
24. Cooke, P.J.; Melchert, T.P.; Connor, K. Measuring Well-Being:A Review of Instruments. *Couns. Psychol.* **2016**, *44*, 730–757. [CrossRef]
25. Boer, D.; Hanke, K.; He, J. On detecting systematic measurement error in cross-cultural research: A review and critical reflection on equivalence and invariance tests. *J. Cross-Cult. Psychol.* **2018**, *49*, 713–734. [CrossRef]

26. Bolier, L.; Ketelaar, S.M.; Nieuwenhuijsen, K.; Smeets, O.; Gartner, F.R.; Sluiter, J.K. Workplace mental health promotion online to enhance well-being of nurses and allied health professionals: A cluster-randomized controlled trial. *Internet Interv.* **2014**, *1*, 196–204. [CrossRef]
27. Mundal, I.; Laake, P.; Mezzich, J.; Bjørkly, S.K.; Lara-Cabrera, M.L. Assessment of the Quality of Life in Parents of Children With ADHD: Validation of the Multicultural Quality of Life Index in Norwegian Pediatric Mental Health Settings. *Front. Psychol.* **2021**, *12*, 638006. [CrossRef]
28. Hajos, T.R.; Pouwer, F.; Skovlund, S.E.; Den Oudsten, B.L.; Geelhoed-Duijvestijn, P.H.; Tack, C.J.; Snoek, F.J. Psychometric and screening properties of the WHO-5 well-being index in adult outpatients with Type 1 or Type 2 diabetes mellitus. *Diabet. Med.* **2013**, *30*, e63–e69. [CrossRef]
29. Ghaheri, A.; Omani-Samani, R.; Sepidarkish, M.; Hosseini, M.; Maroufizadeh, S. The Four-item Patient Health Questionnaire for Anxiety and Depression: A Validation Study in Infertile Patients. *Int. J. Fertil. Steril.* **2020**, *14*, 234–239. [CrossRef]
30. Mokkink, L.B.; Prinsen, C.; Patrick, D.L.; Alonso, J.; Bouter, L.; de Vet, H.C.; Terwee, C.B.; Mokkink, L. COSMIN methodology for systematic reviews of patient-reported outcome measures (PROMs). *User Man.* **2018**, *27*, 1171–1179.
31. Lara-Cabrera, M.L.; Mundal, I.P.; De Las Cuevas, C. Patient-reported well-being: Psychometric properties of the world health organization well-being index in specialised community mental health settings. *Psychiatry Res.* **2020**, *291*, 113268. [CrossRef]
32. Christensen, K.S.; Haugen, W.; Sirpal, M.K.; Haavet, O.R. Diagnosis of depressed young people–Criterion validity of WHO-5 and HSCL-6 in Denmark and Norway. *Fam. Pract.* **2015**, *32*, 359–363. [CrossRef]
33. Mezzich, J.E.; Cohen, N.L.; Ruiperez, M.A.; Banzato, C.E.; Zapata-Vega, M.I. The Multicultural Quality of Life Index: Presentation and validation. *J. Eval. Clin. Pract.* **2011**, *17*, 357–364. [CrossRef] [PubMed]
34. Kroenke, K.; Spitzer, R.L.; Williams, J.B.; Monahan, P.O.; Lowe, B. Anxiety disorders in primary care: Prevalence, impairment, comorbidity, and detection. *Ann. Intern Med.* **2007**, *146*, 317–325. [CrossRef] [PubMed]
35. Kroenke, K.; Spitzer, R.L.; Williams, J.B. The Patient Health Questionnaire-2: Validity of a two-item depression screener. *Med. Care* **2003**, *41*, 1284–1292. [CrossRef] [PubMed]
36. Xu, H.; Tracey, T.J.G. Development of an abbreviated Career Indecision Profile-65 using item response theory: The CIP-Short. *J. Couns. Psychol.* **2017**, *64*, 222–232. [CrossRef]
37. Vandenberg, R.J.; Lance, C.E. A Review and Synthesis of the Measurement Invariance Literature: Suggestions, Practices, and Recommendations for Organizational Research. *Organ. Res. Methods* **2000**, *3*, 4–70. [CrossRef]
38. Greiff, S.; Scherer, R. Still comparing apples with oranges? Some thoughts on the principles and practices of measurement invariance testing. *Eur. J. Psychol. Assess.* **2018**, *34*, 141–144. [CrossRef]
39. Choi, S.W.; Gibbons, L.E.; Crane, P.K. lordif: An R Package for Detecting Differential Item Functioning Using Iterative Hybrid Ordinal Logistic Regression/Item Response Theory and Monte Carlo Simulations. *J. Stat. Softw.* **2011**, *39*, 1–30. [CrossRef]
40. Elosua, P. Evaluación progresiva de la invarianza factorial entre las versiones original y adaptada de una escala de autoconcepto. *Psicothema* **2005**, *17*, 356–362.
41. Satorra, A.; Bentler, P.M. A scaled difference chi-square test statistic for moment structure analysis. *Psychometrika* **2001**, *66*, 507–514. [CrossRef]
42. Faruk, M.O.; Alam, F.; Chowdhury, K.U.A.; Soron, T.R. Validation of the Bangla WHO-5 Well-being Index. *Glob. Ment. Health (Camb)* **2021**, *8*, e26. [CrossRef]
43. Chan, L.; Liu, R.K.W.; Lam, T.P.; Chen, J.Y.; Tipoe, G.L.; Ganotice, F.A. Validation of the World Health Organization Well-Being Index (WHO-5) among medical educators in Hong Kong: A confirmatory factor analysis. *Med. Educ. Online* **2022**, *27*, 2044635. [CrossRef] [PubMed]
44. Schougaard, L.M.V.; de Thurah, A.; Bech, P.; Hjollund, N.H.; Christiansen, D.H. Test-retest reliability and measurement error of the Danish WHO-5 Well-being Index in outpatients with epilepsy. *Health Qual. Life Outcomes* **2018**, *16*, 175. [CrossRef] [PubMed]
45. Chongwo, E.; Ssewanyana, D.; Nasambu, C.; Mwangala, P.N.; Mwangi, P.M.; Nyongesa, M.K.; Newton, C.R.; Abubakar, A. Validation of a Swahili version of the World Health Organization 5-item well-being index among adults living with HIV and epilepsy in rural coastal Kenya. *Glob. Health Res. Policy* **2018**, *3*, 26. [CrossRef] [PubMed]
46. Fung, S.F.; Kong, C.Y.W.; Liu, Y.M.; Huang, Q.; Xiong, Z.; Jiang, Z.; Zhu, F.; Chen, Z.; Sun, K.; Zhao, H.; et al. Validity and Psychometric Evaluation of the Chinese Version of the 5-Item WHO Well-Being Index. *Front. Public Health* **2022**, *10*, 872436. [CrossRef] [PubMed]
47. Roldan-Merino, J.; Hurtado-Pardos, B.; Molina-Raya, L.; Bande, D.; Casas, I.; Farres-Tarafa, M. Psychological impact of the COVID-19 pandemic on nursing students in the first wave: A cross-sectional survey. *Nurs. Open* **2022**, *9*, 2003–2012. [CrossRef]
48. Perera, B.P.R.; Jayasuriya, R.; Caldera, A.; Wickremasinghe, A.R. Assessing mental well-being in a Sinhala speaking Sri Lankan population: Validation of the WHO-5 well-being index. *Health Qual. Life Outcomes* **2020**, *18*, 305. [CrossRef]
49. Omani-Samani, R.; Maroufizadeh, S.; Almasi-Hashiani, A.; Sepidarkish, M.; Amini, P. The WHO-5 Well-Being Index: A Validation Study in People with Infertility. *Iran. J. Public Health* **2019**, *48*, 2058–2064. [CrossRef]
50. Cichon, E.; Kiejna, A.; Kokoszka, A.; Gondek, T.; Rajba, B.; Lloyd, C.E.; Sartorius, N. Validation of the Polish version of WHO-5 as a screening instrument for depression in adults with diabetes. *Diabetes Res. Clin. Pract.* **2019**, *159*, 107970. [CrossRef]
51. Kwon, M.; Kim, H. Psychological Well-Being of Female-Headed Households Based on Age Stratification: A Nationwide Cross-Sectional Study in South Korea. *Int. J. Environ. Res. Public Health* **2020**, *17*, 6445. [CrossRef]

52. Suhaimi, A.F.; Makki, S.M.; Tan, K.A.; Silim, U.A.; Ibrahim, N. Translation and Validation of the Malay Version of the WHO-5 Well-Being Index: Reliability and Validity Evidence from a Sample of Type 2 Diabetes Mellitus Patients. *Int. J. Environ. Res. Public Health* **2022**, *19*, 4415. [CrossRef]
53. Cohen, J. Statistical Power Analysis For The Behavioral Sciences (rev ed.). Hillsdale, NJ: Erlbaum, 1988. *Percept. Mot. Ski.* **1988**, *67*, 1007.
54. Russo, C.; Terraneo, M. Mental Well-being Among Workers: A Cross-national Analysis of Job Insecurity Impact on the Workforce. *Soc. Indic. Res.* **2020**, *152*, 421–442. [CrossRef]
55. Long, D.; Haagsma, J.A.; Janssen, M.F.; Yfantopoulos, J.N.; Lubetkin, E.I.; Bonsel, G.J. Health-related quality of life and mental well-being of healthy and diseased persons in 8 countries: Does stringency of government response against early COVID-19 matter? *SSM Popul. Health* **2021**, *15*, 100913. [CrossRef] [PubMed]
56. Munoz-Rubilar, C.A.; Carrillos, C.P.; Mundal, I.P.; Cuevas, C.L.; Lara-Cabrera, M.L. The duty to care and nurses' well-being during a pandemic. *Nurs. Ethics* **2022**, *29*, 527–539. [CrossRef] [PubMed]
57. Hoang, T.D.; Colebunders, R.; Fodjo, J.N.S.; Nguyen, N.P.T.; Tran, T.D.; Vo, T.V. Well-Being of Healthcare Workers and the General Public during the COVID-19 Pandemic in Vietnam: An Online Survey. *Int. J. Environ. Res. Public Health* **2021**, *18*, 4737. [CrossRef] [PubMed]
58. Saragih, I.D.; Tonapa, S.I.; Saragih, I.S.; Advani, S.; Batubara, S.O.; Suarilah, I.; Lin, C.J. Global prevalence of mental health problems among healthcare workers during the Covid-19 pandemic: A systematic review and meta-analysis. *Int. J. Nurs. Stud.* **2021**, *121*, 104002. [CrossRef]
59. Yang, F.; Yang, B.X.; Stone, T.E.; Wang, X.Q.; Zhou, Y.; Zhang, J.; Jiao, S.F. Stigma towards depression in a community-based sample in China. *Compr. Psychiatry* **2020**, *97*, 152152. [CrossRef]

International Journal of
Environmental Research and Public Health

MDPI

Article

Ultra-Orthodox Nursing Students' Cultural Challenges Inside and Outside Their Community during the COVID-19 Pandemic

Sara Genut [1,*], Yaacov G. Bachner [2], Zvika Orr [3] and Adi Finkelstein [3]

1 Department of Bioinformatics, Faculty of Life and Health Sciences, Jerusalem College of Technology, 7 Beit Hadfus Street, Jerusalem 95483, Israel
2 Department of Epidemiology Biostatistics and Community Health Sciences, Ben-Gurion University of the Negev, Beer Sheva 84105, Israel; bachner@bgu.ac.il
3 Department of Nursing, Faculty of Life and Health Sciences, Jerusalem College of Technology, 7 Beit Hadfus Street, Jerusalem 95483, Israel; orr@g.jct.ac.il (Z.O.); afinkels@g.jct.ac.il (A.F.)
* Correspondence: sarag@jct.ac.il; Tel.: +972-52-2959252

Abstract: In line with findings that nurses from minority groups have an important role in making health services accessible to their community, our study aimed to identify the challenges ultra-Orthodox Jewish nurses faced during COVID-19 in their encounters with patients and health staff from other communities, as well as their own community. The ultra-Orthodox community is a highly religious group that maintains isolation from general society, a phenomenon that affected its member experiences during COVID-19. Our research followed sequential explanatory mixed methods. The quantitative phase included a questionnaire completed by 235 female students (111 ultra-Orthodox and 124 non-ultra-Orthodox), followed by a qualitative phase, which included six focus-groups (n = 15). The quantitative analysis showed that the ultra-Orthodox students felt a higher sense of responsibility toward their community. They used their authority and knowledge to guide their community during the pandemic. The qualitative analysis identified two themes expressed as challenges ultra-Orthodox nursing students encountered within their community and with other sections of Israeli society. Our research shows the important role that transcultural nurses play in mediating updated health information otherwise inaccessible to their community, especially in times of crises. It is important to address dilemmas this group faces inside and outside their respective communities.

Keywords: ultra-Orthodox; transcultural; minority; cultural competence; COVID-19; mixed methods; nursing students

Citation: Genut, S.; Bachner, Y.G.; Orr, Z.; Finkelstein, A. Ultra-Orthodox Nursing Students' Cultural Challenges Inside and Outside Their Community during the COVID-19 Pandemic. *Int. J. Environ. Res. Public Health* **2022**, *19*, 9215. https://doi.org/10.3390/ijerph19159215

Academic Editors: Richard Gray and Sonia Udod

Received: 17 June 2022
Accepted: 25 July 2022
Published: 28 July 2022

1. Introduction

Nurses must recognize patients' needs based on their cultural background [1]. The recommendations of culturally competent baccalaureate nurses to be achieved during nursing education include awareness of personal culture, values, beliefs, attributes, and behaviors; skills in communicating with individuals from other cultures; and cultural knowledge and opportunities for students to interact with different cultures [2–4].

Providing culturally competent healthcare to diverse populations is important for reducing health inequalities and loss of critical information [5,6] and increasing patient satisfaction, which is a key factor in quality of care and correlated with patient compliance [7]. Studies have shown that language barriers [8] and lack of trust in the healthcare system [9] were reasons why minority populations were dissatisfied with the healthcare services they received [10]. Instead, they were likely to be satisfied with the healthcare services received from providers with the same race or ethnicity [11,12].

Considerable research has been performed on transcultural nurses as essential frontline workers providing culturally appropriate services to minority groups [13–16]. Transcultural nursing and ethnic minority nurses are attracting attention because of their central role in making medical care accessible to patients from diverse cultural backgrounds, and especially to patients in their community [14,15,17–19].

One of the goals of the US National Coalition of Ethnic Minority Nurse Associations, specifically highlighted during the COVID-19 pandemic, includes increasing the number of ethnic minority nurses because of their special contribution to society [20]. Dawson (2021) [17] described AA/Black nurses as frontline healthcare providers to patients in hospitals and nursing homes during this pandemic. Given their large network, they were among the first to inform and educate the AA/Black communities regarding COVID-19, working with politicians, social service agencies, healthcare systems, public health departments, etc.

2. The Aim of the Study

Our study aim was to examine the challenges of female Jewish ultra-Orthodox (UO) nursing students in encounters with other communities and their roles within their own community, especially during the COVID-19 pandemic.

Unlike other minorities, the ultra-Orthodox community stays isolated from the general society as part of religious ideology to preserve its traditional beliefs and behavior, a phenomenon that has both social and economic implications [21,22]. These implications influenced the experiences of the community during the COVID-19 pandemic. Ultra-Orthodox people made COVID-19-related decisions based on both health and medical rationalizations and religious considerations, and among them, obedience to their community leaders [23]. This community possesses characteristics typical of minority groups, which make it difficult to cope with the COVID-19 pandemic, such as large families, low socioeconomic status, and crowded living conditions [24]. This was part of the reason why a disproportionately large number of UO people contracted this disease and died [25].

3. Background

3.1. *The Characteristic of the Ultra-Orthodox Community in Israel*

According to the [26] (p. 40), in the general Jewish Israeli population of 2016, 14% defined themselves as UO, 16% as religious or very religious, 25% as traditional, and 45% as secular.

Important factors to consider in relation to religion and health are perceptions, behaviors, and access to health-related information [27]. First, the UO community lives an intense social and community life, built around prayers in synagogues, studying in groups, and multi-participant social events [24,28–30]. To keep themselves isolated from the influence of the so-called secular culture, they object to the use of virtual media and do not use TV or smartphones [31,32]. This factor was crucial in coping with COVID-19 as they lacked access to updated information about the virus and about measures taken by authorities, such as physical distancing. Due to their ideological non-use of the Internet, they were unable to use services remotely, such as food shopping, work, healthcare, and distance learning [33].

Second, there is a science literacy gap between UO and secular education, as sciences are either not taught or taught at a minimal level in UO schools. Moreover, relevant scientific knowledge is accessible nowadays in the media, yet, due to their ideological desire to remain isolated from the secular society, their members forsake the Internet, thereby lacking access to updated scientific knowledge and information [23,34].

Finally, the UO community mistrusts state authorities, which are perceived as interfering with their social isolation [31]. Thus, official instructions regarding COVID-19 were taken by this community with suspicion. Ultra-Orthodox leaders significantly shape believers' perceptions in ways that affect health promotion and use of health services [23]. They influence the health behaviors as well as health-related decisions of individuals, often using "health mediators" between the UO community and professionals and service providers outside the UO world [35].

3.2. *Ultra-Orthodox Jewish Nurses in Israel*

Ultra-Orthodox Jewish nursing students represent a new population in the nursing profession in Israel. This phenomenon derives from the recent changes and needs of the

UO society [36,37]. Women are the main providers in UO households because men devote their lives to religious study [38,39]. These women usually get married young and lack professional qualifications, which results in low-paying jobs. Therefore, for them, nursing studies offer an opportunity to acquire guaranteed employment and a stable source of income [40].

Additionally, there is growing awareness that community clinics and hospital wards must properly meet UO unique needs to maximize cultural competence and gender access [41–43]. This need was also recognized by the government, especially during the COVID-19 pandemic [44], and, therefore, there is a need for both male and female ultra-Orthodox nurses. As part of the national plan for integrating the UO population in academic nursing studies, several schools in Israel provide dedicated, gender-segregated programs to UO men [36] and women [37].

Nevertheless, nursing is not yet an acceptable profession in this community because it challenges a few of their religious norms, and the entry of UO men and women into the nursing profession entails multiple challenges [36,37]: (1) This community generally opposes integrating in academic studies; (2) Nursing is a science-based discipline, and potential students need a strong foundation of science. The elementary and high school programs of the UO education system lack knowledge and skills in many domains; and (3) The *Halakhah* (Jewish law) specifies strict sex-based roles to avoid physical or other connection between men and women [45].

Our study advances the understanding of the experiences of nurses from ethnic minority populations who serve the majority population, and, at the same time, could take advantage of their profession to help their minority community [20]. Research questions include:

1. What are the challenges of UO female nursing students in encounters with patients and health staff who belong to other communities?
2. How were these challenges manifested during the COVID-19 pandemic?
3. What are the challenges of UO female nursing students in their encounter with their community and how did these challenges manifest during the COVID-19 pandemic?

4. Materials and Methods

4.1. Study Settings

All participants were female nursing students at the Jerusalem College of Technology (JCT) [46]. JCT specializes in providing science and technology education to the religious Jewish community and about 45% of JCT's 4700 students are UO Jews; among them, 55% are women. Nursing is the largest department of the institute, and out of the nursing students, 88% were women. Men and women study in separate campuses according to their religious norms. All research participants studied a unit in cultural competence as part of a mandatory first-year academic course named "Sociology of Health and Illness". The course was monitored by the last author; classes were supplemented by theoretical reading and class discussions.

4.2. Study Design

Our main research tools included a questionnaire and focus-group interviews according to sequential explanatory mixed methods [47]. According to this strategy, the analysis of quantitative findings was followed by the analysis of focus-group interviews to explain the quantitative findings.

4.3. Data Collection

4.3.1. Quantitative Phase

For the quantitative phase, we composed a questionnaire comprising 14 items ranked on a 1–10 Likert-scale, (ranging from "strongly disagree" to "strongly agree"). We adopted six items from the Hebrew version of the RCTSH Cultural Competence Assessment Tool (CCATool), student nurse specific, which consists of four sections measuring cultural awareness, cultural knowledge, cultural sensitivity, and cultural practice [48]. The questionnaire focused on the importance accorded by the students to the need of supplying medical information and guidelines with sensitivity to the beliefs, values, and norms of patients of different cultures, specifically in light of the experience during the COVID-19 pandemic. The questionnaire included items to assess the insights of the UO students, who constitute a large proportion of students at the college. Of the 235 female respondents, 111 (47%) were UO.

The questionnaire was administered to nursing students at JCT in June 2020, and 285 of them completed the questionnaire. We statistically analyzed the responses of 235 female students who completed the questionnaire. Fifty questionnaires were omitted from the study because they had a high percentage of missing data.

4.3.2. Qualitative Phase

Six focus group were conducted between January and February 2021, with two to three students in each group ($n = 15$). The participants were all UO female nursing students from all four years of the nursing program at JCT. Each group contained students from the same school year. Purposive sampling was performed and participants were recruited by the first author who knew the participants well and thought that they would contribute to the research. Six students refused to participate in the study.

Each focus group interview lasted 60–90 min, conducted using a script designed under the guidance of the last author, a qualitative research expert. Following our quantitative phase results, the questions were specifically related to participants' dilemmas around the decision to study nursing and their community's response to that decision, as well as students' experiences of encountering different cultures during their clinical rotations, most of which occurred during the COVID-19 pandemic. The first group was a pilot with three students from the second, third, and fourth years; their insights helped finalize the script questions.

All focus group were conducted online (via Zoom) and recorded with the participants' consent. Audio recordings were later fully transcribed by a professional transcriptionist. Transcripts were compared to audiotapes to ensure accuracy by the last author.

4.4. Data Analysis

4.4.1. Quantitative Phase

We conducted factor analysis using a varimax technique to define the categories within the questionnaire items. Twelve of the original fourteen items were categorized into four factors that were significant to the research questions.

Confidence in coping with the effects of racism at work as a nurse; sense of mission as a nursing student in using knowledge and authority in their community; cultural identity and community belonging; and cultural sensitivity. Cronbach's α values for each category showed good internal consistency. Table 1 presents the items of each category, the number of items for each factor, and Cronbach's α.

4.4.2. Qualitative Phase

We chose an inductive approach, which means that the themes identified were closely linked to the data without trying to fit them into an earlier analytic theory [49]. We utilized thematic analysis—a recommended technique for analyzing focus group transcripts [50]. The six phases of thematic analysis as described by Braun and Clarke (2006) [51] were followed: (1) familiarizing with the data; (2) generating initial codes; (3) searching for themes; (4) reviewing themes; (5) defining and naming themes; and (6) producing the report. Phases one and two were conducted individually by the first and the last authors. The initial codes were compared at joint meetings. After comparing the two lists and reaching an agreement, a joint list was prepared. The third and fourth phases were jointly conducted by the two authors and shared with team members for feedback. The fifth and sixth phases were performed by the last author. The analysis was performed manually without the use of any software [52].

Table 1. Categories, Items, and Cronbach's α.

Category	Item Number		Number of Items	Cronbach's α
Confidence in coping with the effects of racism at work as a nurse	13	I am able to incorporate clients' cultural beliefs into the care and treatment I provide	4	0.75
	14	I am very confident to challenge racism and discrimination toward clients		
	15	I am very confident to challenge racism and discrimination toward staff		
	16	I am very confident to challenge racism and discrimination toward me		
Sense of mission as a nursing student in using knowledge and authority in their community	5	The pandemic strengthened my sense of mission and choice in the nursing profession	3	0.75
	7	I used my authority as a nursing student to encourage others in my community to obey the instructions of the Ministry of Health during the pandemic		
	8	I used my knowledge as a nursing student to guide others in my community on how to behave properly during the pandemic		
Cultural identity and community belonging	2	The pandemic taught me that there are differences between my cultural identity and other groups in Israeli society	3	0.65
	3	The pandemic has made me critical of the behavior of members of my community		
	4	The pandemic has made me critical of other people's attitudes towards my community		
Cultural Sensitivity	9	I am very comfortable working with people whose beliefs, values, and practices are different from my own	2	0.61
	10	I am very confident of my ability to establish trust and show respect and empathy to people from other cultures		

4.5. Trustworthiness

To establish the trustworthiness of the present study, we implemented various strategies. *Consistency* was achieved with all focus group sessions being conducted by a single researcher with a single set of questions during a short period [53]. *Credibility* [54] was achieved through practices, including: (1) *a thick description*: we provided in-depth illustrations and abundant details about the culture and social context of our study; (2) *triangulation*: we used multiple coding. Two researchers analyzed the data independently and compared their findings [55]; and (3) *multivocality*: we provided empathic understanding and space for a variety of opinions. To facilitate *transferability* [53], we reported in the article clear descriptions of the research context, selection procedure, characteristics of participants, data collection, and the process of analysis.

5. Results

5.1. Quantitative Phase

A series of independent *t*-tests were conducted to examine any statistically significant differences between the UO students and the general students in the factors identified in the questionnaire. Table 2 presents the results of independent *t*-tests.

Table 2. Independent Samples *t*-Test (Factors).

Category	Ultra-Orthodox n = 111		Non-Ultra-Orthodox n = 124		*t*-Value
	Mean (M)	Std. Deviation (SD)	Mean (M)	Std. Deviation (SD)	
Confidence in coping with the effects of racism at work as a nurse	6.82	1.81	6.47	1.59	1.66
Sense of mission as a nursing student in using knowledge and authority in their community	6.67	2.46	5.93	2.38	2.46 *
Cultural identity and community belonging	6.22	2.31	5.84	2.11	1.58
Cultural sensitivity	7.74	1.76	7.6	1.56	0.68

* $p < 0.05$.

As presented in Table 2, there is a statistically significant difference between the two groups in terms of the *sense of mission as a nursing student in using knowledge and authority in their community* (p = 0.01; t (233) = 2.46). The UO nursing students revealed a higher sense of mission toward their community (M = 6.67, SD = 2.46), compared to other nursing students. Differences related to other factors were not statistically significant between the groups.

Additionally, we conducted the Spearman's correlation coefficient test to examine correlations between the various factors regarding the school year of the female students in the nursing study program. The results are shown in Table 3.

Table 3. Spearman's correlation coefficient between factors according to the school year of the studies.

	School Year	*Confidence in Coping with the Effects of Racism at Work as a Nurse*	*Sense of Mission as a Nursing Student in Using Knowledge and Authority in the Community*	*Cultural Identity and Community Belonging*	*Cultural Sensitivity*
School Year	1	0.02	0.28 **	0.03	−0.01
Confidence in coping with the effects of racism at work as a nurse		1	0.13 *	0.1	0.40 **
Sense of mission as a nursing student in using knowledge and authority in their community			1	0.27 **	0.14 *
Cultural identity and community belonging				1	0.06
Cultural sensitivity					1

* $p < 0.05$, ** $p < 0.01$.

As presented in Table 3, there is a significant positive correlation of the school year with the *sense of mission as a nursing student in using knowledge and authority in their community* factor ($p < 0.01$; r = 0.28). This correlation signifies that as the student advances with nursing studies, the sense of mission toward her community increases. Additionally, there were significant positive correlations between the *sense of mission as a nursing student in using knowledge and authority in their community* factor and the *confidence to cope with the effects of racism at work as a nurse* factor ($p < 0.05$; r = 0.13); the *cultural identity and community belonging* factor ($p < 0.05$; r = 0.27); and the *cultural sensitivity* factor ($p < 0.05$; r = 0.14). Moreover, there was a significant positive correlation between the *confidence in coping with the effects of racism at work as a nurse* factor and the *cultural sensitivity* factor ($p < 0.05$; r = 0.40).

Additional Results

We also conducted Levene's test for equality of variances of each item of the questionnaire to identify any significant statistical differences in specific items between the UO and other students and the non-UO students. The results are presented in Table 4.

Table 4. Independent Samples Test (Items).

	Items	Students		
		Ultra-Orthodox	Non-Ultra-Orthodox	
		$n = 111$	$n = 124$	
No.	**Item**	**Mean**		**Sig. (2-Tailed)**
2	The pandemic taught me that there are differences between my cultural identity and other groups in Israeli society	6.370	6.310	0.859
3	The pandemic has made me critical of the behavior of members of my community	5.950	6.410	0.243
4	The pandemic has made me critical of other people's attitudes towards my community	6.500	4.730	0.000 **
5	The pandemic strengthened my sense of mission and choice in the nursing profession	7.970	7.870	0.233
6	The pandemic raised concerns regarding my exposure to risks, when I become a nurse	4.960	5.580	0.105
7	I used my authority as a nursing student to encourage others in my community to obey the instructions of the Ministry of Health during the pandemic	6.250	5.080	0.004 **
8	I used my knowledge as a nursing student to guide others in my community on how to behave properly during the pandemic	6.000	4.900	0.006 **
9	I am very comfortable working with people whose beliefs, values, and practice are different from my own	7.02	6.96	0.821
10	I am very confident of my ability to establish trust and show respect and empathy to people from other cultures	8.56	8.3	0.170
11	I am aware of my ethnic and cultural identities	8.710	9.000	0.202
12	I am updated regarding the culture and social status of my clients	7.2	7.11	0.710
13	I am able to incorporate clients' cultural beliefs into the care and treatment I provide	6.65	6.25	0.134
14	I am very confident to challenge racism and discrimination toward clients	7.53	6.93	0.029 *
15	I am very confident to challenge racism and discrimination toward staff	6.77	6.51	0.398
16	I am very confident to challenge racism and discrimination toward me	6.530	6.220	0.358

* p-value < 0.05; ** p-value < 0.01.

As presented in Table 4, statistically significant differences exist between the UO and the non-UO students in four items: *The pandemic has made me critical of other people's attitudes towards my community* ($p < 0.001$); *I used my authority as a nursing student to encourage others in my community to obey the instructions of the Ministry of Health during the pandemic* ($p < 0.01$); *I used my knowledge as a nursing student to guide others in my community on how to behave properly during the pandemic* ($p < 0.01$); and *I am very confident to challenge racism and discrimination toward clients* ($p < 0.05$).

5.2. Qualitative Phase

Two themes were identified in the analysis as follows (see Table 5 for quotations):

Table 5. Qualitative results—Selected quotes.

Theme Number	Selected Quotes
Theme 1: Challenges in the encounters Ultra-Orthodox nursing students experience within their community	• *Students had to overcome objections within their community in relation to exercising the students' wish to enter nursing school.* "I know this is not an acceptable step and many look at it as 'What are you doing? Are you going to college? To be a nurse?' But I try not to look at what society now tells me. I went to my rabbi and consulted with him and my parents. Then I decided—I go for it. Of course, I will not do anything that is unacceptable" (C2) " ... I do not see myself as a pioneer ... that's what was right for me ... This profession is a mission. It gives satisfaction ... " (C2) "I felt I had enough resilience to go and do it [study nursing]. That does not mean I would recommend it to anyone else. Each one should think with herself and with her rabbis." (C1) "My high school principal told me I was an educational failure for him ... and that it [nursing] was a bad profession to study, that the learning topics are inappropriate and 'God forbid.' ... it was hard, but I had all the support I needed. It was something I wanted, and no one could move me, so I said to myself 'O.k. we do not have the same worldview' and that's it." (P1) • *Students expressed ambivalence about their role as health information providers to their community.* " ... I also have heard of breast cancer. I called my grandmother and started to publicize it. 'Get examined as soon as you can and do it frequently.' ... I also think that in the future ... the more I am exposed to [medical] cases, and I know what happens, I will warn more people. I don't think I will advise them medically, but I will make recommendations." (B5) " ... Most of the people who asked questions and consulted with me were very UO. They had been turning to me for advice since they heard I had started to study nursing. Even in the first year, when you start to study anatomy, they are convinced you are already a doctor." (D5) "I don't often take the responsibility, but sometimes it is my cousins or other family members or neighbors—people close to me, so I can tell them what I think they should do and whom to consult. They should turn to someone who knows, someone who is qualified." (D5) "We [nursing students] know where and whom to turn to: the Internet, a physician, or a nurse; people constantly ask me." (C5) " ... my brother says, 'I am asking you because ... I don't know the most reliable source, and you know exactly where to look.'" (C4) "Yes, many people turned to me, and it is extremely flattering. I also feel that I know something—maybe not that much, but more than the average person." (B1) " ... It's really amazing when people see you as someone special, not just a child." (B3) • *Students described having mixed feelings in relation to providing care to patients from their community.* "I see the possibility of adapting medical care to the needs of the community. I see this as one of my goals as a nurse and as an UO Jew." (B1) " ... Patients from the UO community understand the nuances. They identify me as one of their own, so we speak differently to each other, and they are happy because I understand them. It is a fact that we need more ultra-Orthodox nurses in the field." (C1) "When they [UO patients] see me taking care of them, they feel more comfortable. I am dressed the same way they are, and I speak their language and feel that they feel more comfortable to approach me. I sit at the nursing station and when they arrive, they turn to me before turning to anyone else." (C5) " ... You really see that UO people are happy to see that there is someone from their community in the field [of nursing] ... It's nice ... I'm also happy to meet patients like me ... the whole 'cultural competence' issue ... if you do not have to do special steps to adapt yourself [to the patient] it is much easier." (P1) " ... Every time an UO patient arrives, especially in my department, it is really difficult to take care of them ... let's say, it is a 20-year-old boy who studies in a yeshiva—I know exactly where he is coming from and that I am the only woman who has ever touched him outside of his family (she grins). Just because I know where he is coming from, it is not so pleasant for me." (C3) " ... As women in the ultra-Orthodox community, we do not touch men ... It is because of 'halakha' roles .... This is how we grew up and this is how we were educated ... I will feel uncomfortable to insert a catheter to a man ... maybe I will choose a women's ward or an emergency room where there is less need to take care of intimate parts of the body" (B1)

Table 5. *Cont.*

Theme Number	Selected Quotes
Theme 1: Challenges in the encounters Ultra-Orthodox nursing students experience within their community	• *Students mediated reliable health and health behavior information to their community at the time of the COVID-19 pandemic.* "You have to know how to approach them [the UO community]. You can't tell them on television ... because they don't watch television. However, as soon as their rabbi tells them to do so, there is a lockdown—then they stay indoors. You have to reach people in a way they prefer." (C1) "My mother's friends call me regarding COVID-19; not that I know what to answer, but they ask. Let's say, they want me to arrange a COVID-19 test for them: when and where they should do it. It is strange that although I am much younger to them, they call and ask." (B3) "The information that reaches the UO community is sometimes confusing, and they don't understand it. Neither do secular people understand these things scientifically. In such situations, I can be a representative and can transmit information." (C2) "More than asking about what happens inside, they [the UO people] ask what happens outside because they don't know what is going on. They lack information ... reliable information. They don't know what is happening outside of their world, if they are missing information. I am a reliable source to them regarding COVID-19." (C2) "I don't feel like I have a mission, but I can make people more aware that if they think they have nothing to be afraid of COVID-19, there is still something to be afraid of." (D2) "Our rabbi said, if someone in the family is sick with COVID-19, the entire family must be in lockdown. You [as a nurse] have to relate to this source of authority and not only to what the Ministry of Health says. It's complicated. All of the responsibility is on you." (B3)
	• *Students appreciated the opportunity to challenge their perceptions about others outside of their community but also mentioned the difficulties involved.* "When you know team members from other communities then you own, your viewpoint changes. We all have prejudices about other societies. If we do not exercise some thinking before, we may judge people automatically by how they look to us. Once you get to know a person a little deeper, stigmas come down" (D1). Now I'm in a clinic where 90% of the patients are Arabs. Really until now, I did not think that I would have to think about their language and culture ... it is important to recognize it as a nurse, ... " (B3) "In high school, you are protected. Those who teach you—these are people from your community. You study with people from your community. Suddenly you come to the academy and the lecturer is, let's say, is a very smart, valued woman, that has a different way of life from you ... It could raise thoughts ... You suddenly meet the world, and it looks a bit different ... very different then what you were told you" (C1) "I had stigmas but when I did my clinical practice, I saw that ... there are no such stigmas. I treat a person, a patient, not his race, his religion. Those stigmas just went down, and I saw it was not an issue" (B5) "This [nursing] also connects me to the rest of the world; the feeling that we are together, united, closer, the minute that I can help them [nonreligious jews]. I think that from this perspective, it is possible that I will succeed in changing the way people look at my community." (B5) " ... telling you how to treat an Arab versus practically take care of an Arab patient is very different. It sounded much harder to me then my experience when it actually happened. I found myself smiling at them, asking 'How are you?' and treat them as human beings." (C1) "I saw this during the COVID-19 pandemic ... patients from other cultural background arrived and they had different opinions than mine. I must know how not to oppose them. I have to treat them in such a way that they accept me taking care of them, regardless of my own UO background." (B3) "When I treat UO patients I feel ... good that I am taking care of them. Now, my work is easier because I know how to relate to UO women ... Arab women—I can only say the few words in Arabic; secular women—it's not that I don't show empathy or concern, but it's just easier for me with UO women as someone who comes from this same background. I think most people are like this. If an Arab is treating an Arab, it will be easier for them than treating a Jew." (C2)
Theme 2: Challenges in the encounters of Ultra-Orthodox nursing students with other sections of Israeli society	

Table 5. *Cont.*

Theme Number	Selected Quotes
Theme 2: Challenges in the encounters of Ultra-Orthodox nursing students with other sections of Israeli society	• *Students encountered racism during the COVID-19 pandemic although they raised criticism towards the behavior of the members of their community.* "There is a remark that I as an UO often hear: 'O.K. You are not like everyone else. You are not the standard UO woman, so it's ok.' They often get me annoyed because none of the UO are 'standard' UO. So, I wonder, what kind of UO people are you talking about?" (B1) "The entire period of the COVID-19 pandemic ... changed what we [UO] thought about the general public because we felt there was immense antagonism against us. Not just against the extremists, but against ordinary people also. It was unfortunate that relations that had developed over years, were upended in one year." (B1) "There is a stigma of mass infection in our community [i.e., UO neighborhoods]; that we live in the most contagious part of the city, and that no one is obeying the lockdown." (B1) "I live in Bnai Brak [the largest UO city in Israel] and I hear a lot of stories about us. I really don't like these stories. So, I feel that I am more critical [toward my community] than others who criticize me as part of this community." (C3) " ... This is something that really bothers me about the UO community: a kind of blocking things out, brainwashing without using their own mind to think. This really gets me angry. Now [during the pandemic] it emerges in more ways." (D1)

5.2.1. Challenges in the Encounters Ultra-Orthodox Nursing Students Experience within Their Community

Students had to overcome objections within their community in relation to exercising the students' wish to enter nursing school.

Most of the participants shared that they faced objections to academic studies from within their close community (high school teachers, friends, cousins, etc.). Some of them specifically faced objections against entering the nursing field and had to keep their plans secret until they began their studies. They all asked for permission from their parents and their rabbi prior to enrolling in nursing school. When asked, participants strongly recommended that other girls from their community study nursing. However, they did not see themselves as activists for social change for girls or women in their community. Rather they emphasized their personal interest in nursing and the mission they see in the nursing profession.

Students expressed ambivalence about their role as health information providers to their community.

Although they encountered objection, participants said that they are highly valued in their community for having studied nursing. Participants noted that people considered them as health authorities and sought their advice regarding health, even though they were still students. Participants explained they were flattered as it raised their confidence and self-pride. They felt obliged to share the health and medical information they acquired in the nursing school with their community. Nevertheless, participants expressed ambivalence since they hesitated to answer medical questions because, as they said, they are still students and preferred to direct such questions to a professional, such as a nurse or physician.

Students described having mixed feelings in relation to providing care to patients from their community.

Participants emphasized their mission as UO nurses familiar with the cultural sensibilities of their community. Participants mention their responsibility to help patients from their community feel comfortable when they arrive at general hospitals and clinics. However, a few of the participants noted that the cultural background they share with patients from their community was not always beneficial. Under certain circumstances, clinical procedures may create situations that conflict with cultural norms and embarrass both parties. For example, in cases where they needed to touch or even talk to young UO men, where both parties were aware of the restrictions about relations between men and women in UO communities. The participants explain how they overcome these difficulties and emphasized that in moments of embarrassment, they focus on their task and remind themselves that everything they are doing is professional with the purpose of helping the patient.

Students mediated reliable health and health behavior information to their community at the time of the COVID-19 pandemic.

The pandemic increased the participants' sense of responsibility for conveying medical information to their community. They described their role during the COVID-19 pandemic amid massive confusion among their community members who have less exposure to smartphones, the Internet, television, and radio. Community members therefore sought and relied on COVID-19-related information from participants. Participants explained that they were surprised to see that the guidelines of the Ministry of Health were often misleading and sometimes contradictory of UO community customs. For example, during the holidays that occurred at the beginning of the epidemic, the directives of the Ministry of Health were to maintain social isolation and the UO people wanted to observe their custom of offering prayers in public. Participants described mediating for their close community between the formal guidelines of the Ministry of Health and those given by community leaders.

5.2.2. Challenges in the Encounters of Ultra-Orthodox Nursing Students with Other Sections of Israeli Society

Students appreciated the opportunity to challenge their perceptions about others outside of their community but also mentioned the difficulties involved.

The experiences of nursing students during their clinical training provided them with the opportunity, sometimes the first opportunity they had experienced, to meet people from other sections of Israeli society, such as nonreligious Jews and non-Jews (i.e., patients from the Arab sector). Participants discussed how this experience was sometimes surprising and made them more open-minded although the encounters were challenging because of exposure to different—sometimes contradictory—values, norms, and customs. Few participants described feeling more comfortable with people from their own community—who they treated more warmly—than other patients, who they treated "by the book".

Students encountered racism during the COVID-19 pandemic, although they raised criticism towards the behavior of the members of their community.

Interactions with patients and staff from various communities of the Israeli society exposed the participants to prejudices toward their community. Participants said that they learned for the first time that the public blames the UO community for the spread of the virus because they did not maintain social distance in the first period of the of the COVID-19 pandemic. The participants said that they are not always comfortable when others see them as representatives of the ultra-Orthodox society. For some participants, the exposure to stigmas about their community increased their sense of identification with their community. These participants were angry with the critical attitude of outsiders, since, as they said, the guidelines did not always reach the ultra-Orthodox community. Some saw their role as nurses as an opportunity to change these prejudices against their community. However, a few criticized the behavior of their community members during the pandemic.

6. Discussion

Previous studies have addressed the factors related to multicultural nurses' experiences in encounters with the general population, as well as factors related to their work with patients from minority groups, especially from their community [14,15,17–19]. This study focused on female UO nursing students, their challenges, and dilemmas in their encounters with the general Israeli population, as well as their own community members, especially during the COVID-19 pandemic.

The nursing profession is noble, as nurses save human lives—a value highly regarded in the Jewish tradition and especially in the UO community [56]. However, the UO female nursing students are exceptional in their community that rejects academic pursuits.

Their vocational nursing training in school, and later their profession, require extensive encounters with different worldviews, which can lead to a clash with their lifestyles [36].

Ultra-Orthodox nursing students' sense of mission

The participants sense of mission was the main finding in both the quantitative and qualitative analyses in our study. Arieli and Hirschfeld (2010) [57] found that, compared to Palestinian–Israeli nursing students, most Jewish students' reason for choosing nursing was an inner desire to serve. Pragmatic considerations for choosing nursing were mentioned but were usually presented by Jewish students as a relatively minor motivation. The quantitative phase of our study showed how the UO nursing students revealed a significantly higher sense of mission toward their community compared to the other nursing students in our study [t (233) = 2.46, 95% confident interval of the difference 0.15–1.39]. In the focus groups, participants emphasized nursing as a mission to help and serve others. They described their mission to provide reliable health-related information to their community. This was especially noticeable during the COVID-19 pandemic, which exposed the trust deficit between their community and health authorities [27].

Entering nursing school gives UO students an opportunity for social mobility [58]. They acquired higher education, and it will help them find a stable and well-paying job in the future, which will improve their social status [59,60]. Nursing education also gives participants in our study a chance for social mobility within their community because they hold valuable social capital: their professional—and potentially lifesaving—knowledge about health issues [14,15,19]. However, although these students are pioneers of their community in terms of entering nursing school, the participants in the focus groups emphasized not regarding themselves as "flag bearers" of social change for other women in their community. They stressed that they entered nursing school after receiving approval from the rabbinical authority and their parents. They reported remaining committed to the values of their community and stated that their choice of the nursing profession was not driven by a desire for social mobility. They were happy to recommend this direction to other UO girls.

Ultra-Orthodox nursing students' culture competence challenges

Our study shows the dilemmas and challenges that the UO nursing students faced in their intercultural encounters with the general society, coming—as they did—from a closed, distinct group that faithfully upholds religious and traditional values and practices [61]. At the same time, they discussed their struggle when facing patients from their own community. Their deep acquaintance with the cultural norms of the UO community brings the UO participants to tread cautiously so as not to offend these patients.

The findings of studies on changes in cultural competence over the years in nursing schools are contradictory. A few studies indicate that there has been no change over the years [62,63], whereas others show that there has been a change [64]. The cultural competence factors examined in our study sample, especially the sense of mission, increased with advances in nursing studies. This was true for the UO participants, as well as the non-UO participants. It is in line with the significant positive correlations between the examined factors, among themselves, and in relation to the school year of the program studies, as it is well confirmed by Spearman's correlation coefficient test.

Utilizing the CCATool [48], Repo et al. (2017) [4] found cultural competence to be positively associated with Finnish nursing students' minority backgrounds and frequency of interacting with different cultures. Following the above finding, we assumed that in our study, as students' progress academically, they perform more practical training in hospitals and in the community and interact with a diverse population both among patients and staff, which enhances their sensitivity toward other cultures. The academic progress of our UO participants also enhances their sense of responsibility toward their community.

Repo et al. (2017) [4] also reported that students with a minority background had higher cultural competence than general Finnish students. This has also been reported by reported by Mesler (2014) [65]. We agree with Repo et al.'s ([4], p. 102) explanation that "this may be due to the fact that minority background students already are culturally aware since they have had to reflect on their own ethnic and cultural identity while living as foreigners in Finland." In our focus groups, the UO participants declared that they believe in equal medical care for all people and that they follow this tenet at work. Compared to other students in our sample, the UO participants were not only more sensitive to the issue of racism toward patients, but they felt more confident in dealing with it. It was manifested in a statistically significant difference between the UO and the non-UO students in the quantitative phase in the item: *I am very confident to challenge racism and discrimination toward clients*. However, they did not state that they were trying to develop awareness or acquire knowledge about patients from other communities.

Ultra-Orthodox nursing students in the COVID-19 pandemic

Their clinical experience, especially when the COVID-19 pandemic first appeared, exposed our study participants to the ignorance of parts of their community members about health issues, their lack of access to the latest and most reliable information due to cultural–religious restrictions, and the serious consequences that all of these had on the community members' health.

Previous studies [14,15,17,18] have noted language and communication problems as barriers, especially for minorities, in gaining access to health services. The UO Jews constitute a minority group in Israeli society, although most of them speak Hebrew, which is the common language of Israel [66]. However, UO communities lack health literacy [27], which refers to "the degree to which individuals have the ability to find, understand, and use information and services to inform health-related decisions and actions for themselves and others" [67].

The participants in the focus groups shared that their community members recognized them as a source of reliable medical information, and they often made the guidelines of the Ministry of Health accessible to their community. It is in line with the findings of the quantitative phase, which showed significant differences between the UO and the non-UO students in the items: *I used my authority as a nursing student to encourage others in my community to obey the instructions of the Ministry of Health during the pandemic; I used my knowledge as a nursing student to guide others in my community on how to behave properly during the pandemic*.

The COVID-19 period accentuated for the participants not only their roles within their community, but also what the public thought about their community. The UO community faced instances of racism during the COVID-19 pandemic. There were cases where people blamed them for spreading the disease by disobeying the official instructions for limiting the spread of the virus [27].

Some of the UO participants in our research were exposed, due to their work as nurses, to the prejudices about their community for the first time, largely because the UO community stays isolated from the general society as part of their religious ideology. The UO students described how patients regarded them as representatives of the UO society, which was not always appropriate, especially when their community was blamed for the spread of the disease. It is in line with the statistically significant difference between the UO and the non-UO students in the quantitative phase in the item: *The pandemic has made me critical of other people's attitudes towards my community*. Moreover, a few participants in the focus groups recounted the comments of the medical staff, especially nurses who worked with them. Iheduru-Anderson et al. (2021) [68] (pp. 122–123) found that "racism in nursing remains under-investigated. There is a collective denial and a culture of silence around racism, which perpetuate systemic racism and its consequences on the nursing profession ... ". Following their experience, the UO participants in our focus groups acknowledged the importance of treating members of their own community with greater warmth because of the difficulties and barriers they face in the society.

Limitations

This study has several limitations. First, the small number of items in the questionnaire limits the number of identified factors in the factor analysis. Hence, significant differences between the UO and the non-UO students in specific items, which are relevant to the research questions, are found in Levene's test for equality of variances of each item but are not revealed in the comparison of the factors between the two groups. Using a larger number of items might define factors, which would include the "missed" items within the categorized groups of items. However, the factors are highly supported by the themes identified in the analysis of the qualitative phase of this study. Second, in the quantitative phase, we compared the UO students—this study's focus—with the non-UO students in the same college. However, the latter are also religious Jews and do not represent the secular section of Israeli society. This might limit the generalization of the study. Our assumption is that because the non-UO participants in the study resemble general Israeli women in terms of their previous education and other social variables, such as participating in the military service (or national service instead) [69], they are integrated into Israeli society, and, therefore, can represent a control group for the UO participants.

7. Conclusions

Our research shows that transcultural nursing students play a decisive role in mediating updated and accurate health information to their community, especially at times of crises, from the initial stages of their training. However, they face dilemmas both inside and outside their respective communities. We believe that insights derived from this study can be utilized to build programs to address the challenges of nurses from minority communities and transcultural nurses. At the policy level, we join the call of Drach-Zahavy et al. (2021) [70] to prepare in advance a crisis plan for nursing schools that could be rapidly implemented, and to incorporate in the nursing curricula crisis-related topics, such as developing flexible coping strategies. We propose that these policies should leverage the substantial potential of transcultural nursing students in working with their communities and consider these students' distinct needs and dilemmas. This will help channelize the social role of transcultural nurses for conveying otherwise inaccessible information to isolated communities.

Author Contributions: Conceptualization, S.G. and A.F.; Methodology, S.G. and A.F.; Validation, S.G., A.F., Y.G.B. and Z.O.; Formal Analysis, S.G., A.F., Y.G.B. and Z.O.; Investigation, S.G. and A.F.; Resources, S.G. and A.F.; Writing—Original Draft Preparation, S.G. and A.F.; Writing—Review & Editing, S.G., A.F., Y.G.B. and Z.O.; Supervision, S.G. and A.F.; Project Administration, S.G. and A.F.; Funding Acquisition, S.G. and A.F. All authors have read and agreed to the published version of the manuscript.

Funding: This work was financed by the Jerusalem College of Technology.

Institutional Review Board Statement: The study was conducted with the approval of the Jerusalem College of Technology Ethics Committee No. 011_20. All participants signed consent forms and were assured of complete confidentiality and anonymity. Participation in the study was voluntary.

Informed Consent Statement: Informed consent was obtained from all subjects involved in the study.

Data Availability Statement: The study did not report any data (all data is reported in the article).

Acknowledgments: The authors would like to acknowledge the nursing students who took part in the study.

Conflicts of Interest: The authors declare no conflict of interest.

References

1. Tosun, B.; BENEFITS Group. Addressing the effects of transcultural nursing education on nursing students' cultural competence: A systematic review. *Nurse Educ. Pract.* **2021**, *55*, 103171. [CrossRef] [PubMed]
2. Calvillo, E.; Clark, L.; Ballantyne, J.E.; Pacquiao, D.; Purnell, L.D.; Villarruel, A.M. Cultural competency in baccalaureate nursing education. *J. Transcult. Nurs.* **2009**, *20*, 137–145. [CrossRef] [PubMed]
3. Campinha-Bacote, J. Delivering patient-centered care in the midst of a cultural conflict: The role of cultural competence. *Online J. Issues Nurs.* **2011**, *16*, 181–184. [CrossRef]

4. Repo, H.; Vahlberg, T.; Salminen, L.; Papadopoulos, I.; Leino-Kilpi, H. The cultural competence of graduating nursing students. *J. Transcult. Nurs.* **2017**, *28*, 98–107. [CrossRef]
5. Schuster, M.; Elroy, I.; Elmakais, I. We are lost: Measuring the accessibility of signage in public general hospitals. *Lang. Policy* **2017**, *16*, 23–38. [CrossRef]
6. Schuster, M.; Elroy, I.; Rosen, B. How culturally competent are hospitals in Israel? *Isr. J. Health Policy Res.* **2018**, *7*, 61. [CrossRef]
7. Govere, L.; Govere, E.M. How effective is cultural competence training of healthcare providers on improving patient satisfaction of minority groups? A systematic review of literature. *Worldviews Evid.-Based Nurs.* **2016**, *13*, 402–410. [CrossRef]
8. Squires, A. Evidence-based approaches to breaking down language barriers. *Nursing* **2017**, *47*, 34–40. [CrossRef]
9. Halbert, C.H.; Armstrong, K.; Gandy, O.H.; Shaker, L. Racial differences in trust in health care providers. *Arch. Intern. Med.* **2006**, *166*, 896–901. [CrossRef]
10. Ume-Nwagbo, P.N. Implications of nursing faculties' cultural competence. *J. Nurs. Educ.* **2012**, *51*, 262–268. [CrossRef]
11. Gaston-Johansson, F.; Hill-Briggs, F.; Oguntomilade, L.; Bradley, V.; Mason, P. Patient perspectives on disparities in healthcare from African-American, Asian, Hispanic, and Native American samples including a secondary analysis of the Institute of Medicine focus group data. *J. Natl. Black Nurses Assoc.* **2007**, *18*, 43–52.
12. Meghani, S.H.; Brooks, J.M.; Gipson-Jones, T.; Waite, R.; Whitfi eld-Harris, L.; Deatrick, J.A. Patient-provider race-concordance: Does it matter in improving minority patients' health outcomes. *Ethn. Health* **2009**, *14*, 107–130. [CrossRef] [PubMed]
13. Lo, M.C.M.; Bahar, R. Resisting the colonization of the lifeworld? Immigrant patients' experiences with co-ethnic healthcare workers. *Soc. Sci. Med.* **2013**, *87*, 68–76. [CrossRef]
14. Lo, M.C.M.; Nguyen, E.T. Caring and carrying the cost: Bicultural Latina nurses' challenges and strategies for working with coethnic patients. *RSF Russell Sage Found. J. Soc. Sci.* **2018**, *4*, 149–171.
15. Lo, M.C.M.; Nguyen, E.T. Resisting the racialization of medical deservingness: How Latinx nurses produce symbolic resources for Latinx immigrants in clinical encounters. *Soc. Sci. Med.* **2021**, *270*, 113677. [CrossRef]
16. Seto, A.; Forth, N.L.A. What is known about bilingual counseling? A systematic review of the literature. *Prof. Couns.* **2020**, *10*, 393–405. [CrossRef]
17. Dawson, M.A. Black nurses collaborative approach to addressing COVID-19 in Black communities. *J. Racial Ethn. Health Disparities* **2021**, *8*, 790–793. [CrossRef]
18. Delgdo-Romero, E.A.; De Los Santos, J.; Raman, V.S.; Merrifield, J.N.; Vazquez, M.S.; Monroig, M.M.; Bautista, E.C.; Duran, M.Y. Caught in the middle: Spanish-speaking bilingual mental health counselors as language brokers. *J. Ment. Health Couns.* **2018**, *40*, 341–352. [CrossRef]
19. Keshet, Y.; Popper-Giveon, A. Work experiences of ethnic minority nurses: A qualitative study. *Isr. J. Health Policy Res.* **2016**, *5*, 18. [CrossRef]
20. Cuellar, N.G.; Aquino, E., Dawson, M.A.; Garcia-Dia, M.J.; Im, E.O.; Jurado, L.F.M.; Lee, Y.S.; Littlejohn, S.; Tom-Orme, L.; Toney, D.A. Culturally congruent health care of COVID-19 in minorities in the United States: A clinical practice paper from the National Coalition of Ethnic Minority Nurse Associations. *J. Transcult. Nurs.* **2020**, *31*, 434–443. [CrossRef]
21. Biale, D.; Assaf, D.; Brown, B.; Gellman, U.; Heilman, S.C.; Rosman, M.; Sagiv, G.; Wodzinsky, M. *Hasidism: A New History*; Princeton University Press: Princeton, NJ, USA, 2018.
22. Rubinstein, A.; Gartner, L.P.; Baskin, J.R.; Morris, B.J.; Jacobs, L.; Shatz-Uffenheimer, R. Hasidism. In *The Encyclopaedia Judaica*, 2nd ed.; Macmillan Reference USA Publisher: New York, NY, USA, 2007; Volume 8, pp. 393–434.
23. Taragin-Zeller, L.; Rozenblum, Y.; Baram-Tsabari, A. Public engagement with science among religious minorities: Lessons from COVID-19. *Sci. Commun.* **2020**, *42*, 643–678. [CrossRef]
24. Malach, G.; Cahaner, L. Statistical Report on Ultra-Orthodox Society in Israel. The Israel Democracy Institute. 2020. Available online: https://www.idi.org.il/books/33367 (accessed on 26 July 2022).
25. Haredi Institute for Public Affairs. The Coronavirus Crisis in the Ultra-Orthodox Population in Israel [Hebrew]. 2020. Available online: https://machon.org.il/wp-content/uploads/2020/06/d79ed7a9d791d7a8-d7a0d792d799d7a3-d794d7a7d795d7a8d795d7a0d794-d795d794d797d7a8d793d799d79d-d791d799d7a9d7a8d790d79c-d7a1d795d7a4d799.pdf (accessed on 26 July 2022).
26. Israeli Central Bureau of Statistics. Society in Israel, Report Number 10: Religion and Self-Definition of Level of Religiosity [Hebrew]. 2018. Available online: https://www.cbs.gov.il/he/publications/DocLib/2018/rep_10/h_print.pdf (accessed on 26 July 2022).
27. Zalcberg, S.; Zalcberg Block, S. COVID-19 amongst the ultra-Orthodox population in Israel: An inside look into the causes of the high morbidity rates. *Contemp. Jew.* **2021**, *41*, 99–121. [CrossRef]
28. Orr, Z.; Unger, S.; Finkelstein, A. Localization of human rights of people with disabilities: The case of Jewish ultra-Orthodox people in Israel. *Hum. Rights Q.* **2021**, *43*, 93–116. [CrossRef]
29. Orr, Z.; Unger, S.; Finkelstein, A. The challenges and dilemmas of local translators of human rights: The case of disability rights among Jewish ultra-Orthodox communities. *J. Hum. Rights* **2021**, *20*, 339–355. [CrossRef]
30. Vardi, M.; Orr, Z.; Finkelstein, A. Civic engagement of students from minority groups: The case of ultra-Orthodox students and communities in Jerusalem. In *Understanding Campus-Community Partnerships in Conflict Zones*; Markovich, D.Y., Golan, D., Shalhoub-Kevorkian, N., Eds.; Palgrave Macmillan: London, UK, 2019; pp. 261–292.
31. Golan, A.; Campbel, H.A. Strategic management of religious websites: The case of Israel's Orthodox communities. *J. Comput.-Mediat. Commun.* **2015**, *20*, 467–486. [CrossRef]

32. Gonen, A.; Sharon, D.; Lev-Ari, L.; Strauss, E.; Segev, R. The impact of nursing students' cultural diversity on the intention and attitudes toward the use of information technology. *J. Transcult. Nurs.* **2016**, *27*, 302–310. [CrossRef]
33. Raz, A.; Keshet, Y.; Popper-Giveon, A.; Karkabi, M.S. One size does not fit all: Lessons from Israel's COVID-19 vaccination drive and hesitancy. *Vaccine* **2021**, *39*, 4027–4028. [CrossRef]
34. Orr, Z.; Erblich, T.; Unger, S.; Barnea, O.; Weinstein, M.; Agnon, A. Earthquake preparedness among religious minority groups: The case of the Jewish ultra-Orthodox society in Israel. *Nat. Hazards Earth Syst. Sci.* **2021**, *21*, 317–337. [CrossRef]
35. Coleman-Brueckheimer, K.; Spitzer, J.; Koffman, J. Involvement of Rabbinic and communal authorities in decision-making by haredi Jews in the UK with breast cancer: An interpretative phenomenological analysis. *Soc. Sci. Med.* **2009**, *68*, 323–333. [CrossRef] [PubMed]
36. Haron, Y.; Azuri, P. Integrating ultra-Orthodox Jewish men in academic nursing training. *J. Transcult. Nurs.* **2016**, *27*, 627–632. [CrossRef]
37. Segev, R.; Strauss, E. Forming an affiliation between two culturally different academic institutions of nursing studies. *Open Nurs.* **2020**, *6*, 1–7. [CrossRef] [PubMed]
38. Kolikant, Y.B.-D.; Genut, S. The effect of prior education on students' competency in digital logic: The case of ultraorthodox Jewish students. *Comput. Sci. Educ.* **2017**, *27*, 149–174. [CrossRef]
39. Buchbinder, E.; Sigad, L.; Strier, R.; Eisikovits, Z. Working poor ultra-Orthodox Jewish women and men: Between economic distress and meaning based on faith. *J. Poverty* **2015**, *19*, 377–398. [CrossRef]
40. Kulik, L. Explaining employment hardiness among women in Israel's ultraorthodox community: Facilitators and inhibitors. *J. Career Assess.* **2016**, *24*, 67–85. [CrossRef]
41. Gabbay, E.; McCarthy, M.W.; Fins, J.J. The care of the ultra-orthodox Jewish patient. *J. Relig. Health* **2017**, *56*, 545–560. [CrossRef]
42. Sharmila, D. Mental health and religion in Israel's ultra-Orthodox Jews. *Lancet* **2005**, *366*, 1516–1517.
43. Snyder, J.; Sommer, B. Special considerations for Orthodox Jewish patients in the emergency departments. *J. Emerg. Nurs.* **1995**, *21*, 569–570. [CrossRef]
44. Waitzberg, R.; Davidovitch, N.; Leibner, G.; Penn, N.; Brammli-Greenberg, S. Israel's response to the COVID-19 pandemic: Tailoring measures for vulnerable cultural minority populations. *Int. J. Equity Health* **2020**, *19*, 71. [CrossRef]
45. Foscarini, G. Ultra-orthodox Jewish women go to work: Secular education and vocational training as sources of emancipation and modernization. *Ann. Di Ca' Foscari Ser. Orient.* **2014**, *50*, 53–74.
46. Finkelstein, A.; Orr, Z. Does volunteering change attitudes towards people with disabilities? A qualitative study of the experience of orthodox Jewish nursing students. *Nurse Educ. Pract.* **2021**, *55*, 103141. [CrossRef]
47. Shorten, A.; Smith, J. Mixed methods research: Expanding the evidence base. *Evid.-Based Nurs.* **2017**, *20*, 74–75. [CrossRef]
48. Papadopoulos, I.; Tilki, M.; Ayling, S. Cultural competence in action for CAMHS: Development of a cultural competence assessment tool and training programme. *Contemp. Nurse* **2008**, *28*, 129–140. [CrossRef]
49. Patton, M.Q. *Qualitative Evaluation and Research Methods*; Sage: Thousand Oaks, CA, USA, 1990.
50. Breen, R.L. A practical guide to focus-group research. *J. Geogr. High. Educ.* **2006**, *30*, 463–475. [CrossRef]
51. Braun, V.; Clarke, V. Using thematic analysis in psychology. *Qual. Res. Psychol.* **2006**, *3*, 77–101. [CrossRef]
52. Basit, T. Manual or electronic? The role of coding in qualitative data analysis. *Educ. Res.* **2003**, *45*, 143–154. [CrossRef]
53. Graneheim, U.H.; Lundman, B. Qualitative content analysis in nursing research: Concepts, procedures and measures to achieve trustworthiness. *Nurse Educ. Today* **2004**, *24*, 105–112. [CrossRef]
54. Tracy, S.J. Qualitative quality: Eight "big-tent" criteria for excellent qualitative research. *Qual. Inq.* **2010**, *16*, 837–851. [CrossRef]
55. Johnson, R.; Waterfield, J. Making words count: The value of qualitative research. *Physiother. Res. Int.* **2004**, *9*, 121–131. [CrossRef]
56. Spiegel, E. *"Talmud Torah is Equivalent to All": The Ultra-Orthodox (Haredi) Education System for Boys in Jerusalem*; JIIS Studies Series No. 405; The Jerusalem Institute for Israel Studies: Jerusalem, Israel, 2011.
57. Arieli, D.; Hirschfeld, M.J. Teaching nursing in a situation of conflict: Encounters between Palestinian-Israeli and Jewish-Israeli nursing students. *Int. Nurs. Rev.* **2010**, *57*, 312–320. [CrossRef]
58. Snee, H.; Goswami, H. Who cares? Social mobility and the 'class ceiling' in nursing. *Sociol. Res. Online* **2021**, *26*, 562–580. [CrossRef]
59. Brown, P. Education, opportunity and the prospects for social mobility. *Br. J. Sociol. Educ.* **2013**, *34*, 678–700. [CrossRef]
60. Payne, G. A new social mobility? The political redefinition of a sociological problem. *Contemp. Soc. Sci.* **2012**, *7*, 55–71. [CrossRef]
61. Kolikant, Y.B.-D.; Genut, S. Change in Order not to Change: Ultraorthodox Hasidic Women's Experience in Studying Computer Science. *Comput. Sci. Educ.* **2021**, 1–26. [CrossRef]
62. Rahma, N.F.; Novieastari, E. Differences in cultural competence between nursing students in academic and professional programs. *Enferm. Clin.* **2019**, *29*, 528–531. [CrossRef]
63. Seidel Glass, P.E. Differences among Undergraduate and Graduate Nursing Students' Cultural Competency. Ph.D. Thesis, Florida International University, Miami, FL, USA, 2013.
64. Witt, A.J. The Impact of Cultural Encounters on the Cultural Competence of Baccalaureate Nursing Students. Ph.D. Thesis, University of North Dakota, Grand Forks, ND, USA, 2016.
65. Mesler, D.M. A comparative study of cultural competence curricula in baccalaureate nursing programs. *Nurse Educ.* **2014**, *39*, 193–198. [CrossRef]

66. Keren-Kratz, M. Westernization and Israelization within Israel's extreme Orthodox Haredi society. *Isr. Stud. Rev.* **2016**, *31*, 101–129. [CrossRef]
67. Center for Disease Control and Prevention What Is Health Literacy? 2021. Available online: https://www.cdc.gov/healthliteracy/learn/index.html (accessed on 26 July 2022).
68. Iheduru-Anderson, K.; Shingles, R.R.; Akanegbu, C. Discourse of race and racism in nursing: An integrative review of literature. *Public Health Nurs.* **2021**, *38*, 115–130. [CrossRef]
69. Genut, S.; Ori, B.; Ben-David Kolikant, Y. Factors influencing women's decision to study computer science: Is it context dependent? *Issues Inf. Sci. Inf. Technol.* **2019**, *16*, 127–141. [CrossRef]
70. Drach-Zahavy, A.; Goldblatt, H.; Admi, H.; Blau, A.; Ohana, I.; Itzhaki, M. A multi-level examination of nursing students' resilience in the face of the COVID-19 outbreak: A cross-sectional design. *J. Adv. Nurs.* **2022**, *78*, 109–120. [CrossRef]

International Journal of
Environmental Research and Public Health

MDPI

Article

A Topic Modeling Analysis of the Crisis Response Stage during the COVID-19 Pandemic

Kyung-Sook Cha and Eun-Man Kim *

Department of Nursing Science, Sun Moon University, 70 Sunmoon-ro 221 beon-gil, Tangjeong-myeon, Asan-si 31460, Korea; chamelda@hanmail.net
* Correspondence: kem7355@hanmail.net; Tel.: +82-41-530-2756

Abstract: The core of disaster management is the ability to respond spontaneously and rapidly to unexpected situations and also to apply planned and adaptable responses that follow manuals and guidelines. This study aimed to observe the changes in information during the COVID-19 pandemic period by collecting and analyzing information announced on a hospital intranet by an infection control team. This study performed text mining of large amounts of data to investigate notices about in-hospital strategies towards COVID-19 to identify changes in the coping strategies during the pandemic. Notices announced within the infection control rooms of 12 university hospitals in South Korea from 1 January to 31 August 2020 were searched. Four representative topics were identified based on the stepwise keywords shown in the topic modeling analysis: (1) "Understanding the new infectious disease", (2) "Preparation of a patient care and management system", (3) "Prevention of spread and securing employee safety" and (4) "Improvement of the management system according to the revision of guidelines". Countries where an infectious disease emerges should provide accurate information on the disease and guidelines to determine how to respond. Medical institutions must revise and complement them while considering their specific circumstances. To efficiently respond to an infectious disease crisis, governments and medical institutions must cooperate closely, and implementing a systematic response is crucial.

Keywords: COVID-19; crisis response; topic modeling

Citation: Cha, K.-S.; Kim, E.-M. A Topic Modeling Analysis of the Crisis Response Stage during the COVID-19 Pandemic. *Int. J. Environ. Res. Public Health* **2022**, *19*, 8331. https://doi.org/10.3390/ijerph19148331

Academic Editors: Richard Gray and Sonia Udod

Received: 8 June 2022
Accepted: 4 July 2022
Published: 7 July 2022

1. Introduction

COVID-19 has been prevalent worldwide since its initial outbreak in China in December 2019 [1], and the World Health Organization (WHO) declared COVID-19 as a pandemic on 11 March 2020 [2]. New infectious diseases are caused by unknown pathogens and have occurred frequently during the 21st century, including severe acute respiratory syndrome and influenza A virus type H1N1. Each new infectious disease outbreak has posed a severe threat to human health. A pandemic exerts enormous adverse effects on health care and various aspects of society such as the economy [3].

Medical institutions are public institutions and are places where many patients who are vulnerable to infection gather. The spread of new infectious diseases can therefore have fatal consequences in these institutions, with cross-infection of new infectious diseases in medical institutions being a severe threat to patient safety. The safety of medical workers taking care of patients on the front line can also not be guaranteed. Barranco et al. [4] reported that the SARS-CoV-2 (severe acute respiratory syndrome coronavirus 2) infection rate attributable to medical institutions reached 12–15%, and according to the International Council of Nurses' analysis data [5], an average of 7% of all COVID-19 patients were receiving care from healthcare workers during the early stages of the COVID-19 pandemic. Preventing hospital transmissions is paramount during an infectious disease outbreak or epidemic, since infections from medical staff lead to medical institution closures, leading to confusion in the medical community [6].

In the event of a pandemic, the predictable costs of not preparing would be huge in human, societal and political terms. Therefore, decision-makers at all levels, including administrators and hospitals, should act as soon as possible [7]. Petak [8] and McLoughlin [9] suggested that the disaster management process has four stages: mitigation and prevention, preparation, planning, and response and recovery. Comfort et al. [10] indicated that both the role of the organization in disaster management and the coping actions taken during disaster management play essential roles. In particular, appropriate responses to infectious disease cases during the epidemic's early stages are more critical than ever since they often occur and spread instantly. The core of disaster management is the ability to respond spontaneously and rapidly to unexpected situations and also to apply planned and adaptable responses that follow manuals and guidelines [11]. In other words, each medical institution must be able to respond in advance appropriately and rapidly to prevent the spread of new infectious diseases within medical institutions. Identifying and organizing the response methods applied during the disaster period can facilitate rapid responses to similar crises.

Despite the importance of responding promptly and appropriately after the outbreak of novel infectious diseases, few studies have been reported. Some studies reported initial responses from the medical institutions after the outbreak of COVID-19 inpatients [7,12]. However, no studies analyzed the response strategies of multiple medical institutions to cope with rapidly changing situations immediately after the influx of new infectious diseases.

When pandemic situations such as COVID-19 occur, coordinated and multidisciplinary management between specialists in infectious diseases, wards, ICUs and infection control teams, as well as the hospital management, is of paramount importance to provide optimal care [12]. In particular, the infection control team is central to establishing an infection control policy in the hospital and delivering it rapidly and accurately to health care workers while also responding to national policy changes. In communicating the policy and information, the team usually uses the hospital's intranet.

This study aimed to collect information announced on a hospital intranet by infection control teams and apply a text network analysis to confirm information changes during the COVID-19 pandemic. The intention was to provide essential data for preparing measures for medical institutions based on the early stages of the pandemic to cope more effectively with a future infectious disease crisis.

This study aimed to characterize the responses of medical institutions according to the time of COVID-19 transmission using text network analysis. This study explored and compared essential keywords based on network centrality indicators (meaning morphemes) provided to medical personnel by the infection control teams of medical institutions. The study also compared changes in those keywords between periods and identified differences between topic groups.

2. Materials and Methods

2.1. Design

This study applied text mining to large amounts of data to analyze the notices on in-hospital strategies towards COVID-19 and to identify changes in the coping strategies of hospitals towards COVID-19 changes.

2.2. Data

Electronic notices were searched that were announced from 1 January to 31 August 2020 by the infection control teams of 12 university hospitals in 5 regions (Seoul, Gyeonggi-do, Daejeon, Chungcheongnam-do, Jeollanam-do) of South Korea. The average number of beds in participating institutions was 940.6 $\pm$ 389.3, and all participating institutions were designated hospitals for infectious diseases designated by the country.

A total of 1653 cases and 50,567 sentences were identified throughout the search.

2.3. Measurements and Data Analysis

This study was conducted in the order of extensive data collection, preprocessing and analysis.

2.3.1. Preprocessing

To extract morphemes—the least meaningful unit—from the unstructured text notices of the infection control teams, each notice was organized into one row of an Excel spreadsheet. Data keywords were extracted using the "Semantic Network Module". NetMiner software (version 4.0, Cyram, Seoul) was used to analyze the relationships between keywords. A co-occurrence matrix was constructed before performing a text network analysis. When extracting keywords, general verbs and nouns unrelated to the content and general terms that are rarely considered key research concepts (e.g., special symbols, additional vocabulary and vocabulary with no direct influence) were removed [13]. The term frequency (TF) indicates the importance of words within a document, and document frequency (DF) indicates how many documents a word appears in. The inverse document frequency (IDF) is the reciprocal of DF and is expressed as a logarithmic value. However, a word with a high TF value is not necessarily a keyword in the document because the same word can also be used in other documents. The IDF value of the words that commonly appear in different sets of documents was calculated and excluded from core word extraction. In other words, the term frequency-inverse document frequency (TF-IDF) indicates the importance of a word in a document as a more significant value multiplied by TF and IDF, meaning the word is frequently used in that document [14].

2.3.2. Centrality Analysis

To determine the frequency of words appearing, we identified the simple frequency of words appearing in the entire network and the number of documents in which words appeared, and then analyzed TF-IDF values. In creating a network where centrality is calculated, the documentation unit was designated a one-day notice when calculating connect lines and simultaneous appearances between words. To understand the relationship between keywords, we used the text network analysis method to form a word network that links the frequency of simultaneous expression between words. To create a word network, we transformed the 2-mode form between word and document into a 1-mode network between word and word, based on this analysis of degree centrality, closeness centrality and betweenness centrality.

2.3.3. Topic Modeling

Topic modeling is a tool used in text mining to identify meaningful patterns between many documents [15,16]. The topic is the probability distribution in which highly associated words are included in the document. In this study, we used latent Dirichlet allocation (LDA)—an algorithm for identifying hidden topics in a document—to model each document's main words and classification [16,17]. Based on prior studies on LDA input options [17,18], a topic analysis was performed by setting the following Markov chain Monte Carlo parameters: alpha = 1.44, beta = 0.001 and 1000 iterations [14,18]. The results of several simulations of the topic analysis were verified by all researchers and infection control specialists, who agreed on a four-stage topic model. A word cloud was created to determine the major words of the determined topics intuitively. The top 100~110 words were extracted according to a topic to identify the core topics. The connectivity degree was analyzed, and the topic-keyword map was visualized using the topic-word two-mode network.

3. Results

3.1. Centrality Analysis

Table 1 lists (in order) words with high TF-IDF values, which indicates the importance of words within the electronic notices announced by the infection control teams.

Table 1. Top 30 keywords extracted from electronic notices over time.

Rank	Stage 1: 1 Jan. to 26 Jan. 2020		Stage 2: 27 Jan. to 22 Feb. 2020		Stage 3: 23 Feb. to 7 May 2020		Stage 4: 8 May to 31 August 2020	
	Sentences (n = 211)		Sentences (n = 523)		Sentences (n = 863)		Sentences (n = 1268)	
	Keywords after Processing (n = 376)		Keywords after Processing (n = 512)		Keywords after Processing (n = 558)		Keywords after Processing (n = 637)	
	Keyword	TF-IDF	Keyword	TF-IDF	Keyword	TF-IDF	Keyword	TF-IDF
1	Person on duty	1.8	Operation	1.1	Hospital inflow	1.4	Caregiver	1.4
2	Nation of occurrence	1.4	Daegu-Gyeongbuk	1	Public health center	1.3	Health	1.3
3	Sore throat	1.4	Texting	0.9	Endoscope	1.2	Cohort ward	1.3
4	Countermeasure	1.2	Case definition	0.9	Level D	1.2	Mobile	1.2
5	Restrict visits	1.2	Travel restrictions	0.9	Schedule	1.2	Texting	1.2
6	Cough	1.1	Management	0.9	Central disaster control headquarters	1.2	Suspected case	1.2
7	Pneumonia of unknown origin	1.1	Visited China	0.9	Infectious disease	1.1	Intensive care unit	1.2
8	Visited China	1.1	Attend	0.9	Resident caregiver	1.1	Commuting to and from work	1.2
9	Respiratory symptoms	1.1	Shutdown	0.9	Convalescent hospital	1.1	Academic conference	1.2
10	Caregiver for the sick	1	Overseas travel	0.9	Support	1.1	Restriction of work	1.1
11	Specimen	1	Drug utilization review (DUR)	0.8	Clinic	1.1	Agency head	1.1
12	Vigilance stage	1	N95 mask	0.8	Within 14 days	1	Asymptomatic	1.1
13	Hospital beds	1	Specimen	0.8	Infectious disease report	1	Public health center	1.1
14	Admission	1	Recommendation	0.8	On duty	1	Resident caregiver	1.1
15	Contact	1	Restrict visits	0.8	Salary	1	Restaurant	1.1
16	Infectious disease response center	0.9	Occurred area	0.8	Target person	1	Meal	1.1
17	Personal protective equipment	0.9	Fever	0.8	Cohabitant	1	Epidemiological investigation	1.1

Table 1. *Cont.*

Rank	Stage 1: 1 Jan. to 26 Jan. 2020		Stage 2: 27 Jan. to 22 Feb. 2020		Stage 3: 23 Feb. to 7 May 2020		Stage 4: 8 May to 31 August 2020	
	Sentences (n = 211)		Sentences (n = 523)		Sentences (n = 863)		Sentences (n = 1268)	
	Keywords after Processing (n = 376)		Keywords after Processing (n = 512)		Keywords after Processing (n = 558)		Keywords after Processing (n = 637)	
	Keyword	TF-IDF	Keyword	TF-IDF	Keyword	TF-IDF	Keyword	TF-IDF
18	Examination	0.9	Caregiver	0.8	Visitor	1	Emergency room	1.1
19	Surgical mask	0.9	Screening questionnaire	0.8	Hospital rooms	1	Attention phase	1.1
20	Management	0.9	Screening clinic	0.8	Seoul or Gyeonggi	1	Organizer	1.1
21	Epidemic	0.9	Unknown origin pneumonia	0.8	Screening questionnaire	1	Central disaster control headquarters	1.1
22	Doctor	0.9	Risk factors	0.8	Health Insurance Review and Assessment Service	1	Clinics	1.1
23	Movement	0.9	Negative result	0.8	National safe clinics	1	Treatment	1.1
24	Entry to country	0.9	Visited Japan	0.8	Risk factors	1	Event	1.1
25	Provide information	0.9	Reception	0.8	Negative results	1	2 m	1
26	Proper use of PPE	0.9	Information	0.8	Healthcare personnel	1	Personal protective equipment	1
27	Entry to hospital	0.9	Restriction	0.8	Self-quarantine	1	Recommendation	1
28	International Traveler Information System (ITS)	0.8	Action	0.8	Transmission	1	Karaoke	1
29	Reinforcement	0.8	Procedure	0.8	Mass outbreak	1	Occupational Safety and Health Management Office	1
30	Upgrade	0.8	Entrance	0.8	Prevention of spread	1	Operation	1
31	Alarm signal	0.8	Statistical Reporting	0.8	Environmental management	1	Approval	1
32	Stages of Interest	0.8	Control	0.8	Drug utilization review (DUR)	0.9	Facility inspection	1
33	Local public health center	0.8	Academic conference	0.8	Polymerase chain reaction (PCR)	0.9	Trainees	1
34	Return to country of origin	0.8	Test results	0.7	Infection controls	0.9	Negative results	1

Table 1. *Cont.*

Rank	Stage 1: 1 Jan. to 26 Jan. 2020		Stage 2: 27 Jan. to 22 Feb. 2020		Stage 3: 23 Feb. to 7 May 2020		Stage 4: 8 May to 31 August 2020	
	Sentences (n = 211)		Sentences (n = 523)		Sentences (n = 863)		Sentences (n = 1268)	
	Keywords after Processing (n = 376)		Keywords after Processing (n = 512)		Keywords after Processing (n = 558)		Keywords after Processing (n = 637)	
	Keyword	TF-IDF	Keyword	TF-IDF	Keyword	TF-IDF	Keyword	TF-IDF
35	Cough etiquette	0.8	Sharing	0.7	Recommendations	0.9	Admission	1
36	Visitor management	0.8	Return to nation	0.7	Confirmed cases	0.9	Religious facilities	1
37	Screening clinic	0.8	Hospital visitor	0.7	Fever	0.9	Attendance	1
38	Risk alert phase	0.8	Visited Southeast Asia	0.7	Fever respiratory clinic	0.9	Control	1
39	Press release	0.8	Visited Macao	0.7	Department head	0.9	Infection controls	0.9
40	Mass outbreak	0.8	Restrict visits	0.7	Screening clinic	0.9	Wearing personal protective equipment	0.9

3.2. Topic Modeling

Based on the stepwise keywords shown in the topic modeling analysis, we identified four representative topics based on consensus among the researchers and in consultation with four infection control experts: (1) "Understanding the new infectious disease", (2) "Preparation of a patient care and management system", (3) "Prevention of spread and securing employee safety" and (4) "Improvement of the management system according to the revision of guidelines" (Table 2). For each topic, a network of keywords for the words with higher probabilities of appearing is visualized in Figure 1a–d.

The important keywords that made up the phase-1 topic were "COVID-19", "Case definition", "Unknown origin pneumonia", and "Korea Disease Control and Prevention Agency". Based on these keywords, this first stage was related to obtaining information on the new infectious disease, such as its definition, methods of transmission, areas of occurrence and legal reporting standards. The first-stage topic was, therefore, "Understanding the new infectious disease". The important keywords that comprised the phase-2 topic were "Screening clinic", "Polymerase chain reaction (PCR)", "Infectious disease report", "Statistical reporting", "Occurrence status" and "Response instruction". These keywords were related to the process of establishing an overall system for patient selection, medical treatment, diagnostic test implementation and confirmation of test results when suspected or confirmed patients visit medical institutions. Based on this interpretation, the second-stage topic was "Preparation of a patient care and management system". The important keywords that comprised the phase-3 topic were "Confirmed case", "Movement path", "Personal protective equipment (PPE)" and "Notice". Based on keywords, the third stage was interpreted as preventing new coronavirus infections from entering medical institutions and strengthening employee safety to avoid faculty members who work on suspected or confirmed coronavirus patients from becoming infected. The third-stage topic was named "Prevention of spread and ensuring employee safety". The important keywords that made up the phase-4 topic were "Entrance", "Changed items", "Medical examination by interview", "Management process" and "Guideline". Based on the keywords, the fourth-step topic was "Improvement of the management system according to the revision of guidelines". As the COVID-19 pandemic continued, the guidelines and standards provided by government agencies in the early stages were continuously revised and supplemented.

Table 2. Topic modeling of four stages.

Keyword	1st	2nd	3rd	4th	5th	6th	7th	8th	9th	10th	11th	12th	13th	14th	15th
Stage 1 (topic 1)	China	COVID-19	Wuhan	Case definition	Unknown origin pneumonia	Korea Centers for Disease Control and Prevention	Expansion	Domestic	DUR (drug utilization review)	Entry to country	Community	Declaration	Information	Response procedure	Announcement
Stage 2 (topic 2)	Clinic	Screening clinic	In hospital	PCR (polymerase chain reaction)	Infectious disease report	Statistical reporting	Consultation details	Occurrence status	Response instructions	Test results	Process	Examination	Doctor	Spread	Negative results
Stage 3 (topic 3)	Confirmed case	Movement path	Personal protective equipment	COVID-19	Notice	Medical examination by interview	Situation room	Level D	Proper use of PPE	Path	Doctor	Support	Specimen	Screening questionnaire	Suspected case
Stage 4 (topic 4)	COVID-19	Entrance	Changed items	Process	Medical examination by interview	Management process	Guideline	Response	Management	Visitor	Notice	Mobile	Spread	Control	Revision

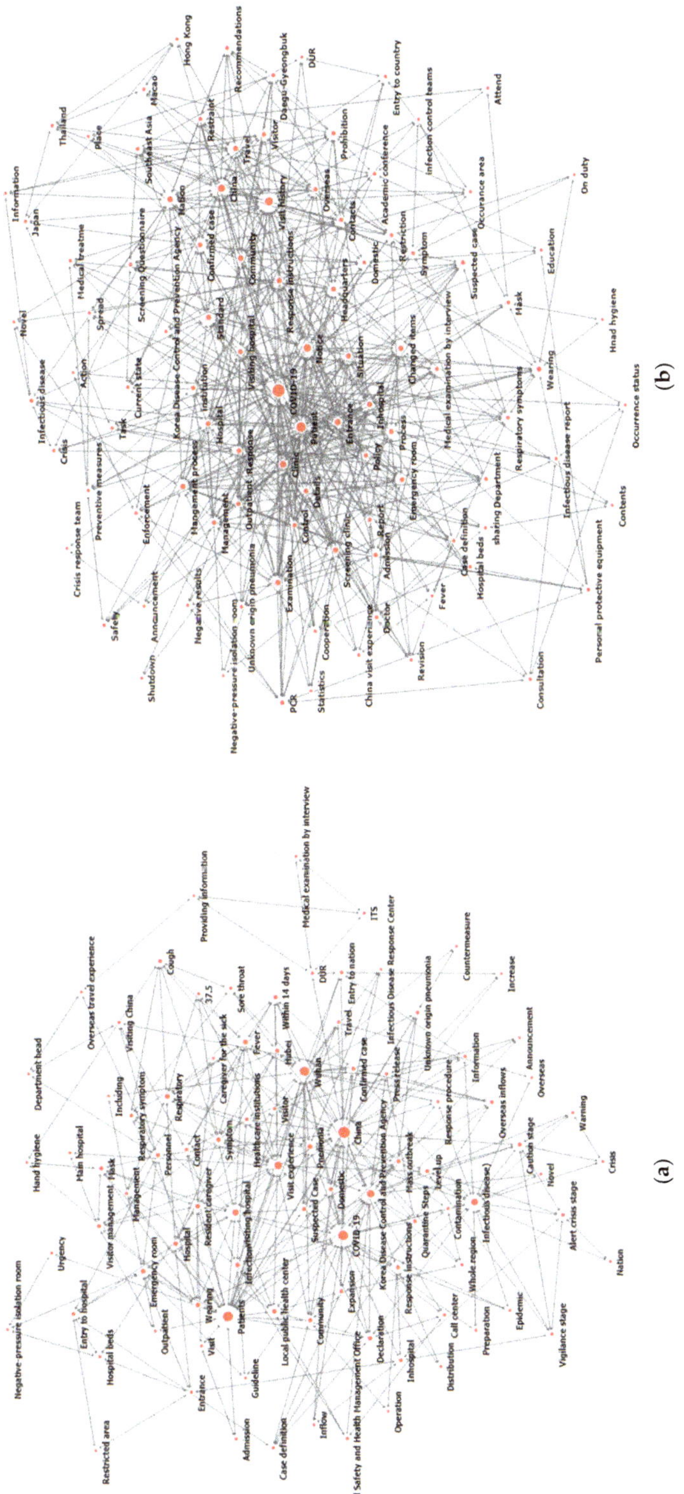

Figure 1. *Cont.*

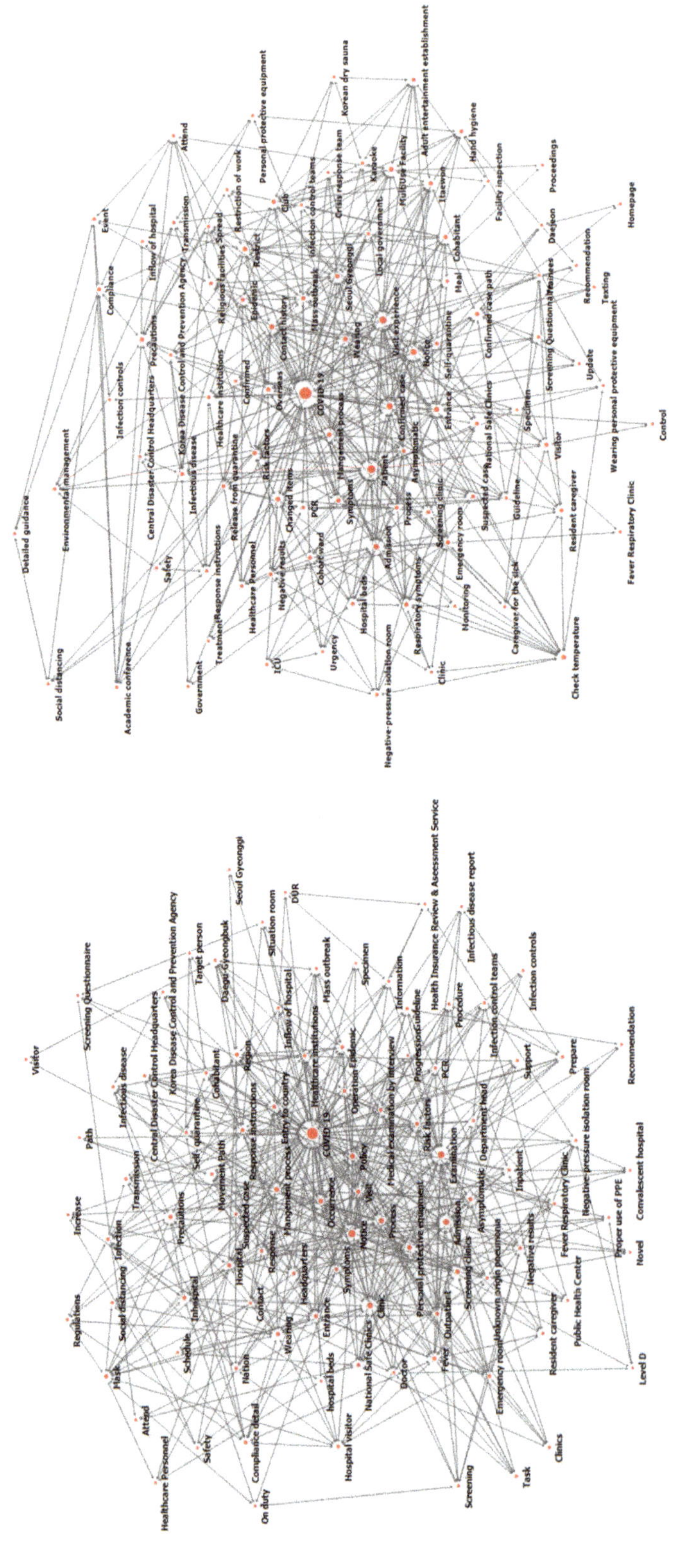

Figure 1. Keyword network of four-step crisis response: **(a)** Stage 1, **(b)** Stage 2, **(c)** Stage 3, **(d)** Stage 4.

4. Discussion

This study attempted to characterize the response strategies of medical institutions during the early stages of the COVID-19 pandemic by applying the topic modeling method to information announced on the intranet by the infection control team of a university hospital in South Korea. The eight months at the beginning of the pandemic were divided into four stages by accounting for the number of confirmed patients in South Korea, the number of confirmed patients overall, the spread pattern and the infectious disease crisis stage declared by the government.

The first stage is "Understanding of the new infectious disease", regarding when Chinese health authorities reported to the WHO that pneumonia was continuously presenting in Wuhan, China and until the first COVID-19 patient occurred in South Korea. There was a lack of information on the infectious disease after its initial outbreak, and the main keywords were "China", "COVID-19", "Wuhan", "case definition", "pneumonia" and "Korea Centers for Disease Control and Prevention". During this time, understanding the disease took precedence in reducing the risk of the disease developing. The Korea Centers for Disease Control and Prevention established COVID-19 case definitions and medical institution response guidelines and has distributed them since January 2020 [19]. Based on guidelines distributed by the Korea Centers for Disease Control and Prevention and related organizations (e.g., Centers for Disease Control and Prevention, WHO), medical institutions prepared for patient occurrences by organizing their knowledge of new infectious diseases, such as knowledge about case definition, diagnosis method, transmission method and patient management method, and providing information via the intranet. As the spread of infectious diseases can be prevented by blocking the transmission path [20], providing appropriate information may help reduce hospital staff's anxiety [21]. COVID-19 is a respiratory infectious disease [22], thus affected patients cannot be distinguished by symptoms alone. COVID-19 initially spread around Wuhan, therefore it was essential to check the history of those who visited the affected area to classify suspected patients. In South Korea, errors could be reduced, and work efficiency could be improved by having the drug utilization review (DUR) system check immigration records.

The second stage is "preparing a patient care and management system". Transmission of COVID-19 into the country is limited. This stage lasted until the first patient occurred in Daegu, when the Ministry of Health and Welfare in South Korea raised the infectious disease crisis alert stage to "alert". South Korea is currently coping with infectious disease epidemics by dividing the crisis warning system into four stages. The first is the stage of interest and refers to the occurrence and epidemic of new infectious diseases abroad. The stage of caution is when new infectious diseases from overseas have moved into South Korea, and the alert stage is when these new infectious diseases have limited transmission. The severe stage (or "Red stage") is the status when the new infectious diseases are introduced and widely spread into the local community or nationwide in South Korea [23]. During the limited spread of infectious diseases in South Korea, medical institutions strengthened their preparedness for the presence of confirmed cases. Medical institutions had to accurately understand the disaster response measures from the government and be familiar with the way to exchange information within medical institutions and how to report to government agencies in the event of a confirmed case so that information sharing could be rapidly performed. It was also necessary at this time to establish a patient treatment and management system to cope with the occurrence of many cases. The main keywords were, therefore, "treatment", "screening clinic", "hospital", "PCR", "infectious disease report", "statistical report", "counselling details", "occurrence status", "response guidelines", "test results", "process" and "test".

The medical institution established an overall response system for patient selection, treatment, diagnostic tests and test result confirmation when a patient visited with suspected or confirmed COVID-19. Operating systems such as patient screening, isolation and management methods were also established to keep confirmed patients from entering medical institutions and prevent cross-infection when patients entered the medical institution.

In 2015, South Korea operated a screening station for people with respiratory diseases at medical institutions during the Middle Eastern respiratory syndrome (MERS) epidemic [24]. The respiratory disease screening clinic allows patients with respiratory symptoms to enter the medical institution only after checking their symptoms and disease history at a separate clinic [25]. This system not only contributes to patient safety by preventing the spread of infectious diseases within the hospital, but also helps to maintain the psychological health of inpatients. Medical institutions should systematize and prepare a response system for the entire disaster system before a confirmed patient presents in the hospital. The Joint Commission on Accreditation of Healthcare Organizations in the United States mandated that medical institutions establish a comprehensive plan for disasters both in and out of hospitals [26]. Medical institutions should form committees that oversee overall decision-making, the establishment of patient care and operation plans, and utilization of physical resources such as preparing related facilities, deploying necessary personnel, allocating specific tasks, and providing and training necessary personnel. Medical institutions that are evaluated by medical institutions in South Korea construct regulations and guidelines for patient management procedures to prepare for infectious disease epidemics and require faculty members to conduct disaster response training once a year. Medical institutions reorganized the existing response system appropriately for the COVID-19 pandemic. Since then, confirmed case numbers exploded around religious facilities in Daegu [27], and the government upgraded the infectious disease crisis alert to the highest level, "Red".

The third stage relates to upgrading to the "Red" level during an outbreak centered in the Itaewon area of Seoul. This period is a stage of "Prevention of spread and securing employee safety". The main keywords were "confirmed patients", "movement routes", "PPE", "new coronavirus infections", "notices", "interviews", "situation rooms", "level D protective equipment", "changing", "moving", "doctors" and "support". Medical institutions strengthened their communication by allowing the active sharing of information related to confirmed patients, such as movement routes. At the same time, faculty members tried to block the inflow of patients with confirmed COVID-19 into medical institutions and prevent the spread throughout the hospital. Another focus was preventing infection via suspected COVID-19 cases or medical workers caring for confirmed patients. Due to the rapid increase in the number of patients with COVID-19 in the community, the occurrence of confirmed cases and cross-infection in hospitals also increased. To prevent the spread of infection throughout the hospital, medical examinations based on visit history to areas in epidemics and the symptoms of these cases were strengthened for visitors, patients and employees. These preliminary examinations are essential to prevent the spread of diseases in medical institutions since they can minimize the risk of infection exposure by rapidly identifying suspected infection cases [28,29]. PPE is a primary and physical defense against exposure to patients' blood and body fluids [29]. To prevent employee infection, selecting PPE appropriate for the situation and wearing and taking it off in the correct way is crucial [30]. Halcomb et al. [31] stated that during the COVID-19 epidemic, a protocol for appropriate PPE supply and the wearing and removing of PPE is needed. During the early stages of the pandemic, medical workers had a high risk of infection due to the severe PPE shortage. In particular, masks are an essential type of PPE for preventing respiratory infections in employees, and N95 masks used in the care of patients with COVID-19 must be fully attached to the face of the user to be effective, thus they should be selected and utilized only after performing a fitting test [32]. Halcomb et al. [31] suggested that nurses must be provided with appropriate PPE and knowledgeable about workplace factors to ensure that patients receive high-quality treatment during the COVID-19 pandemic. Medical institutions, therefore, need to mandate stocking an adequate amount of PPE in preparation for new infectious disease outbreaks, and medical staff should be able to recognize N95 masks suitable for them through regular fitting tests and skillfully wearing and taking off PPE through routine repeated training [33].

The fourth stage is the "Improvement of the management system according to the revision of guidelines" and was based on the spread in Itaewon, Seoul, which changed from a specific regional-oriented trend to a national movement on 31 August 2020. The main keywords for this period were "new coronavirus infections", "entrances", "changes", "processes", "interviews", "management processes", "guidelines", "responses", "operations", "visitors", "notices" and "mobile devices". The response guidelines distributed by the government at the beginning were revised and supplemented as the COVID-19 pandemic progressed. Medical institutions further revised and applied these guidelines to suit their specific situations, and the management and operation systems continuously improved to increase the efficiency of the provided healthcare. For example, the medical institution entrance questionnaire was initially prepared in hardcopy form and was computerized using a mobile authentication method. As the COVID-19 management guidelines and operating systems were repeatedly changed, it was very important to deliver the information rapidly and accurately in a way the subjects could understand.

Information delivery methods used in crises include meetings, the intranet, e-mail, newsletters and text messages [34]. Depending on the situation and subject, there may be differences in their effectiveness, making it necessary to consider and apply appropriate methods. Halcomb et al. [31] suggested the importance of regular delivery of information, such as standardized protocols for clinical treatment and up-to-date information on COVID-19, which requires high levels of communication support during the pandemic. Peiffer-Smadja et al. [12] reported that it is a new challenge to communicate the changed guidelines to all health care workers, as the guidelines very frequently change. Therefore, when communicating large amounts of frequently changed information, it should be communicated in a consistent and clear manner to avoid confusion. In the case of important changes, it is also necessary to consider a method to check whether the health care workers are familiar.

5. Conclusions

New infectious diseases can cause significant losses due to their spread if hospital personnel are not prepared during the early stages of the outbreak. In South Korea, medical institutions in 2015 experienced a disastrous situation regarding infectious diseases as they were the center of the MERS epidemic. With this opportunity, both the government and medical institutions checked and overhauled the problems of the infectious disease crisis management system and organizational structure. This experience served as an essential foundation for the government and medical institutions to respond more quickly and appropriately in the early stages of the COVID-19 pandemic. This study analyzed the preparation and response efforts of medical institutions from the time a COVID-19 case was confirmed in Wuhan until it became prevalent throughout South Korea. These four stages can be applied regardless of the type of infectious disease and the size of medical institutions; therefore, they should be used as reference materials to prepare for the future outbreak of new infectious diseases. However, the generalizability of the study's findings is limited by the analysis only being performed on text information provided by 12 medical institutions through the intranet.

Since it takes considerable time to prepare for various items that are necessary to cope with infectious diseases immediately and quickly (organization of response teams, the establishment of treatment systems, resource allocation, education, training, etc.), it is necessary to efficiently prepare for non-pandemic situations. Novel infectious diseases can be prepared for quickly and effectively by obtaining information on the transmission route and the area of occurrence. Therefore, personnel in charge of sensitively collecting and communicating information related to infectious diseases are needed in a medical institution. More systematic preparation is possible with governmental support.

This study included only crisis preparation and response processes for eight months after the initial outbreak due to the prolonged COVID-19 pandemic period. In the future, it will be necessary to research the process of recovering from the disaster situation after the end of the pandemic. A model that integrates the response strategies of medical institutions' early stages and resilience stages is also recommended.

Author Contributions: K.-S.C. designed the research project and methodology, contributed to the draft of manuscript and revised the final version. E.-M.K. designed the research project, conducted the data analysis and interpreted the data, contributed to the draft of the manuscript and revised the final version of manuscript. All authors have read and agreed to the published version of the manuscript.

Funding: This work was supported by a National Research Foundation of Korea grant funded by the government of South Korea (NRF-2020R1F1A1055437).

Institutional Review Board Statement: Not applicable.

Informed Consent Statement: Not applicable.

Data Availability Statement: The data used and/or analyzed during the current study are available from the corresponding author on request.

Conflicts of Interest: The authors declare no conflict of interest.

References

1. Tian, S.; Hu, W.; Niu, L.; Liu, H.; Xu, H.; Xiao, S.Y. Pulmonary pathology of early-phase 2019 novel coronavirus (COVID-19) pneumonia in two patients with lung cancer. *J. Thorac. Oncol.* **2020**, *15*, 700–704. [CrossRef] [PubMed]
2. World Health Organization. Timeline of WHO's Response to COVID-19. Available online: https://www.who.int/emergencies/diseases/novel-coronavirus-2019/interactivetimeline?gclid=CjwKCAiAnO2MBhApEiwA8q0HYZmGtn5Enkk635nMY238tWplCdqerVcZw4KPxTDAtXDx_203AWCAjBoCJZQQAvD_BwE#event-115 (accessed on 12 November 2021).
3. Cha, K.S.; Shin, M.J.; Lee, J.Y.; Chun, H.K. The role of infection control nurse during emerging infectious disease epidemic: Focusing on the Middle East respiratory syndrome. *Korean J. Healthc. Assoc. Infect. Control Prev.* **2017**, *22*, 31–41. [CrossRef]
4. Barranco, R.; Vallega Bernucci Du Tremoul, L.; Ventura, F. Hospital-acquired SARS-CoV-2 infections in patients: Inevitable conditions or medical malpractice? *Int. J. Environ. Res. Public Health* **2021**, *18*, 489. [CrossRef]
5. International Council of Nurses. More than 600 Nurses Die from COVID-19 Worldwide. Available online: http://www.icn.ch/news/more-600-nurses-die-covid-19-worldwide (accessed on 3 June 2020).
6. Lee, S.Y. Policy directions and tasks for responding to COVID-19. *Issue Focus.* **2020**, *386*, 1–7.
7. Shen, Y.; Cui, Y.; Li, N.; Tian, C.; Chen, M.; Zhang, Y.W.; Huang, Y.Z.; Chen, H.; Kong, Q.F.; Zhang, Q.; et al. Emergency responses to COVID-19 outbreak: Experiences and lessons from a general hospital in Nanjing, China. *Cardiovasc. Interv. Radiol.* **2020**, *43*, 810–819. [CrossRef] [PubMed]
8. Petak, W.J. Emergency management: A challenge for public administration. *Public Adm. Rev.* **1985**, *45*, 3–7. [CrossRef]
9. McLoughlin, D. A framework for integrated emergency management. *Public Adm. Rev.* **1985**, *45*, 165–172. [CrossRef]
10. Comfort, L.K.; Sungu, Y.; Johnson, D.; Dunn, M. Complex system in crisis: Anticipation and resilience in dynamic environments. *J. Contingencies Crisis Manag.* **2001**, *9*, 144–158. [CrossRef]
11. Farazmand, A. Introduction Crisis and emergency management. In *Handbook of Crisis and Emergency Management*; Farazmand, A., Ed.; Marcel Dekker Inc.: New York, NY, USA, 2001; pp. 1–8.
12. Peiffer-Smadja, N.; Lucet, J.C.; Bendjelloul, G.; Bouadma, L.; Gerard, S.; Choquet, C.; Jacques, S.; Khalil, A.; Maisani, P.; Casalino, E.; et al. Challenges and issues about organizing a hospital to respond to the COVID-19 outbreak: Experience from a French reference centre. *Clin. Microbiol. Infect.* **2020**, *26*, 669–672. [CrossRef] [PubMed]
13. Paranyushkin, D. Visualization of text's polysingularity using network analysis. *Comput. Sci.* **2012**, *2*, 256–278.
14. Griffiths, T.L.; Steyvers, M. Finding scientific topics. *Proc. Natl. Acad. Sci. USA* **2004**, *101*, 5228–5235. [CrossRef] [PubMed]
15. Aggarwal, C.C. An introduction to social network data analytics. In *Social Network Data Analytics*; Aggarwal, C.C., Ed.; Springer: Boston, MA, USA, 2011; pp. 1–15.
16. Greene, D.; O'Callaghan, D.; Cunningham, P. How many topics? Stability analysis for topic models. In *Machine Learning and Knowledge Discovery in Databases*; Calders, T., Esposito, F., Hullermeier, E., Meo, R., Eds.; Springer: Berlin/Heidelberg, Germany, 2014; pp. 498–513.
17. Park, E.J.; Kim, Y.J.; Park, C.S. A comparison of hospice care research topics between Korea and other countries using text network analysis. *J. Korean Acad. Nurs.* **2017**, *47*, 600–612. [CrossRef] [PubMed]
18. Lee, S.S. A study on the application of topic modeling for the book report text. *J. Korean Libr. Inf. Sci. Soc.* **2016**, *47*, 1–18.
19. Gyeonggi Infectious Disease Control Center. COVID-19 Guidelines and References. 2021. Available online: http://www.gidcc.or.kr/epvbr/%ec%bd%94%eb%a1%9c%eb%82%98%eb%b0%94%ec%9d%b4%eb%9f%ac%ec%8a%a4%ea%b0%90%ec%97%bc%ec%a6%9d-19covid-19/ (accessed on 23 September 2021).
20. Boly, F.J.; Fraser, V.J.; Kwon, J.H. Basics of healthcare epidemiology and infection prevention. In *Mayhall's Hospital Epidemiology and Infection Prevention*; Weber, D., Talbot, T., Eds.; Lippincott Williams & Wilkins: Philadelphia, PA, USA, 2021; pp. 1–20.
21. Wu, A.W.; Connors, C.; Everly, G.S., Jr. COVID-19: Peer support and crisis communication strategies to promote institutional resilience. *Ann. Intern. Med.* **2020**, *172*, 822–823. [CrossRef] [PubMed]
22. Central Disaster Management Headquarters, Central Disease Control Headquarters. Coronavirus (COVID-19), Republic of Korea: About COVID-19. 2021. Available online: http://ncov.mohw.go.kr/en/ (accessed on 23 November 2021).

23. Ministry of Food and Drug Safety. Infectious Disease Disaster Crisis Response Practical Manual. *Cheongju-si: Ministry of Food and Drug Safety*. 2019. Available online: https://www.mfds.go.kr/brd/m_218/view.do?seq=33284&srchFr=&srchTo=&srchWord=&srchTp=&itm_seq_1=0&itm_seq_2=0&multi_itm_seq=0&company_cd=&company_nm=&page=1 (accessed on 12 November 2021).
24. Lee, S.K.; Lee, S.K.; Kang, K.W. Appropriateness of screening clinic response in proliferation of MERS. *Asia-Pac. J. Multimed. Serv. Converg. Art Humanit. Sociol.* **2017**, *7*, 535–543. [CrossRef]
25. The Korean Society of Infectious Diseases. MERS Response Guidelines: Small and Medium Hospitals. 2015. Available online: https://www.ksid.or.kr/mail/file/MERS04.pdf (accessed on 9 December 2021).
26. Lee, O.C.; Gu, J.A.; Kim, Y.J.; Kim, O.S.; Kim, E.K. *Emergency and Disaster Nursing*, 4th ed.; Hyenmoonsa: Seoul, Korea, 2015; pp. 1–120.
27. Daegu Metropolitan City. Daegu COVID-19. Available online: http://covid19.daegu.go.kr/00937420.html (accessed on 16 November 2021).
28. Palmore, T.N.; Smith, B.A. COVID-19: General Approach to Infection Control in the Health Care Setting. Available online: https://www.uptodate.com/contents/covid-19-general-approach-to-infection-control-in-the-health-care-setting (accessed on 6 August 2021).
29. Sickbert-Bennett, E.E.; Dibiase, L.M. Infectious Disease Surveillance in Healthcare Settings. In *Mayhall's Hospital Epidemiology and Infection Prevention*; Weber, D.J., Talbot, T.R., Eds.; Wolters Kluwer: Alphen aan den Rijn, The Netherlands, 2020; pp. 21–30.
30. Alajmi, J.; Jeremijenko, A.M.; Abraham, J.C.; Alishaq, M.; Concepcion, E.G.; Butt, A.A.; Abou-Samra, A.B. COVID-19 infection among healthcare workers in a national healthcare system: The Qatar experience. *Int. J. Infect. Dis.* **2020**, *100*, 386–389. [CrossRef] [PubMed]
31. Halcomb, E.; Williams, A.; Ashley, C.; McInnes, S.; Stephen, C.; Calma, K.; James, S. The support needs of Australian primary health care nurses during the COVID-19 pandemic. *J. Nurs. Manag.* **2020**, *28*, 1553–1560. [CrossRef] [PubMed]
32. Zhuang, Z.; Bradtmiller, B.; Shaffer, R.E. New respirator fit test panels representing the current U.S. civilian work force. *J. Occup. Environ. Hyg.* **2007**, *4*, 647–659. [CrossRef] [PubMed]
33. Kang, J.H. Simulation results for contamination comparisons by various use protocols of personal protective equipment. *J. Korean Med. Sci.* **2018**, *93*, 41–49. [CrossRef]
34. Johansen, W.; Aggerholm, H.K.; Frandsen, F. Entering new territory: A study of internal crisis management and crisis communication in organizations. *Public Relat. Rev.* **2012**, *38*, 270–279. [CrossRef]

International Journal of
Environmental Research and Public Health

MDPI

Article

Factors Predicting Post-Traumatic Positive and Negative Psychological Changes Experienced by Nurses during a Pandemic COVID-19: A Cross-Sectional Study

Grzegorz Józef Nowicki [1,*], Barbara Ślusarska [1], Bożena Zboina [2], Aneta Jędrzejewska [1] and Marzena Kotus [3]

[1] Department of Family and Geriatric Nursing, Medical University of Lublin, Staszica 6 Str., PL-20-081 Lublin, Poland; basiaslusarska@gmail.com (B.Ś.); jedrzejewska.ab@gmail.com (A.J.)
[2] Department of Pedagogy and Health Sciences, College of Business and Entreprise, Akademicka 20 Str., PL-27-400 Ostrowiec Świetokrzyski, Poland; bozenazboina@poczta.fm
[3] Department of Anaesthesiological and Intensive Care Nursing, Medical University of Lublin, Chodźki 7 Str., PL-20-093 Lublin, Poland; marzenakotus@umlub.pl
* Correspondence: gnowicki84@gmail.com; Tel.: +48-814-486-810

Abstract: It is common knowledge that COVID-19 affects physiopathological changes in all systems of the human body. On the other hand, events related to the COVID-19 pandemic also have a significant impact on the social and mental sphere of human functioning. The aim of this study is to determine the relationship between selected sociodemographic variables and selected subjective cognitive resources, and the positive and negative perception of the consequences of the COVID-19 pandemic in a group of nurses working in Poland. The computer-assisted web interviewing method was conducted between 1 and 15 May 2020. Participants were requested to complete the following questionnaires: The Changes in Outlook Questionnaire (CIOQ), The Impact Event Scale-Revised (IES-R), The Multidimensional Scale of Perceived Social Support (MSPSS), The Safety Experience Questionnaire (SEQ), and The Meaning in Life Questionnaire (MLQ). Three-hundred and twenty fivenurses working all over Poland participated in the study. Their mean age was 39.18 ± 11.16 years. A higher average level was noted among the surveyed nurses in the Positive Change subscale (18.56 ± 4.04). In a multivariate model, taking into account both sociodemographic and cognitive variables, the level of perceived traumatic stress, the level of social support, a sense of security, reflection on safety and a sense of meaning and meaning in life were independent predictors of a positive perception of the consequences of the COVID-19 pandemic. Those variables explained as much as 37% of the dependent variable, and the nature of the relationship was positive. While we are still a long way from understanding the full range of the long-term impact of the COVID-19 pandemic on mental health and psychosocial well-being, it is possible that in this challenging context there are many individual resources available to perceive the effects of the current pandemic positively. Therefore, they should be strengthened through the development and implementation of intervention programs to improve the mental state of nurses.

Keywords: COVID-19; pandemic; nurses; changes in outlook; post-traumatic growth; influencing factors

Citation: Nowicki, G.J.; Ślusarska, B.; Zboina, B.; Jędrzejewska, A.; Kotus, M. Factors Predicting Post-Traumatic Positive and Negative Psychological Changes Experienced by Nurses during a Pandemic COVID-19: A Cross-Sectional Study. *Int. J. Environ. Res. Public Health* **2022**, *19*, 7073. https://doi.org/10.3390/ijerph19127073

Academic Editors: Richard Gray and Sonia Udod

Received: 22 April 2022
Accepted: 2 June 2022
Published: 9 June 2022

1. Introduction

According to the World Health Organization (WHO) [1], the Corona Virus Disease 2019 (COVID-19) pandemic of March 2020 [2] is the most significant global public health threat, placing enormous pressure on healthcare systems. Among the various occupational groups, health care workers (HCW) are most vulnerable to adverse effects related to the pandemic, especially in the field of mental health [3]. Moreover, HCWs represent systemically important professions, which means that their work is necessary, and the demand for it increases in a pandemic.

COVID-19 influences physiopathological changes in all human body systems, especially the immune and respiratory systems. On the other hand, events related to the pandemic also significantly impact the social and mental sphere of human functioning [4,5]. Research shows that HCWs are at high risk of developing mental stress and other adverse mental health symptoms due to exposure to COVID-19 in healthcare settings [6,7]. The results of the available literature reviews also emphasise that fear of infection and transmission of the virus to family members, colleagues and friends is the dominant concern among HCW, limiting their social interactions and the most important risk factor for their physical functioning, as well as well-being and mental health [8]. In addition, there are well-founded concerns about the mental health, mental adjustment, and recovery of HCW caring for COVID-19 patients during and after the pandemic.

Previous studies conducted during epidemics such as the Severe Acute Respiratory Syndrome (SARS) of the 2003 Middle East Respiratory Syndrome (MERS) epidemic of 2013–2016 and Ebola of 2014–2016 indicate adverse psychological effects connected to those epidemics, such as anxiety, depression among HCWs, burnout and post-traumatic stress disorder (PTSD), and their symptoms persist from one to three years [9–11]. On the other hand, a meta-analysis concerning the psychological impact of the COVID-19 pandemic on HCWs showed that the total incidence of depression was 21.7%, anxiety was 22.1%, and PTSD was 21.5% [12]. Another meta-analysis showed that among HCWs, the highest incidence of PTSD was recorded among nurses, followed by physicians and other medical professionals (physiotherapists, medical caregivers) [13]. Furthermore, a metanalysis by Vizheh et al. [14] showed that the mental burden affected 12% to 67% of nurses during the COVID-19 pandemic. In contrast, the meta-analysis by Ślusarska et al. [15] showed that during the COVID-19 pandemic, the prevalence of depression among nurses was 22%, while anxiety disorders were experienced by 29% of them.

Even though a traumatic event can cause post-traumatic symptoms (PTS), it can also become a catalyst for positive change. This phenomenon is called post-traumatic growth (PTG). According to the concept of Calhoun and Tedeschi [16], PTG defines a positive psychological change that follows very stressful and demanding life situations [17]. This means that people have the ability to grow despite experiencing trauma. HCWs have great potential to develop PTG due to their personal and professional characteristics. Olson et al. [18] and Huecker et al. [19] emphasise the great importance of the study of PTG and its predictors among HCW during the COVID-19 pandemic. Despite the high interest of researchers in the negative mental health consequences of the COVID-19 pandemic, research has begun documenting the positive psychological effects of the pandemic. For example, moderately increased levels of PTG have been found in frontline nurses and have been associated with social support [20]. The narrative review showed that HCW working on the frontline had a higher level of PTG compared to HCW away from the frontline [21]. In contrast, studies by Vazquez et al. [22] conducted amongst the general adult population in Spain showed that PTG was associated with primal beliefs about a good world, openness to the future and identification with humanity.

Gathered and analysed research indicates that nurses are the group most at risk of developing PTSD during the COVID-19 pandemic. Therefore, examining the positive and negative perceptions of the COVID-19 pandemic and the predictive factors in this professional group seems to be quite significant. The main mechanisms responsible for the negative consequences of the COVID-19 pandemic may be primarily related to the level of anxiety and depression. Negative feelings can worsen the mental and physical well-being of HCW, undermining their confidence and sense of security and even meaning in life. Personal resources usually play an essential role in risk perception during a pandemic, with its negative consequences, as well as in shaping the well-being and positive consequences of COVID-19 stress in HCW. Personal resources are generally regarded as qualities that are valued by a person and are able to improve their effective functioning in terms of control and impact on the environment [23]. In creative adaptation, subjective personal resources can be used to assist individuals in the effective reinterpretation of challenging and stressful life experiences and ineffective adaptation to professional tasks. The risk of developing COVID-19 increases the occupational requirements of HCWs, leading to a decline in well-being with negative consequences. At the same time, perceptions of social support, security and meaning in life can mitigate the adverse effects and develop positive growth associated with the pandemic.

Studies have shown that meaning in life was positively associated with well-being among American HCW [24], but negatively associated with depression in Turkish HCW [25]. In studies in the Israeli adult population conducted during the COVID-19 pandemic, perceived support from a loved one negatively correlated with the severity of depression, anxiety, obsessive-compulsive disorder (OCD) and PTSD [26]. In contrast, a qualitative study on the protection of HCW against exposure to SARS-CoV-2 during patient care during a pandemic found that the sense of security in terms of confidence in personal protective equipment (PPE) and infection prevention and control (IPC) strategies was associated with a lower level of emotional exhaustion [27]. Given that the COVID-19 pandemic is a prolonged stressful situation, especially for HCWs, the availability of social support, a sense of security, and finding meaning and meaning in life would enable workers to cope with stress and promote well-being and positive functioning.

Therefore, considering the need to understand these phenomena, the aim of this study was to determine the relationship between selected sociodemographic variables and selected subjective cognitive resources, and the positive and negative perception of the consequences of the COVID-19 pandemic in the group of nurses working in Poland. The second goal of the research was to determine which sociodemographic variables and cognitive factors explain the variability of positive and negative perceptions of the consequences of the COVID-19 pandemic. We are particularly interested in factors with a buffer effect for the positive aspects of nurses' perceptions of the aftermath of a pandemic, such as perceived social support, experiencing safety, and a sense of meaning and meaning in life.

2. Materials and Methods

2.1. Study Design and Participants

The analysis was conducted using data collected as part of a cross-sectional study between 1 and 15 May 2020. The detailed study protocol in terms of study stages, participant inclusion and exclusion criteria and data collection methods is described elsewhere [28]. A summary of this analysis is provided below. The research material was collected among 325 nurses using the computer-assisted web interviewing (CAWI) method due to the restrictions related to the COVID-19 pandemic in terms of social isolation.The questionnaire was posted on the "Google Surveys" portal and the link to the questionnaire was promoted twice: on the first and the seventh day of the study on the ten most popular fan pages addressed to nurses on Facebook. Participants were allowed to complete the survey only once.The completion of online questionnaires is an established method in healthcare research [29].

After giving informed consent to participate in the study, in order to verify the respondents, the information that the study was granted to nurses and the question, "Are you a nurse?" appeared on the next page. The respondent could respond "Yes" or "No". In the case of marking the answer "No", the questionnaire was closed automatically, thanking them for their time. To be eligible to participate in the study, respondents had to meet certain inclusion and exclusion criteria. The inclusion criteria included: (1) a nurse working during the COVID-19 epidemic, defined as the period from 20 March 2020; (2) professional activity before the coronavirus epidemic, meaning during January and February 2020; and (3) informed consent to participate in the study by responding "Yes". The exclusion criteria were: (1) being on sick leave, maternity, parental or care leave prior to the announcement of the epidemic in Poland (January and February 2020); (2) being on sick leave, maternity, educational or care leave after the announcement of the epidemic in Poland; (3) withdrawal from work for health reasons; and (4) refusal to give informed consent to participate in the study. There is no target recruitment size. As direct comparisons are not being drawn, a power calculation has not been performed.

2.2. Study Questionnaire

In order to achieve the objectives of the study, a questionnaire consisting of five standardized tools and an original tool were used. All respondents completed the same questionnaire. In the instructional manual concerning each listed tool, the respondents were asked to rate certain factors, taking into account the current epidemiological situation. A detailed description of the questionnaires used is presented in another publication [28], while a short description of the scales is provided below. All the scales used in the study were characterised by optimal internal consistency, presented in our earlier publication in Supplementary Materials [28]. The standardised research scales used in the study include:

- Changes in Outlook Questionnaire (CIOQ). The scale was developed by Joseph et al. [30]. At the same time, in our research, we used the scale in the Polish adaptation of Skalski [31], and it contains 10 statements, five each for two subscales: Positive Change and Negative Change of consequences related to a traumatic event.
- Impact Event Scale-Revised (IES-R). The scale was developed by Weiss and Marmara [32] in the Polish adaptation of Juczyński and Ogińska-Bulik [33] to assess traumatic stress, including disturbing memories and persistent negative emotions related to trauma. In the analysis of the obtained results, we adopted the approach that the diagnosis of PTSD can be suspected only in those people who score above the cross-over point (>1.5) in the overall score and in each of the three dimensions.
- Multidimensional Scale of Perceived Social Support (MSPSS). The scale was developed by Zimeta et al. [34] Inthe Polish adaptation of Buszman and Przybyły-Basista, [35] assesses the perception of social support taking into account three primary sources of support: significant others, family, and friends.
- Safety Experience Questionnaire (SEQ). The scale by Klamut [36] assesses the level of experiencing security. The scale is an operationalization of a two-factor model, in which two subscales have been distinguished: a sense of safety (the level of safety experience related to the current satisfaction of basic needs, having satisfactory living conditions and the ability to act) and reflection on safety (the degree of considering matters related to their own safety, their loved ones' safety, and the safety of the nation and the world in the assessment of life situations and social reality).
- Meaning in Life Questionnaire (MQL). The scale was developed by Steger et al. [37] and the tool used in the research was adapted by Kossakowska et al. [38]. The questionnaire consists of 10 questions and examines two dimensions: presence and search.

The questionnaire was supplemented with a personal information form in order to collect information on several basic sociodemographic data: gender, age, marital status, place of residence, the respondent's cohabitants, whether they have children, education, completed postgraduate education, seniority as a nurse, position held, whether the respondent took care of a suspected or diagnosed patient with SARS-CoV-2 at work, and whether the respondent participated in training on the use of personal protective equipment, and the functioning of the medical facility where they worked during the COVID-19 pandemic.

2.3. Ethical Considerations

Ethical approval was issued by the Bioethics Committee at the Medical University of Lublin (decision number: KE-0254/73/2020). The research was conducted in accordance with the ethical principles contained in Recommendations from the Association of Internet Researchers [39]. Participation in the study was voluntary and anonymous. All study participants gave their informed consent to participate in the study electronically. The informed consent form preceding the questionnaire contained an explanation of the purpose, subject of the research, the approximate duration of the study and the method of answering the questionnaire. After reading the information about the survey, the respondent was asked to express their willingness to participate in the survey by clicking "Yes" or withdrawing from the survey by closing the page in the web browser containing the survey or selecting the "No" option. Only those who chose "Yes" were transferred to the questionnaire page. The respondent could resign from the survey at any time by closing the website with the questionnaire. We have described a detailed method of obtaining informed consent elsewhere [28].

2.4. Statistical Analysis

Continuous variables were presented as means (M) with standard deviation (SD). The Shapiro-Wilk test was used to assess conformity with a normal distribution. Categorical variables were reported as absolute numbers and percentages. Differences between groups were assessed by *t*-test or analysis of variance (ANOVA). Pearson correlation was used to investigate the relationships between numerical variables. Simple and multiple linear regression models were performed to assess the significant predictors of CIOQ—Positive Change or Negative Change. The variables with *p*-value < 0.1 were included in the multiple regression model. Three sets of models were constructed: Model A was performed for each independent variable separately (univariable analysis); Model B, included sociodemographic or cognitive factors, which were significant in the simple model; Model Cincluded all significant variables in simple models. The coefficient of determination (R^2) was provided to describe the adequateness of fit for the performed models. Moreover, in the case of IES-R, MSPSS and MLQ scales, a strong correlation between subscales was observed. One of the subscales—Total Score (which was the strongest related to CIOQ)—was used for each scale to avoid collinearity in multivariable models. Additionally, the analysis restricted to women was performed.Statistical analyses were conducted using IBM Corp. (released in 2017) and IBM SPSS Statistics for Windows, Version 25.0. (IBM Corp, Armonk, NY, USA). Statistical A *p*-value < 0.05 was considered significant for two-tailed tests.

3. Results

3.1. Characteristics of Participants

Three hundred twenty-five nurses working all over Poland participated in the study, most of whom were women (96.7%, *n* = 311). The mean age was 39.18 ± 11.16 years. Most of the respondents lived in a city (66.46%, *n* = 216). 57.75% (*n* = 188) of the respondents were married, while the rest were single, widowed, or divorced. 67.7% (*n* = 220) of the respondents lived with their family, 20.3% with a partner, 3.4% (*n* = 11) with a roommate, and 8.6% (*n* = 28) lived alone. 65.2% (*n* = 212) had children living in their house. 43.7% (*n* = 142) had a master's or higher education (more than a master's). Postgraduate education finished by the surveyed nurses: 44.6% (*n* = 145) completed the specialization training, and 42.2% (*n* = 137) completed a qualification course in the field of nursing. 76% (*n* = 247) of respondents were nurses employed in the ward, 13.6% (*n* = 44) were a two-ward nurse, 4.9% (*n* = 13.6%) were a head nurse, and 5.5% (*n* = 18) were a primary care nurse. 46.5% (*n* = 151) cared for a patient with COVID-19, and 67.4% (*n* = 219) received training concerning the use of personal protective equipment and the functioning of the medical facility in which they work during the COVID-19 pandemic.

3.2. Distribution of the Analysed Features According to Scales CIOQ, IES-R, MSPSS, SEQ and MLQ

Table 1 presents the results of the respondents on the scales used in the study. Among the surveyed nurses, a higher average level was noticed in the subscale of perception of positive consequences of the COVID-19 pandemic (18.56 ± 4.04).

Table 1. Distribution of the analysed features in scales.

Scales	M ± SD
CIOQ—Positive Change	18.56 ± 4.04
CIOQ—Negative Change	14.28 ± 4.49
IES-R—Total score	1.78 ± 0.65
MSPSS—Total score	65.9 ± 13.3
SEQ—Sense of safety	3.23 ± 0.79
SEQ—Reflection on safety	4.21 ± 0.49
MLQ—Total score	5.33 ± 0.87

M: mean; SD: standard deviation; CIOQ: Changes in Outlook Questionnaire; IES-R: Impact Event Scale-Revised; MSPSS: Multidimensional Scale of Perceived Social Support; SEQ: Safety Experience Questionnaire; MLQ: Meaning in Life Questionnaire.

3.3. Relationship between Selected Sociodemographic Variables and the Assessment of Positive and Negative Consequences of the COVID-19 Pandemic

Table 2 presents the relationships between sociodemographic variables and positive and negative consequences related to the traumatic event, which is the COVID-19 pandemic. Age was negatively related to the Positive Change subscale (r = −0.15, p = 0.007), but no significant relationship was observed between age and the Negative Change subscale (r = 0.04, p = 0.48). Respondents living in cities (18.55 ± 4.06) and being widowed or divorced (17.91 ± 3.08) obtained a significantly lower mean value of the Positive Change subscale compared to respondents from rural areas (19.49 ± 3.94) and those who were married (19.41 ± 3.87) or living alone (18.19 ± 4.45). The other analysed variables did not significantly differentiate the mean scores on the Positive Change subscale in the study group.

Table 2. Associations between selected sociodemographic variables on the assessment of positive and negative consequences of the COVID-19 pandemic.

Variable	CIOQ—Positive Change		p	CIOQ—Negative Change		p
M	SD	M		SD		
Age (year)	r = −0.15		0.007	r = 0.04		0.48
Place of residence:						
Urban area Rural area	18.55 19.49	4.06 3.94	0.046	14.12 14.60	4.60 4.28	0.368
Education:						
Bachelor's degree Master's degree or above	18.87 18.87	3.86 4.27	0.99	13.54 14.85	4.30 4.30	0.008
Postgraduate education:						
Postgraduatediploma Qualificationcourse Specialisttrainingcourse	19.25 19.09 18.54	4.30 3.82 4.16	0.42	4.47 15.42 13.28	14.00 4.50 4.27	<0.001
Marital status:						
Married Single Divorced/Separated/Widowed	19.41 18.19 17.91	3.87 4.45 3.08	0.016	13.67 15.42 14.12	3.96 5.27 4.14	0.006

Table 2. *Cont.*

Variable	CIOQ—Positive Change		*p*	CIOQ—Negative Change		*p*
M	SD	M		SD		
			Living arrangements:			
Family	19.11	4.0		14.17	4.55	
Cohabitant/Flat mate/Roommate	18.36	4.31	0.28	14.40	4.41	0.76
Alone	18.32	3.47		14.78	4.37	
			Child(ren) in House:			
No	18.44	4.53	0.166	15.04	5.40	0.025
Yes	19.09	3.74		13.87	3.88	
			Rotating shift schedule:			
No	18.47	4.26	0.234	13.91	4.65	0.316
Yes	19.05	3.93		14.45	4.42	
			Have you nursed a patient diagnosed with COVID-19:			
No	18.69	3.69	0.41	14.09	3.92	0.405
Yes	19.07	4.41		14.50	5.07	
			Was there any training related to the coronavirus epidemic at work:			
No	18.41	4.53	0.16	14.70	4.54	0.244
Yes	19.09	3.76		14.08	4.47	

M. mean; SD: standard deviation; CIOQ: Changes in Outlook Questionnaire.

In the case of the Negative Change subscale, education, completed postgraduate education, marital status and having children, significantly differentiated mean values were obtained. Higher mean values of this subscale occurred among respondents with a master's degree or higher education, respondents who completed aqualification course in postgraduate education, and those living alone and without children.

3.4. Relationship between Positive and Negative Consequences Related to the Traumatic Event Which Is the COVID-19 Pandemic and Selected Cognitive Factors

Table 3 shows the relationship between the CIOQ subscales and selected cognitive variables. Significant and positive relationships were observed between the CIOQ Positive Change subscale and the level of perceived traumatic stress, and reflection on safety, with the strongest relationship between the sense of meaning and meaning in life (r = 0.403, $p < 0.001$) and the sense of social support (r = 0.401, $p < 0.001$). Conversely, there was no significant correlation between the CIOQ Positive Change subscale and the sense of security.

In the case of the second CIOQ Negative Change subscale, it was observed that the level of social support, the sense of security and the sense of meaning and meaning in life were negatively correlated with this subscale, while the level of perceived traumatic stress was positively related. The strongest correlation occurred in the case of experienced traumatic stress (r = 0.481, $p < 0.001$). There was no significant correlation between the CIOQ Negative Change subscale and reflection on safety.

Table 3. The relationship between the CIOQ subscales and selected cognitive variables.

Variable		CIOQ—Positive Change	CIOQ—Negative Change
IES-R—Total score	r	0.147	0.481
	p	0.008	<0.001
MSPSS—Total score	r	0.401	−0.205
	p	<0.001	<0.001
SEQ—Sense of safety	r	0.298	−0.307
	p	0.298	<0.001
SEQ—Reflection on safety	r	0.386	0.021
	p	<0.001	0.704
MLQ—Total score	r	0.403	−0.269
	p	<0.001	<0.001

CIOQ: Changes in Outlook Questionnaire; IES-R: Impact Event Scale-Revised; MSPSS: Multidimensional Scale of Perceived Social Support; SEQ: Safety Experience Questionnaire; MLQ: Meaning in Life Questionnaire; r: correlation coefficient.

3.5. Features Related to the Positive and Negative Perspective of the COVID-19 Pandemic—Multivariable Analysis

Tables 4 and 5 present univariable models (Models A) and multivariable models (Models B) presenting the results of analysis of features significantly related in one-dimensional models for sociodemographic features and cognitive factors, (Model C) taking into account both sociodemographic features and cognitive determinants. In the case of the CIOQ Positive Change subscale, among the analysed sociodemographic features, only marital status was a significant predictor, with age explaining only 3% of the variability of this variable. The cognitive determinants which significantly related to the CIOQ Positive Change subscale included the level of perceived traumatic stress, the level of social support, a sense of security, reflection on safety, and a sense of meaning and meaning in life (Model B), explaining in total 36% of the variability of the dependent variable. In the full multivariable model (Model C), none of the analysed sociodemographic features turned out to be an independent predictor of the CIOQ Positive Change subscale value, and all of the analysed cognitive features explained as much as 37% of the dependent variable, and the nature of the relationship was positive.

In the case of the CIOQ Negative Change subscale, in the multivariable model, among the analysed sociodemographic features, marital status, education and completion of a qualification course in postgraduate education were significantly related to this variable and explained 8% of its variability (Model B). In Model B (among cognitive traits), the level of perceived traumatic stress, the level of social support and the sense of meaning and meaning in life were significantly related to the CIOQ Negative Change subscale, explaining in total 30% of its variability. In the full multivariable model (Model C), variables such as education, completion of a postgraduate qualification course, level of perceived traumatic stress, level of social support, and sense of meaning and meaning in life turned out to be independent predictors of the CIOQ Negative Change subscale (Model C). Together, these features accounted for 38% of the variability of the dependent variable. However, the relationship of such traits as the sense of social support, the sense of security and the sense of meaning and meaning in life in relation to the CIOQ Negative Change variable was negative.

Table 4. Relationship between the positive outlook of the COVID-19 pandemic and selected sociodemographic and cognitive variables.

Variables	Changes in Outlook Questionnaire—Subscale Positive Change										
	Model A			Model B				Model C			
Sociodemographic variables:	b	SE	p	b	SE	p	R^2	b	SE	p	R^2
Age	0.014	0.02	0.483								
Place of residence (reference category: Urban area)	0	0	0	0	0	0		0	0	0	
Rurar area	0.944	0.472	0.046	0.678	0.481	0.160		0.612	0.393	0.121	
Education (reference category: Bachelor's degree)	0	0	0	0	0	0		0	0	0	
Master's degree or above	−0.003	0.452	0.995								
Postgraduate education (reference category: Specialist training course)	0	0	0	0	0	0		0	0	0	
Postgraduate diploma	0.711	0.701	0.311								
Qualification course	0.543	0.481	0.260								
Marital status (reference category: Married)	0	0	0	0	0	0		0	0	0	
Single	−1.217	0.489	0.013	−1.072	0.499	0.032		−0.532	0.411	0.197	
Divorced/Separated/Widowed	−1.500	0.755	0.048	−1.356	0.760	0.076		−0.254	0.626	0.685	
Living arrangements (reference category: Family)	0	0	0	0	0	0	3%	0	0	0	
Cohabitant/Flat mate or Roommate	−0.750	0.534	0.161								
Alone	−0.792	0.809	0.328								
Child(ren) in House (reference category: No)	0	0	0	0	0	0		0	0	0	
Yes	0.652	0.469	0.166								37%
Rotating shift schedule (reference category: No)	0	0	0	0	0	0		0	0	0	
Yes	0.574	0.481	0.234								
Have you nursed a patient diagnosed with COVID-19 (reference category: No)	0	0	0	0	0	0		0	0	0	
Yes	0.371	0.449	0.410								
Was there any training related to the coronavirus epidemic at work? (reference category: No)	0	0	0	0	0	0		0	0	0	
Yes	0.672	0.477	0.160								
Cognitive variables:											
IES-R—Total score	0.917	0.342	0.008	1.756	0.309	<0.001		1.690	0.311	<0.001	
MSPSS—Total score	0.122	0.015	<0.001	0.056	0.016	<0.001		0.059	0.016	<0.001	
SEQ—Sense of safety	1.154	0.262	<0.001	1.354	0.262	<0.001	36%	1.329	0.263	<0.001	
SEQ—Reflection on safety	2.801	0.424	<0.001	1.165	0.424	0.006		1.125	0.424	0.008	
MLQ—Total score	1.868	0.236	<0.001	1.261	0.236	<0.001		1.201	0.237	<0.001	

Model A: univariable analysis; Model B: included significant factors in univariable analysis (performed separately for sociodemographic and cognitive factors); Model C: included all significant factors in univariable analysis; CIOQ: Changes in Outlook Questionnaire; IES-R: Impact Event Scale-Revised; MSPSS: Multidimensional Scale of Perceived Social Support; SEQ: Safety Experience Questionnaire; MLQ: Meaning in Life Questionnaire; b: standardised beta coefficient; SE: standard error.

Table 5. Relationship between the negative perspective of the COVID-19 pandemic and selected sociodemographic and cognitive variables.

Variables	Changes in Outlook Questionnaire—Subscale Negative Change										
	Model A			Model B				Model C			
Sociodemographic variables:	b	SE	*p*	b	SE	*p*	R^2	b	SE	p	R^2
Age	−0.061	0.022	0.007	−0.019	0.033	0.560		−0.031	0.028	0.26	
Place of residence (reference category: Urban area)	0	0	0	0	0	0		0	0	0	
Rular area	0.476	0.528	0.368								
Education (reference category: Bachelor's degree)	0	0	0	0	0	0		0	0	0	
Master's degree or above	−1.310	0.498	0.009	−1.148	0.493	0.02		−0.977	0.410	0.018	
Postgraduate education (reference category: Specialist training course)	0	0	0	0	0	0		0	0	0	
Postgraduate diploma	0.717	0.763	0.348	0.512	0.764	0.503		0.543	0.644	0.400	
Qualification course	2.141	0.523	<0.001	1.592	0.587	0.007		1.305	0.491	0.008	
Marital status (reference category: Married)	0	0	0	0	0	0		0	0	0	
Single	1.748	0.542	0.001	1.626	0.941	0.085		1.558	0.788	0.049	
Divorced/Separated/Widowed	0.446	0.837	0.595	0.802	0.833	0.336	8%	1.097	0.700	0.118	
Living arrangements (reference category: Family)	0	0	0	0	0	0		0	0	0	
Cohabitant/Flat mate or Roommate	0.230	0.596	0.700								
Alone	0.613	0.904	0.498								
Child(ren) in House (reference category: No)	0	0	0	0	0	0		0	0	0	38%
Yes	−1.172	0.520	0.025	0.954	0.957	0.320		0.755	0.799	0.345	
Rotating shift schedule (reference category: No)	0	0	0	0	0	0		0	0	0	
Yes	0.538	0.536	0.316								
Have you nursed a patient diagnosed with COVID-19 (reference category: No)	0	0	0	0	0	0		0	0	0	
Yes	0.417	0.500	0.405								
Was there any training related to the coronavirus epidemic at work? (reference category: No)	0	0	0	0	0	0		0	0	0	
Yes	−0.620	0.531	0.244								
Cognitive variables:											
IES-R—Total score	3.332	0.338	<0.001	2.722	0.358	<0.001		2.757	0.348	<0.001	
MSPSS—Total	−0.069	0.018	<0.001	−0.042	0.018	0.022		−0.05	0.018	0.005	
SEQ—Sense of safety	−1.863	0.308	<0.001	−0.678	0.303	0.026	30%	−0.663	0.294	0.025	
SEQ—Reflection on safety	0.844	0.499	0.092	1.149	0.492	0.02		1.160	0.479	0.016	
MLQ—Total score	−1.388	0.276	<0.001	−0.956	0.274	0.001		−0.783	0.265	0.003	

Model A: univariable analysis; Model B: included significant factors in univariable analysis (performed separately for sociodemographic and cognitive factors); Model C: included all significant factors in univariable analysis; CIOQ: Changes in Outlook Questionnaire; IES-R: Impact Event Scale-Revised; MSPSS: Multidimensional Scale of Perceived Social Support; SEQ: Safety Experience Questionnaire; MLQ: Meaning in Life Questionnaire; b: standardised beta coefficient; SE: standard error.

The results of the analysis restricted to female participants are presented in Supplementary Materials, Tables S1 and S2. Features significant in the analyses conducted on the entire sample (both including women and men) maintained statistical significance as well as the direction and strength of dependence among women.

4. Discussion

The COVID-19 pandemic has severe, multi-faceted consequences for people's psychosocial and mental health [40], especially HCW. Therefore, a better understanding of the underlying protective factors and risks of both negative and positive psychological effects of a pandemic [41] is warranted. Given the need to investigate both the protective factors and risk factors associated with the negative and positive psychological consequences of the current global COVID-19 pandemic, the presented research aimed to identify the relationship between selected socio-demographic variables and cognitive factors, and positive and negative perceptions of the COVID-19 pandemic in the aforementioned group of nurses. Overall, the results of our study indicate that the sociodemographic variables significantly differentiating the surveyed group of nurses in terms of the perception of positive and negative consequences of the COVID-19 pandemic were age, place of residence, education, postgraduate education, marital status, and having children. However, when considering the analysed cognitive variables, it transpired that the majority was associated with a positive and negative perception of the consequences of the COVID-19 pandemic. Although the strongest positive perception of the consequences of the COVID-19 pandemic was associated with the sense of meaning and meaning in life and the perception of social support, the level of perceived traumatic stress was most strongly associated with the negative perception of the consequences of the COVID-19 pandemic. In multivariate models, the analysed sociodemographic and cognitive variables explained 37% of the variable of positive perception of the consequences of the COVID-19 pandemic and 38% of the variable of the negative perception of the consequences of the COVID-19 pandemic, of which, in the analysis of the positive perception of the consequences of the COVID-19 pandemic, none of the analysed sociodemographic features proved to be an independent predictor.

Moreover, the positive perception of the consequences of the COVID-19 pandemic has decreased. Additionally, it was observed that nurses living in rural areas and those who were married were characterised by a higher positive perception of the consequences of the COVID-19 pandemic, whereas a significantly lower level of perception concerning the negative consequences of the COVID-19 pandemic was observed in respondents characterised as having lower education, nurses who completed a qualifying nursing course, and those who were married and those who had children. Cui et al. [42] conducted a study among 167 frontline nurses during the COVID-19 pandemic in China, in Henan and Hubei provinces. In this research, PTG was measured using the Post-traumatic Growth Inventory (PTGI). Their results indicated that, as in our study, married nurses had higher PTG levels.

Conversely, the results of the cited studies indicate that, unlike the authors' research, senior nurses and nurses with a higher level of education had a higher PTG score, while having children did not differentiate the group. Peng et al. [20] conducted a study amongst 116 frontline nurses during the COVID-19 pandemic, where PTG was significantly higher in nurses with children. At the same time, such variables as age, marital status, and education did not differentiate the study group. There are several mechanisms explaining the influence of some sociodemographic variables on the level of PTG. One of the sociodemographic variables which can increase PTG is having children. It relates to the duties and role of the mother, making the woman bolder and stronger in the face of new difficulties and challenges. Psychological research on frontline nurses has shown that identifying with the role of "mother" influences the level of PTG [43]. Updegraff and Taylor [44] proposed an explanation of the impact of being married on a higher level of PTG by linking it with positive mental development after trauma through a support system provided by another close person. However, our research only observed that the respondents remaining in a relationship had a significantly lower level of negative perception of the COVID-19 pandemic.

Another variable is the age of the respondent, which in the case of nurses is associated with longer work experience, therefore some studies indicate that senior nurses had a significantly higher PTG [42] This may be related to the fact that nurses with morework experience show higher levels of critical thinking [45], but the results of our research have not confirmed this. A similar mechanism may apply to the level of education and PTG.

The second group of analysed variables that may influence the positive and negative perceptions of the COVID-19 pandemic were cognitive variables that can be involved in creative adaptation to help individuals effectively reinterpret difficult and stressful situations. In our research, the level of traumatic stress was weakly correlated and positively correlated with the positive perception of the consequences of the COVID-19 pandemic, and moderately correlated and positively correlated with the negative perception of the consequences of the COVID-19 pandemic. It should be emphasised that in both analysed situations, the correlations are positive, although the higher strength of the correlation of traumatic stress associated with COVID-19 was associated with a negative perception of the consequences of this pandemic. This discovery was partially in line with our expectations, because the PTG theory was proposed as a possible positive psychological consequence of the encountered traumatic events [46,47], and the individual's perception of a traumatic event becomes a necessary condition for development [48,49]. On the basis of the obtained research results, it can be hypothesized that too high an intensity of traumatic stress causes a negative perception of the consequences of a pandemic. Chen et al. [50] obtained similar results amongst nurses, while Park et al. [51] confirmed this relationship among Amazon MTurk employees. Thus, PTG is associated with the symptoms of post-traumatic stress disorder and can be treated as a coping mechanism in the face of persistent suffering from trauma [52].

Tedeschi and Calhoun [53] stressed the great importance of social support as a direct predictor of PTG. People who experienced a traumatic event with a high level of social support more often received emotional or material support from family members, friends, or various social groups [54]. Conversely, one of the ways to combat the spread of the SARS-CoV-2 virus was the introduction of social isolation rules, limiting social support through face-to-face contact. This was especially truein the case of nurses, who were more exposed to the virus and became more isolated than the rest of society due to the nature of their work. The authors' results showed that the sense of social support was positively correlated with a positive and negatively correlated with a negative perception of the COVID-19 pandemic. Obtained results were confirmed in previous studies among nurses during the COVID-19 pandemic [55–57]. One possible explanation is that high perceived social support can provide a sense of having a safe environment, emphasize feelings of belonging, serve as a buffer against stress, provide new meaning, and generate more positive perceptions, which endorse growth [58].

Safety is one of the most important categories which allows a description of the context of human life and the way people function [59]. In the context of experiencing security, the emotional aspect is feeling, while the rational, cognitive aspect is a reflection on security [60]. During the COVID-19 pandemic, especially at its beginning, nurses faced numerous problems that disturbed their sense of security and influenced their reflection on safety. These problems include, among others, a shortage of personal protective equipment, nursing staff shortages, fear for the health of oneself and relatives, etc. The authors' research revealed the sense of security and reflection on safety as positively correlated with a positive perception of the COVID-19 pandemic, while the feeling of safety negatively correlated with a negative perception of the COVID-19 pandemic. Other research has confirmed that fear of infection and awareness of the risks are associated with PTG, but the relationship between the availability of personal protective equipment and PTG has not been confirmed [42,61]. Unfortunately, there are no studies assessing the impact of the sense of security on PTG among health care workers on the level of PTG. Therefore, further research is required to assess this aspect considering many intermediary variables, such as the availability of personal protective equipment, the workplace, the level of knowledge about the virus and many others.

According to the literature, the confrontation of an individual with stressful life events accompanied by various losses poses a challenge to the desire to perceive the world as meaningful and predictable, and thus may contribute to a search for meaning [62]. Earlier studies have shown a positive relationship between the presence of meaning in life and PTG [63,64]. Our research confirmed this fact, which showed a positive relationship between the search for meaning in life and a positive and negative relationship between the negative perception of the consequences of the COVID-19 pandemic. Unfortunately, there are few studies assessing the impact of meaning in life on PTG during the COVID-19 pandemic. Interesting observations about the sense of meaning and importance of life and other elements of psychological functioning during the COVID-19 pandemic were made by Baños et al. [65]. They assessed, inter alia, the meaning in life in various periods of the COVID-19 pandemic and found that its level was stable over time in the assessed periods of the lockdown. On the other hand, Trzebiński et al. [66] showed that the level of meaning and meaning in life positively correlates with lower anxiety and lower stressrelated to COVID-19. The explanatory mechanism may be that the search for meaning and meaning in life allows the individual to positively reassess traumatic events, strengthen the psychological resources needed to rediscover themselves, restore the individual to a basic, complex world, and be oriented towards future goals [67].

4.1. Implications for Nursing Practice and Education

The practical implications of our research indicate the importance of social support, a sense of security, reflection on safety and a sense of the meaning and meaning of life as protective factors in creating post-traumatic positive psychological changes in the face of this and future pandemics. Accordingly, we recommend that healthcare leaders provide support from their supervisors and develop safe practice procedures. Highly engaged and participatory leadership facilitates dealing with group problems, sharing and processing ideas, and empathetic team leaders can provide an understanding of nurses' needs and awareness of the thoughts and feelings of the nursing staff [68]. Another aspect of the practical implications in creating post-traumatic positive psychological changes should include conducting psychological interventions in nurses working in environments with high stress related to contact with an infected patient. Both psychologists, as well as direct close associates, can provide psychological first aid [69].

As for the educational aspects, they apply not only to the nurses themselves, working in direct contact with the infected patient but also to healthcare leaders in understanding the problem and organizational support in solving new problems that arise in the face of a pandemic. Our research indicates the critical role of cognitive variables in mitigating the adverse psychological effects of a pandemic. Therefore, it is vital to develop cognitive resources during both undergraduate and postgraduate education to be easier for nurses, with the participation of nursing leaders, to cope with the adverse psychological consequences of a pandemic. Nurses who can cope well with the adverse psychological effects of a pandemic will contribute to helping individuals in society cope with stress when an epidemiological emergency occurs. This research can contribute to the development of the nursing practice by identifying some significant cognitive resources contributing to the protection of the mental health of oneself, one's family and the community, which can be developed during training on how to deal with a pandemic.

4.2. The Strengths and Limitations

The strengths and weaknesses of this study deserve consideration. Firstly, to our knowledge, it is one of the few studies which assesses, inter alia, the impact of the sense of security, reflection on safety and the meaning and meaning of life on the positive and negative perception of the consequences of the COVID-19 pandemic carried out with a group of nurses. Secondly, in our research we used standardised questionnaires which had good reliability coefficients and were adapted to the assessment for the COVID-19 pandemic [28]. Thirdly, the nurses we studied worked in Poland, where they had not participated in combating the COVID-19 pandemic for many decades.

Our research has several limitations. First, the study's cross-sectional design is a constraint from which we can infer correlation, not construct causation. Our sample of nurses is not a nationwide representative sample. The average age of the respondents was lower than the average age of nurses in Poland. In our sample, the mean age was 39.18 ± 11.16, while the mean age of nurses in Poland, according to the statistics of the Supreme Chamber of Nurses and Midwives, in 2020, was 53.16 years [70]. The age difference between the group we studied and nurses in general, is particularly visible in the overrepresentation of the youngest age group of 21–30 years.

Nevertheless, the research results may be helpful in modeling research hypotheses and recommendations in the implementation of psychological care during a pandemic, especially among the younger age group of nurses. It is worth emphasizing that the study was conducted at the beginning of the COVID-19 pandemic in conditions of epidemic restrictions. The only chance to obtain data was to conduct CAWI studies, which was associated with more frequent participation in the study by younger people. Secondly, we adopted an online dissemination strategy due to the limitations of social contacts. Therefore, it was not possible to collect data on people who refused to participate in the study, and no percentage of refusals was recorded. In addition, when recruiting participants in the study, we relied on access to social networking sites, which is why the surveyed population does not include participants who do not have access to social networking sites and nurses who do not use these sites. Third, the study was conducted at the beginning of the COVID-19 pandemic, and as some authors suggest, PTG measured shortly after contact with a traumatic event may be an initial coping strategy [22]. Nevertheless, the results of our study can provide a valuable reference point for the discussion of PTG studies conducted in later or post-pandemic periods. Fourth, the research subject was Polish nurses, whose cultural context may cause their responses to differ from those of nurses working in other countries. Fifthly, filling in the questionnaire on their own could cause the respondents to underestimate or exaggerate the severity of certain symptoms to minimize or exacerbate their problems.

5. Conclusions

The COVID-19 pandemic quickly altered the working conditions for nurses in Poland, increasing the level of traumatic stress related to the pandemic. The authors' observations revealed the prevalence of positive post-traumatic psychological changes among nurses. It has been observed that younger nurses living in rural areas and are married more often perceive the consequences of a pandemic positively. Whereas respondents with a higher education, with a qualification in the field of nursing, single people and those without children perceive the negative effects of the COVID-19 pandemic significantly more often. In a multivariate analysis, lower levels of perceived traumatic stress and higher levels of social support, a sense of security, reflection on safety, and a sense of meaning and meaning in life are the main sources of a 37% buffering explaining the variability of the prospect of positive consequences of the COVID-19 pandemic among nurses. Factors predicting post-traumatic negative psychological changes experienced by nurses during the COVID-19 pandemic in a multidimensional model reveal 38% of variability of negative consequences, and, among them, apart from sociodemographic features, a high level of perceived traumatic stress and low levels of social support, sense of security and sense and importance are important.

Our research clarifies the insufficient knowledge concerning the predictors of post-traumatic positive and negative psychological changes experienced by nurses during the COVID-19 pandemic. Moreover, we were able to identify the importance of the level of perceived traumatic stress, social support, sense of security, reflection on safety, and the sense of meaning and importance of life as protective factors in the mechanisms of creating post-traumatic positive psychological changes.

Supplementary Materials: The following supporting information can be downloaded at: https://www.mdpi.com/article/10.3390/ijerph19127073/s1, Table S1: Relationship between the positive outlook of the COVID-19 pandemic and selected sociodemographic and cognitive variables in woman; Table S2. Relationship between the negative perspective of the COVID-19 pandemic and selected sociodemographic and cognitive variables in woman.

Author Contributions: Conceptualized the design and the data analysis, conducted the experimental procedure, interpreted the data and drafted, finalized the manuscript, contributed to the design of the analysis, conducted the statistical analysis and contributed to the draft manuscript, G.J.N. and B.Ś.; interpreted the data and contributed to the draft manuscript, B.Z. and A.J.; contributed to the draft manuscript and revised the final version, M.K. All authors have read and agreed to the published version of the manuscript.

Funding: This research received no external funding. The article processing charge was funded by the Medical University of Lublin.

Institutional Review Board Statement: The study was conducted in accordance with the HelsinkiDeclaration (updated in 2013). The study was approved by the Bioethics Committee of the MedicalUniversity of Lublin (decision number: KE-0254/73/2020).

Informed Consent Statement: Informed consent was obtained from all subjects involved in the study.

Data Availability Statement: The datasets used and/or analyzed during the current study areavailable from the corresponding author on reasonable request.

Acknowledgments: The authors would like to express our gratitude to Maciej Polak, DHSC for his assistance inpreparing statistical analyses.

Conflicts of Interest: The authors declare that they have no conflicts of interest.

References

1. World Health Organization. Director-General's Opening Remarques at the Media Briefing on COVID-19—11 March 2020. Available online: https://www.who.int/director-general/speeches/detail/who-director-general-s-opening-remarks-at-the-media-briefing-on-covid-19---11-march-2020 (accessed on 20 January 2022).
2. Lai, J.; Ma, S.; Wang, Y.; Cai, Z.; Hu, J.; Wei, N.; Wu, J.; Du, H.; Chen, T.; Li, R.; et al. Factors associated with mental health outcomes among health care workers exposed to coronavirus disease 2019. *JAMA Netw. Open* **2020**, *3*, e203976. [CrossRef] [PubMed]
3. World Health Organization. COVID-19 Continues to Disrupt Essential Health Services in 90% of Countries. Available online: https://www.who.int/news/item/23-04-2021-covid-19-continues-to-disrupt-essential-health-services-in-90-of-countries (accessed on 20 January 2022).
4. Badahdah, A.; Khamis, F.; Al Mahyijari, N.; Al Balushi, M.; Al Hatmi, H.; Al Salmi, I.; Al Bulushi, Z.; Al Noomani, J. The mental health of health care workers in Oman during the COVID-19 pandemic. *Int. J. Soc. Psychiatry* **2021**, *67*, 90–95. [CrossRef] [PubMed]
5. Clay, J.M.; Parker, M.O. Alcohol use and misuse during the COVID-19 pandemic: A potential public health crisis? *Lancet Public Health* **2020**, *5*, e259. [CrossRef]
6. Benfante, A.; Di Tella, M.; Romeo, A.; Castelli, L. Traumatic stress in healthcare workers during COVID-19 pandemic: A review of the immediate impact. *Front. Psychol.* **2020**, *11*, 569935. [CrossRef] [PubMed]
7. Sun, N.; Wei, L.; Shi, S.; Jiao, D.; Song, R.; Ma, L.; Wang, H.; Wang, C.; Wang, Z.; You, Y.; et al. A qualitative study on the psychological experience of caregivers of COVID-19 patients. *Am. J. Infect. Control* **2020**, *48*, 592–598. [CrossRef] [PubMed]
8. Franklin, P.; Gkiouleka, A. A Scoping Review of Psychosocial Risks to Health Workers during the Covid-19 Pandemic. *Int. J. Environ. Res. Public Health* **2021**, *18*, 2453. [CrossRef]
9. Temsah, M.H.; Al-Sohime, F.; Alamro, N.; Al-Eyadhy, A.; Al-Hasan, K.; Jamal, A.; Al-Maglouth, I.; Aljamaan, F.; Al Amri, M.; Barry, M.; et al. The psychological impact of COVID-19 pandemic on health care workers in a MERS-CoV endemic country. *J. Infect. Public Health* **2020**, *13*, 877–882. [CrossRef]
10. Maunder, R.G.; Lancee, W.J.; Balderson, K.E.; Bennett, J.P.; Borgundvaag, B.; Evans, S.; Fernandes, C.M.; Goldbloom, D.S.; Gupta, M.; Hunter, J.J.; et al. Long-term psychological and occupational effects of providing hospital healthcare during SARS outbreak. *Emerg. Infect. Dis.* **2006**, *12*, 1924–1932. [CrossRef]

11. Kisely, S.; Warren, N.; McMahon, L.; Dalais, C.; Henry, I.; Siskind, D. Occurrence, prevention, and management of the psychological effects of emerging virus outbreaks on healthcare workers: Rapid review and meta-analysis. *BMJ* **2020**, *369*, m1642. [CrossRef]
12. Li, Y.; Scherer, N.; Felix, L.; Kuper, H. Prevalence of depression, anxiety and post-traumatic stress disorder in health care workers during the COVID-19 pandemic: A systematic review and meta-analysis. *PLoS ONE* **2021**, *16*, e0246454. [CrossRef]
13. Yunitri, N.; Chu, H.; Kang, X.L.; Jen, H.J.; Pien, L.C.; Tsai, H.T.; Kamil, A.R.; Chou, K.R. Global prevalence and associated risk factors of post-traumatic stress disorder during COVID-19 pandemic: A meta-analysis. *Int. J. Nurs. Stud.* **2022**, *126*, 104136. [CrossRef] [PubMed]
14. Vizheh, M.; Qorbani, M.; Arzaghi, S.M.; Muhidin, S.; Javanmard, Z.; Esmaeili, M. The mental health of healthcare workers in the COVID-19 pandemic: A systematic review. *J. Diabetes Metab. Disord.* **2020**, *19*, 1–12. [CrossRef] [PubMed]
15. Ślusarska, B.; Nowicki, G.J.; Niedorys-Karczmarczyk, B.; Chrzan-Rodak, A. Prevalence of depression and anxiety in nurses during the first eleven months of the COVID-19 pandemic: A systematic review and meta-analysis. *Int. J. Environ. Res. Public Health* **2022**, *19*, 1154. [CrossRef] [PubMed]
16. Calhoun, L.G.; Tedeschi, R.G. Positive aspects of critical life problems: Recollections of grief. *OMEGA J. Death Dying* **1990**, *20*, 265–272. [CrossRef]
17. Tedeschi, R.G.; Calhoun, L.G. Posttraumatic growth: Conceptual foundations and empirical evidence. *Psychol. Inq.* **2004**, *15*, 1–18. [CrossRef]
18. Olson, K.; Shanafelt, T.; Southwick, S. Pandemic-driven post-traumatic growth for organizations and individuals. *JAMA* **2020**, *324*, 1829–1830. [CrossRef]
19. Huecker, M.; Shreffler, J.; Danzl, D. COVID-19: Optimizing healthcare provider wellness and post-traumatic growth. *Am. J. Emerg. Med.* **2021**, *46*, 693–694. [CrossRef]
20. Peng, X.; Zhao, H.Z.; Yang, Y.; Rao, Z.L.; Hu, D.Y.; He, Q. Post-traumatic growth level and its influencing factors among frontline nurses during the COVID-19 pandemic. *Front. Psychiatry* **2021**, *12*, 632360. [CrossRef]
21. Finstad, G.L.; Giorgi, G.; Lulli, L.G.; Pandolfi, C.; Foti, G.; León-Perez, J.M.; Cantero-Sánchez, F.J.; Mucci, N. Resilience, coping strategies and post-traumatic growth in the workplace following COVID-19: A narrative review on the positive aspects of trauma. *Int. J. Environ. Res. Public Health* **2021**, *18*, 9453. [CrossRef]
22. Vazquez, C.; Valiente, C.; García, F.E.; Contreras, A.; Peinado, V.; Trucharte, A.; Bentall, R.P. Post-traumatic growth and stress-related responses during the COVID-19 pandemic in a national representative sample: The role of positive core beliefs about the world and others. *J. Happiness Stud.* **2021**, *22*, 2915–2935. [CrossRef]
23. Hobfoll, S.E.; Johnson, R.J.; Ennis, N.; Jackson, A.P. Resource loss, resource gain, and emotional outcomes among inner city women. *J. Pers. Soc. Psychol.* **2003**, *84*, 632–643. [CrossRef] [PubMed]
24. Shiri, S.; Wexler, I.; Marmor, A.; Meiner, Z.; Schwartz, I.; LevzionKorach, O.; Azoulay, D. Hospice care: Hope and meaning in life mediate subjective well-being of staff. *Am. J. Hosp. Palliat. Care* **2020**, *37*, 785–790. [CrossRef] [PubMed]
25. Güngör, A.; Uçman, A.G. Depression and hopelessness in Turkish healthcare workers: The moderating and mediating roles of meaning in life. *Glob. Public Health* **2020**, *15*, 236–246. [CrossRef] [PubMed]
26. Ferber, S.G.; Weller, A.; Maor, R.; Feldman, Y.; Harel-Fisch, Y.; Mikulincer, M. Perceived social support in the social distancing era: The association between circles of potential support and COVID-19 reactive psychopathology. *Anxiety Stress Coping* **2022**, *35*, 58–71. [CrossRef]
27. Ehrenzeller, S.; Durovic, A.; Kuehl, R.; Martinez, A.E.; Bielser, M.; Battegay, M.; von Rotz, M.; Fringer, A.; Tschudin-Sutter, S. A qualitative study on safety perception among healthcare workers of a tertiary academic care center during the SARS-CoV-2 pandemic. *Antimicrob. Resist. Infect. Control* **2022**, *11*, 30. [CrossRef]
28. Nowicki, G.J.; Ślusarska, B.; Tucholska, K.; Naylor, K.; Chrzan-Rodak, A.; Niedorys, B. The severity of traumatic stress associated with COVID-19 pandemic, perception of support, sense of security, and sense of meaning in life among nurses: Research protocol and preliminary results from Poland. *Int. J. Environ. Res. Public Health* **2020**, *17*, 6491. [CrossRef]
29. Buchanan, E.A.; Hvizdak, E.E. Online survey tools: Ethical and methodological concerns of human research ethics committees. *J. Empir. Res. Hum. Res. Ethics* **2009**, *4*, 37–48. [CrossRef]
30. Joseph, S.; Williams, R.; Yule, W. Changes in outlook following disaster: The preliminary development ofa measure to assess positive and negative responses. *J. Trauma. Stress* **1993**, *6*, 271–279. [CrossRef]
31. Skalski, S. New Perspective Questionnaire to measure positive and negative trauma effects. Polish adaptationof the Short Form of the Changes in Outlook Questionnaire. *Ann. UMCS Sect. J.* **2019**, *32*, 307–317.
32. Weiss, D.; Marmar, C. The Impact of Event Scale-Revised. In *Assessing Psychological Trauma and PTSD: A Handbook for Practitioners*; Wilson, J., Keant, T., Eds.; Guildford Press: New York, NY, USA, 1997; pp. 341–399.
33. Juczyński, Z.; Ogińska-Bulik, N. Measurement of post-traumatic stress disorder-Polish version of Impact Event Scale-Revised. *Psychiatry* **2009**, *6*, 15–25.
34. Zimet, G.; Dahlem, N.; Zimet, S.; Farley, G. The Multidimensional Scale of Perceived Social Support. *J. Pers. Assess.* **1988**, *52*, 30–41. [CrossRef]
35. Buszman, K.; Przybyła-Basista, H. The polish adaptation of the Multidimensional Scale of Perceived Social Support. *Pol. Forum Psychol.* **2017**, *22*, 581–599.
36. Klamut, R. Two-factor model of safety experience-Theoretical assumptions and empirical verification: Safety Experience Questionnaire. *Pol. Forum Psychol.* **2019**, *24*, 308–323.

37. Steger, M.F.; Frazier, P.; Oishi, S.; Kaler, M. The Meaning in Life Questionnaire: Assessing the Presence of and Search for meaning in life. *J. Couns. Psychol.* **2006**, *53*, 80–93. [CrossRef]
38. Kossakowska, M.; Kwiatek, P.; Stefaniak, T. Meaning in life. The Polish version of Meaning in Life Questionnaire MLQ (PL). *Psychologia Jakości Życia* **2013**, *12*, 111–131.
39. Markham, A.; Buchanan, E. Ethical Decision-Making and Internet Research: Recommendations from the AoIR Ethics Working Committee (Version 2.0). Available online: https://aoir.org/reports/ethics2.pdf2012 (accessed on 30 April 2020).
40. De Pierro, J.; Lowe, S.; Katz, C. Lessons learned from 9/11: Mental health perspectives on the COVID-19 pandemic. *Psychiatry Res.* **2020**, *288*, 113024. [CrossRef]
41. Holmes, E.A.; O'Connor, R.C.; Perry, V.H.; Tracey, I.; Wessely, S.; Arseneault, L.; Ballard, C.; Christensen, H.; Cohen Silver, R.; Everall, I.; et al. Multidisciplinary research priorities for the COVID-19 pandemic: A call for action for mental health science. *Lancet Psychiatry* **2020**, *7*, 547–560. [CrossRef]
42. Cui, P.P.; Wang, P.P.; Wang, K.; Ping, Z.; Wang, P.; Chen, C. Post-traumatic growth and influencing factors among frontline nurses fighting against COVID-19. *Occup. Environ. Med.* **2021**, *78*, 129–135. [CrossRef]
43. Xu, M.; Zhang, Y. Psychological survey of the first batch of clinical frontline support nurses to fight against COVID-19 epidemic. *Nurs. Res.* **2020**, *34*, 368–370.
44. Updegraff, J.A.; Taylor, S.E. *From vulnerability to growth: Positive and negative effects of stressful life events.InLoss and Trauma: General and Close Relationship Perspectives*; Harvey, J.H., Miller, E.D., Eds.; Brunner-Routledge: Philadelphia, PA, USA, 2000; pp. 3–28.
45. Zuriguel-Pérez, E.; Falcó-Pegueroles, A.; Agustino-Rodríguez, S.; Gómez-Martín, M.D.C.; Roldán-Merino, J.; Lluch-Canut, M.T. Clinical nurses's critical thinking level according to sociodemographic and professional variables (Phase II): A correlational study. *Nurse Educ. Pract.* **2019**, *41*, 102649. [CrossRef]
46. Schubert, C.F.; Schmidt, U.; Rosner, R. Posttraumatic growth in populations with post-traumatic stress disorder-a systematic review on growth-related psychological constructs and biological variables. *Clin. Psychol. Psychother.* **2016**, *23*, 469–486. [CrossRef] [PubMed]
47. Wu, X.; Kaminga, A.C.; Dai, W.; Deng, J.; Wang, Z.; Pan, X.; Liu, A. The prevalence of moderate-to-high post-traumatic growth: A systematic review and meta-analysis. *J. Affect. Disord.* **2019**, *243*, 408–415. [CrossRef] [PubMed]
48. Helgeson, V.S.; Reynolds, K.A.; Tomich, P.L. A meta-analytic review of benefit finding and growth. *J. Consult. Clin. Psychol.* **2006**, *74*, 797–816. [CrossRef] [PubMed]
49. Zoellner, T.; Maercker, A. Posttraumatic growth in clinical psychology—A critical review and introduction of a two component model. *Clin. Psychol. Rev.* **2006**, *26*, 626–653. [CrossRef] [PubMed]
50. Chen, R.; Sun, C.; Chen, J.J.; Jen, H.J.; Kang, X.L.; Kao, C.C.; Chou, K.R. A Large-scale survey on trauma, burnout, and post-traumatic growth among nurses during the COVID-19 pandemic. *Int. J. Ment. Health Nurs.* **2021**, *30*, 102–116. [CrossRef] [PubMed]
51. Park, C.L.; Wilt, J.A.; Russell, B.S.; Fendrich, M.R. Does perceived post-traumatic growth predict better psychological adjustment during the COVID-19 pandemic? Results from a national longitudinal survey in the USA. *J. Psychiatr. Res.* **2022**, *146*, 179–185. [CrossRef]
52. Nishi, D.; Matsuoka, Y.; Kim, Y. Posttraumatic growth, post-traumatic stress disorder and resilience of motor vehicle accident survivors. *Biopsychosoc. Med.* **2010**, *4*, 7. [CrossRef]
53. Tedeschi, R.G.; Calhoun, L.G. The Posttraumatic Growth Inventory: Measuring the positive legacy of trauma. *J. Trauma Stress* **1996**, *9*, 455–471. [CrossRef]
54. Hu, R.; Wang, X.; Liu, Z.; Hou, J.; Liu, Y.; Tu, J.; Jia, M.; Liu, Y.; Zhou, H. Stigma, depression, and post-traumatic growth among Chinese stroke survivors: A longitudinal study examining patterns and correlations. *Top Stroke Rehabil.* **2022**, *29*, 16–29. [CrossRef]
55. Zhang, X.T.; Shi, S.S.; Qin Ren, Y.; Wang, L. The traumatic experience of clinical nurses during the COVID-19 pandemic: Which factors are related to post-traumatic growth? *Risk Manag. Healthc. Policy* **2021**, *14*, 2145–2151. [CrossRef]
56. Mo, Y.; Tao, P.; Liu, G.; Chen, L.; Li, G.; Lu, S.; Zhang, G.; Liang, R.; Huang, H. Post-traumatic growth of nurses who faced the COVID-19 epidemic and its correlation with professional self-identity and social support. *Front. Psychiatry* **2022**, *12*, 562938. [CrossRef] [PubMed]
57. Zhai, H.K.; Li, Q.; Hu, Y.X.; Cui, Y.X.; Wei, X.W.; Zhou, X. Emotional creativity improves post-traumatic growth and mental health during the COVID-19 pandemic. *Front Psychol.* **2021**, *12*, 600798. [CrossRef] [PubMed]
58. Tedeschi, R.G.; Shakeaspere-Finch, J.; Takn, K.; Calhoun, L.G. *Posttraumatic Growth: Theory, Research, and Applications*; Routledge: London, UK, 2018.
59. Schwartz, S.H. An overview of the Schwartz theory of basic values. *Online Read. Psychol. Cult.* **2012**, *2*, 1–20. [CrossRef]
60. Klamut, R. Security experience and civic activity in the context of sex. *Humanit. Soc. Sci.* **2014**, *21*, 67–81.
61. Moreno-Jiménez, J.E.; Blanco-Donoso, L.M.; Demerouti, E.; BeldaHofheinz, S.; Chico-Fernández, M.; Moreno-Jiménez, B.; Garrosa, E. The role of healthcare professionals' passion in predicting secondary traumatic stress and post-traumatic growth in the face of COVID-19: A longitudinal approach. *Int. J. Environ. Res. Public Health* **2021**, *18*, 4453. [CrossRef] [PubMed]
62. Davis, C.G.; Wortman, C.B.; Lehman, D.R.; Silver, R.C. Searching for meaning in loss: Are clinical assumptions correct. *Death Stud.* **2000**, *24*, 497–540.
63. Kashdan, T.B.; Kane, J.Q. Post-traumatic distress and the presence of post-traumatic growth and meaning in life: Experiential avoidance as a moderator. *Pers. Individ. Dif.* **2011**, *50*, 84–89. [CrossRef]

64. Triplett, K.N.; Tedeschi, R.G.; Cann, A.; Calhoun, L.G.; Reeve, C.L. Posttraumatic growth, meaning in life, and life satisfaction in response to trauma. *Psychol. Trauma Theory Res. Pract. Policy* **2012**, *4*, 400–410. [CrossRef]
65. Baños, R.M.; Garcés, J.J.; Miragall, M.; Herrero, R.; Vara, M.D.; Soria-Olivas, E. Exploring the heterogeneity and trajectories of positive functioning variables, emotional distress, and post-traumatic growth during strict confinement due to COVID-19. *J. Happiness Stud.* **2021**, *2*, 1–26. [CrossRef]
66. Trzebiński, J.; Cabański, M.; Czarnecka, J.Z. Reaction to the COVID-19 pandemic: The influence of meaning inlife, life satisfaction, and assumptions on world orderliness and positivity. *J. Loss Trauma* **2020**, *25*, 544–557. [CrossRef]
67. Updegraff, J.A.; Silver, R.C.; Holman, E.A. Searching for and finding meaning in collective trauma: Results from a national longitudinal study of the 9/11 terrorist attacks. *J. Pers. Soc. Psychol.* **2008**, *95*, 709–722. [CrossRef] [PubMed]
68. Zhou, H.; Jin, M.; Ma, Q. Remedy for work stress: The impact and mechanism of ethical leadership. *Cent. Eur. J. Public. Health* **2015**, *23*, 176–180. [CrossRef] [PubMed]
69. Levin, J. Mental health care for survivors and healthcare workers in the aftermath of an outbreak. In *Psychiatry of Pandemics. A Mental Health Response to Infection Outbreak*; Huremović, D., Ed.; Springer: Cham, Switzerland, 2019; pp. 127–141.
70. Main Chamber of Nurses and Midwives. Analyzes and Reports. Available online: https://nipip.pl/dane-statystyczne/ (accessed on 18 May 2022).

International Journal of
Environmental Research and Public Health

MDPI

Article

Effect of Job Stress on Burnout among Nurses Responding to COVID-19: The Mediating Effect of Resilience

Yoon Jung Cha [1,2], Kang-Sook Lee [1,3,*], Jeong Hee Cho [2], Ik Soon Choi [2] and Dahyeon Lee [1,3]

[1] Department of Health Promotion, Graduate School of Public Health and Healthcare Management, The Catholic University of Korea, Seoul 06591, Korea; chayj44@gmail.com (Y.J.C.); dada2020@catholic.ac.kr (D.L.)
[2] Seoul National University Bundang Hospital, Seongnam 13620, Korea; nrcjh72@gmail.com (J.H.C.); ischoi66@snubh.org (I.S.C.)
[3] Department of Preventive Medicine, College of Medicine, The Catholic University of Korea, Seoul 06591, Korea
* Correspondence: leekangs@catholic.ac.kr; Tel.: +82-10-2289-1938

Abstract: Background: This study was conducted to evaluate the relationship of job stress, burnout, and resilience of 271 nurses who worked alternately at a university hospital in South Korea Province and a state-designated inpatient ward for COVID-19 in Korea. Methods: The study sample included nurses who worked at a university hospital in South Korea, during the period between February 2020 and May 2021. The participants (n = 271) responded to an online survey between April 2021 and 12 May 2021. The questionnaire included information related to job stress, burn out, and resilience. Results: In phase 1 of regression, job stress had a significant negative effect on resilience of recovery ($\beta = -0.397$, $p < 0.001$). In phase 2, job stress had a significant positive effect on burnout ($\beta = 0.513$, $p < 0.001$). In phase 3, resilience had a significant negative effect on burnout ($\beta = -0.459$, $p < 0.001$). Seventy-five percent of burnout was directly associated with job stress, while 25% of burnout was indirectly associated through mediated effects, through resilience. Conclusions: The promotion of resilience would not only serve as the basis for active coping in situations where burnout and stress are severe, but also serve as a basic driving force for actively overcoming them. Further study to cope with stress and reduce burnout at the organizational level should be conducted.

Keywords: COVID-19; novel infectious disease; burnout; job stress; resilience

Citation: Cha, Y.J.; Lee, K.-S.; Cho, J.H.; Choi, I.S.; Lee, D. Effect of Job Stress on Burnout among Nurses Responding to COVID-19: The Mediating Effect of Resilience. *Int. J. Environ. Res. Public Health* **2022**, *19*, 5409. https://doi.org/10.3390/ijerph19095409

Academic Editors: Richard Gray and Sonia Udod

Received: 16 February 2022
Accepted: 26 April 2022
Published: 29 April 2022

1. Introduction

The occurrence of emerging infectious diseases has been increasing due to frequent overseas exchanges and changes in the environment and ecosystems worldwide [1]. A case in point is the novel coronavirus disease, which has been the most recently occurring infectious disease that was first detected in December 2019 in Wuhan, Hubei Province, China.

The coronavirus disease-19 (COVID-19) has spread worldwide due to its continued proliferation [2]. Initially known only as an infectious respiratory disease with an unknown cause, on 9 January 2020, the World Health Organization (WHO) revealed that the disease is caused by a heretofore undetected RNA virus pathogen belonging to the *Coronaviridae* family. COVID-19 is an infectious respiratory disease caused by SARS-CoV-2. There are various respiratory symptoms of COVID-19 such as fever, cough, dyspnea, and pneumonia. Although there are asymptomatic and mild cases, it can be viewed as a potentially fatal infectious disease. As of May 2021, the accumulated number of confirmed COVID-19 patients was 162,208,643 worldwide. In particular, the accumulated number of confirmed COVID-19 patients in Korea was 132,290, the death toll was 1903, and the number of confirmed patients per day was 597, without a significant decrease [3].

COVID-19 continues to spread rapidly in clusters across various places in the community. This raised the necessity for active responses from medical personnel. Among them, the presence of nursing personnel is required the most in various healthcare units, from screening clinics for COVID-19 response to intensive care units [4].

It has been reported that the occurrence of an emerging infectious disease causes severe stress among nurses [5]. Nurses working with emerging infectious diseases must treat diseases more severely than those of ordinary patients and comply with rules concerning special clothes and infection guidelines instead of wearing general nursing uniforms. The severity and intensity of the work of nurses responding to COVID-19 are higher than those of nurses working in general wards [6]. In general, the number of patients per nurse in the general ward is 10–15, and they typically work for 8 h. For intensive care unit nurses, the number of patients per nurse is two to three critical patients and two to three with mild symptoms, and the length of their working hours is also eight. The number of patients per two nurses in the COVID isolation ward is one to two and two to three patients with mild symptoms, and their work is carried out in shifts of two hours for a total of eight hours.

Job stress occurs when individual needs and organizational goals are imbalanced in the process of communicating within and beyond the organization. Nurses experience psychological burnout due to an increased demand for professional knowledge and skills, role conflicts with other medical staff, poor working environments, conflicts with management and employees of other departments, and various other needs of nurses [7]. Moreover, research has reported that nurses working in the intensive care unit, who must meet the complex needs of patients in critical situations, experience a greater sense of burnout and mental distress than nurses in general wards [8].

Psychological capital refers to utilizing constructive psychological strengths to improve one's performance in a given environment to embody progressive thinking and attitudes [9]. A previous study defined psychological capital as four dimensions: efficacy, resilience, hope, and optimism. Among them, resilience has begun to be widely studied in the field of positive psychology [10]. Resilience is the ability to recover from and overcome distress caused by problems and obstacles in achieving goals [10]. Moreover, resilience enables the achievement of goals and the improvement of performance based on individuals' positive psychological states.

In response to the emerging COVID-19 pandemic, the Central Disaster and Safety Countermeasure Headquarters in Korea designated hospitals dedicated to infectious disease prevention and public hospitals, to share roles in isolating and treating infected persons in negative pressure isolation rooms [11]. Moreover, Designated Public Relief Hospitals in Korea diagnose and treat respiratory and non-respiratory patients separately to protect them from infection within the facility [12]. Nurses working in state-designated inpatient treatment rooms provide care, to patients diagnosed with new infectious diseases or suspected patients, in a single-room negative pressure isolation ward, wearing Level-D protective equipment [13].

So far, there have been studies to find the influencing factors of burnout in emergency room nurses, cancer ward nurses and intensive care unit nurses. A previous study about COVID-19 response nurses wrote about the association of the sub-factors of job stress and resilience with burnout, but that study did not examine the mediating effect of resilience [14].

This study examines how factors of job stress relate to burnout among nurses working at Designated Public Relief Hospitals in Korea during the COVID-19 outbreak. Moreover, this study determines the mediating effect of resilience on the relationship between factors of job stress in response to COVID-19 and burnout. This study aims to prove such a correlation. Job stress will have a positive correlation with job burnout and a negative correlation with resilience. Resilience will affect job stress and job burnout. The greater the resilience, the better it is expected to be able to respond to job stress and burnout. This study highlights the importance of enhancing the resilience of medical personnel responding to COVID-19.

2. Subjects and Methods

2.1. Study Sample and Data Collection

The study sample included nurses who worked at a university hospital in South Korea during the period between February 2020 and May 2021. The sample also included nurses working in state-designated inpatient treatment wards in hospitals located in the southern regions of South Korea where confirmed or suspected COVID-19 patients were hospitalized or treated (COVID-19 isolation ward, COVID-19 isolation intensive care unit, and COVID-19 suspect patient isolation ward). A poster containing a QR code was displayed at the hospital so that those interested in participating in the study could gain access to the online survey, which had been prepared in Google Forms. A total of 300 people worked at the hospital dedicated to COVID-19. Twenty-nine nurses did not participate, so the total number of participants was two hundred and seventy one. The use of an online survey for data collection was rather effective given the ongoing pandemic. This allowed us to contact participants by phone to answer any questions related to the study, which eliminated the need for any face-to-face interaction.

This study was approved by the Institutional Review Board of Seoul National University Bundang Hospital (IRB NO. B-2012/652-305).

2.2. Measures

2.2.1. Socio-Demographic Variables

Participants responded to a survey regarding their socio-demographic characteristics such as gender, age, years of service, educational background, and annual salary. Gender was classified into "male" and "female". Age was classified at 10-year intervals from the "20s" to the "60s". The number of years of service at the current hospital was categorized as "less than one year", "less than one to three years", "less than three to five years", "less than five to ten years", and "more than ten years". Educational background was classified as "high school education or lower", "associate degree", "bachelor's degree", "master's degree", and "doctoral degree", while the annual salary level was classified at intervals of 16,000 dollars into five groups, from "less than 16,000 dollars" to "more than 65,000 dollars".

2.2.2. Korean Occupational Stress Scale (KOSS)

A previous study developed a scale to measure and identify factors causing job stress among the Korean population [15]. Considering the number of questions in the entire survey, an abridged version of the scale was used, which excluded factors of job climate and job insecurity and reduced the number of questions constituting each sub-factor. KOSS consists of 30 questions on a 5-point Likert scale ranging from of "strongly disagree", to "strongly agree". Items (Cronbach's α) were included such as physical environment (0.313), on-job demands (0.828), lack of job autonomy (0.205), relationship conflicts (0.757), organizational system (0.878), and inadequate compensation (0.790).

2.2.3. Scale of Burnout

Burnout was measured using a scale consisting of 15 questions, adapted and validated by Shin [16] for Korean workers. This scale is based on the Maslach Burnout Inventory-General Survey (MBI-GS) developed by [17]. Shin's study secured the validity of the 15-item scale by deleting one question on impersonalization with the lowest internal consistency [16]. Thus, the scale included a total of 15 questions with five questions on emotional exhaustion, four on cynicism (impersonalization), and six on job achievement reduction. Participants responded on a five-point Likert scale ranging from "not at all" to "very much so". Since the orientation of the items regarding job achievement reduction is described in a positive manner, responses to these items were reverse scored to facilitate interpretation. Cronbach's α for each item was emotional exhaustion 0.890, cynicism (impersonalization) 0.788, and job achievement reduction 0.817.

2.2.4. Korean-Connor-Davison Resilience Scale (K-CD-RISC)

Resilience was measured using a self-reporting scale measuring one's stress coping capability. The Connor–Davison Resilience Scale (CD-RISC) was developed by [18] and adapted by [19]. This study used the Korean version of the CD-RISC that consists of a total of twenty-five questions, including nine for toughness, eight for patience, four for optimism, two for control, and two for spirituality. Participants responded on a five-point Likert scale. Cronbach's α for each item was toughness 0.823, patience 0.872, optimism 0.704, control 0.653, spirituality 0.636.

2.3. *Data Analysis*

The SPSS 25.0 program (IBM Corporation, Armonk, NY, USA) was used to analyze the data and calculate the Cronbach's α for each scale to confirm their reliability. Descriptive statistical analysis was conducted to determine the levels of the research variables, and a correlation analysis was conducted to identify the correlation between the research variables. To determine the relationship between job stress and burnout, regression analysis was conducted according to the mediation effect verification procedure proposed by [6] and re-verified by bootstrapping using SPSS Process Macro. Statistical significance was determined based on a 5% significance level.

3. Results

3.1. *General Characteristics of the Study Sample*

Of the participants, 33 men and 238 women were selected and analyzed as subjects. Of the 271 participants, 226 (87.8%) identified as female, 125 (46.1%) were in their 20s, 70 (25.8%) had served for less than 1 to 3 years, 226 (83.4%) nurses had a bachelor's degree, and 151 (55.7%) received an annual salary of between 32,000 dollars and less than 48,000 dollars (Table 1).

Table 1. General characteristics of the study participants.

Variables	Categories	n	%
Gender	Male	33	12.2
	Female	238	87.8
Age(year)	20–29	125	46.1
	30–39	91	33.6
	40–49	43	15.9
	50–59	12	4.4
Duration of service(year)	1<	54	19.9
	1–3	70	25.8
	3–5	59	21.8
	5–10	41	15.1
	≥10	47	17.3
Academic background	High school diploma	3	1.1
	Associate degree	30	11.1
	Bachelor	226	83.4
	Master	12	4.4
Annual income (thousand dollars/year)	16–32	73	26.9
	32–48	151	55.7
	48–65	44	16.2
	≥65	3	1.1

3.2. *Correlation Analysis*

Pearson's correlation analysis was conducted to determine the relationship between the variables in this study.

Job stress and burnout demonstrated a statistically significant positive correlation (r = 0.499, $p < 0.001$). Job stress and resilience demonstrated a significant negative correlation (r = −0.420, $p < 0.001$). Burnout and resilience demonstrated a significant negative correlation (r = −0.589, $p < 0.001$).

Furthermore, the absolute value of the correlation coefficient between the measurement variables was less than 0.80, whereby there was no issue of multicollinearity (Table 2).

Table 2. Correlation analysis of job stress, burnout and resilience.

	Average	Standard Deviations	Job Stress	Burnout	Resilience
Job stress	3.08	0.46	1		
Burnout	2.91	0.52	0.499 ($p < 0.001$)	1	
Resilience	3.52	0.56	−0.420 ($p < 0.001$)	−0.589 ($p < 0.001$)	1

3.3. Verification of the Mediating Effect of Resilience in the Relationship between Job Stress and Burnout

In Step 1, gender, a control variable, was found to have a statistically significant negative effect on resilience ($\beta = -0.145$, $p < 0.05$). Resilience among females was lower than that of males. Job stress, an independent variable, had a significant negative effect on resilience ($\beta = -0.397$, $p < 0.001$). The explanatory power of the control variables and job stress for resilience were 21.6% (F = 12.114, $p < 0.001$).

In Step 2, it was found that job stress had a significantly positive effect on burnout, a dependent variable ($\beta = 0.513$, $p < 0.001$). The explanatory power of the control variables and job stress for burnout was 26.9% (F = 16.166, $p < 0.001$).

Finally, in Step 3, it was found that job stress had a significantly positive effect on burnout ($\beta = 0.331$, $p < 0.001$). Moreover, resilience had a significant negative effect on burnout ($\beta = -0.459$, $p < 0.001$). The explanatory power of the control variables, job stress, and resilience for burnout was 43.4% (F = 28.758, $p < 0.001$).

Therefore, job stress directly relates to burnout and indirectly relates to burnout through resilience (Table 3).

Table 3. Results of mediated effectiveness verification of resilience.

Model	Dependent Variable	Independent Variable	B	SE	β	T	p	F(R2)
1	Resilience	Gender (female)	−0.248	0.101	−0.145	−2.465	0.014	12.114 (0.216) $p < 0.001$
		Age	0.034	0.046	0.053	0.736	0.462	
		Duration of service	−0.004	0.033	−0.009	−0.113	0.910	
		Academic background	0.099	0.072	0.077	1.365	0.173	
		Annual income	0.066	0.059	0.080	1.118	0.265	
		Job stress	−0.486	0.072	−0.397	−6.776	<0.001	
2	Burnout	Gender (female)	0.062	0.090	0.039	0.692	0.489	16.166 (0.269) $p < 0.001$
		Age	−0.027	0.041	−0.045	−0.647	0.518	
		Duration of service	−0.021	0.030	−0.057	−0.716	0.475	
		Academic background	−0.028	0.065	−0.024	−0.440	0.660	
		Annual income	−0.045	0.052	−0.060	−0.865	0.388	
		Job stress	0.579	0.064	0.513	9.063	<0.001	
3	Burnout	Gender (female)	−0.043	0.080	−0.027	−0.536	0.592	28.758 (0.434) $p < 0.001$
		Age	−0.012	0.036	−0.021	−0.338	0.736	
		Duration of service	−0.023	0.026	−0.061	−0.873	0.384	
		Academic background	0.013	0.057	0.011	0.235	0.814	
		Annual income	−0.017	0.046	−0.023	−0.378	0.706	
		Job stress	0.373	0.061	0.331	6.119	<0.001	
		Resilience	−0.423	0.048	−0.459	−8.749	<0.001	

Zero is not included between the lower and upper limits of the 95% confidence interval for the estimate of the indirect effects of job stress on burnout mediated through resilience. Thus, it may be stated that the mediating effect of resilience on the relationship between job stress and burnout is statistically significant (Table 4).

Table 4. Validate the mediated effectiveness of resilience with bootstrapping.

Path	B	SE	95% CI	
			LLCI	ULCI
Job stress → Resilience → burnout	0.205	0.047	0.126	0.305

3.4. *Summary of the Results of Hypothesis Testing*

The results of the hypothesis test conducted earlier are summarized in Table 5.

Table 5. Summary of hypothesis validation results.

	Hypothesis	Result
1.1	*Job stress will have a significant negative correlation to resilience.*	Adoption
1.2	*Job stress will have a significant positive correlation with burnout.*	Adoption
1.3	*Resilience will have a significant negative correlation to burnout.*	Adoption
2.1	*Resilience will play a role in the relationship between job stress and burnout.*	Adoption

4. Discussion

This study attempted to examine the relationship between factors of job stress, burnout, and resilience among nurses responding to COVID-19. Further, it verified the mediating effects of resilience on the relationship between job stress and burnout.

Factors of job stress had a significant negative effect on resilience. This is consistent with a previous finding where job stress and resilience were negatively related [20]. Moreover, Baek confirmed that the input of resilience offsets negative effects in the presence of job stress [6]. Therefore, while it is necessary to create optimal job environments and forms of work to reduce job stress for nurses responding to COVID-19, it is also important to improve individual resilience to effectively reduce stress.

Job stress is positively associated with burnout among nurses working against COVID-19. This is consistent with findings from a previous study by [21], who investigated the effects on the burnout of state-designated inpatient treatment ward nurses with a focus on job stress [21]. Oh's study made use of Parker and DeCotiis's study job stress measurement tool to determine the level of job stress of intensive care unit nurses. The results showed that their stress level was higher than that of general ward nurses [8,22]. On the basis of this finding, it can be inferred that the job stress and burnout of intensive care unit nurses working against emerging infectious diseases are also higher than those of general ward nurses. Increased job stress also leads to an increase in job burnout. Therefore, it is necessary to constantly monitor the professional environment, rest system for the staff, availability of enough manpower, and the individual state of work overload to reduce the job stress of nurses responding to COVID-19.

The study by [21] presented research results where the job stress of intensive care unit nurses was higher than that of general ward nurses, using a job stress measurement tool developed by [8,22]. This demonstrates that the job stress and burnout of intensive care unit nurses working against emerging infectious diseases are higher than those of nurses working in general wards. Most of the participants in this study are in their 20s, and there is no significant difference from 3 to 5 years of continuous work. In previous studies, superiors have a higher job stress due to the burden of role as middle managers [14]. After more than nine years, job stress is less felt as the opportunity to judge independently increases due to the increase in proficiency and position [23].

According to a previous study by [7] that examined the effect of resilience on burnout with a focus on the experience of clinical nurses, burnout among clinical nurses decreases with higher resilience. This finding supports the results of the current study—resilience has a significant negative effect on burnout [7]. This study highlights the need for individuals to improve resilience on their own and at the organizational level, as well as to become a supporting basis thereof. A nurse's career, work type management, character content activity, resilience enhancement program, and enjoyment of leisure activities are required. These activities can improve the resilience of nurses [24].

Resilience plays a partially mediating role in the relationship between job stress and burnout among nurses responding to COVID-19. Job stress relates burnout through resilience, indicating that burnout decreases with low job stress and a high level of resilience. This is consistent with the results of a previous study by [25], which states that methods of improving resilience should be sought out to reduce burnout [25]. Accordingly, the promotion of resilience would not only serve as the basis for active coping in situations where burnout and stress are severe, but also serve as a basic driving force for actively overcoming them.

Infection control fatigue of nurses affects job stress. In order to improve this, it is necessary to improve the working environment and provide customized training programs for each career [26]. As the risk and workload from unpredictable emerging infectious diseases and various disastrous situations increase for medical personnel, including those responding to COVID-19, there is an increased need for personnel in the medical sector. A previous study suggested that changing personal and organizational situations might help to prevent job burnout of medical personnel coping with emerging infectious diseases. Personal situations refer to increasing the ability to personally overcome burnout through education, while changes in organizational situations refer to changes in the job environment and organizational members [27].

Sufficient medical personnel should be replaced when they take a break by preparing appropriate standards for the intensity of work and rest areas of medical personnel responding to COVID-19. Spaces for them to rest during breaks must be created in the hospitals. This can be accomplished by acquiring enough extra manpower. These measures pertain to the aspects of providing adequate control and resources in the job demands-resources model to for alleviating psychological factors such as job stress, burnout, tension, and anxiety in the job demand resource model [28].

Hospitals must minimize mental and physical damage to medical personnel who are unfairly treated due to overwork. Instead, hospitals need to improve the treatment of medical personnel before focusing on being patient centered. This will positively reduce the effect of factors associating job stress and job burnout among medical personnel. Nurses' job stress and burnout were found to be higher as the social support was lower. Applying this, social support is expected to have an important effect on resilience [29]. A study on the development of a coaching program to improve the resilience of new nurses was conducted in 2018 [30].

5. Conclusions

Based on this study, a personal-level measure was proposed to improve the resilience among individual medical personnel and reduce job stress. However, support from hospitals and organizations is also important. This is because while there is no limit to internalizing resilience from the perspective of medical staff practicing medicine, resilience is influenced by factors responsible for buffering, such as social support and resources possessed by organizations, superiors, and colleagues [31]. Therefore, a wider range of studies must be conducted on organizational-level countermeasures to alleviate job stress in the future.

6. Limitation

Since the survey was conducted only in the southern regions of South Korea, generalizing the findings of this study will be limited. It has limitations as only male and female without other in the gender classification were investigated. Future studies should include a larger and more diverse sample of nurses responding to COVID-19, and further compare the degree of job stress and job burnout among nurses working in general wards. As this is a cross-sectional study, it is difficult to determine a causal relation.

Author Contributions: Conceptualization, K.-S.L. and Y.J.C.; methodology, Y.J.C.; software, D.L.; validation, Y.J.C., J.H.C. and I.S.C.; formal analysis, Y.J.C.; investigation, J.H.C.; resources, J.H.C.; data curation, I.S.C.; writing—original draft preparation, Y.J.C.; writing—review and editing, D.L.; visualization, D.L.; supervision, K.-S.L.; project administration, K.-S.L. All authors have read and agreed to the published version of the manuscript.

Funding: This research received no external funding.

Institutional Review Board Statement: This study was approved by the Institutional Review Board of Seoul National University Bundang Hospital (IRB NO. B-2012/652-305).

Informed Consent Statement: This study is a survey study and received a written consent from during the questionnaire.

Data Availability Statement: This study is a self-reported survey, and information was obtained from the subject oneself.

Acknowledgments: We thank Seoul National University Bundang Hospital and hospitals located in the southern regions of Gyeonggi-do.

Conflicts of Interest: The authors declare no conflict of interest.

References

1. Lee, M.A. Diagnosis for Imported Cases of Emerging and Reemerging Infectious Diseases in Korea. *Ewha Med. J.* **2016**, *39*, 37–44. [CrossRef]
2. Korea Centers for Disease Control and Prevention; National Institute of Health. COVID-19 Virus Characterictic | COVID-19 | Research. Available online: http://www.kdca.go.kr/contents.es?mid=a40509010000 (accessed on 4 May 2021).
3. Korea Centers for Disease Control and Prevention. COVID-19>Occurrence Trend>Domestic Occurrences. Available online: http://ncov.mohw.go.kr/bdBoardList_Real.do?brdId=1&brdGubun=11&ncvContSeq=&contSeq=&board_id=&gubun= (accessed on 4 May 2021).
4. Cha, Y.-K. The Revision of the 「Medical Service Law」 in 2015 and Proposal for Post-COVID-19 World—Focusing on Nurse-Related Regulations. *Law Rev.* **2021**, *21*, 295–339.
5. Lehmann, M.; Bruenahl, C.A.; Löwe, B.; Addo, M.M.; Schmiedel, S.; Lohse, A.W.; Schramm, C. Ebola and psychological stress of health care professionals. *Emerg. Infect. Dis.* **2015**, *21*, 913–914. [CrossRef] [PubMed]
6. Baron, R.M.; Kenny, D.A. The moderator–mediator variable distinction in social psychological research: Conceptual, strategic, and statistical considerations. *J. Personal. Soc. Psychol.* **1986**, *51*, 1173–1182. [CrossRef]
7. Kang, J.-S.; Lim, J.Y. Effects of clinical nurses' resilience on job stress and burnout. *Korea Contents Assoc.* **2015**, *15*, 263–273. [CrossRef]
8. Oh, E.-W.; Yang, S.-M.; Kim, S.-H.; You, H.N.; Chin, E.Y.; Kim, Y.J.; Kim, Y.H. Compare the level of job stress, burn-out and job satisfaction between intensive care unit nurses and general unit nurses. *J. Korea Inst. Orient. Med. Inform.* **2016**, *22*, 27–36.
9. Luthans, F. The need for and meaning of positive organizational behavior. *J. Organ. Behav.* **2002**, *23*, 695–706. [CrossRef]
10. Luthans, F.; Youssef, C.M. Human, social and now positive psychological capital management: Investing in people for competitive advantage. *Organ. Dyn.* **2004**, *33*, 143–160. [CrossRef]
11. Ministry of Health and Welfare & Korea. Management of Medical Institutions with Confirmed Cases of COVID-19 (3.4.). Available online: http://ncov.mohw.go.kr/guideBoardView.do?brdId=3&brdGubun=35&dataGubun=&ncvContSeq=988&contSeq=988&board_id=&gubun= (accessed on 4 May 2021).
12. Ministry of Health and Welfare & Korea. Designated Public Relief Hospitals in Korea—Ministry of Health and Welfare & Korea. Available online: https://www.mohw.go.kr/react/popup_200128.html (accessed on 4 May 2021).
13. Lee, J.-W.; Kim, W.S.; Yoon, M.J. Nurses' experiences of nursing cohort-isolated psychiatric patients with emerging infectious diseases. *J. Korean Acad. Nurs.* **2020**, *10*, 289.
14. Shin, R.; Baek, H.-J.; Ahn, D.-B. Influence of Job Stress and Resilience on the Burnout of Nurses Who Works at the Designated Public Relief Hospital. *J. Korea Contents Assoc.* **2021**, *21*, 595–608.

15. Chang, S.J.; Koh, S.B.; Kang, D.; Kim, S.A.; Kang, M.G.; Lee, C.G.; Chung, J.J.; Cho, J.J.; Son, M.; Chae, C.H.; et al. Developing an Occupational Stress Scale for Korean Employees. *Ann. Occup. Environ. Med.* **2005**, *17*, 297–317. [CrossRef]
16. Shin, K.-H. The Maslach Bunout Inventory-General Survey (MBI-GS): An Application in South Korea. *Korean J. Ind. Organ. Psychol.* **2003**, *16*, 1–17.
17. Maslach, C.; Jackson, S.E.; Leiter, M.P.; Schaufeli, W.; Schwab, R. Maslach Burnout Inventory–General Survey. *Maslach Burn. Inventory-Test Man.* **1996**, *1*, 19–26.
18. Connor, K.M.; Davidson, J.R. Development of a new resilience scale: The Connor-Davidson Resilience Scale (CD-RISC). *Depress. Anxiety* **2003**, *18*, 76–82. [CrossRef] [PubMed]
19. Baek, H.-S.; Lee, K.-U.; Joo, E.-J.; Lee, M.-Y.; Choi, K.-S. Reliability and validity of the Korean Version of the Connor-Davidson Resilience Scale. *Psychiatry Investig.* **2010**, *7*, 109–115. [CrossRef]
20. Baek, Y.-S.; Jang, Y.H.; Kin, Y.J.; Lim, J.K. The effects of resilience on job stress—Focusing on the mediating effect BWF. *Korean Acad. Soc. Bus. Adm.* **2016**, *11*, 1644–1660. [CrossRef]
21. Lim, Y.-H.; Cho, Y.-C. Effects of job stress, fatigue, burnout, and job satisfaction on turnover intention among general hospital nurses. *J. Korea Acad. Ind. Coop. Soc.* **2018**, *19*, 264–274.
22. Parker, D.F.; DeCotiis, T.A. Organizational determinants of job stress. *Organ. Behav. Hum. Perform.* **1983**, *32*, 160–177. [CrossRef]
23. Kwon, K.J.; Lee, S.H. Occupational Stress and Coping Styles as Factors Affecting the Burnout of Clinical Nurses. *J. Korean Acad. Nurs. Adm.* **2012**, *18*, 383–393. [CrossRef]
24. Kim, S.-E. Influence of Clinical Nurses' Personality and Resilience on Happiness Index. *J. Digit. Converg.* **2019**, *17*, 357–365.
25. Ryu, J.L.; Ju, J.S.; Kim, S.H. The Convergence factors of nurses' character on the burnout: Focused on the mediating effects of resilience. *J. Korea Acad. Ind. Coop. Soc.* **2021**, *22*, 354–362.
26. Jun, S.H.; Lee, M.H.; Choi, M.J. COVID-19 Infection Control-Related Fatigue, Job Stress, and Burnout in Nurses. *J. Korean Acad. Soc. Home Health Care Nurs.* **2021**, *28*, 16–25.
27. Maslach, C.; Schaufeli, W.B.; Leiter, M.P. Job burnout. *Annu. Rev. Psychol.* **2001**, *52*, 397–422. [CrossRef] [PubMed]
28. Chung, M.H.; Park, I.H.; Lee, H.J. The Study of the Effects of Customer Related Social Stressors on the Job Burnout of the Airline Flight Attendants -Focused on the Moderating Effects of the Resilience. *J. Aviat. Manag. Soc. Korea* **2013**, *11*, 173–192.
29. Park, M.-Y. *Effect on Nurse's Burnout in Isolation Unit of Nationally Designated Hospitals: Focusing on Job Stress, Job Satisfaction, and Social Support*; Graduate School of Nursing, Gachon University: Seongnam, Korea, 2018; Volume 8.
30. Han, M.; Do, M.-H. Basic Research for the Development of a Coaching Program for Improving the Resilience. *J. Korean Coach. Res.* **2018**, *11*, 165–182. [CrossRef]
31. Luthans, F.; Avolio, B.J., Avey, J.B.; Norman, S.M. Positive psychological capital: Measurement and relationship with performance and satisfaction. *Pers. Psychol.* **2007**, *60*, 541–572. [CrossRef]

International Journal of
Environmental Research and Public Health

MDPI

Article

Early Nurse Management Experiences from Finnish COVID-19 Hubs: An In-Action Review

Mari S. Nevala * and Satu Vuorela

Laurea University of Applied Sciences, 01300 Vantaa, Finland; satu.vuorela@laurea.fi
* Correspondence: mari@nevala.com

Abstract: Primary healthcare (PHC) clinics are the point of access for many COVID-19 patients; however, the focus of crisis response work has been in securing hospital capacities. The purpose of this study was to describe the early nurse management experiences from PHC clinics within Greater Helsinki dedicated to caring for all ambulatory patients with possible COVID-19 symptoms. The study objectives were to make PHC crisis response contributions known and to provide an in-action review (IAR) of crisis response efforts. Nurse managers from the four COVID-19 hubs in Greater Helsinki were interviewed using thematic pair interviews. The data were analyzed inductively using thematic analysis, by which four main themes emerged: (1) capacity development led to a state of flux, (2) infection prevention control (IPC) was critical, (3) management of staff was essential in facilitating crisis response, and (4) respondents' personal experiences. The state of flux stressed the provision of PHC services, but quick developments in telemedicine eased that burden. Conversation surrounding IPC was extensive, though discrepancies suggest that global efforts to standardize IPC practices must begin locally. Leadership was adjusted to accommodate for the crisis, especially regarding the motivation of staff. A vision to aspire toward in crisis recovery is needed.

Keywords: nurse management; crisis management; primary healthcare; COVID-19 ambulatory care; in-action review

Citation: Nevala, M.S.; Vuorela, S. Early Nurse Management Experiences from Finnish COVID-19 Hubs: An In-Action Review. *Int. J. Environ. Res. Public Health* **2022**, *19*, 4885. https://doi.org/10.3390/ijerph19084885

Academic Editors: Richard Gray and Sonia Udod

Received: 20 February 2022
Accepted: 14 April 2022
Published: 17 April 2022

1. Introduction

In December 2019, an outbreak of pneumonia with an unknown etiology occurred in the city of Wuhan, China. Scientists later identified the cause of the viral disease now known as the coronavirus disease 2019 (COVID-19) to be a novel strain of coronavirus (SARS-CoV-2) [1]. On 11 March 2020, the World Health Organization (WHO) declared COVID-19 a pandemic. At that time, Finland had confirmed a total of 40 COVID-19 cases and zero deaths associated with the disease [2]. Though Finland had a relatively small number of cases early in the pandemic, examples of overwhelmed healthcare systems in China and Italy provided data to model pandemic situations and their effects on healthcare capacities [3]. The Finnish Institute for Health and Welfare (THL) had predicted that the peak of the first pandemic wave could potentially result in over 900 simultaneously hospitalized COVID-19 patients in Finland, of which 280 would need intensive care unit (ICU) level care [4]. Before the crisis, Finland had a total of 259 ICU beds, of which 70 were in the capital region [5]. According to the models, COVID-19 could have become a substantial threat to healthcare capacity in Finland [3].

The government of Finland declared emergency conditions on the 16 March 2020, based on the fifth exceptional situation defined by Finnish law, in which a dangerous and contagious pathogen is widespread [6,7]. In order to slow the spread of the virus within the population, the government implemented nationwide restrictions. The Finnish government also defined crisis standards of care, by which healthcare organizations postponed non-essential services and prioritized urgent care. The Ministry of Social Affairs and Health (STM) published guidelines for surge capacity development in emergency and ICU services, requiring 1.5–2 times the normal ICU capacity. During the peak of the first pandemic wave, there were consistently over 40 (<50) COVID-19 patients in the ICUs within the capital region, meaning that the increase in ICU capacity was more than sufficient [5].

Countries that have been successful in slowing the progression of the COVID-19 pandemic have implemented healthcare systems that include diagnosing and treating mild cases [8]. However, the focus of crisis response work has primarily been on hospital capacities. The STM had instructed municipalities to dedicate an ambulatory access point, referred to as COVID-19 hubs in this study, for suspected and confirmed cases of COVID-19 [9,10]. The three cities within Greater Helsinki each dedicated entire primary healthcare (PHC) clinics as their COVID-19 hubs [11].

Primary health care is the frontline defense for COVID-19 crisis response work at the community level [12–14]. The WHO defines PHC to be health care that accounts for the whole of society, considering both the proximity and equitable distribution of healthcare services [15]. The Finnish Health Care Act divides Finland's healthcare system into two distinct areas, provincial and municipal, or specialized and PHC services [16]. Before the PHC development in 1972, 90% of healthcare costs in Finland were due to specialized services. Now, even with just 0.7 physicians in PHC per 1000 inhabitants, specialized health care accounts for just 5% of total healthcare costs. Nurses' roles in PHC are important, as nurses held a total of 28% of urgent care-related PHC appointments [17]. These numbers highlight the importance of PHC and PHC nurses in the Finnish healthcare system and, ultimately, the significance of their contribution to the national COVID-19 crisis response as well.

Literature Review

The WHO has classified all three coronavirus diseases as priority diseases for research and development because of their risk to public health, which makes infection prevention and control (IPC) critical [18]. The WHO defines IPC to be a practical discipline that aims at preventing infections in healthcare settings, and for which implementation depends upon the transmission mode of a given pathogen [19]. COVID-19 is defined as being transmissible through droplets, meaning that it spreads through infected liquid respiratory particles [20]. Transmission risk management is the mitigation of transmission risk to as low as reasonably possible without unintentional repercussions, and a hierarchy of controls identifies relevant interventions, which are, in the descending order: elimination, substitution, engineering, administrative, and personal protective equipment (PPE) controls [21,22].

Elimination, within the hierarchy of controls, is the most effective and means removing the risk altogether—for instance, through physical isolation of symptomatic patients. Substitution refers to replacing the risk with another risk [22–24]. Engineering controls remove or reduce the hazard at its source, such as by maintaining physical distance through seating arrangements, improving ventilation and air filtration, and using physical barriers such as plexiglass partitions [20,22,25]. Administrative controls change working patterns to reduce or eliminate transmission risk, and leaders within health care are responsible for creating, communicating, and implementing clear IPC policies, such as policies for managing ill staff utilizing syndromic surveillance [19,22,25–28]. Personal protective equipment is the least effective at protecting healthcare workers (HCW) from risk and there has been much discussion about the level of PPE needed to mitigate nosocomial COVID-19 transmissions [21,23,29]. According to the THL, HCWs are to comply with universal, contact, and droplet precautions when caring for suspected and confirmed cases of COVID-19 [30]. The National Emergency Supply Agency was responsible for securing PPE when shortages threatened to put HCWs at risk [31].

Frontline HCWS are susceptible to both unprecedented physical and psychological stress related to the crisis, and many nursing platforms are worried about the wellbeing of nurses [32–37]. The COVID-19 healthcare crisis has underscored the need for effective leadership within health care, and understanding what motivates and empowers HCWs to work during public health emergencies, despite the risks involved, is an important aspect of preparedness [32,38]. One review of nurses' experiences in working during acute respiratory infection (ARI) epidemics found that nurses have a personal sense of professional obligation to work despite the risks, but are supported through professional camaraderie, adequate PPE and staffing, clear and timely communication of information, organizational preparedness, and effective leadership [39]. Nurse leaders identified that the most challenging aspect of COVID-19 leadership is responding to the increase in emotional health needs of nurses, stating that leadership in nursing may face challenges, such as distrust, in the future due to COVID-19 experiences [40]. Servant leadership, which is a leadership style in which leaders are defined by their desire to serve others and by their intent to empower their followers, can be argued to be an effective leadership style in healthcare crises, as frontline HCWs are served by their leaders in order to continue to provide quality patient care [41,42]. It is also an effective leadership method in building trust between leaders and followers [41].

Crisis management is the development and implementation of an organization's capability to respond to and recover from crises, as insufficient crisis recovery efforts can lead to a new crisis [43]. The WHO identifies PHC to be a gatekeeper in the COVID-19 healthcare crisis by reducing the need for hospital services via the identification, triage, and diagnosis of COVID-19 patients and by addressing the fear of COVID-19 within the community [12]. Primary health care has been immeasurably burdened by the crisis, due to factors such as the prioritization of COVID-19-related care [44,45]. The PHC contribution to the COVID-19 crisis response is seen in the literature through after-action reviews, which show both the resilience and weaknesses of our healthcare systems [10,14,44,46,47]. Frontline PHC nursing experiences are less represented in the literature, though one study found issues concerning employment insecurity and inadequate PPE to be elements of the PHC nursing COVID-19 experience [48]. There are very few, if any, publications on the experiences of nurses and/or nurse managers working within COVID-19 hubs.

In order to evaluate and improve public health response, both after-action reviews (AAR) and in-action reviews (IAR) of crisis response efforts are essential [49–51]. The purpose of this study was to describe the early nurse management experiences from PHC clinics within Greater Helsinki dedicated to caring for all ambulatory patients with possible COVID-19 symptoms. The research question was: "What were the early experiences of nurse managers of PHC clinics dedicated to caring for patients with possible COVID-19 symptoms?" The objectives were to make PHC crisis response contributions known and to provide an IAR of crisis response efforts. Nurse managers from the four COVID-19 hubs within Greater Helsinki were interviewed using thematic pair interviews. Data were analyzed inductively using thematic analysis. This study was conducted as the first author's master's thesis in Global Health and Crisis Management [52].

2. Materials and Methods

Both AAR and IAR guidelines were utilized for the purposes of this study [49–51]. The data were collected through thematic pair interviews of key informants using telecommunication. The study was designed to use minimal staff resources and to reduce the role of the interviewer to lessen the impact of possible bias. Thematic interviewing is defined to be conversation encompassing predefined themes, for which the structure of the interview framework is essential [53]. In generating the themes for this interview, a semi-structured literature search was conducted on the topic with the help of information retrieval guidance services provided by the university library. Themes were extracted by categorizing information into possible background information and potential interview themes. Potential interview themed notes were coded, and the codes were then categorized into five themes: capacity development, management of staff, infection prevention, emerging issues, and overall experiences. Possible questions were then derived from the codes.

A clear purposive strategy for respondent recruitment was applied using the defined target group from the purpose of the study [53]. The term "early" is defined by the time between the activation of the Emergency Powers Act and the last conducted interview

(16 March 2020–2 February 2021). The respondents were all working as nurse managers of the four COVID-19 hubs in Greater Helsinki during this time. Greater Helsinki is defined by the three separate municipalities of Espoo, Helsinki, and Vantaa. Espoo and Vantaa each had one COVID-19 hub, while Helsinki had two. The four respondents were identified as the most relevant sources of information because including respondents from other parts of Finland would have diluted the context of the study. The first author contacted the respondents directly using the names and email addresses listed on municipal websites [53]. All communication with the respondents, including the interviews, was conducted in Finnish. All three cities gave their approval for the study and all four targeted nurse managers participated in the study. To better triangulate the data, the two managers from Helsinki were each paired with a manager from either Espoo or Vantaa.

In line with general data protection regulations (GDPR), each respondent gave their written and informed consent to the collection, usage, and storage of the data produced by the interviews. Only the first author had access to the original data from the interviews. After the thesis report was published in December 2021, the original data from the interviews (recordings, transcriptions, and original paper codes) were destroyed due to the high risk of being able to identify respondents and their contributions. The original mind maps are retained by the first author. Respondents were made aware of the extent of their contribution through member checking and participation was voluntary throughout the duration of the study [53,54]. This study was exempt from an ethical statement from the Human Sciences Ethics Committee of the Helsinki Region of Universities of Applied Sciences; however, the first author retains the study permits obtained from the municipalities and the informed consent letters signed by the respondents [55].

2.1. Data Analysis

The data were analyzed and coded inductively using thematic analysis. Thematic analysis is a qualitative research analysis method that can be used to identify, analyze, organize, describe, and report themes within data. The thematic analysis process can be described in six phases [56].

2.1.1. Phase 1: Familiarize with the Data

This phase requires an immersion into the data, which is achieved through active rereading of the data [56]. After the data were collected, the recorded interviews were listened to by the first author multiple times before, during, and after transcription. The transcription process itself engendered active familiarization with the data, as the first author transcribed both interviews herself. Throughout the analysis process, the first author would return to the full transcriptions and/or interview recordings as needed. This was done when the context of authentic separated data was in question.

2.1.2. Phase 2: Form Codes from the Data

Coding happens after an in-depth familiarization of the data and is a reflective process that simplifies data characteristics [56]. This second phase was completed by hand [53]. Two copies of each interview transcription were printed at the university library. Initial codes were identified and documented on one copy by identifying sections of text belonging to a certain code. These sections were then cut out of the second copy of the transcriptions and labeled for temporal placement in the interview. The cut-out text sections were attached by paper clips to index cards labeled with the identifying codes. The index cards were placed in front of the first author as she continued to code, making it easier to add text sections to codes because the data included four similar accounts of experiences. In this way, the coding was not entirely inductive but contained deductive properties as well. Initially, the unit of analysis was keywords and phrases, but due to fragmentation, the data were later recoded using meaning units.

2.1.3. Phase 3: Form Themes from the Codes

Themes combined single components of data and were generated inductively by arranging and rearranging the codes into groups of similar codes [56]. The author continued to refamiliarize herself with the authentic data, and mind maps were utilized in linking codes together into themes. The mind maps produced hierarchies of codes, categories, themes, and main themes.

2.1.4. Phase 4: Review the Themes

The coded data was then compared to the themes to make sure there was a coherent connection between them [56]. The author refamiliarized herself with the authentic data in the form of the full transcriptions and interviews, while asking the data "What belongs under this theme?" Some themes expanded or collapsed, though always in reference to the authentic data. This phase was conducted until successful member checking and theoretical saturation were reached.

2.1.5. Phase 5: Name and Define the Themes

The fifth phase involved defining and naming themes. This was completed by determining what parts of the data were captured within each theme [56]. Once all relevant sections of the data were included within themes, the analysis was complete. The four main themes that emerged from the analysis are state of flux, infection prevention, management of staff, and personal experiences.

2.1.6. Phase 6: Writing the Results

The data analysis was conducted in the original language of the content. Results were translated by the first author during the writing of the report. The translation from Finnish to English was delayed for as long as possible due to its ontological significance [57]. The results were written utilizing the final mind maps of the four main themes. Each direct quote has been used with the permission of the corresponding respondent.

3. Results

The purpose of this study was to describe the early nurse management experiences from PHC clinics within Greater Helsinki dedicated to caring for all ambulatory patients with possible COVID-19 symptoms. The research question was: "What were the early experiences of nurse managers of PHC clinics dedicated to caring for patients with possible COVID-19 symptoms?". Two thematic pair interviews were conducted by the first author on 10 November 2020 and on 2 February 2021. The interviews were 56 min and 35 s, and 61 min and 55 s long, respectively. The interviews ended when respondents reached a point of saturation. Four main themes emerged from the data, which can be used to answer the research question: capacity development created a state of flux, infection prevention was a crucial component to COVID-19 crisis response work, the management of staff was an essential facilitation of crisis response work, and the respondents' personal experiences. Table 1 shows a summary of these results, depicting the themes under each main theme.

Table 1. Themes and main themes.

Themes	Main Themes
Changes to patient flow Changes to nurses' roles Changes to communication between stakeholders	State of flux created by capacity development
Stakeholders involved in IPC Planning of IPC Protocols for IPC Equipment for IPC	IPC as a crucial component of COVID-19 crisis work

Table 1. *Cont.*

Themes	Main Themes
Recruiting staff to COVID-19 work Motivation of staff Leadership skills needed	Management of staff as an essential facilitation of crisis work
How COVID-19 hubs were born Personal experiences	Respondents' personal experiences

3.1. *State of Flux*

The nurse managers spoke unanimously of how their PHC clinics had been in a state of flux for the duration of the crisis. Each respondent spoke of how their clinics functioned as large PHC providers within their communities before the crisis. They experienced changes to patient flow, nurses' roles, and communication, as portrayed by Table 2, which includes themes and examples of original quotes.

Table 2. Examples of original quotes depicting state of flux.

Example of Original Quote	Themes
… we had been a big urgent care clinic … all patients needing urgent care came straight through the door and to the nurses … we used to have eight frontline nurses on Mondays receiving urgent care patients so the mass of patients was pretty big … informing the community … how could we reach at least some of them so that everybody doesn't rush in [on Monday] … … for sure the biggest burden … is how do we get the burden from the non-essential care handled when we at some point get to that work … there is a large number of non-essential appointments waiting clients are waiting impatiently … and what kind of bombs will we get there … the thousands, no thousands is no longer sufficient, but tens of thousands of clients in the queue …	Changes to patient flow
… if there is a [mild case] then they go straight to the nurse, so essentially the same as during normal urgent care operations … a large portion of patients do not necessarily see a physician at all … the nurse assesses the need for care, of course with a low physician consultation threshold …	Changes to nurses' roles
… normally meetings were around [the city] and now [I] don't need to drive every day in different directions as everything happens on [telecommunication channel] …	Changes to communication between stakeholders

Each respondent told of how, in setting up their COVID-19 hubs, they directed their regular patients to other municipal PHC clinics. Provision of non-essential PHC services declined and, as treatment queues grew, the nurse managers were increasingly concerned for their local communities. One respondent said that it was unclear to her whether other PHC clinics served their regular patients in numbers that would reflect successful continuation of care. Telemedicine services helped ease the burden of the crisis on PHC provision and created opportunities for nurses to work remotely. Overloaded telephone services, however, highlighted the importance of equitable need-for-care assessments.

In one COVID-19 hub, nurses were responsible for work in supportive roles while physicians saw all patients alone. Another hub operated utilizing physician and nurse pair work, in which physicians saw all patients but had nurses documenting and assisting in the exam room. The last COVID-19 hubs operated somewhat normally, in that patients classified as mild cases were seen independently by nurses, with a low physician consultation threshold. According to most respondents, communication between different stakeholders had improved drastically, though capacity development and IPC initially paused certain organizational structures such as non-essential meetings and trainings. Only one respondent told of how she had her staff trained to treat ARI and COVID-19 patients during initial capacity development. The respondent who had provided this training to her nurses also had her nurses working independently.

3.2. Infection Prevention

Conversation surrounding IPC was extensive and included the following themes (depicted in Table 3): stakeholders involved in IPC, planning of IPC measures, protocols in IPC, and equipment used in IPC. Nurse managers identified both experts and staff as stakeholders in IPC. They identified the patient's role in IPC indirectly when they identified triage nurses as crucial stakeholders because they guided patients on IPC. The experts involved were the municipalities' epidemiological departments and infection control nurses, with whom the respondents collaborated. The nurse managers followed and communicated new IPC guidelines that their staff were then responsible for receiving and implementing. Strict sick leave protocols were crucial to mitigating exposure among staff, though syndromic surveillance was not mentioned. Three respondents firmly declared that they had not had nosocomial infections, while one respondent did not confirm or deny either way. As an example of the creative IPC solutions that nurse managers implemented, each had organized lunch breaks differently. One respondent implemented staggered lunch breaks but did not elaborate further. To facilitate potential contact tracing, one respondent had everyone eating in the same groups of six and one had their staff reserve their lunch times on a spreadsheet every morning. The fourth strategy was to organize lunch so that staff used different break rooms according to their daily work assignments. This required turning meeting rooms into break rooms containing refrigerators, microwaves, and water dispensers.

Table 3. Examples of original quotes depicting IPC.

Example of Original Quote	Themes
... when a patient comes through the door ... we have a nurse receiving them ... takes hand sanitizer and patient puts on a mask and then hand sanitizer again and then they are directed to sit ...	Stakeholders involved in IPC
... changed the placement of the chairs and tables and removed extra chairs ... so that gathering restrictions are implemented ...	Planning of IPC
... we have three [break rooms] at the moment and it is very clearly divided that when you are working here, then you go there to eat and when you are working over there, you eat over here ...	Protocols for IPC
... we received from the security-of-supply centers these so-called supplies which were stored there at some point for this purpose but it became apparent that they too were slightly outdated ... and masks smelled a bit like cellar ...	Equipment for IPC

Equipment for IPC included PPE, disposable utensils, and ionic air purifiers. One municipality provided lunch to its COVID-19 hub HCWs, along with disposable utensils as an IPC measure. Only one respondent mentioned utilizing ionic air purifiers, which were placed in each exam room. The topic of PPE, on the other hand, was brought up numerous times, as respondents noted they were worried for the safety of their staff when the availability and effectiveness of PPE were uncertain. Neither interview included a discussion about the specifics of how frontline HCWs used PPE. All nurse managers mentioned receiving PPE stock from the National Emergency Supply Agency. One respondent said the supplies that came from there were outdated and smelled of cellar. The municipalities lifted the COVID-19 hubs onto a list of critical operations, which meant that they received necessary supplies before other clinics did.

Each room was cleaned and items that had accumulated over the years, such as books, were removed. The strategic restocking of rooms, flow of people, time spent within the facility, clean/dirty sides, separate areas for donning/doffing PPE, and separate entrances for COVID-19 hub patients were carefully considered. There were notable differences in how respondents had organized their waiting areas and in how they handled confirmed COVID-19 cases. One respondent said that confirmed cases waited in an empty room, from which they were escorted to the exam room. Another said that their confirmed cases were all seen in one exam room but did not mention if they were waiting in a separate area. One respondent had separate waiting areas for patients over the age of 70 and for younger patients, which was notable because this interview took place before the equitable administration of vaccines began. Another respondent had arranged for patients to wait in separate areas according to their triage status.

3.3. Management of Staff

Nurse managers needed strong leadership skills and the ability to adjust their leadership styles, as they led, motivated, and recruited staff during an unprecedented global crisis. Table 4 shows examples of original quotes pertaining to the management of staff. In setting up the COVID-19 hubs, the very first thing respondents did was recruit the necessary nursing staff and address their concerns. Though all respondents considered working at the COVID-19 frontline as voluntary, some light contradictions to the voluntary nature of the work were evident. For instance, the authors use the term "recruit" lightly, as one respondent did not agree with the context of the term when verifying the results, though she too spoke of transferring at-risk staff to other PHC clinics. Need for further recruitment was at times exacerbated by low work motivation and the burnout of nursing staff. A shortage of nurses and workspaces affected the recruitment process as well.

Table 4. Example quotes depicting motivation of staff.

Example of Original Quote	Themes
… at our clinic everyone is [there] purely voluntarily … they have been asked and they have volunteered …	Recruiting staff to COVID-19 work
… not in any monetary way have we been able to motivate because … there is no promise of extra vacation or anything like that … it comes from within the staff and from [when] we try to support them to … trust themselves and others …	Motivation of staff
… I noticed that a leadership style in which I speak to the nurses as one team and where I treat nurses somehow equally … I had to change it … I end up individually taking and considering each nurse kind of like according to their personality … it somehow feels like I have developed sensory antenna which are still extremely sensitive to … who is burning out …	Leadership skills needed

At the point of the interviews, the respondents considered motivating staff to be their single biggest task and for this they relied heavily upon their own leadership skills, as one respondent stated clearly that she had not been provided with additional resources. The respondents stated that their nurses were motivated by occasional refreshments provided by municipalities, patients, and pharmaceutical companies. All respondents spoke highly of their staff and of how team spirit was high among frontline nurses. As managers, they were able to delegate responsibilities without hesitation, which also had a motivational impact. According to the majority of respondents, the most challenging time for staff motivation was after the summer of 2020 and into the fall, as their staff began losing hope. Both internal and external work rotations were the most utilized and most effective way to motivate staff.

Respondents told of how they had to adjust their leadership styles to better accommodate the complex needs of their staff, especially at the beginning of the crisis. One respondent told of how she had to strengthen her ability to recognize individual needs among her staff, as experienced nurses suddenly had more reservations than new nurses. Leading crisis response work at the COVID-19 hubs required skills such as mindful presence, openness, and listening, which all communicated availability. Clear communication skills quickly became critical, as respondents had to consistently communicate new information in a manner that was clear and easy to understand. By focusing on the clarity and transparency of communication, respondents were able to reassure nursing staff in times of uncertainty.

3.4. Personal Experiences

The general storyline to the "birth" of COVID-19 hubs states that the respondents had a few days' time to first dismantle normal PHC operations and then set up COVID-19 hub operations. One original quote depicting this story is below in Table 5, under the theme of how COVID-19 hubs were born. One respondent heard of the decision to dedicate her clinic as a COVID-19 hub through the local newspaper. She lightly criticized her city's timeliness in communication, though she ultimately had a few more days to prepare than her interview partner had. The urgency and stress involved in setting up operations over a short period was emphasized in each interview.

Table 5. Example quotes depicting respondents' personal experiences.

Example of Original Quote	Theme
… we got the information on Friday afternoon the 13th of the third [month] that on Monday operations had to be completely different and we had until then to cancel or move all of Monday's appointments from this facility to elsewhere … [reiterates] there was the weekend's time … and all spaces needed to be handled again, all rooms had to be organized … we had the time to warn staff that afternoon that Monday would be new operations and everyone was asked to come in early to work … it was a big job over the weekend … and also all the procedures like how do we … actually handle and what and where … and how do we organize the whole [city's] operations anew …	How COVID-19 hubs were born
I can say that it has been a unique experience … I would not have believed a year ago that we would be in this kind of a situation that the entire world has gotten this virus … pretty cool that I have been able to experience this on the frontline …	Personal experiences

The respondents spoke openly about the big emotions and concerns they experienced, of which uncertainty was most prevalent. The feeling of uncertainty was present even during the interviews, as some respondents noted that they did not know what the vision for crisis recovery work was. The respondents and their staff also experienced fear of the virus, disbelief and hopelessness due to PPE shortages, and worry about the effectiveness of PPE. One respondent went so far as to say that she felt responsible for the health of her staff. On the flip side, crisis response work had also been rewarding. All respondents spoke of how, together with their nurses, they did not want to give up or give in. Two respondents noted they felt honored to have had the once-in-a-lifetime experience of leading the frontline of such a global crisis.

4. Discussion

The purpose of this study was to describe the early nurse management experiences from PHC clinics within Greater Helsinki dedicated to caring for all ambulatory patients with possible COVID-19 symptoms. The objectives were to make PHC crisis response contributions known and to provide an IAR of crisis response efforts. Together with the emerging literature, the results reflect that the COVID-19 crisis has immeasurably burdened PHC, the extent of which is yet unknown [14,44,45]. Primary health care is the frontline defense for COVID-19 response work at the community level, though the contribution is underrepresented in the literature [5,9,10,12,14,46,48].

Nurse managers of COVID-19 hubs described capacity development as a rapid and hectic process. They had a few days' time to develop COVID-19 hub services for their communities. This process led to a state of flux that has lasted over a year and continues to stress the provision of non-essential, yet necessary, PHC services [45]. While the one respondent's comment regarding the number of patients waiting in treatment queues is subjective experience, it is clear that a vision for crisis recovery work is needed as nurses begin to face the tremendous treatment queues with limited healthcare services to offer [43]. The COVID-19 crisis can be our best opportunity to develop our healthcare systems to be more resilient and to better address healthcare inequities overall [10,14,44,46,47].

Infection prevention was a major topic within both interviews, as the purpose of the COVID-19 hubs was to prevent infection. The implementation of IPC required creativity from the nurse managers as they planned and orchestrated different methods for the practical implementation of IPC measures within their own COVID-19 hubs. As the COVID-19 crisis has increased our understanding of the holistic consequences of uncontrolled pandemics, it has also created a fantastic opportunity for increasing IPC awareness globally [58]. Awareness comes at a critical point in global health, as the WHO has identified its first-ever list of priority pathogens, for which it recommends increasing and standardizing IPC practices, along with better coordination of surveillance [59]. Discrepancies within IPC, as seen in the literature and in this study, suggest that our efforts to standardize IPC practices must begin within our local communities [21,23,29,30].

The nurse managers of the four COVID-19 hubs spoke openly about their experiences during the interviews, often modeling servant leadership characteristics [41,42]. They have been on the frontline of the crisis and appreciate the unique opportunity it has afforded them. The respondents' experiences, together with the literature, highlight the importance of leadership skills within COVID-19 response work [39,40,42]. Respondents spoke of how their single most important job has been and continues to be in motivating staff in the continued crisis response and recovery work, which is an experience supported by the literature as well [40]. As leadership in nursing faces new challenges brought forth by the crisis, nurse managers need more support in motivating nursing staff in order to mitigate the so-called COVID-19 effect, which may result in nurses leaving the profession [34–37,40].

Limitations

Limitations to this study are related to the nature of the prolonged COVID-19 crisis and the possible language barrier. As a non-native Finnish speaker, the first author held both interviews in Finnish between 8 and 10 months into the crisis, with a 10-week gap between the two interviews due to the time required to secure research permits and schedule interviews. Neither the possible language barrier nor the contextual difference between the two interviews were seen to be of significance in the collected data. While piloting the interview is essential in thematic interviewing, this interview was not piloted due to the narrow target group, nature of the crisis, and the context of IARs [53]. Including respondents outside of the target group would have diluted the contextual base and this study would also have used more resources [60]. The results of this study are dependent upon the context. Trustworthiness for thematic analysis is determined through concepts of credibility, transferability, dependability, and confirmability. The engagement period was short, though data triangulation, respondent saturation, and member checking aided in achieving credibility [56].

5. Conclusions

This study is significant in that it is an IAR of PHC crisis response in Greater Helsinki from a nursing perspective. Nurse managers have stood in the face of fear and uncertainty and have led their staff through the beginning of an unprecedented global health crisis. Primary healthcare leaders can utilize the results of IARs and AARs to critically analyze and strengthen crisis preparedness in PHC for future and inevitable pandemics [14].

Author Contributions: Conceptualization, M.S.N.; data curation, M.S.N.; formal analysis, M.S.N.; methodology, M.S.N. and S.V.; project administration, M.S.N.; supervision, S.V.; validation, S.V.; writing—original draft, M.S.N.; writing—review and editing, S.V. All authors have read and agreed to the published version of the manuscript.

Funding: This research received no external funding.

Institutional Review Board Statement: Not applicable.

Informed Consent Statement: Informed consent was obtained from all subjects involved in the study.

Data Availability Statement: The data presented in this study are available on request from the corresponding author. The data are not publicly available due to the risk of compromised anonymity of respondents and their employers.

Acknowledgments: Many thanks to the respondents of the study for their participation and openness in telling their stories. Thanks to Maria Lowe for her contribution to language editing.

Conflicts of Interest: The author has been employed by two of the four targeted PHC clinics during normal operations and knew one respondent personally. This may have influenced the author's interest in the study but is not considered to have a role in the design of the study; in the collection, analyses, or interpretation of data; in the writing of the manuscript; or in the decision to publish the results.

References

1. Wang, C.; Horby, P.W.; Hayden, F.G.; Gao, G.F. A novel coronavirus outbreak of global health concern. *Lancet* **2020**, *395*, 470–473. [CrossRef]
2. World Health Organization. Coronavirus Disease 2019 (COVID-19) Situation Report 51. Available online: https://www.who.int/docs/default-source/coronaviruse/situation-reports/20200311-sitrep-51-covid-19.pdf?sfvrsn=1ba62e57_10 (accessed on 20 May 2020).
3. Kattainen, S.; Kiiski, O.; Bendel, S.; Jokinen, J.; Reinikainen, M.; Varpula, T. Koronaviruspandemiaan liittynyt tehohoidon tarve ja hoitotulokset Suomessa kevään ja kesän 2020 aikana. *Duodecim* **2021**, *137*, 375–382. Available online: https://www.duodecimlehti.fi/duo15980 (accessed on 26 March 2021).
4. Finnish Institute for Health and Welfare. Koronaepidemian Tämän Hetken Ennuste: Noin 11300 Ihmistä Tarvitsee Sairaalahoitoa Ja Heistä 3600 Tehohoitoa. Available online: https://thl.fi/fi/-/koronaepidemian-taman-hetken-ennuste-noin-11-300-ihmista-tarvitsee-sairaalahoitoa-ja-heista-3-600-tehohoitoa (accessed on 1 September 2021).
5. Finnish Government. Koronakriisin Vaikutukset Ja Suunnitelma Epidemian Hallinnan Hybridistrategiaksi. Available online: https://valtioneuvosto.fi/documents/10616/21411573/VN_2020_12.pdf (accessed on 6 June 2020).
6. Finnish Government. Hallitus Totesi Suomen Olevan Poikkeusoloissa Koronavirustilanteen Vuoksi. Available online: https://valtioneuvosto.fi/artikkeli/-/asset_publisher/10616/hallitus-totesi-suomen-olevan-poikkeusoloissa-koronavirustilanteen-vuoksi (accessed on 20 May 2020).
7. Finnish Law. Valmiuslaki. Available online: https://finlex.fi/fi/laki/ajantasa/2011/20111552?search%5Btype%5D=pika&search%5Bpika%5D=valmiuslaki (accessed on 8 June 2020).
8. World Health Organization. Covid-19 Strategy Update. *Wkly. Epidemiol. Rec.* **2020**, *95*, 185–208. Available online: https://apps.who.int/iris/bitstream/handle/10665/332018/WER9519-eng-fre.pdf?ua=1 (accessed on 27 May 2020).
9. Ministry of Social Affairs and Health. Kunnalla on Oikeus Poiketa Terveydenhuollon Kiireettömän Hoidon Määräajoista Ja Sosiaalihuollon Palvelutarpeen Arvioinnista Koronavirustilanteen Takia. Available online: https://stm.fi/-/kunnalla-on-oikeus-poiketa-terveydenhuollon-kiireettoman-hoidon-maaraajoista-ja-sosiaalihuollon-palvelutarpeen-arvioinnista-koronavirustilanteen-takia (accessed on 10 September 2021).
10. Majeed, A. Addressing COVID-19 Proactively through Primary Care in England's National Health Service. In *Primary Care in the COVID-19 Pandemic*; Basu, S., Alpert, J.L., Phillips, R.S., Applebaum, W., Eds.; Available online: http://info.primarycare.hms.harvard.edu/primary-care-during-covid-0 (accessed on 25 March 2022).
11. Valtanen, T. Pääkaupunkiseudulle Perustetaan Erillisiä Koronaterveysasemia—Ylilääkäri: Myös Muut Sairastuneet on Kyettävä Hoitamaan, Vaikka Palvelut Ruuhkautuvat. Available online: https://yle.fi/uutiset/3-11257695 (accessed on 26 March 2021).
12. World Health Organization. Role of Primary Care in the COVID-19 Response. Available online: https://apps.who.int/iris/bitstream/handle/10665/331921/Primary-care-COVID-19-eng.pdf?sequence=5&isAllowed=y (accessed on 25 March 2022).
13. Mughal, F.; Mallen, C.D.; Mckee, M. The impact of COVID-19 on primary care in Europe. *Lancet* **2021**, *6*. [CrossRef] [PubMed]
14. Plagg, B.; Piccoliori, G.; Oschmann, J.; Engl, A.; Eisendle, K. Primary Health Care and Hospital Management during COVID-19: Lessons learned from Lombardy. *Risk Manag. Healthc. Policy* **2021**, *14*, 3987–3992. [CrossRef] [PubMed]
15. World Health Organization; United Nations Children's Fund. A Vision for Primary Health Care in the 21st Century. Available online: https://apps.who.int/iris/bitstream/handle/10665/328065/WHO-HIS-SDS-2018.15-eng.pdf?sequence=1&isAllowed=y (accessed on 10 September 2021).
16. Finnish Law. Terveydenhuoltolaki 30.12.2010/1326. Available online: https://www.finlex.fi/fi/laki/ajantasa/2010/20101326 (accessed on 8 June 2020).
17. Lehtomäki, L. Valtakunnallisia Suosituksia Terveyskeskuksen Talon Tavoiksi. Doctoral Dissertation, University of Tampere, Tampere, Finland, 28 August 2009. Available online: https://trepo.tuni.fi/bitstream/handle/10024/66495/978-951-44-7758-4.pdf?sequence=1&isAllowed=y (accessed on 10 April 2022).
18. World Health Organization. Prioritizing Diseases for Research and Development in Emergency Contexts. Available online: https://www.who.int/activities/prioritizing-diseases-for-research-and-development-in-emergency-contexts (accessed on 25 August 2021).

19. World Health Organization. Infection Prevention and Control of Epidemic- and Pandemic- Prone Acute Respiratory Infections in Health Care. Available online: https://www.who.int/publications/i/item/infection-prevention-and-control-of-epidemic-and-pandemic-prone-acute-respiratory-infections-in-health-care (accessed on 20 August 2021).
20. World Health Organization. Infection Prevention and Control during Health Care When Coronavirus Disease (COVID-19) Is Suspected or Confirmed. Available online: https://www.who.int/publications/i/item/WHO-2019-nCoV-IPC-2021.1 (accessed on 31 August 2021).
21. Hospital Onset COVID-19 Working Group; Environmental Modelling Group. Masks for Healthcare Workers to Mitigate Airborne Transmission of SARS-CoV-2. Available online: https://assets.publishing.service.gov.uk/government/uploads/system/uploads/attachment_data/file/979441/S1169_Facemasks_for_health_care_workers.pdf (accessed on 27 August 2021).
22. National Institute for Occupational Safety and Health. Hierarchy of Controls. Available online: https://www.cdc.gov/niosh/topics/hierarchy/ (accessed on 31 August 2021).
23. Morris, G.A.; Cannady, R. Proper Use of the Hierarchy of Controls. *Prof. Saf.* **2019**, *64*, 37–40. Available online: https://www.proquest.com/scholarly-journals/proper-use-hierarchy-controls/docview/2269008352/se-2?accountid=12003 (accessed on 31 August 2021).
24. Khan, R.F. How Does the Hierarchy of Controls Integrate with the Epidemiologic Triangle to Help Address and Understand Transmission of SARS-CoV-2? *J. Occup. Environ. Med.* **2020**, *62*, 665–668. [CrossRef]
25. Dehghani, F.; Omidi, F.; Yousefinejad, S.; Taheri, E. The Hierarchy of Preventive Measures to Protect Workers against the COVID-19 Pandemic: A Review. *Work* **2020**, *67*, 771–777. [CrossRef]
26. Madad, S.; Moskovitz, J.; Boyce, M.R.; Cagliuso, N.V.; Katz, R. Ready or not, patients will present: Improving urban pandemic preparedness. *Disaster Med. Public Health Prep.* **2020**, *15*, 267–270. [CrossRef]
27. Wee, L.E.; Sim, X.Y.J.; Conceicao, E.P.; Aung, M.K.; Goh, J.Q.; Yeo, D.W.T.; Gan, W.H.; Chua, Y.Y.; Wijaya, L.; Tan, T.T.; et al. Containment of COVID-19 cases among healthcare workers: The role of surveillance, early detection, and outbreak management. *Infect. Control Hosp. Epidemiol.* **2020**, *41*, 765–771. [CrossRef]
28. World Health Organization. COVID-19 Strategic Preparedness and Response Plan: Operational Planning Guideline. Available online: https://www.who.int/publications/m/item/covid-19-strategic-preparedness-and-response-plan-operational-planning-guideline (accessed on 1 September 2021).
29. Jackson, T.; Deibert, D.; Wyatt, G.; Durand-Moreau, Q.; Adisesh, A.; Khunti, K.; Khunti, S.; Smith, S.; Chan, X.H.S.; Ross, L.; et al. Classification of aerosol-generating procedures: A rapid systematic review. *BMJ Open Respir. Res.* **2020**, *7*. [CrossRef] [PubMed]
30. Finnish Institute for Health and Welfare. Toimenpideohje Epäiltäessä Koronaviruksen (SARS-CoV-2) Aiheuttamaa COVID-19-Infektiota. Available online: https://thl.fi/fi/web/infektiotaudit-ja-rokotukset/taudit-ja-torjunta/taudit-ja-taudinaiheuttajat-a-o/koronavirus-covid-19/toimenpideohje-epailtaessa-koronaviruksen-covid-19-aiheuttamaa-infektiota (accessed on 25 August 2021).
31. National Emergency Supply Agency. Suojavarusteiden Riittävyys Varmistetaan Koko Maassa. Available online: https://www.huoltovarmuuskeskus.fi/a/suojavarusteiden-riittavyys-varmistetaan-koko-maassa (accessed on 26 March 2021).
32. Wong, A.H.; Pacella-LaBarbara, M.L.; Ray, J.M.; Ranney, M.L.; Chang, B.P. Healing the Healer: Protecting Emergency Health Care Workers' Mental Health during COVID-19. *Ann. Emerg. Med.* **2020**, *76*, 379–384. [CrossRef] [PubMed]
33. García-Fernández, L.; Romero-Ferreiro, V.; López-Roldán, P.D.; Padilla, S.; Calero-Sierra, I.; Monzó-García, M.; Pérez-Martín, J.; Rodriguez-Jimenez, R. Mental health impact of COVID-19 pandemic on Spanish healthcare workers. *Psychol. Med.* **2020**, *30*, 42–50. [CrossRef] [PubMed]
34. Finnish Nurses' Union. Yli Puolet Sairaanhoitajaliiton Koronakyselyn Vastaajista Miettii Alanvaihtoa Koronapandemia Aikana. Available online: https://sairaanhoitajat.fi/yli-puolet-sairaanhoitajaliiton-koronakyselyn-vastaajista-mietti-alanvaihtoa-koronapandemian-aikana/ (accessed on 30 March 2021).
35. International Council of Nurses. The Global Nursing Shortage and Nurse Retention. Available online: https://www.icn.ch/sites/default/files/inline-files/ICN%20Policy%20Brief_Nurse%20Shortage%20and%20Retention.pdf (accessed on 20 March 2021).
36. Japanese Nursing Association. Survey Results on the Actual Status of Nurses' Responses to COVID-19. Available online: https://www.2020yearofthenurse.org/uploads/2021/03/JNA-News-Release-2021-Vol.34.pdf (accessed on 20 March 2021).
37. American Nurses Association. Provision 5: Self-Care & COVID-19. 2020. Available online: https://www.nursingworld.org/~{}4a1fea/globalassets/covid19/provision-5_-self-care--covid19-final.pdf (accessed on 30 March 2021).
38. Devnani, M. Factors associated with the willingness of health care personnel to work during influenza public health emergency: And integrative review. *Prehospital Disaster Med.* **2012**, *27*, 551–566. [CrossRef] [PubMed]
39. Fernandez, R.; Lord, H.; Halcomb, E.J.; Moxham, L.; Middleton, R.; Alananzeh, I.; Ellwood, L. Implications for COVID-19: A systematic review of nurses' experiences of working in acute care hospital settings during a respiratory pandemic. *Int. J. Nurs. Stud.* **2020**, *111*. [CrossRef]
40. Joslin, D.; Joslin, H. Nursing Leadership COVID-19 Insight Survey. *AONL* **2020**, *18*, 527–531. [CrossRef]
41. Aij, K.H.; Rapsaniotis, S. Leadership requirements for Lean versus servant leadership in health care: A systematic review of the literature. *J. Healthc. Lead.* **2017**, *9*, 1–14. [CrossRef]
42. Sanders, J.; Balcom, C. Clinical leadership during the COVID-19 pandemic: Reflections and lessons learned. *Healthc. Manag. Forum* **2021**, *34*, 316–319. [CrossRef]
43. British Standards Institute. *Crisis Management—Guidance and Good Practice*; BSI Standards Limited: London, UK, 2014.

44. Lim, J.; Broughan, J.; Crowley, D.; O'Kelly, B.; Fawsitt, R.; Burke, M.C.; McCombe, G.; Lambert, J.S.; Cullen, W. COVID-19's impact on primary care and related mitigation strategies: A scoping review. *Eur. J. Gen. Pract.* **2021**, *27*, 166–175. [CrossRef]
45. Rissanen, P.; Parhiala, K.; Kestilä, L.; Härmä, V.; Honkatukia, J.; Jormanainen, V. COVID-19-Epidemian Vaikutukset Väestön Palvelutarpeisiin, Palvelujärjestelmään Ja Kansantalouteen—Nopea Vaikutusarvio. Available online: https://www.julkari.fi/bitstream/handle/10024/139694/URN_ISBN_978-952-343-496-7.pdf?sequence=1&isAllowed=y (accessed on 20 April 2021).
46. Kim, J.-H.; Takahashi, K.; Funato, M.; Negishi, K.; Schwarz, D.; Higuchi, M.; Ouichi, K.; Bitton, A. Public Health Centers in Japan's COVID-19 Response and Recovery. In *Primary Care in the COVID-19 Pandemic*; Basu, S., Alpert, J.L., Phillips, R.S., Applebaum, W., Eds.; Available online: http://info.primarycare.hms.harvard.edu/primary-care-during-covid-0 (accessed on 25 March 2022).
47. Xu, Z.; Wang, Y.; Qian, Y.; Lu, Y. Primary Care Practitioners' Barriers to and Experience of COVID-19 Epidemic Control in China: A Qualitative Study. *J. Gen. Intern. Med.* **2020**, *35*, 3278–3284. [CrossRef]
48. Halcomb, E.; McInnes, S.; Williams, A.; Ashley, C.; James, S.; Fernandez, R.; Stephen, C.; Calma, K. The experiences of Primary Healthcare Nurses during the COVID-19 Pandemic in Australia. *J. Nurs. Scholarsh.* **2020**, *52*, 553–563. [CrossRef] [PubMed]
49. International Health Regulations. Monitoring and Evaluation Framework. 2005. Available online: http://apps.who.int/iris/bitstream/handle/10665/276651/WHO-WHE-CPI-2018.51-eng.pdf?sequence=1&isAllowed=y (accessed on 8 March 2021).
50. World Health Organization. Guidance for after Action Review (AAR). Available online: https://apps.who.int/iris/bitstream/handle/10665/311537/WHO-WHE-CPI-2019.4-eng.pdf?sequence=1&isAllowed=y (accessed on 8 March 2021).
51. European Center for Disease Prevention and Control. Conducting In-Action and After-Action Reviews of the Public Health Response to COVID-19. 2020. Available online: https://www.ecdc.europa.eu/sites/default/files/documents/In-Action-and-After-Action-Reviews-of-the-public-health-response-to-COVID-19.pdf (accessed on 7 June 2020).
52. Nevala, M. Early Nurse Management Experiences from Finnish Primary Health Care Clinics Functioning as COVID-19 Care Sites. Available online: https://urn.fi/URN:NBN:fi:amk-2021122190318 (accessed on 25 March 2022).
53. Hirsjärvi, A.; Hurme, H. *Tutkimushaastattelu*; Gaudeamus Helsinki University Press: Helsinki, Finland, 2008.
54. European Parliament; The Council of the European Union. Regulations. *Off. J. Eur. Union* **2016**. Available online: https://eur-lex.europa.eu/legal-content/EN/TXT/PDF/?uri=CELEX:32016R0679&qid=1637135435524&from=EN (accessed on 3 May 2020).
55. Metropolia University of Applied Sciences. The Human Sciences Ethics Committee of the Helsinki Region Universities of Applied Sciences. Available online: https://www.metropolia.fi/en/rdi/ethics-committee (accessed on 25 March 2022).
56. Nowell, L.S.; Norris, J.M.; White, D.E.; Moules, N.J. Thematic Analysis: Striving to Meet the Trustworthiness Criteria. *Int. J. Qual. Methods* **2017**, *16*. [CrossRef]
57. Temple, B.; Young, A. Qualitative research and translation dilemmas. *Qual. Res.* **2004**, *4*, 161–178. [CrossRef]
58. World Health Organization. Global Shortage of Innovative Antibiotics Fuels Emergence and Spread of Drug-Resistance. 2021. Available online: https://www.who.int/news/item/15-04-2021-global-shortage-of-innovative-antibiotics-fuels-emergence-and-spread-of-drug-resistance (accessed on 25 August 2021).
59. World Health Organization. WHO Publishes List of Bacteria for Which New Antibiotics Are Urgently Needed. Available online: https://www.who.int/news/item/27-02-2017-who-publishes-list-of-bacteria-for-which-new-antibiotics-are-urgently-needed (accessed on 25 August 2021).
60. Kvale, S. *Interviews: An Introduction to Qualitative Research Interviewing*; Sage Publications: Thousand Oaks, CA, USA, 1996.

International Journal of
Environmental Research and Public Health

MDPI

Article

Impact of SARS-CoV-2 Pandemic on Psychosocial Burden and Job Satisfaction of Long-Term Care Nurses in Poland

Katarzyna Tomaszewska [1,*], Bożena Majchrowicz [2] and Marek Delong [3]

1 Department of Nursing, Institute of Health Protection, The Bronisław Markiewicz State Higher School of Technology and Economics, 37-500 Jarosław, Poland
2 Department of Nursing, Institute of Social and Health Sciences, East European State Higher School, 37-700 Przemyśl, Poland; bozenam4@op.pl
3 Department of Management, University of Technology, 35-959 Rzeszów, Poland; m.delong@prz.edu.pl
* Correspondence: tomka8@wp.pl; Tel.: +48-795-580-108

Abstract: Psychosocial consequences of the coronavirus pandemic are severe for health care workers due to their higher levels of exposure. Nurses often experience tremendous psychological pressure as a result of their workload in a high-risk environment. The purpose of this study was to determine the impact of the SARS-CoV-2 pandemic on the psychosocial burden and job satisfaction of nurses employed in long-term care. One hundred thirty-eight nurses employed in long-term care participated in the study. The respondents were 96.4% female and 3.6% male. The mean age of the respondents was 53.99 (standard deviation—4.01). The study was conducted between February and June 2021. The research tool was a standardized psychosocial risk scale questionnaire, which is a scientifically validated diagnostic tool with high reliability and accuracy coefficients. The primary tests used during the statistical analyses were non-parametric Mann–Whitney U (for two samples) and Kruskal–Wallis (for more than two samples) tests for assessing differences. During these analyses, in addition to standard statistical significance, appropriate *p*-values were calculated using the Monte Carlo method. Correlations between ordinal or quantitative variables were made using Spearman's rho coefficient. The results obtained allow us to conclude that the respondents rated the characteristics present in the workplace that constitute psychosocial risks at an average level. Emotional commitment and continuance-type commitment to the respondents' job position were also at a medium level. Respondents' self-rated ability to work for nurses employed in long-term care during the SARS-CoV-2 pandemic and commitment to patient care was high at 4.0 and 4.18, with a maximum of 5 points.

Keywords: nurse; long-term care; psychosocial burden; SARS-CoV-2; psychosocial risk scale

Citation: Tomaszewska, K.; Majchrowicz, B.; Delong, M. Impact of SARS-CoV-2 Pandemic on Psychosocial Burden and Job Satisfaction of Long-Term Care Nurses in Poland. *Int. J. Environ. Res. Public Health* **2022**, *19*, 3555. https://doi.org/10.3390/ijerph19063555

Academic Editor: Paul B. Tchounwou

Received: 12 February 2022
Accepted: 15 March 2022
Published: 17 March 2022

1. Introduction

COVID-19 is a disease caused by a coronavirus infection (SARS-CoV-2), with the first cases diagnosed in 2019 in China. Due to the rapid spread of the disease, the World Health Organization (WHO) declared it a pandemic in March 2020. According to Johns Hopkins University, as of 17 August 2020, there were 21,901,102 laboratory-confirmed cases of coronavirus, including 774,299 deaths worldwide. The International Council of Nurses (ICN) reported that more than 600 nurses worldwide had died from COVID-19 by 3 June 2020. [1]. As of today (December 2021), the SARS-CoV-2 coronavirus outbreak continues, with the daily number of cases increasing, and the fourth wave of the pandemic refuses to subside. On New Year's Day, 1 January 2022, the Ministry of Health reported another 12,032 cases of coronavirus infection in the country; 505 have died. Poland is approaching the alarming number of 100,000 deaths from the epidemic (currently 97,559) [2].

The COVID-19 pandemic, like any health crisis, negatively affects the well-being of individuals, thereby affecting groups and entire societies. In a pandemic, people experience a range of negative emotions such as feelings of danger, fear, uncertainty, frustration or anger; they tend to be sad, lonely and confused. These emotions lead to suffering and destroy well-being, satisfaction and satisfaction with life. The emotions not only reduce the quality of life but also lead to mental health problems. The most important source of anxiety in a pandemic is, of course, the disease itself and its consequences: we fear for our own health and that of our loved ones, and these fears are often accompanied by a fear of death. Anxiety can also involve isolation, distancing, prohibition of movement, obligation to wear masks and often limits cognitive and social functioning [3].

Statistics maintained by the Supreme Council of Nurses and Midwives (NRPiP) show that there were more than 230,000 active nurses in Poland in 2021. There were about 5.1 nurses per 1000 inhabitants, and their average age was 52.59, which is not a satisfactory result when compared with the data of OECD countries (Organization for Economic Cooperation and Development). In the next 4 years, about 25% of all nurses will reach retirement age and will be entitled to a pension. Currently, in Poland, "the retirement age is 60 years for women and 65 years for men". Considering the fact that in a pandemic, people experience a range of negative emotions such as a sense of threat, fear, uncertainty, frustration or anger, which leads to suffering, destroys well-being, satisfaction and satisfaction with life, reduces its quality and leads to mental health problems, the number of active nurses may still decrease [4].

The COVID-19 pandemic has placed a significant burden on the health care system. WHO has called for action to reduce its impact on the mental and physical health of health workers. Previous experience with viral outbreaks demonstrates that those delivering health services directly in inpatient care, as well as in-home care, are at increased risk of infection, depression and stress symptoms [5]. In 1984, the International Labor Organization defined psychosocial risks as a kind of interaction between job content, work organization, management systems, conditions and competences, needs and individual characteristics of a worker. The International Labor Organization's approach is the source of the most current and widely accepted definition of psychosocial occupational hazards, indicating that "psychosocial occupational hazards are those aspects of work organization and management, together with their social and environmental context, that have the potential to cause psychological, social or physical harm" [6].

Since the beginning of the pandemic, nurses have been exposed to a high emotional burden due to longer and closer contact with patients with COVID-19 and at the same time more exposure to the infection than other health care workers, which negatively affects their mental health, occurrence of anxiety and depression. Findings from multiple authors show that a higher mental burden was more prevalent during the first period of the pandemic (spring 2020), decreasing during the second period (fall 2020). This decrease in the second period may be due to the fact that at the beginning of the pandemic (the "first wave"), there was a lot of confusion, lack of information, lack of training of these professionals, lack of PPE, high number of infections in both groups and lack of diagnostic testing. In the second period, the training improved, as well as the level of knowledge of nurses about the COVID-19 virus [7].

Nurses often face tremendous psychological pressure as a result of overwhelming workloads, 12 h on-call schedules (also at night) and working in high-risk environments [8], not only in hospitals or clinics, but also in long-term care [9]. Given the increasing demands on those employed in health care, it is crucial to understand and address the psychosocial burden on staff. These efforts must seek to alleviate major sources of anxiety among health care workers during the SARS-CoV-2 pandemic. Some of these concerns include access to personal protective equipment, balancing one's own mental and physical health with patient care, fear of exposing family members to the virus, supporting other family members, fear of developing symptoms and increased work demands [10–12]. Moral damage or "psychological distress" resulting from actions or lack thereof has been highlighted during the pandemic as a particular threat to health care providers. As Greenberg et al. eloquently articulated, health care personnel "will be the heroes of the day, but we will need them for tomorrow." Health care workers must receive the support necessary to reach their full potential over the long term [13]. Risks associated with working with patients during the

SARS-CoV-2 pandemic, fear of infection, unpredictability of events, feelings of helplessness and anxiety about performing existing job duties are just a few of the elements that nurses currently face while working [14]. Therefore, the mental health of nurses working with COVID-19 infected patients must be monitored and maintained during the outbreak [15]. The services provided will only be of high quality if the work environment provides nurses with the right conditions to support them [16].

According to recent reports, nurses are the health care workers who had the most psychological problems as a result of the COVID-19 outbreak. Although the initial impact on their mental health is evident, at some point, they seem to have adapted to the "new normal" [17]. However, the reporting of mental health problems among nurses during the COVID-19 pandemic worldwide is very low. According to WHO, the COVID-19 pandemic may have both long- and short-term effects on mental health; therefore, it is necessary to address the impact of COVID-19 on nurses' mental health [18].

In our study, we aimed to assess the impact of the SARS-CoV-2 pandemic on the psychosocial burden and job satisfaction of nurses working in long-term care, as well as to determine to what extent the fulfillment of professional tasks and shift work affects job satisfaction and whether the stress associated with contact with patients infected with coronavirus may cause the desire to change jobs.

2. Materials and Methods

2.1. Research Design

In the present study, a survey was conducted among nurses employed in inpatient and residential long-term care in Podkarpackie Voivodeship (Poland) who were providing work during the survey. Its aim was to assess the impact of the SARS-CoV-2 pandemic on the psychosocial burden and job satisfaction of nurses working in long-term care. The survey was conducted between February and June 2021.

2.2. Methods

The study of psychosocial risks at work and their consequences in the study group was carried out using the Psychosocial Risk Scale (SRP), which is a scientifically validated diagnostic tool and is characterized by high coefficients of reliability and accuracy. The SRP makes it possible to assess the presence of work characteristics that can be potentially threatening and to evaluate their level of stressfulness. It also takes into account such aspects of employees' functioning as absenteeism at work, frequency of accidents at work, health condition and ability to work, satisfaction with seven aspects of work, involvement in work and willingness to change work. The scale consists of four parts. Part A includes demographic data; Part B contains questions related to health and occupational functioning; Part C consists of 50 statements related to job characteristics that represent potential psychosocial risks. These characteristics are grouped into three main factors: job content, job context and interpersonal pathologies, which in turn consist of bundles of questions belonging to the nine psychosocial dimensions of the work environment listed in Cox's theory (job content, temporal frame of work, workload, control, organizational culture and functions, interpersonal relationships, role in organization/responsibility, career development, work-home relationship). Part D is a set of statements related to job characteristics specific to occupations in a given economic sector, with reference to our study in the health care sector. The psychometric properties of Parts B and C of the Psychosocial Risk Scale were determined by surveying 7623 respondents. The value of α-Cronbach's internal consistency coefficient for the whole scale was 0.94 [19].

2.3. Participants

The study group consisted of 138 nurses employed in long-term inpatient and in-home care. Inclusion criteria were employment in long-term care with the same provider for at least 1 year and occupation as a nurse. The exclusion criteria were lack of consent to participate in the study and employment of less than 1 year in long-term care. The questionnaires were handed out to the nurses and, after completion, were personally collected by the authors of the study, who clarified any doubts on an ongoing basis.

2.4. Statistical Analysis

The primary tests used during the statistical analyses were the non-parametric Mann–Whitney U test (for 2 samples) and Kruskal–Wallis test (for more than 2 samples) to assess differences. During these analyses, in addition to standard statistical significance, the corresponding p-values were also calculated using the Monte Carlo method. This is indicated by (b) next to the significance result for the Mann–Whitney U test and by (c) for the p-value result of the Kruskal–Wallis test. Correlations between ordinal or quantitative variables were made using Spearman's rho coefficient, which indicates the intensity of the relationship and its direction—positive or negative. The resulting value ranges from −1 to 1, with (−1) indicating a perfect negative correlation and (1) a perfect positive correlation. The Monte Carlo method, in most cases, is based on a sample of 10,000 tables with the starting number of random number generator 2,000,000. The analysis was performed using the IBM SPSS 26.0 package (IBM, New York City, NY, USA) with the Exact Tests module. All relationships were considered statistically significant when $p \leq 0.05$.

2.5. Ethical Procedures

The participation of nurses in the study was voluntary and anonymous. The study was conducted in accordance with the ethical standards of the Declaration of Helsinki (64th WmA General Assembly, Fortaleza, Brazil, October 2013) and in accordance with Polish legal regulations. The study was approved by the Bioethics Committee (KB/PWSW/1/2022).

3. Results

The survey was conducted among 138 randomly selected nurses employed in long-term inpatient and residential care in Podkarpackie voivodeship. All respondents correctly completed the survey questionnaire; the rate of correct answers was $N = 138$. The characteristics of the study group are shown in Table 1.

Table 1. Characteristics of the study group of nurses.

Variable		Respondents (N = 138)	
Sex	Female	133	96.4%
	Male	5	3.6%
Position	Nurse	138	100.0%
Education	Secondary and post-secondary education	47	34.1%
	Higher	91	65.9%
Type of contract	Employment contract for an indefinite period	133	96.4%
	Contract of mandate/contract for specific work	5	3.6%
Shift work	No	50	36.2%
	Yes	88	63.8%

The data in Table 2 represent the results of Part A of the questionnaire, which includes questions on demographic data such as gender, age, education, job title, length of service, form of employment, shift work performed and number of persons in the household.

Table 2. Results of Part A of the Psychosocial Risk Scale questionnaire.

Group	Mean *	Median **	Standard Deviation	Minimum	Maximum
Age (years)	53.99	54.00	4.01	34	64
Total length of service	33.75	32.50	27.95	4	352
Length of service in current position	23.52	25.00	10.59	1	43
Number of persons in the household	3.22	3.00	1.54	0	10
Number of children in the household	1.03	1.00	1.15	0	5

* Mean value obtained in individual data in 138 respondents. ** The value of a feature in an ordered series, above and below which there are an equal number of observations.

Questionnaire Results

Results obtained during statistical analysis were related to mean scores for the prevalence of health-care-specific psychosocial risks (Part D of the Psychosocial Risk Scale). In our own study, 96% of the respondents believed that the workplace in which the services were provided fully provided employees with personal protective equipment and staff shortages resulted in increased hours of work. Despite the increased workload, the number of sick leave did not increase, averaged 0.87, and the number of days absent from work in the past year was ±8.46. Self-assessment of ability to work during the SARS-CoV-2 pandemic and commitment to work among the surveyed nurses was high at 4.0 and 4.18, with a maximum of 5 points. The overall mean of the psychosocial risk characteristics present in the workplace was found to be low (0.42 ± 0.17). The emotional involvement of the respondents was at a mean level of 2.14 with a maximum of 4 points, as well as the involvement of the "persistence" type in the occupation, which averaged 2.32 with a maximum of 4 points.

Table 3 shows those job characteristics that are health-care-specific, belonging to the job content category and industry-specific included in Part D of the Social Risk Scale.

Table 3. The most common characteristics of nurse work in health care (N = 138).

Characteristics of Nurse Work	Mean	Median	Standard Deviation	Minimum	Maximum
My work requires the use of modern technology.	1.87	2.00	0.538	1	4
My work requires readiness to respond quickly most of the time.	2.05	2.00	0.424	1	4
My work requires adherence to strictly defined procedures.	2.12	2.00	0.499	1	4
My work is often controlled (internal and external audits, visits, quality control, etc.).	1.99	2.00	0.656	1	4
There is an employee evaluation system at my work.	2.03	2.00	0.672	1	4
My work requires constant improvement of qualifications.	1.97	2.00	0.672	1	4
At work I am exposed to psychological aggression from patients (shouting, verbal abuse, blackmail, threats, etc.).	1.40	1.00	0.788	1	4
I am required to be available at work.	2.01	2.00	0.598	1	4
I work under particularly difficult physical conditions.	1.79	1.00	1.000	1	4
At work I am exposed to physical aggression from patients (beating, pushing, pulling, using dangerous tools).	1.08	1.00	0.402	1	4
My work requires a lot of physical effort.	2.22	2.00	1.025	1	4

Table 3. *Cont.*

Characteristics of Nurse Work	Mean	Median	Standard Deviation	Minimum	Maximum
My work is connected with responsibility for health and life of other people.	2.32	2.00	0.683	1	4
My work requires close cooperation in a team.	1.98	2.00	0.330	1	3

Among nurses who cared for coronavirus-positive patients, statistically significant negative correlations were found between the mean of occurring workplace characteristics that constitute psychosocial hazards and global job satisfaction and job satisfaction scores on a scale of 1 to 5. The significant strength of the relationship indicates that a higher mean of psychosocial hazards present in the workplace is associated with lower global job satisfaction. On the other hand, a slightly less pronounced correlation coefficient value indicates that respondents experiencing higher psychosocial risks have lower job satisfaction scores on a scale of 1 to 5 (Table 4).

Table 4. Correlation of sociodemographic data with Psychosocial Risk Scale scores (N = 138).

Spearman's Rho		Age	Total Length of Service	Length of Service in Current Position	Number of Persons in the Household	Number of Children in the Household
Global job satisfaction (total satisfaction 7–28)	Correlation coefficient	0.078	0.119	−0.014	−0.173 *	−0.226 **
	Relevance (two-sided)	0.360	0.163	0.874	0.042	0.008
Average of workplace characteristics that constitute psychosocial risks (0–1)	Correlation coefficient	−0.145	−0.106	0.038	0.081	0.091
	Relevance (two-sided)	0.089	0.217	0.661	0.344	0.287
Satisfaction with current job (1–5)	Correlation coefficient	0.042	0.050	−0.135	−0.076	−0.134
	Relevance (two-sided)	0.624	0.558	0.114	0.377	0.117

* Correlation significant at the 0.05 level (two-sided). ** Correlation significant at the 0.01 level (two-sided).

Comparing the number of people and number of children in the household with global job satisfaction showed negative statistically significant correlations, which were characterized by weak strengths of association. A higher number of people and higher number of children in the household were associated with lower global job satisfaction due to stress and risk of COVID-19 virus transmission to the home environment. Considering age, total job tenure and tenure in the current job, there were no statistically significant correlations with global job satisfaction, the average of job characteristics present in the workplace that constitute psychosocial risks and satisfaction ratings with the current job on a scale of 1 to 5. When analyzing global job satisfaction during the SARS-CoV-2 pandemic, the average of job characteristics present in the workplace that constitute psychosocial risks, and satisfaction ratings on a scale of 1 to 5, only the results of the latter variable varied significantly by gender as evidenced by the p-values of the Mann–Whitney U test. It is women who, in comparison to men, rated the level of job satisfaction higher. The analysis of the Mann–Whitney U test showed that the level of global job satisfaction, the average of job characteristics constituting psychosocial risks at work and the evaluation of satisfaction with the current job on a scale from 1 to 5 were not statistically significant, as differentiated by the level of education. The results of global job satisfaction, the mean of job characteristics constituting psychosocial hazards in the workplace and the rating of satisfaction with current job performance on a scale of 1 to 5 were not statistically significant, as differentiated by the form of employment, as evidenced by the p-values of the Mann–Whitney U test.

Shift work significantly differentiated global job satisfaction, the average level of psychosocial hazards present in the workplace and satisfaction with current job on a scale from 1 to 5, as evidenced by the Mann–Whitney U test results. Respondents who work shifts, compared to others, had lower global job satisfaction, experienced higher levels of psychosocial hazards and rated their job satisfaction lower (Table 5).

Table 5. Job characteristics constituting psychosocial risks and satisfaction levels of shift nurses.

Shift Work		Global Job Satisfaction (Total Satisfaction 7–28)	Average of Workplace Characteristics That Constitute Psychosocial Risks (0–1)	Satisfaction with Current Job (1–5)
No	Average	21.24	0.35	3.92
	Median	21.00	0.34	4.00
	Average rank	83.07	52.65	84.74
	N	50	50	50
	Standard deviation	3.73	0.13	0.80
Yes	Average	19.52	0.46	3.41
	Median	20.00	0.46	3.50
	Average rank	61.79	79.07	60.84
	N	88	88	88
	Standard deviation	3.17	0.18	0.83
Total	Average	20.14	0.42	3.59
	Median	20.00	0.39	4.00
	N	138	138	138
	Standard deviation	3.47	0.17	0.85
Mann–Whitney U		1521.500	1357.500	1438.000
p		0.003	0.000	0.000
p (Monte Carlo)		0.002	0.000	0.000

4. Discussion

Our study investigated the impact of the SARS-CoV-2 pandemic on the psychosocial burden and job satisfaction of nurses employed in long-term care in Poland. Surprisingly, in the obtained results of the statistical analysis of the survey questionnaire, nurses showed less work-related stress than we expected. Of the nurses surveyed, 87.0% stated that their job position had procedures for dealing with patients during a pandemic. For 71.7% of the respondents, responsibility for human health and life or readiness to react quickly (86.2% of the respondents) were not a problem. In our study, according to the respondents, the overall mean of the psychosocial risk factors at work was 0.42 ± 0.17. Emotional commitment of the respondents was at the mean level of 2.14 with a maximum of 4 points, as well as commitment at the occupied workstation, which was at the mean level of 2.32 with a maximum of 4 points. Studies by other authors have confirmed the relationship between psychosocial risk factors [20], which included high job demands, low job autonomy, low control, high effort-reward imbalance, interpersonal conflict, low social support, low trust and employee anxiety and stress [21].

According to Mlokosiewicz, more than a quarter of Polish employees experienced stress at work every day, with almost one-third of employees (32%) believing that the company was not interested in their psychological well-being. According to the employees' assessment, stress related to psychosocial hazards ranked first among other hazards (physical, chemical and biological) in the workplace (indicated by up to 72% of respondents) [22]. In the study by Kowalczuk et al., the nurses rated the demands of their jobs high (mean score about 3.5). The ability to control their work and the level of social support were rated at an average level (mean score of 3.01 and 3.06, respectively). Respondents rated satisfaction with life rather high (mean score of 3.62). The scale of desirable changes (3.57 points) that should take place in their work was rated high [23]. Based on the results of the review conducted by Al Thobaity and Alshammari, most of the problems faced by nurses in dealing with patients with COVID-19 could be divided into two types. The first consists of staffing shortages, depression due to anxiety and fear of infection, lack of communication with patients and exhaustion due to long hours without adequate food. The second type includes lack of medical supplies and materials, such as personal protective equipment [24]. In our study, 96% of the respondents believed that the workplace where the services were provided fully provided personal protective equipment to the employees and staff shortages resulted in increased hours of work. Working more hours was moderately correlated with fear and anxiety ($p \leq 0.012$). In the study by Lin et al., almost half of the students surveyed (49.1%) would give up their choice of nursing as a career. The analysis showed that fear of COVID-19 ($\beta = 0.226$, $p < 0.001$) influenced the intention to change the field of study [25]. Alnazly and Hjazeen's study showed that nurses had moderate levels of anxiety (mean score: 24.34 $\pm$ 13.43) and depression (43.8% of the sample) and severe anxiety (73.8%) and stress (45.4%). Nurses who cared for patients who tested positive for coronavirus in 2019 and those who had friends or family members who tested positive had higher levels of anxiety and distress ($p < 0.001$ and $p = 0.010$) [26].

Increasing psychological problems of medical workers, mainly nurses and more often women than men, concern increased levels of anxiety, depression, insomnia, chronic fatigue and stress. They especially fear for their own health and that of their families, bear the burden of emotional contact with patients and are subject to occupational overload due to staff shortages and inadequate personal protective equipment. In a state of mental decompensation, they require reliable information support, stress and tension reduction and rest. In the case of continuous work for many hours, they should be guaranteed a place for solitary rest and relaxation and their daily needs such as food, sleep, protective clothing and contact with family [13]. Cengiz et al. showed that the level of participants' effort in complying with personal protective equipment (PPE) was very high (more than 84.0%). The analysis showed that only 61.1% of the participants could sleep well and regularly. It was found that 85.0% of the participants followed the quarantine rules, 75.7% paid attention to social distancing while working and 81.7% followed the social distance rule in the places where they ate. It was found that 46.7% of the participants feared that they might be carriers of COVID-19 and 38.9% feared COVID-19 infection [27]. In a study by Sikaras et al., 52.4% of the respondents worked in COVID-19 units, the results of 67.9% and 42.9%, respectively, suggested the occurrence of fatigue and burnout among them and showed a strong positive correlation ($p < 0.01$, $r = 0.70$) [28]. The findings of Alameddine et al. showed that 67.8% of the nurses were satisfied with their jobs and most of the nurses stated that they were unlikely to quit their jobs in the coming year (76.2%). Nurses' resilience was directly related to job satisfaction ($p < 0.05$) [29]. Similarly, in our study, women compared to men rated job satisfaction higher. Higher mean psychosocial risks at work are associated with lower overall job satisfaction. Studies by Najder and Potocka have shown that the mere presence of psychological workload in the work environment, even if their presence is not stressful for employees, significantly correlates with health and occupational functioning [30], which has not been confirmed by our study.

Prevention of occupational stress, which is becoming an increasingly common health risk for those working with COVID-19 patients, is a major challenge, mainly for occupational health services. Improving psychosocial working conditions and reducing the stress experienced by workers contributes to maintaining and improving their health, as well as maintaining their ability to work. This is particularly important in a coronavirus pandemic situation. In addition, a friendly environment, as well as the fact that the employer cares about the health of employees, promotes greater work engagement [31].

Limitations of the Study

Nurses in this study working in long-term care were aware that the patients either tested positive for COVID-19 or were suspected cases. The questionnaire used is a self-report instrument; that is, current psychological well-being influenced the respondents' assessment of the situation. In addition, due to the nature of the long-term residential and home care services provided, the study had a small sample size and large sex bias, which means that the generalizability of the findings is limited.

5. Conclusions

A survey of nurses providing inpatient and residential long-term care services in the Podkarpackie Voivodeship (Poland) provides insight into the impact of the SARS-CoV-2 pandemic on their psychosocial burden and job satisfaction. Self-assessment of work ability of surveyed nurses employed in long-term care during the SARS-CoV-2 pandemic and involvement in patient care was high at 4.0 and 4.18 with a maximum of 5 points. The results indicate that the overall average psychosocial distress in the workplace was below health norms. The emotional involvement of the respondents was at an average level, and the higher the level of psychosocial risks present, the lower the global job satisfaction of the respondents.

The results of the presented study allow us to assume that since the onset of the COVID-19 pandemic, the nurses interviewed, along with the gained experience and greater knowledge, have changed their relationships with patients infected with the coronavirus and the level of fear and anxiety was reduced, which positively affects the quality of nursing care. Additionally, introduced vaccinations and mutation of the virus (currently OMICRON) influence severity, in many cases, being asymptomatic COVID-19 among nurses and patients covered by long-term care.

Author Contributions: Study design, K.T.; data collection, K.T. and B.M.; statistical analysis, K.T. and B.M.; interpretation of data, K.T. and B.M.; manuscript preparation, K.T. and M.D.; literature review, K.T., B.M. and M.D. All authors have read and agreed to the published version of the manuscript.

Funding: This research received no external funding.

Institutional Review Board Statement: Not applicable.

Informed Consent Statement: Informed consent was obtained from all subjects involved in the study.

Conflicts of Interest: The authors declare no conflict of interest.

References

1. Mekonen, E.; Shetie, B.; Muluneh, N. The Psychological Impact of COVID-19 Outbreak on Nurses Working in the Northwest of Amhara Regional State Referral Hospitals, Northwest Ethiopia. *Psychol. Res. Behav. Manag.* **2021**, *13*, 1353–1364. [CrossRef] [PubMed]
2. Service of the Republic of Poland. Coronavirus: Information and Recommendations. Available online: https://www.gov.pl/web/koronawirus/wykaz-zarazen-koronawirusem-sars-cov-2 (accessed on 11 October 2021).
3. Duszyński, J.; Afelt, A.; Ochab-Marcinek, A.; Owczuk, R.; Pyrć, K.; Rosińska, M.; Rychard, A.; Smiatacz, T. Zrozumieć COVID-19 Opracowanie Zespołu ds. COVID-19 Przy Prezesie Polskiej Akademii Nauk. Available online: https://informacje.pan.pl/images/2020/opracowanie-covid19-14-09-2020/ZrozumiecCovid19_opracowanie_PAN_interactive.pdf (accessed on 12 January 2022).
4. Supreme Chamber of Nurses and Midwives. Analyzes and Reports. Available online: https://nipip.pl/dane-statystyczne/ (accessed on 24 January 2022).
5. Muller, A.E.; Hafstad, E.V.; Himmels, J.P.W.; Smedslund, G.; Flottorp, S.; Stensland, S.Ø.; Stroobants, S.; Van De Velde, S.; Vist, G.E. The mental health impact of the covid-19 pandemic on healthcare workers, and interventions to help them: A rapid systematic review. *Psychiatr. Res.* **2020**, *293*, 113441. [CrossRef] [PubMed]
6. Cox, T.; Griffiths, A.; Rial-González, E. *Research on Work-Related Stress*; European Agency for Safety and Health at Work: Luxembourg, 2000.

7. Sánchez-Sánchez, E.; García-Álvarez, J.; García-Marín, E.; Gutierrez-Serrano, M.; Alférez, M.; Ramirez-Vargas, G. Impact of the COVID-19 Pandemic on the Mental Health of Nurses and Auxiliary Nursing Care Technicians—A Voluntary Online Survey. *Int. J. Environ. Res. Public Health* **2021**, *18*, 8310. [CrossRef] [PubMed]
8. Healy, S.; Tyrrell, M. Stress in emergency departments: Experiences of nurses and doctors. *Emerg. Nurse* **2011**, *19*, 31–37. [CrossRef]
9. Chen, S.-C.; Lai, Y.-H.; Tsay, S.-L. Nursing Perspectives on the Impacts of COVID-19. *J. Nurs. Res.* **2020**, *28*, e85. [CrossRef]
10. Shanafelt, T.; Ripp, J.; Trockel, M. Understanding and Addressing Sources of Anxiety Among Health Care Professionals During the COVID-19 Pandemic. *JAMA J. Am. Med. Assoc.* **2020**, *323*, 2133–2134. [CrossRef]
11. Fathiariani, L.; Nassimbwa, J. Investigating the burden of mental distress among nurses at a provincial COVID-19 referral hospital in Indonesia: A cross-sectional study. *BMC Nurs.* **2021**, *20*, 76. [CrossRef]
12. Xu, X.; Manzoor, F.; Jiang, S.; Mumtaz, A. Unpacking the Mental Health of Nurses during COVID-19: Evidence from Pakistan. *J. Clin. Med.* **2021**, *10*, 3546. [CrossRef]
13. Frawley, T.; van Gelderen, F.; Somanadhan, S.; Coveney, K.; Phelan, A.; Lynam-Loane, P.; De Brún, A. The impact of COVID-19 on health systems, mental health and the potential for nursing. *Ir. J. Psychol. Med.* **2020**, *38*, 1–7. [CrossRef]
14. Tomaszewska, K.; Majchrowicz, B.; Ratusznik, D. Rationing of Nursing Care on Example of Selected Health Care Facility. *Int. J. Environ. Res. Public Health* **2021**, *18*, 12824. [CrossRef]
15. Liu, Y.; Long, Y.; Cheng, Y.; Guo, Q.; Yang, L.; Lin, Y.; Cao, Y.; Ye, L.; Jiang, Y.; Li, K.; et al. Psychological Impact of the COVID-19 Outbreak on Nurses in China: A Nationwide Survey During the Outbreak. *Front. Psychiatry* **2020**, *11*, 598712. [CrossRef] [PubMed]
16. Llop-Gironés, A.; Vračar, A.; Llop-Gironés, G.; Benach, J.; Angeli-Silva, L.; Jaimez, L.; Thapa, P.; Bhatta, R.; Mahindrakar, S.; Scavo, S.B.; et al. Employment and working conditions of nurses: Where and how health inequalities have increased during the COVID-19 pandemic? *Hum. Resour. Health* **2021**, *19*, 1–11. [CrossRef] [PubMed]
17. Sampaio, F.; Sequeira, C.; Teixeira, L. Impact of COVID-19 outbreak on nurses' mental health: A prospective cohort study. *Environ. Res.* **2021**, *194*, 110620. [CrossRef] [PubMed]
18. Varghese, A.; George, G.; Kondaguli, S.V.; Naser, A.Y.; Khakha, D.C.; Chatterji, R. Decline in the mental health of nurses across the globe during COVID-19: A systematic review and meta-analysis. *J. Glob. Health* **2021**. [CrossRef] [PubMed]
19. Mościcka-Teske, A.; Potocka, A. *Psychosocial Risk Scale—Building and Application Principles*; Komisja Krajowa NSZZ Solidarność: Łódź-Gdańsk, Poland, 2014.
20. Heitzman, J. Impact of COVID-19 pandemic on mental health. *Psychiatr. Polska* **2020**, *54*, 187–198. [CrossRef]
21. Mátó, V.; Tarkó, K.; Lippai, L.; Nagymajtényi, L.; Paulik, E. Psychosocial work environment risk factors among university employees—A cross-sectional study in Hungary. *Slov. J. Public Health* **2020**, *60*, 10–16. [CrossRef]
22. Młokosiewicz, M. Stres w miejscu pracy a potencjał pracowników. *Studia Pr. WNEiZ US* **2018**, *51*, 235–247. [CrossRef]
23. Kowalczuk, K.; Krajewska-Kułak, E.; Rolka, H.; Kondzior, D.; Sarnacka, E. Psychosocial working conditions of nurses. *Hygeia Public Health* **2015**, *50*, 621–629.
24. Al Thobaity, A.; Alshammari, F. Nurses on the Frontline against the COVID-19 Pandemic: An Integrative Review. *Dubai Med. J.* **2020**, *3*, 87–92. [CrossRef]
25. Lin, Y.; Hu, Z.; Danaee, M.; Alias, H.; Wong, L.P. The Impact of the COVID-19 Pandemic on Future Nursing Career Turnover Intention Among Nursing Students. *Risk Manag. Health Policy* **2021**, *14*, 3605–3615. [CrossRef]
26. Alnazly, E.K.; Hjazeen, A.A. Psychological Distress and Coping Strategies among Nurses during the COVID-19 Pandemic: A Cross-Sectional Online Survey. *Open Nurs. J.* **2021**, *15*, 262–272. [CrossRef]
27. Cengiz, Z.; Isik, K.; Gurdap, Z.; Yayan, E.H. Behaviours and experiences of nurses during the COVID-19 pandemic in Turkey: A mixed methodsstudy. *J. Nurs. Manag.* **2021**, *29*, 2002–2013. [CrossRef] [PubMed]
28. Sikaras, C.; Ilias, J.; Tselebis, A.; Pachi, A.; Zyga, S.; Tsironi, M.; Rojas Gil, A.P.; Panagiotou, A. Nursing staff fatigue and burnout during the COVID-19 pandemic in Greece. *AIMS Public Health* **2021**, *9*, 94–105. [CrossRef] [PubMed]
29. Alameddine, M.; Bou-Karroum, K.; Ghalayini, W.; Abiad, F. Resilience of nurses at the epicenter of the COVID-19 pandemic in Lebanon. *Int. J. Nurs. Sci.* **2021**, *8*, 432–438. [CrossRef] [PubMed]
30. Najder, A.; Potocka, A. Psychospołeczne Zagrożenia Zawodowe i ich Związek ze Zdrowiem oraz Funkcjonowaniem Zawodowym Pracowników Ochrony Zdrowia. Available online: http://www.pielegniarstwo.ump.edu.pl/uploads/2015/3/313_3_57_2015.pdf (accessed on 12 February 2022).
31. Waszkowska, M.; Wężyk, A.; Merecz-Kot, D. Psychosocial risk management in occupational health. *Med. Ogólna Nauk. Zdrowiu* **2013**, *19*, 445–452.

International Journal of
Environmental Research and Public Health

MDPI

Article

A Phenomenological Study of Nurses' Experience in Caring for COVID-19 Patients

Hye-Young Jang [1], Jeong-Eun Yang [2] and Yong-Soon Shin [1,*]

1 School of Nursing, Research Institute of Nursing Science, Hanyang University, Seoul 04763, Korea; white0108@hanyang.ac.kr
2 Department of Nursing, Jesus University, Jeonju-si 54989, Korea; elfyang@jesus.ac.kr
* Correspondence: ysshin2k@hanyang.ac.kr; Tel.: +82-2-2220-0798

Abstract: This study aimed to understand and describe the experiences of nurses who cared for patients with COVID-19. A descriptive phenomenological approach was used to collect data from individual in-depth interviews with 14 nurses, from 20 October 2020 to 15 January 2021. Data were analyzed using the phenomenological method of Colaizzi. Five theme clusters emerged from the analysis: (1) nurses struggling under the weight of dealing with infectious disease, (2) challenges added to difficult caring, (3) double suffering from patient care, (4) support for caring, and (5) expectations for post-COVID 19 life. The findings of this study are useful primary data for developing appropriate measures for health professionals' wellbeing during outbreaks of infectious diseases. Specifically, as nurses in this study struggled with mental as well as physical difficulties, it is suggested that future studies develop and apply mental health recovery programs for them. To be prepared for future infectious diseases and contribute to patient care, policymakers should improve the work environment, through various means, such as nurses' practice environment management and incentives.

Keywords: nursing; infectious diseases; caregiving; SARS-CoV-2; qualitative research

Citation: Jang, H.-Y.; Yang, J.-E.; Shin, Y.-S. A Phenomenological Study of Nurses' Experience in Caring for COVID-19 Patients. *Int. J. Environ. Res. Public Health* **2022**, *19*, 2924. https://doi.org/10.3390/ijerph19052924

Academic Editor: Paul B. Tchounwou

Received: 23 January 2022
Accepted: 1 March 2022
Published: 2 March 2022

1. Introduction

As the novel coronavirus disease (COVID-19) spreads worldwide and becomes more serious, the World Health Organization (WHO) has declared it a global epidemic. In Korea, the first case of COVID-19 was confirmed on 20 January 2020; as of 29 June 2021, the total number of patients was 156,167, of which 6882 were quarantined and treated, with a fatality rate of 1.29% [1].

COVID-19 is caused by a novel coronavirus—severe acute respiratory syndrome coronavirus-2 (SARS-CoV-2)—and manifests in clinical symptoms, such as cough (74.9%), fever (68.0%) and dyspnea (60.9%) among hospitalized patients [2]. In the case of SARS-CoV-2, it has been reported that if patients are isolated within 5 days of the onset of clinical symptoms, secondary infections occur less frequently; transmission can be effectively blocked by isolating immediately after the onset of symptoms [3]. However, hospitalizations in negative pressure isolation rooms, to block airborne infections, create a more isolated environment than the general intensive care unit environment; mandate medical personnel to wear unfamiliar and uncomfortable protective equipment; prohibit family visits and outside contact. Isolation affects patients as well, as it has been reported that many patients were insufficiently informed about the isolation environment and period, and this uncertainty caused them to experience depression [4]. These circumstances increase the importance of caring for patients in isolation.

Caring is an important concept within the field of nursing, as it affects the health of the patient as a whole [5]. In particular, in the early stages of outbreaks of new infectious diseases, all aspects, such as the pathology, transmission route, and effective treatment of the disease are uncertain [6]. Even the effectiveness of protective equipment is uncertain. It has been found that healthcare providers' anxiety and fear in such conditions affects their ability to care for patients [7,8]. In the context of the COVID-19 pandemic, many scholars predict that the time before and after the pandemic will be very different and are asking if we are ready for post- or the 'with COVID-19 era' [9–11]. Even in nursing, this change is difficult to ignore, and nursing professionals and researchers should answer whether we are preparing the 'with COVID-19 era'. In order to identify the reality of nursing in the 'with COVID-19 era', it is necessary to understand what nursing and caring experiences were like for nurses who have been care professionals during the unprecedented COVID-19 pandemic. During the pandemic, nurses played a positive role in the rapid reorganization of the nursing system, improvement of team communication, coordination materials for emergency and continuous care, improvement of efficiency of nursing performance as a front-line caregiver, and caring for other nurses [12]. However, nurses are starting to experience burnout, having been unaware that the pandemic would soon change health professions universally [13]. For this, it is necessary to examine the experiences of nurses who have been, and are, caring for quarantined patients.

Studies on the nursing experience of patients with COVID-19 are underway in countries in various trajectories of the COVID-19 pandemic, such as Spain [14], Italy [15], Canada [16], the United States [17], and China [18], and these previous studies are focused on the lived nursing experience itself or the ethical aspect. Experiences of nursing care reported so far are summarized as providing nursing care [14–16], psychosocial and emotional aspects [14,15,18,19], resource management [14,16], struggling on the frontline [19,20], personal growth [18,19] and adapting to changes [18,20].

In the context of the COVID-19 pandemic, the Korean government responded using the K-Quarantine, also known as 3T–Test (diagnosis/confirmation), Trace (epidemiological survey/trace) and Treat (isolation/treatment) [21]. In particular, since February 2020, COVID-19 hospitals have been designated and operated for safe isolation beds for hospitalization of COVID-19 patients [22]. As patients diagnosed with COVID-19 are transferred to a designated hospital, operating a medical system that receives intensive treatment and care, the nurses at the hospitals are facing a high level of depression, anxiety, and stress [23,24].

However, the nursing experience of Korean nurses is only a small part of the research done in the early stage of the pandemic, and that knowledge is not enough to understand the essence of nursing in the special nursing environment of COVID-19. Therefore, this study was conducted to understand the lived nursing experience of the nurses at COVID-19-designated hospitals during the third wave [25] of the COVID-19 pandemic in Korea. The nursing experience of Korean COVID-19-dedicated hospital nurses could provide a unique opportunity to develop long-term sustainable response strategies under a long-lasting pandemic.

Phenomenological research focuses on vivid experiences, perceived or interpreted by participants, and aims to view and describe the world of their consciousness as a real world. In addition, exploring the experiences of others can discover insights that were previously unavailable, so it is considered a useful method for the purpose of this study. Particularly, Colaizzi's [26] method focuses on deriving a collection of common attributes and themes from multiple responses, rather than individual attributes. This method will facilitate an in-depth understanding of how nurses experienced caregiving for patients with COVID-19, and further contribute to the literature, regarding high-quality nursing care for quarantined patients. Therefore, the purpose of this study is to investigate the meaning and essence of nurses' experiences of caring for COVID-19 patients, using a phenomenological research method.

2. Materials and Methods

2.1. Study Design

The philosophical framework and study design of this study were guided by phenomenology. The philosophical aim of phenomenology is to provide an understanding of the participant's lived experiences [27]. In order to reveal the true essence of the 'living experience', it is first necessary to minimize the preconceived ideas that researchers may have about the research phenomenon (bracketing). Through such a phenomenological attitude, the participant's experience can be explored as it is [28]. From a phenomenological point of view, objectivity is obtained by being faithful to the phenomenon, and it can be secured by paying attention to the phenomenon itself rather than explaining what it is. As such, phenomenology seeks to reveal meaning and essences in the participant's experiences of the participant to facilitate understanding [28].

This study is an inductive study, applying the phenomenological research method of Colaizzi [26], in order to gain an in-depth understanding of the essence of nurses' experience in caring for COVID-19 patients, and it followed the guideline for qualitative research, established by the Consolidated Criteria for Reporting Qualitative Research [29]. The question of this study is, "What is the meaning and essence of the care experience of nurses who directly cared for COVID-19 patients?"

2.2. Participants and Settings

Participants were nurses working at a COVID-19 Infectious Disease Hospital in Seoul and Gyeonggi Province. The COVID-19 Infectious Disease Hospital was established and is operated by the Ministry of Health and Welfare, one of the central government ministries of South Korea, to respond to infectious diseases during the COVID-19 pandemic. It is dedicated to managing infected patients.

The inclusion criteria were as follows: nurses who had directly cared for confirmed or suspected COVID-19 patients in an isolation ward for at least 1 month; could communicate well and comprehend the purpose of this study; had voluntarily consented to participate. Nurses who had cared for COVID-19 patients for less than 1 month, had not participated in direct care, or had not been released from isolation, were excluded. Fourteen nurses participated in in-depth interviews individually (Table 1).

Table 1. General Characteristics of Participants (N = 14).

Variables		N
Sex	Male	2
	Female	12
Age (years)	<30	5
	30–39	3
	40–49	6
Education	College	11
	Graduate School	3
Number of patients per nurse	3	1
	4	6
	5	4
	6	2
	7	-
	8	-
	9	1
Period of working in isolation ward, (months)	<3	1
	3–<6	4
	6–<9	5
	9–<12	3
	12≤	1

Table 1. *Cont.*

Variables	N
Change of place of residence during working in the isolation ward, yes	4
Infection control education on COVID-19, yes	12

Note. COVID-19 = coronavirus disease-2019.

2.3. Data Collection

Data were collected through in-depth interviews from 20 October 2020 to 15 January 2021 using purposive sampling (n = 12) and snowball sampling (n = 2). The sample size was determined by data saturation [30]. Data saturation was considered achieved when no new themes were revealed in the interviews of participants. Data saturation was determined by two researchers after the fourteenth case interview. Interviews were conducted either online or face-to-face by one well-trained researcher, depending on participants' convenience. During face-to-face interviews, we created a comfortable atmosphere by beginning with everyday conversations. Interviews began with an open-ended question: "Tell me about your experience of caring for patients with COVID-19", so that participants could elaborately and spontaneously describe their experiences. The interviews lasted about 60–120 min, and data collection and analysis were conducted simultaneously.

2.4. Data Analysis

The interview content was transcribed verbatim within 24 h of each interview by the researcher. Transcripts of each participant's interview and the memos were used to analyze data. Two researchers with doctoral degrees independently analyzed and discussed findings.

Data analysis was guided by Colaizzi's seven-step descriptive phenomenological method [26]: (1) researchers read all accounts multiple times to understand the overall flow of participants' experiences in caring for COVID-19 patients; (2) we extracted significant statements from each description, focusing on meaningful statements related to participants' caring experiences; (3) we formulated meanings from those significant statements, trying to discover the latent meaning in the context; (4) we organized those formulated meanings into themes and theme clusters; (5) the phenomenon under study was exhaustively described by integrating all the research results; (6) we identified the fundamental structure of the phenomenon; (7) finally, we validated this study by receiving feedback from two participants.

In the entire process of data analysis, we tried to keep a distance from the researcher's thoughts and feelings, and point of view about the phenomenon, as well as the content of the data, while being conscious of Husserl's 'bracketing' [28]. In this way, we tried to avoid data distortion, reduction, and exaggeration by the researcher, and we tried to confirm and understand the perspective, attitude, and feeling of the participant as much as possible in the participant's statement.

2.5. Rigor

To ensure trustworthiness of this study, the four criteria established by Lincoln and Guba [31] were used. For enhancing truth-value, we tried to obtain a rich set of data by selecting participants who would like to express the research phenomenon well and making it as comfortable as possible for the participants to state their experiences. We showed the study results to two participants to verify whether the derived results reflected the participants' experiences.

To ensure applicability, we provided the general characteristics of participants and tried to provide a thick description of the research phenomenon.

To establish consistency, Colaizzi's analysis method was adhered to, and the detailed research process and original data for each theme were presented to enhance the reader's understanding of the research results. The researcher conducted the research while taking a neutral attitude throughout the research process, excluding bias, prejudices, assumptions (bracketing), so that the participant's experience distortion by the researcher was minimized. In other words, in order to establish neutrality, which means freedom from prejudice about research results, at the beginning of the study, the researcher explicated any assumptions that could influence data collection and analysis [32] (ex. participants will mostly have negative emotions while caring for patients without any preparation. Participants will be withdrawn from the social perspective because they are taking care of infected patients.) The other researcher reviewed data analysis to ensure that the researcher's assumptions did not influence data interpretation.

2.6. Ethical Considerations

This study was approved by the Institutional Review Board of the researcher's affiliated institution (HYUIRB-202009-009). Participants were informed about the purpose of the study, reporting of study results, and interview recordings. We obtained written informed consents from all participants before data collection. In addition, it was explained that even after consenting, participants could withdraw from the study at any time without any harm if they wished. All participants were provided with a small reward as appreciation for their participation in the study.

3. Results

The essential structure of the phenomenon was identified as 'Going beyond the double suffering tunnel of taking charge of infected patients into the future'. The essence of the phenomenon is presented as five theme clusters, and twelve themes emerged from analyzing nurses' experiences with caring for COVID-19 patients: (1) nurses struggling under the weight of dealing with infectious disease, (2) challenges added to difficult caring, (3) double suffering from patient care, (4) support for caring, and (5) expectations for post-COVID-19 life (Table 2).

Table 2. Theme Clusters and Themes.

Theme Clusters	Themes
1. Nurses struggling under the weight of dealing with infectious disease	Anxiety and fear accompanying patient care Dignity ignored due to the fear of infectious diseases
2. Challenges added to difficult caring	The burden of triple distress for everyone's safety; Wearing PPE Work loaded solely on nurses Confusing and uncertain working conditions
3. Double suffering from patient care	Self-isolation: anxiety becomes a reality A contrasting perception of nurses: heroes of society versus subjects of avoidance
4. Support for caring	Companionship and sharing difficulties Support and appreciation from patients and people A sense of satisfaction and self-esteem
5. Expectations for post-COVID-19 life	Restoring everyday life Preparing for the future

3.1. Nurses Struggling under the Weight of Dealing with Infectious Disease

Participants felt fear and anxiety while caring for COVID-19 patients, as they have remained unaware of any definitive treatments. Consumed by thoughts of contracting the disease, they reported feeling unable to remain calm and dutifully serve their patients. In particular, it was shocking, as well as saddening, for them to be unable to provide respectful end of life care toward patients who could not recover.

3.1.1. Anxiety and Fear Accompanying Patient Care

The anxiety and fear at the heart of the thought that they could also be infected became an invisible chain, binding the participants. According to them, nursing without being guaranteed safety was challenging. When facing the reality of nursing while fearing patients' diseases, it felt unfamiliar for participants to worry about their own and their patients' safety simultaneously, rather than completely immersing themselves in patients' recovery. They were uncertain of whether their feelings were normal; although they tried their best to provide quality care, they found it challenging to do so while dealing with their persistent anxiety.

> *To be honest, that was the hardest for me. Since we were constantly exposed to the risk of infection, it was hard to care for patients due to anxiety rather than due to physical challenges while caring for the patient.* (Participant J)

3.1.2. Dignity Ignored Due to the Fear of Infectious Diseases

Having to watch patients struggling alone and in isolation, without the support and comfort of their family members during their final moments, made participants feel extremely sorry and heartbroken. The most distressing aspect of caring for patients on their deathbed was that patients and nurses were faced with the reality that patients' families would not be allowed to be with them during their moment of dying; the fact that they would pass away without receiving appropriate treatment was secondary. "Patients who died during the COVID-19 period were the most pitiful" does not just indicate the limitations of medical treatment. It highlights dignity, which is be protected even in the worst circumstances, but was disregarded due to the fear of contracting infectious diseases. Participants experienced unimaginable shock and ethical anguish as they witnessed patients being taken to crematoriums without being seen by their family members, with their bodies in bags without having their clothing changed. As these uncontrollable experiences kept repeating, participants made a paradoxical resolve to prevent patients from dying.

> *Patients who die while I work in the ward usually have their families come to see them and hold their hands. However, for those who die of COVID-19, families come and check their patients on the monitor. I think that's the most heartbreaking and sad thing.* (Participant L)

> *The post-death process was really shocking. I feel like it didn't treat people like human beings. Thus, that hurt me the most. I think that's hard while working in the ward. When patients die, I know how they will be treated. I am so sorry, and my heart hurts. That's why I really want to discharge them. Seriously, I think I'm getting desperate for this kind of feeling.* (Participant B)

3.2. *Challenges Added to Difficult Caring*

Participants struggled every day, and factors that made their lives more challenging are as follows: the personal protective equipment (PPE) that had to be worn for patient care, working in chaotic conditions without clear instructions, and being overburdened with tasks.

3.2.1. The Burden of Triple Distress for Everyone's Safety; Wearing PPE

Participants had to endure a significant amount of pain and discomfort for safety purposes, especially while nursing patients in PPE. Less than 10 min after wearing them, the inside of the protective clothing would become warm and fill with sweat, and the eye goggles would become foggy. In these situations, participants experienced difficulties in certain activities, such as communicating with patients, securing intravenous (IV) lines, or drawing blood. Occasionally, they had to wear gloves that did not fit well due to a lack of proper supplies, making their practice more difficult.

> *I think the hardest thing was to wear Level D and go inside. At first, I did the intubation wearing protective clothing. At that time, my body became sluggish, and my vision*

became narrower because I was wearing goggles. So, even if I moved a little, it got too hot and I would sweat too much, and it was really hard to deal with something in there. Because it was too hot. (Participant D)

3.2.2. Work Loaded Solely on Nurses

To prevent the spread of COVID-19, hospitals implemented policies to minimize the number of family members and caregivers in contact with patients, which increased the burden of caregiving on participants. Blood collections and portable X-ray imaging that radiological technologists performed also became nurses' duties. In addition, nurses had to prepare documents for the hospital transfers of patients, and were also responsible for checking, storing, and delivering parcels to patients. Nurses were gradually exhausted as most duties, especially those outside their purview, were delegated to them.

To be honest, there are not just nurses in the hospital. However, it's a situation where we have to take on everything that other employees have done. I feel like they're giving all their work to the nurses. We have to prepare everything that the radiology department had to do on their own before. For the meal distribution for COVID-19 patients, nurses have to do everything that the nutrition team previously did. For blood collection, we have to do all the things that the laboratory medicine department used to do. It's overwhelming that nurses have to do most of the work. (Participant F)

3.2.3. Confusing and Uncertain Working Conditions

Participants' routine caring for COVID-19 patients has been as uncertain as COVID-19 patients' conditions. Due to the number of confirmed cases increasing daily and sudden confirmations of the infection in colleagues, situations such as the operation of additional negative pressure wards or temporary closures of wards occurred unexpectedly. Consequently, participants were frequently relocated, and their work schedules and wards were changed, creating confusion. In particular, unclear guidelines and insufficient training made their jobs more difficult.

It's tough to get the work schedule on a weekly basis. Actually, I don't know my work schedule for Tuesday even on Monday, so I don't know which shift I will work on the next day. Hence, it's really very stressful. (Participant E)

3.3. Double Suffering from Patient Care

Participants experienced not only physical difficulties but also mental and social challenges while caring for COVID-19 patients. They endured self-isolation along with their families, and were uncomfortable with causing their family members to experience isolation. In addition, unlike the usual positive public perception of nurses, participants felt a social disconnection from the negativity and stigma surrounding them, which was also hurtful and uncomfortable.

3.3.1. Self-Isolation: Anxiety Becomes a Reality

Participants contracted the virus while caring for patients or had to enter complete self-isolation due to coming in contact with infected colleagues. They endured the anxiety and fear of being infected and suddenly became subjects of self-isolation, leading to concerns about having their personal information exposed, and the social stigma of being confirmed COVID-19 patients. Those who tested negative felt "uncomfortable relief", even as their colleagues were testing positive during self-isolation.

When being in self-isolation, as you know, I must contact my child's school. I had to contact a homeroom teacher of my child. Actually I didn't really do anything wrong, but I really, really felt bad. Wouldn't the image appear strange to my child? Because of that thought, every time I thought about that, I thought if I should resign. (Participant N)

3.3.2. A Contrasting Perception of Nurses: Heroes of Society versus Subjects of Avoidance

Even with the "Thank you Challenge" campaign spreading among the public, to express gratitude and respect towards health care professionals who responded to COVID-19, nurses did not feel particularly gratified. In a pandemic, the true heroes fighting COVID-19 could only work efficiently in isolation from other people. Close neighbors viewed participants as dangerous sources of pollution or pathogens that threatened their safety. Unlike the warm gaze of the public to see the nurses, participants felt judged by those around them, which made their jobs more uncomfortable.

> *Above all, the most challenging thing is the social perspective of "these people are working in an isolation hospital now". People close to me have this kind of perspective ... When one of the nurses is reported on the news or the media as a confirmed patient, we also feel like cringing. Such social perspectives were very hard for us because we've become people that the public wants to avoid rather them feeling appreciation for us and thinking of us like we are working hard and trying our best.* (Participant M)

3.4. *Support for Caring*

Sympathetic colleagues, and supportive and appreciative patients, encouraged participants to care for patients despite their difficulties. In addition, participants felt rewarded and proud of their care when they witnessed patients recovering, which further drove them to fulfill their duties.

3.4.1. Companionship and Sharing Difficulties

Participants endured difficult working routines with the support of colleagues, who best understood their struggles. In experiencing and sharing the same difficulties, participants found comfort with their colleagues. As nurses cannot quit, as that would mean additional pressures for their colleagues, they rely on each other for support.

> *To be honest, I think I'm being able to endure hard times thanks to my companionship. It's hard for us all. And fortunately, all colleagues are friendly, and many colleagues are so considerate of each other. We're not pushing each other to go in, but we are voluntarily working. Even though COVID-19 is hard for me, this companionship has helped me learn and endure with them until now.* (Participant I)

3.4.2. Support and Appreciation from Patients and People

While struggling, words of support and appreciation from patients, family, and friends helped participants withstand their difficult situations.

> *A patient wrote a very long letter. "Thank you. Thank you so much for taking care of me, and I was moved by the hard work you did. And even in the heat, you never got annoyed". Well, because the patient wrote a lot of appreciative words like this, I was really grateful. Somehow, apart from the money, I thought it was terrific to work.* (Participant A)

3.4.3. A Sense of Satisfaction and Self-Esteem

The sense of satisfaction and self-esteem felt while caring for COVID-19 patients became an essential incentive for participants to remain in nursing. When patients hospitalized in severe conditions were able to recover, participants felt rewarded by their occupation, and their self-esteem was increased.

> *At first, the patient's condition was so bad. So, we thought the patient would actually die, but it turned out that the patient improved so much and was discharged later. We felt like we were being compensated for the hard work. I had pride that we did an excellent job in nursing.* (Participant D)

3.5. *Expectations for Post-COVID-19 Life*

As COVID-19 keeps persisting in everyday life, expectations for life after COVID-19 are gradually blurring. Participants are unsure if there will ever be a time when they can care for their patients without protective clothing. Much of what participants wanted to accomplish after COVID-19 has been delayed for at least a year, but they have some expectations and are preparing for another future.

3.5.1. Restoring Everyday Life

Even in the current uncertain situation, participants have sincerely performed their nursing duties, while dreaming of restoring daily life. They recognized the importance of everyday social activities, such as eating together, watching movies, capturing bright smiles on camera, and realized that these activities were all they wished to do. Conversely, along with these wishes, there are also concerns about being able to return to the past sense of normalcy.

> *Returning to normality is what I want the most, and I think the next step is to think about it together with the management team and the government. I believe our request should be reviewed to combat physical exhaustion, and psychotherapists need to be involved and actively work on recovering. It's not just that we get rest. Professional intervention is necessary.* (Participant M)

3.5.2. Preparing for the Future

Participants encountered COVID-19, which occurred several years after the Middle East respiratory syndrome (MERS) epidemic, as another infectious disease that was able to threaten society at any time. In addition, chaotic situations in the hospital were not promptly managed, as the effects of the virus were so severe and fast that the experience of nursing MERS patients became insignificant. The MERS experience was inadequate in training healthcare providers to respond to similar future emergencies. Accordingly, efforts have been made to incorporate the vivid nursing experiences of COVID-19 into protocols against bracing for other diseases in the future.

> *That's why even though I don't know when the COVID-19 pandemic will end, once it's over, I think the protocol needs to be more complete. Furthermore, I think we should regularly stockpile a certain amount of items for the future. And, we need to plan a little more neatly how to manage nursing staff systematically.* (Participant K)

> *Since we don't know when another infectious disease will afflict us, we have to prepare a lot for response training to infectious diseases, facilities and personnel of institutions, and locations for care facilities. To reduce certain mistakes, I think we should prepare well now.* (Participant M)

4. Discussion

This study was conducted to understand the meanings and essence of the experiences of nurses who cared for COVID-19 patients, using a descriptive phenomenological method. As a result of this study, 5 theme clusters and 12 themes were extracted.

The first theme cluster indicated that the nurses struggled under the weight of dealing with infectious diseases. Participants expressed anxiety and fear in the absence of a definitive treatment for COVID-19. This is similar to the results of previous studies that reported that the lack of information and knowledge about unfamiliar diseases leads to ambiguity in nursing services, resulting in nurses feeling fearful and anxious [33]. The anxiety and fear accompanying patient care may be the result of rushing to the battlefield without any preparation [19]. In addition, participants appeared to have persistent fears of unintentional exposure and of transmitting the virus to co-workers [34]. Nurses who performed shift work during COVID-19 had a significantly increased association between COVID-19-related work stressors and anxiety disorder [24]. These physiological and psychological conditions are reported to create high stress and further lead to post-traumatic stress [35]. Hence, nurses caring for COVID-19 patients require continuous evaluation and management to sustain their mental wellbeing.

In the COVID-19 pandemic, nurses are experiencing ethical anguish in the face of unique situations that they have never experienced before. In particular, watching patients pass away alone, in isolation, without the support and comfort of family members, causes unimaginable shock and anguish. Moral distress between patient dignity and infection control is a similar experience to nurses in other countries, reported in previous studies. Nurses are known to experience contradictory feelings [18] as they experience the pressure of having to coordinate their responsibilities for the prevention of COVID-19 infection, along with other moral responsibilities [16].

Therefore, we need to create an ethically supportive environment [36], not just alleviate the ethical distress experienced by nurses [37]. In addition, it is necessary to find ways to guarantee both infection control and dignified death; for instance, family members can wear protective clothing and safely participate in their relatives' end-of-life processes. Other measures to ensure a dignified death include minimal post-mortem medical interference, and respect for and adherence to cultural customs [38].

The second theme cluster was participants' aggravated caring difficulties. Participants in this study were uncomfortable with the heat and sweat caused by wearing sealed PPE. This seems to be a slightly different experience than the Italian nurses who raised some concerns about the lack of PPE, the inadequacy of PPE, and the lack of guidelines for proper use [15]. In Korea, where resources, such as PPE, were relatively abundant since the COVID-19 pandemic declaration, wearing PPE acted as a triple pain burden on the safety of all people rather than the problem of lack of equipment.

It is similar to a previous study, demonstrating that these devices make it difficult to communicate with patients and perform basic tasks [34]. The appropriate wearing of PPE has been reported to protect medical staff from burnout [39]. However, continuous wearing of PPE can cause tissue damage or skin reactions, and prolonged wearing of goggles has been found to increase discomfort and fatigue due to abrasive straps and visual distortion [38]. Therefore, compliance with the PPE-wearing guidelines should be monitored and shift work should be assigned, taking into account the maximum period during which nurses are allowed to wear protective equipment.

It has also been found that medical workload has been excessively delegated to nurses taking care of COVID-19 patients. Policies to minimize social contact with patients have burdened nurses with extra tasks, causing exhaustion [40]. The excessive increase in work burden is in line with the results of qualitative research on the experience of nurses in other countries. A study by Liu et al. [34], in the early days of the COVID-19 pandemic, reported that nurses had done a lot of work. Recent studies also reported that COVID-19 caused a lot of work for nurses [20], and the treatment characterized by many isolated patients increased the work of nurses exponentially [14]. Nurses are constantly aware of new knowledge and skills associated with evolving pandemics and viruses, and receive new training, in preparation for adapting to the situation and providing care for suspected or identified patients [20]. In addition, frequent changes of working locations and wards, changes in work schedules, and confusion over working guidelines, have made nurses' lives uncertain.

The final theme of the challenge with difficult care was the confusing and uncertain working conditions, partly related to nursing staffing [14]. However, it was more difficult for the participants in this study to be able to predict their work schedule, rather than the shortage of nursing personnel. This may be due to the difficulty in predicting the hospitalization rates of infected patients and the problems caused by frequent and rapid relocation of nurses, depending on the number of hospitalized patients. In this study, the uncertainty in working conditions is consistent with the report by Liang et al. [20], that there was uncertainty among nurses about being transferred to the areas where the epidemic was most serious. Moreover, the ambiguity surrounding COVID-19 and whether patients have contracted it have been shown to increase nurses' stress [33]. Even in such situations, thoroughly preparing for and predicting potential emergency situations, based on comprehensive data analysis, knowledge accumulation, and education, can reduce the uncertainty and anxiety surrounding infectious diseases.

The third theme cluster was double suffering from patient care. Despite continuing to monitor self-health to avoid infecting others, nurses contracted the virus or had to self-isolate due co-workers' positive diagnoses. Sabetian et al. [41] found that 273 out of a total of 4854 cases contracted the virus while caring for COVID-19 patients, of which 51.3% were nurses. The fear of self-reliance approaching reality is a reflection of the situation at the time, when nurses were not allowed to return home after cohort isolation for two weeks as their colleagues were diagnosed with COVID-19 [19].

Notably, participants felt that they were subjected to dual perceptions, both as national heroes and as contagions. In Korea, the "Thank You Challenge" campaign encouraged expressing gratitude and respect to medical staff. The Korean people were deeply impressed by the situation of nurses and care protection, as they knew that they could not care for patients infected with COVID-19 without the sacrifice and compassionate mission of the nurses [42]. However, nurses have reported preferring forms of recognition and support other than hero worship [37], indicating that the campaign alone was insufficient in improving their morale. Participants also felt that their community members wanted to avoid them and considered them as dangerous contagions, threatening public safety. Previous studies reported that nurses were treated as viruses [19] or suffered from stigma [20], and conversely, were motivated to work harder through public support [19]. However, there are few research reports that nurses experience double suffering from patient care due to the coexistence of such contrasting perceptions. These experiences corroborate previous findings that disease uncertainty and social anxiety have caused nurses to be perceived as carriers and spreaders of the virus [33].

The fourth theme cluster was supporting caring. Participants endured their situations because quitting would have overburdened their colleagues. While participants found it awkward to work with nurses from different wards at the beginning of the COVID-19 pandemic, their relationships improved and became encouraging and supportive [19]. It is worth noting that, even in situations of extreme stress and emotional exhaustion, support from colleagues and teams can positively impact recovery [43]. In addition, this study found that support and appreciation from patients and families encouraged participants to endure their difficult situations [19,35]. In previous studies, negative emotions, such as fatigue, helplessness, and fear of infections, prevailed in the early stages of COVID-19, but coping strategies were created with adaptation, support from others, and expressions of positive emotions [44]. International researchers reported that nurses dealt with and attempted to overcome their challenges and feelings and emotional responses by coping during the pandemic. Nurses in the United States [17] and India [45] used teamwork and peer support, and used personal coping strategies, such as relationship development, play, exercise, meditation, and distractions.

In the face of unknown diseases and unpredictable dangers, participants took responsibility and devoted themselves to their mission. Despite nurses and healthcare staff demonstrating professional devotion [33,34], a social atmosphere that demands sacrifice should be avoided to decrease their experiences of stress and fatigue.

The last theme cluster encompassed expectations for post-COVID-19 life. The participants had been doing their best to care for patients, while dreaming of returning to their regular lives, despite working in uncertain conditions. To instill a sense of normalcy in their lives, it is imperative to provide physical and mental health support to exhausted nurses. Even after the impact of COVID-19 has diminished, it is necessary to fully recognize the inherent stress and emotional burden experienced by nurses and support recovery with routine procedures and systems [44]. This aspect of the pandemic has been reported by Italian nurses to have obvious psychological trauma, which is quite similar to that reported in China [46,47]. As COVID-19 cases begin to decline, research into resilience, particularly post-traumatic stress syndrome in nursing staff, will be needed [48]. Although new epidemic outbreaks cannot be prevented, risk awareness can direct attention to emerging epidemics and promote capacity development toward disease management and control [19,49]. As seen from this study, experience alone did not prepare nursing staff to deal with novel disease outbreaks. Hence, specific protocols and standard operating procedures, targeting different disease risk scenarios, should be established to support nursing work, with ample resources.

Limitations of This Research

In this study, we applied a phenomenological approach to understanding nurses' experiences of COVID-19 patient caring, and the participants were the nurses who involuntarily cared for COVID-19 patients. Accordingly, there is a limitation in that the nursing experience of the nurses who voluntarily participated in COVID-19 patient nursing could not be presented. We conducted online or face-to-face interviews, depending on the participants' preferences, but the online interview had limitations, in that it did not fully grasp the vivid experiences contained in the non-verbal expressions of the participants and did not describe their experiences in more depth. Participants were in a vulnerable situation; not only were they at risk of infection, but were also responsible for covering the duty of their colleagues with confirmed COVID-19, and the work of other health care assistants because they were wearing PPE. Despite these limitations, it is significant that this study gained a deeper understanding of nurses' experiences of caring for COVID-19 patients and came a little closer to the essence of nursing.

5. Conclusions

This study is significant as it explored and organized nurses' experiences of caring for COVID-19 patients, using a descriptive phenomenological research method. The findings of this study are useful primary data for developing appropriate measures for health professionals' wellbeing during outbreaks of infectious diseases.

A limitation of this study is that, because data were collected before the participants were vaccinated against COVID-19, negative emotional aspects, such as anxiety and fear about caring for patients, were drawn as the main results. In the future, it is necessary to balance this perspective by incorporating experiences of healthcare providers who have been vaccinated against COVID-19. In addition, as nurses in this study struggled with mental as well as physical difficulties, it is suggested that future studies develop and apply mental health recovery programs for them.

Author Contributions: H.-Y.J., J.-E.Y. and Y.-S.S. conceived and designed the study; H.-Y.J. acquired data; H.-Y.J. and Y.-S.S. analyzed the data; H.-Y.J. and J.-E.Y. wrote the first draft. All authors contributed to revisions of the manuscript and critical discussion. All authors have read and agreed to the published version of the manuscript.

Funding: This research received no external funding.

Institutional Review Board Statement: The study was conducted in accordance with the Declaration of Helsinki, and approved by the Institutional Review Board of Hanyang University (HYUIRB-202009-009-1, 30 September 2021).

Informed Consent Statement: Informed consent was obtained from all subjects involved in the study.

Data Availability Statement: The data presented in this study are available on request from the corresponding author.

Conflicts of Interest: The authors declare no conflict of interest.

References

1. Korean Disease Control and Prevention Agency. Current Status of COVID-19 Outbreak and Vaccination in Korea. Available online: http://ncov.mohw.go.kr/tcmBoardView.do?contSeq=355174 (accessed on 29 June 2021).
2. Suleyman, G.; Fadel, R.A.; Malette, K.M.; Hammond, C.; Abdulla, H.; Entz, A.; Demertzis, Z.; Hanna, Z.; Failla, A.; Dagher, C.; et al. Clinical characteristics and morbidity associated with coronavirus disease 2019 in a series of patients in metropolitan Detroit. *JAMA Netw. Open.* **2020**, 3, e2012270. [CrossRef] [PubMed]

3. Park, S.E. Epidemiology, virology, and clinical features of severe acute respiratory syndrome-coronavirus-2 (SARS-CoV-2; Coronavirus Disease-19). *Clin. Exp. Pediatr.* **2020**, *63*, 119–124. [CrossRef] [PubMed]
4. Yang, I.; Kim, H.; Jang, Y.; Kang, Y.A. Associations among uncertainty, depression, and anxiety in isolated inpatients. *J. Korean Acad. Psychiatr. Ment. Health Nurs.* **2019**, *28*, 216–225. [CrossRef]
5. Hwang, H.L.; Tu, C.T.; Wang, H.H. Development and psychometric evaluation of the Caring Scale for Institutionalized Elders. *J. Nurs. Res.* **2017**, *25*, 140–148. [CrossRef] [PubMed]
6. Kim, D.H. Supply status of negative pressure isolation rooms: Focused on the neighborhood unit. *HIRA Policy Trends* **2020**, *14*, 29–42.
7. Hwang, S.; Kim, S. Health care professional's duty of care in a public health emergency. *J. Korean Bioeth. Assoc.* **2019**, *20*, 29–43. [CrossRef]
8. Heo, Y.J.; Kim, J.H.; Jeong, J.; Lee, S. Nurses' experience in caring for patients with infectious diseases in a hospital isolated unit. *J. Korean Assoc. Qual. Res.* **2019**, *4*, 32–39. [CrossRef]
9. Das, N. Psychiatrist in post-COVID-19 era—Are we prepared? *Asian J. Psychiatr.* **2020**, *51*, 102082. [CrossRef]
10. Lee, S.M.; Lee, D.H. Opportunities and challenges for contactless healthcare services in the post-COVID-19 era. *Technol. Forecast. Soc. Chang.* **2021**, *167*, 120712. [CrossRef]
11. Simons, G.; Bald, D.S. A critical review of the definition of 'wellbeing' for doctors and their patients in a post COVID-19 era. *Int. J. Soc. Psychiatry* **2021**, *67*, 984–991. [CrossRef]
12. Lee, J.; Cho, H.S.; Shin, S.R. Nursing strategies for the post-COVID-19 era. *Int. Nurs. Rev.* **2021**, *68*, 149–152. [CrossRef] [PubMed]
13. Thompson, D.R.; Darbyshire, P.D. Nightingale's year of nursing: Rising to the challenges of the COVID-19 era. *BMJ* **2020**, *370*, m2721. [CrossRef] [PubMed]
14. Fernández-Castillo, R.; González-Caro, M.; Fernández-García, E.; Porcel-Gálvez, A.; Garnacho-Montero, J. Intensive care nurses' experiences during the COVID-19 pandemic: A qualitative study. *Nurs. Crit. Care* **2021**, *26*, 397–406. [CrossRef] [PubMed]
15. Catania, G.; Zanini, M.; Hayter, M.; Timmins, F.; Dasso, N.; Ottonello, G.; Aleo, C.; Sasso, L.; Bagnasco, A. Lessons from Italian front-line nurses' experiences during the COVID-19 pandemic: A qualitative descriptive study. *J. Nurs. Manag.* **2021**, *29*, 404–411. [CrossRef] [PubMed]
16. Peter, E.; Mohammed, S.; Killackey, T.; MacIver, J.; Variath, C. Nurses' experiences of ethical responsibilities of care during the COVID-19 pandemic. *Nurs. Ethics* **2022**, 1–14. [CrossRef] [PubMed]
17. Kelley, M.; Zadvinskis, I.M.; Miller, P.S.; Monturo, C.; Norful, A.A.; O'Mathúna, D.; Roberts, H.; Smith, J.; Tucker, S.; Sills, G.; et al. United States nurses' experiences during the COVID-19 pandemic: A grounded theory. *J. Clin. Nurs.* **2021**, 1–14. [CrossRef] [PubMed]
18. Pei, J.; Luo, D.; Yang, B.X.; Zhang, H.; Zhu, X.; Chen, J. Nurses' experiences of providing care to patients with COVID-19 in the ICU in Wuhan: A descriptive phenomenological research. *BMJ Open* **2021**, *11*, e045454. [CrossRef]
19. Lee, N.; Lee, H.J. South Korean nurses' experiences with patient care at a COVID-19-designated hospital: Growth after the frontline battle against an infectious disease pandemic. *Int. J. Environ. Res. Public Health* **2020**, *17*, 9015. [CrossRef] [PubMed]
20. Liang, H.; Wu, Y.; Wu, C. Nurses' experiences of providing care during the COVID-19 pandemic in Taiwan: A qualitative study. *Int. J. Ment. Health Nurs.* **2021**, *30*, 1684–1692. [CrossRef] [PubMed]
21. Shim, H. Seoul Unveils Roadmap to Make "K-Quarantine" Global Standard. Available online: http://www.koreabiomed.com/news/articleView.html?idxno=8479 (accessed on 20 August 2020).
22. Ministry of Health and Welfare. Financial Support of Krw 39 Billion for 69 COVID-19 Designated Hospitals. Available online: http://www.mohw.go.kr/react/al/sal0301vw.jsp?PAR_MENU_ID=04&MENU_ID=0403&CONT_SEQ=353539 (accessed on 21 May 2020).
23. Kim, M.; Yang, Y. Mental health status and its influencing factors: The case of nurses working in COVID-19 hospitals in South Korea. *Int. J. Environ. Res. Public Health* **2021**, *18*, 6531. [CrossRef]
24. Park, S.; Lee, Y.; Kim, T.; Jung, S.J. Anxiety and COVID-19 related stressors among healthcare workers who performed shift work at four COVID-19 dedicated hospitals in Korea. *J. Occup. Environ. Med.* **2021**, *63*, 875–880. [CrossRef] [PubMed]
25. Central Disaster Management Headquarters & Central Disease Control Headquarters. Updates on COVID-19 in Republic of Korea. Available online: http://ncov.mohw.go.kr/tcmBoardView.do?brdId=&brdGubun=&dataGubun=&ncvContSeq=361268&contSeq=361268&board_id=140&gubun=BDJ (accessed on 24 November 2020).
26. Colaizzi, P.F. *Psychological Research as the Phenomenologist View It*, 1st ed.; Valle, R.S., Mark, K., Eds.; Oxford University Press: New York, NY, USA, 1978; pp. 48–71. ISBN 10-0195023153.
27. Cohen, M.Z. A historical overview of the phenomenologic movement. *Image J. Nurs. Sch.* **1978**, *19*, 31–34. [CrossRef] [PubMed]
28. McConnell-Henry, T.; Chapman, Y.; Francis, K. Husserl and Heidegger: Exploring the disparity. *Int. J. Nurs. Pract.* **2009**, *15*, 7–15. [CrossRef] [PubMed]
29. Tong, A.; Sainsbury, P.; Craig, J. Consolidated criteria for reporting qualitative research (COREQ): A 32-item checklist for interviews and focus groups. *Int. J. Qual. Health Care* **2007**, *19*, 349–357. [CrossRef] [PubMed]
30. Morse, J.M. Determining sample size. *Qual. Health Res.* **2000**, *10*, 3–5. [CrossRef]
31. Guba, E.G.; Lincoln, Y.S. *Effective Evaluation: Improving the Usefulness of Evaluation Results through Responsive and Naturalistic Approaches*; Jossey-Bass: San Francisco, CA, USA, 1981; p. 104.

32. Streubert, H.J.; Carpenter, D.R. (Eds.) *Qualitative Research in Nursing. Advancing the Humanistic Imperative*, 2nd ed.; Lippincott: Philadelphia, PA, USA, 1999.
33. Kalateh Sadati, A.; Zarei, L.; Shahabi, S.; Heydari, S.T.; Taheri, V.; Jiriaei, R.; Ebrahimzade, N.; Lankarani, K.B. Nursing experiences of COVID-19 outbreak in Iran: A qualitative study. *Nurs. Open* **2021**, *8*, 72–79. [CrossRef]
34. Liu, Q.; Luo, D.; Haase, J.E.; Guo, Q.; Wang, X.Q.; Liu, S.; Xia, L.; Liu, Z.; Yang, J.; Yang, B.X. The experiences of health-care providers during the COVID-19 crisis in China: A qualitative study. *Lancet Glob. Health* **2020**, *8*, e790–e798. [CrossRef]
35. Wang, Y.; Guo, H.; Du, X.; Song, W.; Lu, C.; Hao, W. Factors associated with post-traumatic stress disorder of nurses exposed to corona virus disease 2019 in China. *Medicine* **2020**, *99*, e20965. [CrossRef] [PubMed]
36. Corley, M.C.; Minick, P.; Elswick, R.K.; Jacobs, M. Nurse moral distress and ethical work environment. *Nurs. Ethics* **2005**, *12*, 381–390. [CrossRef] [PubMed]
37. Silverman, H.J.; Kheirbek, R.E.; Moscou-Jackson, G.; Day, J. Moral distress in nurses caring for patients with COVID-19. *Nurs. Ethics* **2021**, *28*, 1137–1164. [CrossRef] [PubMed]
38. World Health Organization. Rational Use of Personal Protective Equipment for COVID-19 and Considerations during Severe Shortages. Available online: https://www.who.int/publications/i/item/rational-use-of-personal-protective-equipment-for-coronavirus-disease-(covid-19)-and-considerations-during-severe-shortages (accessed on 29 June 2021).
39. Morgantini, L.A.; Naha, U.; Wang, H.; Francavilla, S.; Acar, Ö.; Flores, J.M.; Crivellaro, S.; Moreira, D.; Abern, M.; Eklund, M. Factors contributing to healthcare professional burnout during the COVID-19 pandemic: A rapid turnaround global survey. *PLoS ONE* **2020**, *15*, e0238217. [CrossRef] [PubMed]
40. Yoon, K.J. Changes and tasks in Korea's healthcare system in times of the COVID-19 pandemic. *Health Welf. Pol. Forum* **2020**, *290*, 34–49.
41. Sabetian, G.; Moghadami, M.; Hashemizadeh Fard Haghighi, L.; Shahriarirad, R.; Fallahi, M.J.; Asmarian, N.; Moeini, Y.S. COVID-19 infection among healthcare workers: A cross-sectional study in southwest Iran. *Virol. J.* **2021**, *18*, 58. [CrossRef] [PubMed]
42. Kang, Y.; Shin, K.R. COVID-19: Korean nurses' experiences and ongoing tasks for the pandemic's second wave. *Int. Nurs. Rev.* **2020**, *67*, 445–449. [CrossRef]
43. Maben, J.; Bridges, J. COVID-19: Supporting nurses' psychological and mental health. *J. Clin. Nurs.* **2020**, *29*, 2742–2750. [CrossRef] [PubMed]
44. Lee, S.H. Mental health impacts in health care workers during the COVID-19 pandemic. *J Korean Neuropsychiatr. Assoc.* **2021**, *60*, 19–22. [CrossRef]
45. George, C.E.; Inbaraj, L.R.; Rajukutty, S.; de Witte, L.P. Challenges, experience and coping of health professionals in delivering healthcare in an urban slum in India during the first 40 days of COVID-19 crisis: A mixed method study. *BMJ Open* **2020**, *10*, e042171. [CrossRef]
46. Xiao, H.; Zhang, Y.; Kong, D.; Li, S.; Yang, N. The effects of social support on sleep quality of medical staff treating patients with coronavirus disease 2019 (COVID-19) in January and February 2020 in China. *Med. Sci. Monit.* **2020**, *26*, e923549. [CrossRef]
47. Huang, C.; Wang, Y.; Li, X.; Ren, L.; Zhao, J.; Hu, Y.I.; Zhang, L.I.; Fan, G.; Xu, J.; Gu, X.; et al. Clinical features of patients infected with 2019 novel coronavirus in Wuhan, China. *Lancet* **2020**, *395*, 497–506. [CrossRef]
48. Duncan, L.D. What the COVID-19 pandemic tells us about the need to develop resilience in the nursing workforce. *Nurs. Manag.* **2020**, *27*, 22–27. [CrossRef]
49. Cui, P.P.; Wang, P.P.; Wang, K.; Ping, Z.; Wang, P.; Chen, C. Post-traumatic growth and influencing factors among frontline nurses fighting against COVID-19. *Occup. Environ. Med.* **2021**, *78*, 129–135. [CrossRef] [PubMed]

International Journal of
Environmental Research and Public Health

MDPI

Article

Good Care during COVID-19: A Narrative Approach to Care Home Staff's Experiences of the Pandemic

Marleen D. W. Dohmen [1,2,*], Charlotte van den Eijnde [1,2], Christina L. E. Thielman [1], Jolanda Lindenberg [1,2], Johanna M. Huijg [1,2] and Tineke A. Abma [1,2]

1 Leyden Academy on Vitality and Ageing, 2333 AA Leiden, The Netherlands; eijnde@leydenacademy.nl (C.v.d.E.); thielman@leydenacademy.nl (C.L.E.T.); lindenberg@leydenacademy.nl (J.L.); huijg@leydenacademy.nl (J.M.H.); abma@leydenacademy.nl (T.A.A.)
2 Department of Public Health and Primary Care, Leiden University Medical Center, 2333 ZA Leiden, The Netherlands
* Correspondence: dohmen@leydenacademy.nl

Abstract: Due to its major impact on Dutch care homes for older people, the COVID-19 pandemic has presented care staff with unprecedented challenges. Studies investigating the experiences of care staff during the COVID-19 pandemic have shown its negative impact on their wellbeing. We aimed to supplement this knowledge by taking a narrative approach. We drew upon 424 personal narratives written by care staff during their work in a Dutch care home during the COVID-19 pandemic. Firstly, our results show that care staff have a relational-moral approach to good care. Residents' wellbeing is their main focus, which they try to achieve through personal relationships within the triad of care staff–resident–significant others (SOs). Secondly, our results indicate that caregivers experience the COVID-19 mitigation measures as obstructions to relational-moral good care, as they limit residents' wellbeing, damage the triadic care staff–residents–SOs relationship and leave no room for dialogue about good care. Thirdly, the results show that care staff experiences internal conflict when enforcing the mitigation measures, as the measures contrast with their relational-moral approach to care. We conclude that decisions about mitigation measures should be the result of a dialogic process on multiple levels so that a desired balance between practical good care and relational-moral good care can be determined.

Keywords: COVID-19; mitigation measures; care homes; wellbeing; care ethics; relational care; narratives

Citation: Dohmen, M.D.W.; van den Eijnde, C.; Thielman, C.L.E.; Lindenberg, J.; Huijg, J.M.; Abma, T.A. Good Care during COVID-19: A Narrative Approach to Care Home Staff's Experiences of the Pandemic. *Int. J. Environ. Res. Public Health* **2022**, *19*, 2106. https://doi.org/10.3390/ijerph19042106

Academic Editors: Richard Gray and Sonia Udod

Received: 7 January 2022
Accepted: 10 February 2022
Published: 13 February 2022

1. Introduction

Like many care homes around the world, Dutch care homes for older people have been severely affected by the coronavirus disease 2019 (COVID-19) pandemic. In the Netherlands, within one month after the onset of the pandemic, care home residents represented approximately 10% of all reported COVID-19 cases [1] whilst making up less than 1% of the total Dutch population [2]. After the first wave of the pandemic, from March to June 2020, care home residents were greatly overrepresented in the mortality figures, comprising nearly 46% of all COVID-19-related deaths [3]. During the second wave, from July 2020 to January 2021, this number remained alarmingly high, rising slightly to 50% [4].

The COVID-19 pandemic presented care home staff with unprecedented challenges. The novelty of the disease resulted in great uncertainty about its spread and effects. Since there were shortages of personal protective equipment (PPE), care staff felt pressured to work without protection. This added to the fear of both contracting and spreading the novel coronavirus [5], a fear that became reality, as many residents were infected with and died from COVID-19. It was not only the disease itself, but also the related mitigation measures that were challenging for care staff. For instance, they were required to enforce room isolation for residents suspected of having a COVID-19 infection, as well as a temporary visiting ban, excluding residents' significant others (SOs) and other informal caregivers from the care home.

In the past two years, many studies have been published about the experiences of care staff during the COVID-19 pandemic. The results show that doctors and nurses are traumatized from working on the front line [6,7]. They were confronted with dire situations and dilemmas due to the limited capacity of the health system and limited resources [8,9], all the while balancing their duty to care with their own safety and that of their families [6]. In several instances, staff shortages, limited resources and the following of COVID-19 mitigation protocols resulted in negative medical outcomes and sometimes even death for those receiving care [10]. Moreover, many care workers on the front line died as a result of COVID-19 infection [11]. In addition, the COVID-19 pandemic amplified existing disparities in the care sector. Firstly, COVID-19 mitigation measures reinforced an existing valuation of *cure* over *care*, as short-term care settings were given priority over long-term care settings with regard to COVID-19 testing and the distribution of PPE [12–14]. Secondly, freelance care workers in care homes were exposed to more dangerous situations than permanent staff, as they had less access to PPE and were more often required to work risky shifts [15]. The challenging circumstances that care staff faced during the COVID-19 pandemic are reflected in the results of a systematic review investigating the impact of COVID-19 on care staff's mental health. The results included increased depressive symptoms, anxiety, stress and poor sleep quality (for detailed information see [16]). Similar results have been found for Dutch care home staff in particular, with reports of increased work and emotional loads and decreased wellbeing since the onset of the COVID-19 pandemic [5,17].

The studies published about experiences of care staff during COVID-19 thus far have mainly relied on surveys and interviews that use pre-defined topics. We aim to supplement the knowledge gained from these studies by taking a more explorative approach. In January 2020, we started an action research project collecting narratives from care home staff about their daily experiences providing care. Care home staff were free to share narratives about whichever topic in their work was important to them and they continued to share these narratives throughout the COVID-19 pandemic, allowing us to collect a large amount of data foregrounding care home staff's own perspectives during this time. To our knowledge, there is no prior study that has taken this approach. In addition, the research methods used to investigate the experiences of care staff during the pandemic have thus far been mainly retrospective. Our study aims to capture care staff's lived experience as closely as possible by asking them to share their daily experiences during their work shift soon after the fact.

An explorative approach centered on the emic perspectives of care staff could help us gain a deeper understanding of the experiences of care staff during the COVID-19 pandemic. Further knowledge about this is needed to mitigate the negative effects of the pandemic on care staff, especially in the long run. Previous studies have highlighted the risks and prevalence of moral injury and compassion fatigue for care staff due to the dire situations and moral dilemmas they encounter during the COVID-19 pandemic [18–20]. Dilemmas in this context do not only revolve around life and death, but also around everyday ethics, as was found in an international study on the ethical challenges faced by care staff during the COVID-19 pandemic [21]. By taking an explorative approach, we may gain better insight into the dilemmas care staff encounter during the COVID-19 pandemic, perhaps especially those that occur in everyday work. These insights can then serve as a knowledge base to counter moral injury and compassion fatigue for care staff. In addition, learning more about the experiences of care staff during the COVID-19 pandemic can help us prepare for any similar scenarios in the future, as the intention of care staff to care in a public health crisis has been linked to their experiences during previous public health crises [22].

We aim to contribute to existing knowledge by answering the following research question: Which experiences did Dutch care home staff describe in their narratives during their work shifts in the COVID-19 pandemic? We draw upon original data from 424 brief personal narratives, written by care home staff members during the first and second waves of the COVID-19 pandemic in the Netherlands. Within these narratives, it is shown that care staff have a relational-moral approach to care and that the COVID-19 mitigation measures obstruct their efforts to deliver care in the relational-moral sense.

2. Materials and Methods

2.1. Ethical Approval

This study was reviewed and declared not subject to the law on research involving human subjects by the Institutional Review Board of the Medical Ethical Committee Leiden-Den Haag-Delft for observational studies and was registered under number N20.095. The protocol was assessed and considered compliant with scientific due diligence.

2.2. Context of the Study

Data collection for this study took place as part of a larger study examining the possibilities of using narratives about personal experiences with care to account for its quality. The study took place from January 2020 to December 2021 on the psychogeriatric ward of two care homes in the Netherlands. During this time, care staff captured many brief personal narratives about whichever topic in their work was important to them using the digital application SenseMaker® [23]. Consequently, we collected many narratives during the COVID-19 pandemic in the Netherlands. These narratives took place in the context of COVID-19, but their content was not restricted to COVID-19.

2.3. Design

The larger study had an action research design and was conducted in close collaboration with the stakeholders in practice. The sub-study presented here had a qualitative design, in which we analyzed narrative data through open coding.

2.4. Sampling

Sampling was restricted to the two care homes partaking in the larger study. For the current study, only data from one of the two care homes was included. The care staff in this care home continued to share their narratives throughout both the first and the second waves of the COVID-19 pandemic. Care staff in the other care home stopped sharing narratives because of the increased workload due to the COVID-19 pandemic, resulting in not enough data for analysis.

The psychogeriatric ward included in the study had two units, separated by a hallway. Both units had individual rooms for each of their 13 residents and a main living room. There were two shifts a day and three care workers present on each unit during a shift. These were vocational nurses and certified nursing assistants. During some shifts, there were also an activity worker and a hostess present. The care staff working on the ward were predominantly female. The residents living on the ward all had a diagnosis of dementia and were generally in an advanced state of the disease. They required complex care due to multimorbidity, low mobility and frailty, and their dementia brought about cases of challenging behavior such as shouting, wandering and aggression. During the studied period, there was one reported case of a COVID-19 infection on the ward.

During the study, the entire care team on the ward had access to the digital application SenseMaker®. Six of the 25 team members were enthusiastic about using it regularly and partaking in research activities. Among these six active participants were two activity workers and four vocational nurses. These participants were between 35 and 57 years old and were all female. The six individuals were also the ones who received coaching (see Section 2.6). The digital application remained open to other care team members, who used it sporadically. Employees of the care home organization who were not part of the care team of the specific psychogeriatric ward were excluded from participation.

2.5. Data Collection and Materials

Data was collected using the SenseMaker® application, a distributed ethnography tool suitable for complex environments [23]. Participants had access to this application via smartphone, computer and tablet. Participants captured their narratives as a written answer to the following open-ended questions: 'What did you do or experience during your shift that stuck with you? What happened and how did this affect you?' Participants were free to share narratives about whichever topic or experience was important to them, not restricted to COVID-19. Within the narratives, care staff described a specific experience they had, in about 3–10 sentences. They described what happened and how this affected them and others. They captured their narratives during their work shifts or shortly after. The use of this explorative method contributed to the collection of data that closely resembled participants' lived experiences.

In total, 723 narratives were captured by care staff during the course of the project. To answer the research question, only narratives submitted during the first (March through June 2020) and second (July 2020 through January 2021) waves of the COVID-19 pandemic in the Netherlands were included. All narratives shared during this period were included, from the six active participants as well as from the other care team members. This led to the inclusion of 424 narratives.

2.6. Procedure

Over the course of four months, the six active participants received individual coaching by authors MD and CE in becoming aware of their experiences and capturing their narratives of them. The coaching consisted of four exercises carried out by the participants, each followed by a telephone conversation with either MD or CE to discuss the exercise. Participants' feedback and remaining learning needs served as input for the content of each following coaching round.

In this coaching process, we followed an action-reflection learning approach [24]. Participants worked together in small groups to develop the skills necessary for this project and to reflect on the situations they encountered in their work. For the first exercise, participants were asked to take a picture of (a moment with) a resident that, to them, said something about that resident specifically. For the second exercise, participants were asked to reflect on a written narrative of a fictive experience and to discuss whether the experience was described in a useful and complete manner. The third exercise encouraged participants to learn from each other's experiences. Participants reflected on narratives shared by their colleagues and discussed how sharing narratives could serve as a source of inspiration in their work. The fourth exercise focused on becoming more aware of one's own qualities. Participants discussed which of their qualities they utilize to contribute to positive experiences for a particular resident. After each coaching round, a newsletter with reflections on the exercise and a selection of that month's captured narratives was shared with the entire care team.

There were no requirements as to the amount of narratives care staff had to share. We stimulated the capturing of narratives by verbally encouraging the care staff, by being regularly present on the ward (outside the period of the visiting ban), by distributing posters and newsletters around the ward and by celebrating milestones. Participants also engaged in peer-to-peer coaching, encouraging their colleagues to capture narratives.

2.7. Analysis

Given the explorative nature of our study, and our goal to follow the content of the experiences of the participants, the narratives were analyzed using thematic analysis [25] by the authors CE and CT independently. MAXQDA (version 20) qualitative data analysis software was used for analysis. Through coding, the authors CE and CT identified themes and patterns in the data. The coding authors then compared and discussed the codes and after discussion merged them into one code book. When data was coded differently, the codes were discussed until a consensus was reached between the authors CE and

CT. In addition, the coding authors indicated in which narratives the participants' work during COVID-19 was described in general terms and in which narratives they shared the specific impact of COVID-19 on their work. These codes were compared and discussed with MD, resulting in a final set of general narratives and COVID-19 specific narratives. Next, the process of constant comparison was initiated [26], in which authors CE, CT and MD compared codes to discover relations and patterns within the general themes. In this phase, several meetings were held between the first author and the coding authors CE and CT. The first meetings were focused on descriptive findings, whereas the following meetings focused on identifying relations and patterns within the general themes.

The narratives presented in Section 3 have been translated from Dutch to English by the authors, anonymized and edited for clarity.

3. Results

From the 424 narratives care staff shared during their work shifts in the COVID-19 pandemic, the vast majority (362) are about experiences that took place during the pandemic but were not explicitly related to COVID-19. From these narratives, we gain insight into care staff's general approach to care in times of COVID-19. Below, we first describe care staff's approach to care, based on these general narratives. Thereafter, we describe the specific impact of COVID-19 on care staff's approach to care, the wellbeing of residents and their own wellbeing, based on 62 narratives specifically about COVID-19 and related measures. An overview of results can be found in Table 1.

Table 1. Overview of themes emerging from care staff's narratives.

Emerging Themes	Emerging Sub-Themes	Relationships Involved
Care staff's approach to care during COVID-19	Focus on residents' wishes and desires	care staff–resident
	Knowledge of the resident's identity to tailor care	care staff–resident
	Care staff–resident relationship as inherently valuable	care staff–resident
	Complexity of caring for people with dementia	care staff–resident
	Valuing the resident–SO relationship	Resident–SO
	Facilitating the resident–SO relationship	care staff–resident–SO
	Need for appreciation from residents' SOs	care staff–SO
	Conversation about dissatisfaction from residents' SOs	care staff–SO
	Focus on residents' wishes and desires	care staff–resident
	Knowledge of the resident's identity to tailor care	care staff–resident
	Care staff–resident relationship as inherently valuable	care staff–resident
	Complexity of caring for people with dementia	care staff–resident
Mitigation measures alter care staff's approach to care	Turning down appeals to care and support	Care staff–resident
	Actively contributing to negative experiences	Care staff–resident
	Tensions between residents on the ward	Resident–resident
	Mediating conflicts between residents	Care staff–resident
	Face masks as a physical barrier to contact with residents	Care staff–resident
	Residents prone to blame care staff for mitigation measures	Care staff–resident
	Enabling remote contact between residents and SOs	Care staff–resident–SO
	Facilitation turns from supportive to crucial	Care staff–resident–SO
	Partly taking on the role of the SO	Care staff–resident–SO
	Being the bearer of bad news towards SOs	Care staff–SO
	Facing SO's frustration over mitigation measures	Care staff–SO
	Adhering to the mitigation measures in a strict manner	Care staff–resident–SO
The impact of COVID-19 on residents' wellbeing	Restricted freedom for residents	
	Limited contact between residents and SOs	
	Positive effect of remote contact on residents' wellbeing	
	Remote contact no replacement for face-to-face contact	

Table 1. *Cont.*

Emerging Themes	Emerging Sub-Themes	Relationships Involved
The impact of COVID-19 on care staff's wellbeing	Wellbeing of care staff linked to wellbeing of residents	
	Enforcing mitigation measures leads to internal conflict	

3.1. Care Staff's Approach to Care during COVID-19

The wellbeing of residents plays a central role in the narratives that care staff shared about their work during the COVID-19 pandemic. Specifically, the narratives show a strong focus on residents' wishes and desires, rather than their needs and limitations. Care staff described how they offered small daily activities to residents and how this lightened up their mood. Care staff also described how they used knowledge of the resident's identity to tailor these activities to personal wishes and desires.

> *"A resident's happy face during the daily care. I know that this resident used to teach English and loves music very much. During the daily care, I started talking English to her and my colleague joined in. We spontaneously started singing a song in English and the resident sang along at the top of her lungs. After the song, she said how much she liked it. A wonderful and beautiful experience, so much happiness."*

A relational approach to care is important for getting to know the resident's identity. In addition, the narratives show that care staff see their relationship with residents as inherently valuable as well. They wrote about one-on-one moments with residents and described these to have had a direct positive effect on the wellbeing of both residents and care staff.

> *"Smoking a cigarette together with a resident of whom I know enjoys this enormously. A moment with just the two of us, a quiet chat. Enjoying being outside for a moment, away from the rest of the ward. A moment of one-on-one attention during the day, moments to cherish. I enjoy seeing him enjoying himself in these moments. He also says this himself, very beautiful and inspiring."*

Furthermore, care staff described feelings of frustration and powerlessness when they encountered difficulties in easing a resident's agitation, sadness or aggression. These types of narratives emphasize the complexity of caring for and contributing to the wellbeing of people with dementia.

> *"It's hard when you don't understand someone's behavior and have to deal with their frustrations every day. You want everyone to enjoy themselves and be well, but there are some aspects over which you have no control and I find that difficult at times."*

Within the narratives, care staff described the value of the relationship between residents and their SOs for the wellbeing of residents. To enhance residents' wellbeing, care staff try to facilitate this relationship, both practically, e.g., ensuring that the resident is out of bed and dressed when SOs arrive to visit, and emotionally, e.g., supporting SOs in making contact with their loved one who has dementia.

> *"A resident's wife asked me for additional guidance during her visit. I explained to her that her husband just likes to sit and listen to his wife talking. Indeed, the resident sat and listened with a smile. His wife told me she felt so much more at ease now that she had seen her husband smile during the visit."*

The narratives show that care staff desired appreciation from SOs for the work they do. On the one hand, care staff shared narratives about how happy they were when SOs expressed their gratitude. On the other hand, they also shared narratives about how it affected them when SOs were dissatisfied with the care provided. Furthermore, care staff described how they handled dissatisfaction from SOs. They tried to resolve it by engaging in conversation and explaining their way of working. Generally, these conversations ended with an agreement to approach things differently next time, whether it be by the care staff or by the SO.

> *"A resident's wife came to me during the physical exercise hour. She was upset that she was not informed about this activity and she would like her husband to participate. I told her that her husband always participates when there are no visitors. I had also told her twice before that there was an exercise hour every Thursday afternoon. I let her talk and cry. After she had calmed down a bit I told her that I would inform her daughter when the exercise hour would take place and I would put it in the resident's agenda. She was happy about this and said that she knows I am doing my best, but that she hates it when her husband is not involved and just sits there by himself. I can understand that. I put the appointment in the agenda for next week and informed her daughter by email. These kinds of conversations are quite difficult but also quite exhausting because it never seems to be good enough for this family."*

3.2. The Impact of COVID-19

From the 62 narratives about COVID-19 specifically, the vast majority (59) were about the impact of the mitigation measures. The other three were about the impact of the disease itself. Temporally, the 62 narratives specifically about COVID-19 were concentrated on changes in the mitigation measures. The mitigation measures care staff described most were: (i) ward isolation for all residents; (ii) room isolation for residents suspected of having a COVID-19 infection; (iii) wearing PPE; (iv) the visiting ban and (v) required supervision during visits after the ban was lifted. Enforcing these mitigation measures was part of care staff's duties during the COVID-19 pandemic. Care staff described the impact of the mitigation measures on their approach to care, the wellbeing of residents and their own wellbeing. These findings are presented below.

3.2.1. COVID-19 Mitigation Measures Alter Care Staff's Approach to Care

Care staff's approach to care was impacted by COVID-19 mitigation measures in both the first and second waves of the COVID-19 pandemic in the Netherlands.

Within the narratives, care staff wrote about having to turn down appeals to care and support from dependent residents, hindering them from meeting residents' wishes and desires. In addition, there were several cases in which the mitigation measures required care staff to actively contribute to negative experiences for residents, for instance when they had to physically guard residents from leaving their room when in isolation.

> *"A resident grabbed my hand and asked me not to leave her. She wanted to come with me to the other ward. Unfortunately that is not possible during corona. Such a difficult moment. I truly had a hard time having to leave her behind!"*

With everyone isolated on the ward, care staff described high tensions between residents and how they had to serve as mediators. They shared how residents were quickly annoyed with each other and how small incidents led to verbal aggression, threats and physical altercations. Due to the residents' dementia, keeping the peace by explaining the situation to residents did not always work.

> *"Mrs. Schwarz is not in a good mood. She is short-tempered. One of the residents is yelling 'help me, help me' and this has been going on for a long time. Mrs. Schwarz rolls towards her. 'Shut up, stupid woman! If you don't, I'll slap you or throw you out!' She has a threatening attitude. I addressed her on her behavior, but 10 min later the above-mentioned repeated itself."*

Furthermore, the narratives indicate that the mitigation measures negatively impacted on the relationships between care staff and residents. Firstly, care staff described how wearing a face mask formed a physical barrier to making contact with residents. Moreover, they wrote that residents were confused as to why care staff were wearing masks and why they were refusing to take them off.

> "*Several times a day a resident asks me: 'take off that mask, don't be silly. I think it's nonsense, I can't see you now.*"

Secondly, care staff wrote that residents were frustrated by the limited contact they could have with their SO's because of the visiting ban. Since care staff members were the ones required to enforce the visiting ban, residents had difficulties understanding why this measure was taken and were prone to blame the care staff personally.

> "*A resident is standing at the window. Her husband has come to wave to her from outside. As a result of the corona restrictions, no visitors are allowed. The resident gestures to her husband: 'come upstairs.' I explain to her that that's not possible. 'Then I'll go to him.' I tell her that's not possible either. 'You are so mean', she tells me.*"

Regarding the contact between residents and SOs, the narratives show that care staff's facilitation changed from supportive to crucial during the visiting ban. Without the help of care staff, no contact would have been possible at all between those inside and those outside the care home. Care staff wrote about enabling remote contact between residents and SOs by helping residents to video call with their SOs and by guiding residents to the window when their SOs were standing on the terrain of the care home, wanting to wave to their loved one inside. In addition, there were instances where care staff took on part of the role that the SO usually had.

> "*A resident asked her daughter: can you bring me some eel? Daughter is not allowed to do this because of COVID. Therefore, I took it upon myself to bring some eel for her. The resident was totally surprised and became emotional. She kissed and hugged me. We sent a picture to her daughter.*"

Meanwhile, care staff's own contact with residents' SOs took on a predominantly negative tone. Due to COVID-19, care staff often had to be the bearer of bad news towards SOs, whether it was by communicating new restrictions or by enforcing existing ones. Care staff wrote how they were apprehensive to convey these messages, as they did not want to hurt SOs and were anxious about their reactions.

> "*There are visitors in the living room, even though that is not allowed during this corona time. A colleague is afraid to point out the rules to them and asks if I will do it. With jitters in my stomach I approach the family. I ask them to leave the living room. They react somewhat resentfully and choose to break off the visit. The residents at the tables find it ridiculous and are angry. The cheerful mood has clearly turned. The resident for whom the visitors stopped by is shouting that this is no way to treat people.*"

As the first point of contact, care staff were frequently confronted with SOs' frustration over the mitigation measures. They wrote about SOs expressing their grief over the measures, urging them to relieve the measures, blaming them for enforcing the measures and reacting angrily when they held them to the measures.

> "*I received a call from the family of a resident. I'm getting a lot of blame. They don't agree with the visiting rules. They think it's ridiculous. 'Grandma doesn't need to be accompanied, can't she just visit him alone?' It's not allowed, I tell them. Besides, there is a supervisor in the visiting area, supervising everyone. We get accused of giving grandma a second heart attack. It feels like they're blackmailing us.*"

Furthermore, the narratives show that care staff strictly adhered to the mitigation measures, despite the challenges this posed (e.g., dissatisfaction from SOs). Care staff's adherence to the rules shows that they saw no room for conversation with residents and SOs over the measures. This differed from their usual approach to care, in which they engaged in conversation to dissolve dissatisfaction, as shown under Section 3.1.

3.2.2. Residents' Wellbeing: Restricted Freedom and Limited Contact with SOs

Care staff's narratives about the impact of the mitigation measures on residents' wellbeing focused strongly on two mitigation measures from the first wave of the COVID-

19 pandemic in the Netherlands: the visiting ban and the isolation of residents on the ward. Another mitigation measure that was often described in this context was room isolation for residents suspected to have a COVID-19 infection, which was a measure in place in both the first and second waves.

The narratives show that residents' restricted freedom due to ward and room isolation had a negative impact on their wellbeing. Care staff described how the isolation caused confusion, agitation, sadness, anger and despair.

> *"Mr. Silva is isolated in his room due to suspected COVID. I am accompanying him in his room this morning. I am in protective gear, safety goggles, face mask. Mr. Silva is very emotional. He has lost all hope. He misses his wife and he is in pain. He rolls to the window and wants to open it. He tries to stand up and says: I'd rather end things. This gets to me. Luckily, his test result is negative and the room isolation is lifted."*

Due to the visiting ban, there was only limited contact between residents and their SOs, which care staff described as having a negative effect on residents' wellbeing. Residents missed their SOs and did not understand why they did not visit anymore. Care staff indicated the restrained contact with SOs led to increased apathy, agitation and challenging behavior in residents.

> *"Mr. Spears tells me he is in a bad place. He is not seeing his loved ones. Not his wife, not his children. I explain to him that visitors are not allowed right now. He says that it's ridiculous."*

To remain in touch, SOs sought other ways of making contact during the visiting ban. The most common of these were conducting video calls and standing on the terrain of the care home, waving to their loved ones inside. Care staff described the positive effect of remote contact on residents' wellbeing.

> *"During the outdoor performance Mr. Simon was partying hard. After two gloomy days, it was beautiful to see how he was uplifted by the music and his wife and son who were downstairs dancing along! Really wonderful to see!"*

However, the narratives also show that remote contact was no replacement for face-to-face contact. Remote contact was one-dimensional, did not allow for intimacy and was sometimes mentioned to be confusing for residents.

3.2.3. Care Staff Wellbeing: Experiencing Dire Situations and Internal Conflict

Care staff were confronted with dire situations on the ward in both the first and second waves of the COVID-19 pandemic. Their own wellbeing appeared to be linked to residents' wellbeing, as they described how the negative effects of mitigation measures on residents in turn affected them.

> *"I was emotionally very affected by the despair of a resident who had to be isolated in his room. I found it difficult to be confronted with such visible suffering. Especially since there wasn't much I could do besides lend an ear and be physically present. I sat in the office and cried for a while afterwards."*

Furthermore, care staff described how having to enforce mitigation measures led to internal conflict. The narratives show that care staff experienced large contrasts between what they were required to do (enforcing and adhering to mitigation measures) and what was in their hearts (contributing to positive experiences for residents).

> *"I accompanied a resident to the first visit from his wife [since the visiting ban was lifted]. They have to stay 1.5 m apart. They can't touch each other. No hug, no kiss. Not even when saying goodbye. Both the resident and his wife are having a hard time with this. His wife calls it degrading. I find it so sad it has to go like this. I would really love to just allow it."*

4. Discussion

By taking an explorative approach in which care staff were free to share narratives about whichever topics in their work were important to them, we have gained an insight into their approach to care during the COVID-19 pandemic in general terms, as well as into the specific impact of COVID-19 on their approach to care, the wellbeing of residents and their own wellbeing.

The results show that within care staff's narratives, residents' wellbeing was the main focus during the COVID-19 pandemic. Furthermore, care staff see their relationships with residents as important way in the context of contributing to their wellbeing. As a consequence, they invest in getting to know the residents to attune care to their personal wishes and desires, although this is at times challenging due to the complexity of caring for people with dementia. Moreover, care staff aim to facilitate the relationships between residents and their SOs, as they see this as an important influence on residents' wellbeing. Within their own relationship with SOs, care staff engage in dialogue to come to a mutual understanding of good care, whilst desiring appreciation from SOs for the work they do.

The way of working that is foregrounded in care staff's narratives is in line with the relational-moral approach to good care in care ethics, which states that the definition of good care is shaped in and by the relationship between the caregiver and care receiver. In good care, it is not the rules and procedures that are most prominent, but the nature of the caregiver –care receiver relationship. Accordingly, Tronto [27] states that good care is a two-way affair: it is the outcome of a dialogic process between caregiver and care receiver and adjusted to personal needs, wishes and desires [28]. Our data clearly shows that the relational approach does not only concern the resident–care staff relationship, but extends to SOs in a reciprocal interaction of appreciation, value and meaningful engagement.

In 62 narratives, care staff explicated the impact of COVID-19 on their experiences, predominantly in terms of the impact of the COVID-19 mitigation measures. Due to the effects of these measures on care staff's approach to care and residents' wellbeing, the mitigation measures can be seen as obstructions to good care in the relational-moral sense in several ways.

Firstly, the mitigation measures limited care staff's ability to attune care to residents' personal wishes and desires, and sometimes even required care staff to contribute to negative experiences for residents. This was in stark contrast to their preferred approach to care. Moreover, the mitigation measures formed a serious threat to residents' autonomy by isolating them from the outside world [29,30]. The fact that the mitigation measures focused on adding days to residents' lives rather than adding life to residents' days, shows the dominancy of thinking about good care in a practical sense rather than in a relational-moral sense. Indeed, research shows that in situations of environmental pressure, practical care often prevails over relational-moral care [31].

Secondly, the mitigation measures put pressure on the relationship between care staff and residents. Care staff had to enforce the mitigation measures, which frustrated residents. Moreover, care staff frequently had to turn down appeals for care and support from residents. Importantly, a relationship of trust is a requirement for relational-morally good care [32]. Tronto [27] describes how trust between caregiver and care receiver is developed in a cyclical process of four phases. In the first phase, the caregiver is attentive and recognizes the need for care in the care receiver. In the second phase, the caregiver accepts the responsibility to meet the identified care needs and determines how to do this. The third phase consists of the caregiver using her expertise to directly meet the care needs. In the fourth and last phase, the care receiver responds to the received care, to which the caregiver is once again attentive, constituting a cycle. It is plausible that the imposing of mitigation measures diminished the trust residents had in their caregivers, especially since it was often unclear to residents why care staff were acting in this way. The narratives show that the mitigation measures mainly intervened in the second and third phase of Tronto's cyclical care process. Caregivers were still attentive to residents' needs but were no longer able to take responsibility and actions to meet these needs, causing moral distress [18,19,21].

Instead, they had to take responsibility for a different aspect of care (i.e., physical health and safety), which did not directly match residents' explicit wishes and desires. The residents' responses to the safety measures (i.e., Tronto's fourth phase) confirms this mismatch, as their sadness, frustration, desperation and challenging behavior increased.

Lastly, the safety measures put a strain on the contact between care staff and SOs, as communication over the mitigation measures resulted in their interactions becoming primarily negative. In addition, the foregrounding of life itself over living, and with that practical care, left no room for dialogue. This differed greatly from care staff's usual way of engaging with SOs, which involves conversation and compromise, as they describe in their narratives. As the care staff put forward, they have a relational-moral approach to care, meaning they view good care as an intersubjective understanding reached through a dialogic process. Therefore, not being able to align value perspectives about the mitigation measures forms an obstruction to delivering relational-morally good care. The strained relationships between care staff with SOs during the COVID-19 pandemic is incongruent with previous findings showing that people cooperate rather than compete in times of crisis, but may be explained through an important determinant of this cooperation: an emerging sense of identity [33]. The mitigation measures emphasized the boundaries between those inside and those outside the care home, creating an ingroup and an outgroup. As such, the shared identity that emerged within the care home may have differed notably from that outside the care home, hampering cooperation.

The finding that mitigation measures posed obstructions in terms of a relational-moral approach to care is in line with findings from an international study into the experiences of social workers during the COVID-19 pandemic [21]. The study found that social workers had to work harder to establish and maintain relationships of trust with those receiving care, whilst only being partially able to meet care needs.

Importantly, the narratives also show that being confronted with dire situations due to the COVID-19 mitigation measures had a negative impact on the wellbeing of care staff themselves. This is in line with several studies showing an increase in emotional load, depression, anxiety and stress for care staff due to COVID-19 [5,17]. Furthermore, we found that having to enforce mitigation measures led care staff to experience internal conflict. The internal conflict described by care staff is in line with a recent finding showing that care staff experiences feelings of guilt when enforcing the mitigation measures [34]. The internal conflict experienced by care staff may be viewed in terms of moral distress. As practical care was foregrounded over relational-moral care, care staff had to repeatedly take actions that violated their moral code. Ultimately, this could result in moral injury, a risk that several studies have highlighted [18–20].

The COVID-19 pandemic is and has been an evolving situation. Given its temporal dynamics, we compared narratives from the first and second waves of the COVID-19 pandemic in the Netherlands. There were no specific temporal changes in the impact of COVID-19 on care staff's approach to care other than changes in mitigation measures. Although different measures presented different challenges, they each presented challenges for the triadic relationship between care staff, residents and SOs. Regarding the impact of COVID-19 on the wellbeing of residents, the narratives centered around mitigation measures promoting isolation, which were stricter in the first wave of the COVID-19 pandemic in the Netherlands than in the second wave. Narratives about the impact of COVID-19 on the wellbeing of care staff did not present specific temporal changes. Care staff wellbeing was affected by the negative effect of mitigation measures on residents' wellbeing and by the internal conflict they experienced when enforcing mitigation measures; both factors were present throughout the first and second waves of the COVID-19 pandemic in the Netherlands.

4.1. Strengths and Limitations

The two strengths of our study are the explorative approach, in which care staff were able to share narratives about whichever topic was important to them, and the capturing of data shortly after the experience took place. By taking such an approach, we were able to capture care staff's lived experiences during the COVID-19 pandemic as closely as possible. In addition, the narrative approach highlighted the impact of COVID-19 in terms which cannot be expressed by numbers. Future studies may include the perspectives of care staff to a further degree by involving them in the process of data interpretation as well.

One possible limitation of our study is that we have no way of comparing the narratives shared during the COVID-19 pandemic with narratives outside of the context of COVID-19, and so we cannot be sure whether or not COVID-19 affected care staff's approach to care in more ways than they explicitly stated by themselves. The strong focus on residents' wellbeing may have been a way to elicit positive emotions, which is an effective coping strategy in times of stress [35]. The desire for appreciation from residents' SOs may have also been a result of the extra pressure COVID-19 put on care staff as intermediaries and bridges to the outside world.

Another limitation is that our study had a small sample size. Narratives from care staff stemmed from one psychogeriatric ward only. When it comes to the generalizability of our findings, there are several factors to consider. Firstly, care staff on the ward included in the study worked according to the Enjoying Life approach, a narrative approach focused on residents' personal wellbeing and desires rather than their needs and limitations [36]. The impact of the COVID-19 pandemic on care staff's approach to care may be different for care staff working on wards where the approach to care differs to begin with. Secondly, there was one case of COVID-19 on the ward included in the study during the studied period, reported on the last day of the second wave (31 January 2021). A different image of the impact of COVID-19 may have emerged on wards where care staff experienced more COVID-19 infections and COVID-19-related deaths. Thirdly, individual differences are likely to play a role in one's wellbeing and approach to care during the COVID-19 pandemic. These may include socioeconomic status [37], job type (e.g., a nurse whose daily tasks focus on medical procedures or an activity therapists whose work is focused on residents' mental wellbeing) [38], fear of COVID-19 [39,40] and level of resilience [41]. Comparing narratives between the two care homes included in the larger study may have provided us with a more diverse understanding of the experience of care home staff during the COVID-19 pandemic. However, data from the second care home was too limited for analysis.

Lastly, we used the SenseMaker® application in a longitudinal fashion, while it was developed to be used in a cross-sectional one. SenseMaker is suitable for gaining an understanding of complex systems, which suits the context of the care home better than research methods that assume linearity. Testing the applicability of SenseMaker® to collect and use narratives about personal experiences with care to account for its quality was part of the goals of our larger study. Whilst we worked together with the developers of SenseMaker® to adjust the application to this goal and context, the method has not yet been validated for longitudinal use. For more information on SenseMaker® as a research tool see [23].

4.2. Implications

Dichter and colleagues [29] described the importance of balancing infection prevention and person-centered care during the COVID-19 pandemic to maintain the wellbeing of older people living in German care homes, as did Verbeek and colleagues [42] in the Dutch context. By stemming from the direct experiences of care staff, our findings underline and stress the importance of finding this balance.

Furthermore, our findings underline the importance of a relational-moral approach for the wellbeing of all involved in the triad of care staff–residents–SOs. This finding is in line with developments in the Dutch long-term care sector, as the focus has shifted over the past few years from physical health, protocols and evidence-based practice to relationships, wellbeing and attuning care to personal wishes and desires [43]. Our findings also show that care staff value this relational-moral approach to care, and yet they had to adhere to COVID-19 mitigation measures that foregrounded practical care. Finding the right balance in such a situation is extremely difficult. The notion of democratic care may offer guidance in this context [28,44]. Democratic care foregrounds an ongoing dialogic process within the triad of care staff–residents–SOs. Through this dialogic process, all parties collaboratively determine what good care is. In a previous study, we extended the notion of democratic care to include dialogue about good care on multiple levels: on a micro-level (between care staff, residents and SOs), on a meso-level (between care staff and managers) and on a macro-level (for internal policy and the reporting of quality of care to supervisory bodies) [44]. Mitigation measures and their implications for good care may be discussed and decided upon through an ongoing dialogic process between those involved on multiple levels. In this process, those in power should actively create space for the voices of people in vulnerable situations, as this constitutes the democratic potential of a care home [44].

However, creating room for such a dialogue in a crisis situation has been proven difficult. In the Netherlands, many decisions about handling the COVID-19 pandemic were taken in a top-down manner. Consequently, our study shows that care staff encountered situations of moral distress, where the actions they had to take (i.e., mitigation measures) violated their moral codes. In turn, care staff felt that they had no room to engage in a conversation about good care with residents and SOs. In a previous publication, we highlighted the importance of a structure and a culture for engaging in dialogue to enhance the democratic potential of care homes. Ensuring a structure and a culture of listening to a variety and voices and discussing differences under normal circumstances may help create more space for dialogue on multiple levels in a crisis situation as well.

Furthermore, our findings underline the importance of ongoing mental support for care staff during the pandemic. This is not only needed to protect their wellbeing, but also to retain care workers in the care sector. The Dutch care sector has been experiencing a large outflow of workers regardless of COVID-19, mainly due to lack of opportunities for personal development. The resulting personnel shortages lead to high levels of time pressure and workload, leading others to leave the sector as well [45]. The extra pressure COVID-19 puts on care staff has increased the already problematic outflow of care workers from the sector [45]. Our findings show that measures to retain and attract care staff may focus on creating more opportunities to deliver care in a relational-moral way, as care staff views this as fundamental to good care. The notion of democratic care as described above, in which dialogue between those involved in the care process plays an important role, may offer further guidance in this context.

5. Conclusions

In the study presented here, we have shown that residents' wellbeing has been Dutch care home staff's central focus during the COVID-19 pandemic. They aimed to achieve this by forming and maintaining relationships within the triad of care staff–residents–SOs. Their way of working is in line with relational-moral approach to good care in care ethics, where good care is a two-way affair: its definition is the outcome of a dialogic process, shaped in and by the caregiver–care receiver relationship [27,28]. Importantly, we find reciprocal appreciation is essential in the triadic relationship between care staff, residents and SOs and therewith extend Tronto's caregiver–care receiver relationship to include SOs.

When it comes to the impact of COVID-19, care staff are primarily concerned with the mitigation measures and moral distress related to these measures, rather than the disease itself. We have found that care staff see the mitigation measures as obstructions to good care, as they harm residents' wellbeing, limit the ability of care staff to contribute to residents' wishes and desires, damage the care staff–resident relationship in terms of trust, sour the contact between care staff and SOs and leave no room for dialogue about the definition of good care in different situations.

In addition, we have shown that COVID-19 mitigation measures have a negative impact on care staff's own wellbeing. Enforcing mitigation measures leads care staff to be confronted with dire situations and emotionally charged responses from both residents and SOs. In enforcing the mitigation measures, care staff experience internal conflict, as what they are required to do differs from what they see as good care.

Our findings underline the importance of finding a balance between good care in a practical sense and a relational-moral sense. Prioritizing life over living itself, as happened during the COVID-19 pandemic, is often not in line with care staff's, residents' and SOs' views on good care. Our way of handling COVID-19 in care homes should therefore be a process of ongoing dialogue on multiple levels about the type of good care those involved value most. Care home organizations should acknowledge a variety of voices and ensure that there is a structure and culture in place which can accommodate the discussion of differences. Those in power should actively make space for the voice of people in vulnerable situations, on multiple levels.

Author Contributions: Conceptualization, M.D.W.D., C.v.d.E., C.L.E.T., J.L. and J.M.H.; Data curation, C.v.d.E. and C.L.E.T.; Formal analysis, M.D.W.D., C.v.d.E. and C.L.E.T.; Funding acquisition, J.M.H.; Investigation, M.D.W.D. and C.v.d.E.; Methodology, M.D.W.D., C.v.d.E., C.L.E.T. and J.M.H.; Project administration, J.M.H.; Supervision, J.M.H.; Writing—original draft, M.D.W.D.; Writing—review & editing, M.D.W.D., C.v.d.E., C.L.E.T., J.L., J.M.H. and T.A.A. All authors have read and agreed to the published version of the manuscript.

Funding: This study was funded by the Dutch Ministry of Health, Welfare and Sport under number 329327. The funding source was not involved in writing this manuscript nor in the decision to submit for publication.

Institutional Review Board Statement: The study was conducted in accordance with the Declaration of Helsinki, was reviewed by the Institutional Review Board of the Medical Ethical Committee Leiden-Den Haag-Delft for observational studies and registered under number N20.095. The protocol was assessed and considered compliant with scientific due diligence.

Informed Consent Statement: Informed consent was obtained from all subjects involved in the study.

Data Availability Statement: Data available on request due to privacy restrictions.

Acknowledgments: We would like to extend our grateful thanks to all the care home workers who contributed to this study, whether it was by sharing their narratives with us, by encouraging their colleagues to do so or simply by opening their world to us in the challenging times of COVID-19. We also want to thank our colleagues and team members for their contributions to the larger study which enabled us to write this manuscript.

Conflicts of Interest: The authors declare no conflict of interest.

References

1. Dutch Central Government, Committee on Public Health, Welfare and Sports, Taskforce Infection Disease Control. Report of a Technical Briefing. Dutch Federal Government, 2020. Available online: https://www.tweedekamer.nl/debat_en_vergadering/commissievergaderingen/details?id=2020A01496 (accessed on 10 November 2021).
2. COVID-19 Dashboard. Available online: https://coronadashboard.rijksoverheid.nl/landelijk/verpleeghuiszorg (accessed on 10 November 2021).
3. Epidemiological Situation COVID-19 in the Netherlands, 2020. Rijksinstituut voor Volksgezondheid en Milieu (RIVM) (Dutch National Institute of Public Health and Environment). Available online: https://www.rivm.nl/sites/default/files/2020-08/COVID-19_WebSite_rapport_wekelijks_20200707_1251.pdf (accessed on 10 November 2021).
4. Kruse, F.M.; Van Tol, L.; Vrinzen, C.; Van der Woerd, O.; Jeurissen, P.P.T. The Impact of COVID-19 on Long-Term Care in the Netherlands: The Second Wave, 2020. LTCcovid, International Long-Term Care Policy Network. Available online: https://ltccovid.org/wp-content/uploads/2020/11/COVID-19-Long-Term-Care-situation-in-the-Netherlands-_-the-second-wave-25-November-2020-2.pdf (accessed on 10 November 2021).
5. Member Poll Corona Nursing Home, 2020. Verpleegkundigen & Verzorgenden Nederland (V&VN) (Nurses & Caregivers Netherlands). Available online: https://www.venvn.nl/media/el0asgfw/01_peiling_corona_verpleeghuis.pdf (accessed on 29 November 2021).
6. McDougall, R.J.; Gillam, L.; Ko, D.; Holmes, I.; Delany, C. Balancing health worker well-being and duty to care: An ethical approach to staff safety in COVID-19 and beyond. *J. Med. Ethics* **2021**, *47*, 318–323. [CrossRef] [PubMed]
7. McKenna, H. Covid-19: Ethical issues for nurses. *Int. J. Nurs. Study* **2020**, *110*, 103673. [CrossRef] [PubMed]
8. Emanuel, E.J.; Persad, G.; Upshur, R.; Thome, B.; Parker, M.; Glickman, A.; Zhang, C.; Boyle, C.; Smith, M.; Philips, J.P. Fair allocation of scarce medical resources in the time of covid-19. *N. Engl. J. Med.* **2020**, *382*, 2049–2055. [CrossRef] [PubMed]

9. White, D.B.; Lo, B. A framework for rationing ventilators and critical care beds during the COVID-19 pandemic. *JAMA* **2020**, *323*, 1773–1774. [CrossRef] [PubMed]
10. Nioi, M.; Napoli, P.E.; Finco, G.; Demontis, R.; Fossarello, M.; D'aloja, E. Fear of the COVID-19 and medical liability. Insights from a series of 130 consecutives medico-legal claims evaluated in a single institution during SARS-CoV-2-related pandemic. *Signa Vitae.* **2021**, *17*, 79–85.
11. Erdem, H.; Lucey, D.R. Healthcare worker infections and deaths due to COVID-19: A survey from 37 nations and a call for WHO to post national data on their website. *Int. J. Infect. Dis.* **2021**, *102*, 239–241. [CrossRef]
12. Dutch Central Government. Test Capacity Quadrupled, Corona Testing Possible for all Healthcare Personnel. 2021. Available online: https://www.rijksoverheid.nl/onderwerpen/coronavirus-tijdlijn/nieuws/2020/03/31/testcapaciteit-verviervoudigd-coronatests-mogelijk-voor-al-het-zorgpersoneel (accessed on 29 January 2022).
13. V&VN. Working without Personal Protective Equipment? Unacceptable! 2020. Available online: https://www.venvn.nl/nieuws/werken-zonder-beschermende-middelen-onacceptabel/ (accessed on 29 January 2022).
14. V&VN. V&VN poll: Masks Shortages Persist, Psychological Pressure High. 2020. Available online: https://www.venvn.nl/nieuws/peiling-v-vn-tekorten-maskers-houden-aan-psychische-druk-hoog/ (accessed on 29 January 2022).
15. Duijs, S.E.; Haremaker, A.; Bourik, Z.; Abma, T.A.; Verdonk, P. Pushed to the margins and stretched to the limit: Experiences of freelance eldercare workers during the Covid-19 pandemic in the Netherlands. *Fem. Econ.* **2021**, *27*, 217–235. [CrossRef]
16. Vindegaard, N.; Benros, M.E. COVID-19 pandemic and mental health consequences: Systematic review of the current evidence. *Brain Behav Immun.* **2020**, *89*, 531–542. [CrossRef]
17. Kruse, F.M.; Abma, I.; Jeurissen, P.P.T. The Impact of COVID-19 on Long-Term Care in the Netherlands. LTCcovid, International Long-Term Care Policy Network. Available online: https://ltccovid.org/wp-content/uploads/2020/05/COVID19-Long-Term-Care-situation-in-the-Netherlands-25-May-2020-1.pdf (accessed on 29 November 2021).
18. Litam, S.D.A.; Balkin, R.S. Moral injury in health-care workers during COVID-19 pandemic. *Traumatology* **2021**, *27*, 14–19. [CrossRef]
19. Alharbi, J.; Jackson, D.; Usher, K. The potential for COVID-19 to contribute to compassion fatigue in critical care nurses. *J. Clin. Nurs.* **2020**, *29*, 2762–2764. [CrossRef]
20. Čartolovni, A.; Stolt, M.; Scott, P.A.; Suhonen, R. Moral injury in healthcare professionals: A scoping review and discussion. *Nurs. Ethics.* **2021**, *28*, 590–602. [CrossRef] [PubMed]
21. Banks, S.; Cai, T.; de Jonge, E.; Shears, J.; Shum, M.; Sobočan, A.M.; Strom, K.; Truell, R.; Uriz, M.S.; Weinberg, M. Practising ethically during COVID-19: Social work challenges and responses. *Int. Soc.* **2020**, *63*, 569–583. [CrossRef]
22. Oh, N.; Hong, N.; Ryu, D.H.; Bae, S.G.; Kam, S.; Kim, K.Y. Exploring nursing intention, stress, and professionalism in response to infectious disease emergencies: The experience of local public hospital nurses during the 2015 MERS outbreak in South Korea. *Asian Nurs Res.* **2017**, *11*, 230–236. [CrossRef] [PubMed]
23. Van der Merwe, S.E.; Biggs, R.; Preiser, R.; Cunningham, C.; Snowden, D.J.; O'Brien, K.; Jenal, M.; Vosloo, M.; Blignaut, S.; Goh, Z. Making Sense of Complexity: Using SenseMaker as a Research Tool. *Systems* **2019**, *7*, 25. [CrossRef]
24. Marsick, V.J.; Cederholm, L.; Turner, E.; Pearson, T. Action-reflection learning. *Train. Dev.* **1992**, *46*, 63–67.
25. Braun, V.; Clarke, V. Using thematic analysis in psychology. *Qual. Res. Psychol.* **2006**, *3*, 77–101. [CrossRef]
26. Glaser, B.; Strauss, A. *The Discovery of Grounded Theory: Strategies for Qualitative Research*; Sociology Press: Mill Valley, CA, USA, 1967.
27. Tronto, J.C. *Moral Boundaries. A Political Argument for an Ethic of Care*; Routledge: Abingdon-on-Thames, UK, 1993.
28. Tronto, J.C. Protective Care or Democratic Care? Some Reflections on Terrorism and Care. In Proceedings of the SIGNAL, Cifas, Belgium, 23 September 2016. Available online: https://vimeo.com/185843576 (accessed on 31 December 2021).
29. Dichter, M.N.; Sander, M.; Seismann-Petersen, S.; Köpke, S. COVID-19: It is time to balance infection management and person-centered care to maintain health of people living in German nursing homes. *Int. Psychogeriatr.* **2020**, *32*, 1157–1160. [CrossRef]
30. Gordon, A.L.; Goodman, C.; Achterberg, W.; Barker, R.O.; Burns, E.; Hanratty, B.; Martin, F.C.; Meyer, L.; O'Neill, D.; Schols, J.; et al. Commentary: COVID in care homes—Challenges and dilemmas in healthcare delivery. *Age Ageing* **2020**, *49*, 701–705. [CrossRef]
31. Johannessen, A.K.; Werner, A.; Steihaug, S. Work in an intermediate unit: Balancing between relational, practical and moral care. *J. Clin. Nurs.* **2014**, *23*, 586–595. [CrossRef]
32. Sevenhuijsen, S. Caring in the third way: The relation between obligation, responsibility and care in Third Way discourse. *Crit. Soc. Policy* **2000**, *20*, 5–37. [CrossRef]
33. Drury, J. The role of social identity processes in mass emergency behaviour: An integrative review. *Eur. Rev. Soc. Psychol.* **2018**, *29*, 38–81. [CrossRef]
34. Smaling, H.J.A.; Tilburgs, B.; Achterberg, W.P.; Visser, M. The Impact of Social Distancing Due to the COVID-19 Pandemic on People with Dementia, Family Carers and Healthcare Professionals: A Qualitative Study. *Int. J. Environ. Res. Public Health* **2022**, *19*, 519. [CrossRef] [PubMed]
35. Ong, A.D.; Bergeman, C.S.; Bisconti, T.L.; Wallace, K.A. Psychological resilience, positive emotions, and successful adaptation to stress in later life. *J. Pers Soc. Psychol* **2006**, *91*, 730–749. [CrossRef]
36. Huijg, J.M. Personal stories improve standard care and resident wellbeing. *NRC* **2019**, *21*, 505–509. [CrossRef]

37. Wanberg, C.R.; Csillag, B.; Douglass, R.P.; Zhou, L.; Pollard, M.S. Socioeconomic status and well-being during COVID-19: A resource-based examination. *Am. J. Appl. Psychol.* **2021**, *105*, 1382–1396. [CrossRef]
38. Islam, M.S.; Baker, C.; Huxley, P.; Russell, I.T.; Dennis, M.S. The nature, characteristics and associations of care home staff stress and wellbeing: A national survey. *BMC Nurs.* **2017**, *16*, 22. [CrossRef]
39. Coelho, C.M.; Suttiwan, P.; Arato, N.; Zsido, A.N. On the nature of fear and anxiety triggered by COVID-19. *Front. Psychol.* **2020**, *11*, 581314. [CrossRef]
40. Troisi, A.; Nanni, R.C.; Riconi, A.; Carola, V.; Di Cave, D. Fear of COVID-19 among healthcare workers: The role of neuroticism and fearful attachment. *J. Clin. Med.* **2021**, *10*, 4358. [CrossRef]
41. Killgore, W.D.S.; Taylor, E.C.; Cloonan, S.A.; Dailey, N.S. Psychological resilience during the COVID-19 lockdown. *Psychiatry Res.* **2020**, *291*, 113216. [CrossRef]
42. Verbeek, H.; Gerritsen, D.L.; Backhaus, R.; de Boer, B.S.; Koopmans, R.T.C.M.; Hamers, J.P.H. Allowing visitors back in the nursing home during the COVID-19 crisis: A Dutch national study into first experiences and impact on well-being. *J. Am. Med. Dir. Assoc.* **2020**, *21*, 900–904. [CrossRef]
43. Verbeek-Oudijk, D.; Koper, I. Het leven in Een Verpleeghuis: Landelijk Overzicht van de Leefsituatie, Ervaren Kwaliteit van Leven en Zorg van Oudere Verpleeghuisbewoners in 2019 [Life in a Nursing Home: National Survey of the Living Situation, Perceived Quality of Life and Care of Older Nursing Home Residents in 2019]. The Netherlands Institute for Social Research. Available online: https://www.scp.nl/publicaties/publicaties/2021/02/19/het-leven-in-een-verpleeghuis (accessed on 29 November 2021).
44. Dohmen, M.D.W.; Huijg, J.H.; Abma, T.A. Democratic Care in Nursing Homes: Responsive Evaluation to Mutually Learn about Good Care. In *Institutions and Organizations as Learning Environments for Participation and Democracy—Opportunities, Challenges, Obstacles*; Spannring, R., Ed.; Springer Publishing: New York, NY, USA, 2022; in press.
45. CBS. Mobility of Employees; Labor Market Care and Welfare (Broad), Inflow, Outflow, Balance, Region. 2021. Available online: https://azwstatline.cbs.nl/#/AZW/nl/dataset/24050NED/table?ts=1591279185724 (accessed on 27 January 2022).

International Journal of
Environmental Research and Public Health

MDPI

Article

Assessment of Psychosocial Functioning of Polish Nurses during COVID-19 Pandemic

Kamila Rachubińska [1], Anna Maria Cybulska [1,*], Joanna Sołek-Pastuszka [2], Mariusz Panczyk [3], Marzanna Stanisławska [1], Przemysław Ustianowski [1] and Elżbieta Grochans [1]

1 Department of Nursing, Pomeranian Medical University in Szczecin, 71-210 Szczecin, Poland; kamila.rachubinska@pum.edu.pl (K.R.); stamarz@pum.edu.pl (M.S.); przemyslaw.ustianowski@gmail.com (P.U.); elzbieta.grochans@pum.edu.pl (E.G.)

2 Department of Anaesthesiology and Intensive Therapy in Szczecin, Pomeranian Medical University, 71-242 Szczecin, Poland; joanna.pastuszka@pum.edu.pl

3 Department of Education and Research in Health Sciences, Faculty of Health Science, Medical University of Warsaw, 00-581 Warsaw, Poland; mariusz.panczyk@wum.edu.pl

* Correspondence: anna.cybulska@pum.edu.pl

Abstract: (1) The COVID-19 pandemic has significantly affected the psychological well-being of people around the world. The aim of this study was to assess the levels of psychological distress of nurses (anxiety, depression, stress, insomnia) in relation to sociodemographic variables and psychosocial variables: self-assessment of health, quarantine, psychological support, presence of chronic diseases and the Impact of Events Scale (IES-R). (2) A total of 207 nurses working with COVID-19 patients at the Independent Public Clinical Hospital No. 1 of the Pomeranian Medical University in Szczecin participated in the study. The study was conducted with the diagnostic survey method, using the Athens Insomnia Scale, the Generalized Anxiety Disorder questionnaire, the Impact of Event Scale—Revised, the Patient Health Questionnaire-9, The Perceived Stress Scale and a questionnaire of our authorship. (3) Among the respondents, 40.58% suffered sleep disturbance, 36.71% had mild anxiety, 71.95% had high stress according to the PSS-10 and 31.88% had depression according to the PHQ-9. The study observed that the chances of insomnia decreased with the age of the respondents. Moreover, the form of employment of nurses significantly affected the levels of depression, anxiety and stress. (4) Education, gender and age were variables that significantly affected the severity of anxiety, depression and insomnia in the surveyed nurses working with patients with COVID-19.

Keywords: public health; COVID-19; pandemic; depression; anxiety; insomnia; nursing

Citation: Rachubińska, K.; Cybulska, A.M.; Sołek-Pastuszka, J.; Panczyk, M.; Stanisławska, M.; Ustianowski, P.; Grochans, E. Assessment of Psychosocial Functioning of Polish Nurses during COVID-19 Pandemic. *Int. J. Environ. Res. Public Health* **2022**, *19*, 1435. https://doi.org/10.3390/ijerph19031435

Academic Editors: Richard Gray and Sonia Udod

Received: 22 December 2021
Accepted: 24 January 2022
Published: 27 January 2022

1. Introduction

The COVID-19 pandemic has affected the well-being of people around the world, and from the beginning of the pandemic, specialized bodies have emphasized the importance of protecting the health of those that are particularly vulnerable to SARS-CoV-2 infection, including medical workers. The changes that occurred as a result were multifaceted and affected not only society as a whole but, more importantly, each individual. In a very short period, almost every person had to reorganize their daily functioning, and the chaos in the public space translated into the loss of daily routine activities. The very fact of being threatened by the danger of infection with an unknown and dangerous pathogen and the complete change in daily functioning undoubtedly became a source of stress. The fear of losing one's own and one's family's health and life, the vision of potential life and economic problems and the periods of forced isolation negatively influenced the well-being of most of us. It seems that the stress associated with new conditions of functioning may have significantly affected people for whom everyday professional activity was a potential source of infection with an unknown virus. Working in healthcare during this specific period became particularly difficult. The lack of reliable information and detailed procedures, limitations related to the scarcity of protective measures and, perhaps most importantly, initial diagnostic difficulties resulting from the lack of access to virus-confirming tests and long waiting periods for their results caused tension, fatigue and a sense of overload. These elements may have resulted in symptoms of anxiety, depression, sadness and insomnia [1,2].

The definition of anxiety is not unequivocal in the literature, although the descriptive characteristics are well circumscribed and easily identifiable. The American Psychiatric Association defines anxiety as the anticipation of future danger or a negative event, accompanied by feelings of dysphoria or physical symptoms of tension [3]. The term "depression" is used to describe a particular type of mood and emotion disorder, recognized as a disease phenomenon. In fact, there is no fully sharp line between "ordinary" depression and "true" depression. Depression is characterized by the presence of sadness and despair for a long period that affects the disorganization of complex activity [4]. Stress is the process by which environmental factors threaten or disturb the body's balance and by which the body responds to the threat. The environmental factors in question are often referred to as stressors. They activate complex mechanisms of both physiological and psychological responses and significantly affect the health status of an individual [5].

Presumably, exposure to deep, prolonged stress during the COVID-19 pandemic will have a negative impact on the mental health of the public, including healthcare workers. Workers in direct contact with COVID-19 patients are particularly vulnerable to symptoms such as depression, anxiety, stress and poor sleep quality, and their mental health may require special attention. In the fight against the COVID-19 pandemic, medical workers often have to live with the risk of infection, often inadequately protected, overworked, exhausted, sleep-deprived, isolated and lacking contact with loved ones. The difficult situation often has a negative impact on their levels of psychological distress, which may result in a decrease in the quality of their work. In the face of these threats, it is necessary to implement a comprehensive mental health plan, especially among workers who have direct contact with the infected [6]. The aim of the study was to assess the levels of psychological distress of nursing staff (anxiety, depression, stress, insomnia) in relation to sociodemographic and psychosocial variables: self-rated health status, quarantine, psychological support, presence of chronic diseases and experience of traumatic events according to the Impact of Events Scale (IES-R) during the COVID-19 pandemic.

2. Materials and Methods

2.1. Settings and Design

A diagnostic survey method utilizing a questionnaire technique was used to assess the levels of psychological distress of nurses. Due to the COVID-19 pandemic and the recommendations of the Polish government to minimize contact with other people, potential respondents were invited via email to participate in the study. Volunteers completed the survey questionnaires in Polish via an online platform (https://docs.google.com/ (accessed on 20 November 2021)) (Table S1).

Respondents were recruited from among nursing staff working directly with patients diagnosed with SARS-CoV-2 infection in the Independent Public Clinical Hospital No. 1 of the Pomeranian Medical University named Prof. Tadeusz Sokołowski in Szczecin.

The inclusion criteria for the study were a current license to practice as a nurse, aged >18 years and informed consent to participate in the study. The study was conducted according to the guidelines of the Declaration of Helsinki and approved by the Ethics Committee of the Pomeranian Medical University in Szczecin (KB-0012/25/04/2020/Z). Our study was conducted taking into account ethical considerations. Informed consent was required, and participation in the study was voluntary. Moreover, the participants were assured of anonymity and confidentiality, and were free to withdraw from the study at any stage.

The results of the study were presented to the Chief Nurse of SPSK 1 in Szczecin. Due to the anonymity of the study participants, we requested a more complete analysis of psychological disorders and psychological nurses for psychological support.

2.2. Research Instruments

Standardized survey instruments were used to assess the psychosocial functioning of nursing staff during the COVID-19 pandemic:

- **The Impact of Event Scale (IES-R, Impact of Event Scale—Revised)** [7] is a questionnaire designed to determine the extent of psychological impact following exposure to a public health crisis within one week of exposure. The Impact of Event Scale consists of 22 statements describing symptoms of perceived stress in the last 7 days in relation to the traumatic event experienced. It is rated on a 5-point Likert-type scale (0–4). It captures three dimensions of PTSD: intrusion (expressing recurrent images, dreams, thoughts or perceptual impressions associated with the trauma), arousal (characterized by increased alertness, anxiety, impatience and difficulty concentrating) and avoidance (manifested by efforts to rid oneself of thoughts, emotions or conversations associated with the trauma). Cronbach's alpha coefficient for the entire scale, which finally included 12 items, was 0.77. A three-factor structure of the tool was demonstrated, explaining 60.04% of the variance. This analysis revealed moderate-to-high values of the factor loadings of all items that form subscales, with the exception of the fifth subject. On this basis, it was decided to reject the fifth item. The Polish version of the PDI is a relevant and reliable distress assessment tool.
- **The Generalized Anxiety Questionnaire** (GAD-7, Generalized Anxiety Disorder) is a screening tool used to determine feelings associated with generalized anxiety syndrome. The survey consists of 7 questions. Each question has a score from 0 to 3 points, the sum of which indicates the severity of anxiety: 0–4 points (no anxiety), 5–9 (mild anxiety), 10–14 (moderate anxiety) and 15–21 (severe anxiety). Using the threshold score of 10, the GAD-7 has a sensitivity of 89% and a specificity of 82% for generalized anxiety disorder. It is also moderately good at screening for other anxiety disorders: panic disorder (sensitivity 74%, specificity 81%), social anxiety disorder (sensitivity 72%, specificity 80%) and post-traumatic stress disorder (sensitivity 66%, specificity 81%) [8].
- **The PHQ-9** (Patient Health Questionnaire-9) is a questionnaire that was designed to screen for depression. It was developed based on the diagnostic criteria for depression contained in the Diagnostic and Statistical Manual of Mental Disorders (DSM-IV). The maximum number of points possible is 27, which indicates the highest possible severity of depression. A score of less than five indicates normal, 5 to 9 points indicates mild depression, 10 to 14 points indicates moderate depression, 15 to 19 points indicates moderately severe depression and 20 to 27 points indicates severe depression. The PHQ-9 showed significant positive internal consistency (Cronbach's alpha = 0.7) and the scores of each of its nine items positively correlated (0.31–0.68; $p < 0.05$) with the total score. The convergent validity was significantly positive ($r = 0.58$; $p < 0.05$). Using >6 points as the cutoff point, the sensitivity and specificity of the PHQ-9 for recognizing a major depression episode were found to be 70.4% and 78.2% respectively [9].
- **The Athens Insomnia Scale** (AIS) is a short, eight-item scale that allows for quantitative measurement of insomnia symptoms based on ICD-10 criteria. The total score of the scale ranges from 0 to 24 points. The first five items relate to sleep-related symptoms (difficulty falling asleep, waking up during the night, waking up early in the morning, sleep duration and quality) and correspond to criterion A of the ICD-10 diagnosis of inorganic insomnia. A symptom should be marked if it occurred at least three times a week for at least a month, which is consistent with the duration and frequency of symptoms required for the ICD-10 diagnosis of insomnia (criterion B). The other three items relate to daytime functioning (mood, physical and mental performance, sleepiness) and correspond to criterion C of the ICD-10 diagnosis of insomnia,

which includes complaints about the consequences of insomnia during the day. The Athens Insomnia Scale is the first tool for assessing insomnia-related symptoms, which has achieved Polish validation. The study confirmed the good psychometric properties of the scale. The internal consistency (Cronbach's alpha = 0.90) and the test–retest reliability (r^2 = 0.92) of the AIS were found to be very satisfactory. These values remained practically unchanged when any of the items were removed from the analysis [10].

- **The Perceived Stress Scale PSS-10** (PSS-10, The Perceived Stress Scale) is an instrument that is used to assess the severity of stress related to the subject's situation in the last 4 weeks in the context of subjective feelings and personal life problems. Interpretation is carried out by analyzing the ten-point norms that indicate the severity of stress: low score (1–4 points), average score (5–6 points) and high score (7–10 points). The Polish adaptation of the scale was made in 2009 by Juczyński and Ogińska-Bulik. The reliability of the Polish adaptation of the PSS-10 scale (Cronbach's α coefficient) ranges from 0.72 to 0.90 [11].
- **Self-administered questionnaire—including questions about sociodemographic data** (age, education, place of residence, marital status, employment status, parental status), physical symptoms over the past 14 days (included fever, chills, headache, muscle aches, cough, difficulty breathing, dizziness, sore throat and persistent fever, as well as persistent fever and cough or difficulty breathing), history of contact with COVID-19 (close contact with a person with confirmed COVID-19).

2.3. *Statistical Analysis*

Quantitative and categorical variables were described with descriptive statistics methods. For the quantitative variables, the following measures were determined: central tendency (mean, M) and dispersion (standard deviation, SD). For the categorical variables, the following measures were determined: number (N) and frequency (%).

The influences of selected sociodemographic and health-related factors and the psychological impact after exposure on insomnia according to the IES-R were estimated using a non-linear estimation for the logistic regression model. The Rosenbrock and quasi-Newton methods of estimation were applied, appointing asymptotic standard errors. The accuracy of the data adjustment to the suggested logit was checked using the Hosmer–Lemeshow test. The model fit was also tested using V-fold cross-validation. For each factor, the odds ratio (OR) was determined, together with a 95% confidence interval.

The influence of selected sociodemographic and health-related factors, as well as the psychological impact after exposure according to IES-R, on the levels of psychological distress of nurses (anxiety, depression, stress) was estimated using a multivariate linear regression model. The least-squares method of estimation was applied to calculate the parameters of the regression model. For each factor, which was an independent variable tested in the regression model, the following indicators were determined: unstandardized (b) and standardized regression ($\beta_{stand.}$) coefficients, 95% confidence interval (CI), t-test and *p*-value. The proportion of the variance for a dependent variable that was explained by the independent variables was calculated with the adjusted R-squared ($R^2_{adj.}$).

All the calculations were performed with STATISTICATM 13.3 software (TIBCO Software, Palo Alto, CA, USA). For all analyses, a *p*-level of <0.05 was considered statistically significant.

3. Results

3.1. *Characteristics of Respondents*

A total of 312 respondents working directly with patients diagnosed with COVID-19 were invited to participate in the survey between 1 January and 1 April 2021. Only 207 nurses correctly completed the surveys (completion rate: 66%). The mean age of the respondents was 37.87 years. The vast majority of the respondents were female (83.09%), in a formal relationship (52.66%), achieved higher education (79.23%) and living in a city of more than 100 thousand residents (66.67%). The most frequently chosen forms of employment were employment contract (67.15%) and non-shift work (68.60%). Half of the respondents had children (50.24%). A majority of the respondents did not have any chronic disease (68.60%), 12.56% had chronic hyperthyroidism or hypothyroidism and 7.25% had hypertension (Table S2).

3.2. Pandemic-Related Variables

Most of the respondents (65.70%) rated their health as good and had not been quarantined (80.68%). Almost all (98.55%) respondents stated the presence of personal protective equipment, while more than half of the respondents (57.49%) indicated a lack of psychological support in the workplace. Less than half of the respondents (48.79%) indicated close contact with a person with confirmed COVID-19 infection in the past 4 weeks. The most common symptom (40.10%) in the past 4 weeks was a headache.

3.3. Psychological Variables

Selected psychological variables (sleep disturbance, anxiety, stress severity, depression) of the respondents were analyzed in this study.

Based on the results obtained according to the Athens Insomnia Scale (AIS), it was found that 40.58% of the respondents had sleep disorders. When anxiety was examined according to the Generalized Anxiety Questionnaire (GAD-7), it was observed that the vast majority of the respondents experienced anxiety of varying severities: 36.71% had mild anxiety, 19.81% had moderate anxiety and 9.18% had severe anxiety. Moreover, it was shown that a majority of the respondents (71.95%) experienced a high level of stress according to PSS-10, while in the case of depression, according to the PHQ-9, it was shown that only 37.2% of the respondents had no symptoms.

The psychological impact of the COVID-19 pandemic was assessed using the results obtained according to the IES-R. It was observed that the mean total score was 34.25 points (SD = 19.65). For the subscales, the respondents scored 12.34 points, 11.58 points and 12.12 points for intrusion, arousal and avoidance, respectively (Tables S3 and S4).

3.4. Assessment of Nurses' Levels of Psychological Distress (Anxiety, Depression, Stress, Insomnia) in Relation to Sociodemographic Variables

This study analyzed the influence of selected sociodemographic variables (age, gender, marital status, place of residence, education, form of employment) on the psychological variables of nurses during the SARS-CoV-2 pandemic.

Based on the collected data, it was observed that the chance of experiencing insomnia decreased with the age of the subjects (OR = 0.959, $p = 0.023$) (Table 1).

Table 1. Influence of sociodemographic variables on the occurrence of insomnia according to the AIS.

Factor		b	OR	−95% CI	+95% CI	t	*p*
Intercept		0.031	1.031	0.093	11.458	0.001	0.980
Gender	Female (ref.)						
	Male	−0.745	0.475	0.197	1.145	2.751	0.097
Age		−0.042	0.959	0.924	0.994	5.170	0.023
Marital status	Single (ref.)						
	Formal relationship	−0.409	0.664	0.287	1.541	0.908	0.341
	Casual relationship	−0.411	0.663	0.275	1.600	0.835	0.361

Table 1. *Cont.*

Factor		b	OR	−95% CI	+95% CI	t	*p*
Place of residence	Rural area (ref.)						
	Small town	0.203	1.225	0.384	3.908	0.118	0.732
	Big city	−0.241	0.786	0.275	2.249	0.201	0.654
Education	Secondary/ post-secondary education (ref)						
	Higher	0.098	1.103	0.459	2.652	0.048	0.826
Number of children	None (ref.)						
	One	0.553	1.738	0.750	4.025	1.663	0.197
	Two and more	0.479	1.614	0.595	4.382	0.884	0.347
Type of employment	Employment contract	1.180	3.254	0.931	11.374	3.416	0.065
	Self-employment	0.675	1.964	0.527	7.323	1.011	0.315
	Contract of mandate	0.976	2.655	0.937	7.518	3.379	0.066
Shift work	No (ref.)						
	Yes	0.360	1.434	0.749	2.745	1.182	0.277

b—regression coefficient, OR—odds ratio, CI—confidence interval, ref.—reference level.

Model I explained approximately 9% of the variance in the Generalized Anxiety Disorder (GAD-7) anxiety variable ($F(13, 193) = 2.614$, $p = 0.002$). Respondents with a college education had significantly higher levels of anxiety according to GAD-7 compared with those with secondary/post-secondary education ($\beta_{stand.} = 0.190$, $p = 0.014$). Respondents employed under a contract of employment had significantly higher levels of anxiety as measured by the GAD-7 compared with people without such a form of employment ($\beta_{stand.} = 0.400$, $p = 0.002$), while those employed under a contract of employment also had significantly higher levels of anxiety as measured by the GAD-7 compared with persons without such a form of employment ($\beta_{stand.} = 0.328$, $p = 0.015$). Respondents employed on the basis of a contract of mandate showed a significantly higher level of anxiety according to GAD-7 in comparison with persons without this form of employment ($\beta_{stand.} = 0.169$, $p = 0.037$) (Table S5).

In the case of model II, which explained more than 7% of the variation in depression using the Patient Health Questionnaire-9 (PHQ-9) ($F(13, 193) = 2.105$, $p = 0.015$), men had a significantly lower level of depression compared with women ($\beta_{stand.} = -0.154$, $p = 0.030$). Respondents employed under a contract of employment had significantly higher levels of depression according to the PHQ-9 compared with those without this form of employment ($\beta_{stand.} = 0.415$, $p = 0.002$). Respondents employed under a contract had significantly higher levels of depression compared with those without this form of employment ($\beta_{stand.} = 0.299$, $p = 0.029$), while those employed under a contract of mandate had significantly higher levels of depression compared with those without this form of employment ($\beta_{stand.} = 0.218$, $p = 0.008$) (Table S6).

Model III explained only 0.2% of the variation in the stress level variable according to The Perceived Stress Scale (PSS-10) ($F(13, 193) = 1.309$, $p = 0.050$). Respondents employed under a contract of employment had significantly higher levels of stress compared with those without this form of employment ($\beta_{stand.} = 0.347$, $p = 0.011$) (Table S7).

3.5. Assessment of Levels of Psychological Distress of Nurses (Anxiety, Depression, Stress, Insomnia) in Relation to Self-Assessment of Health, Quarantine, Psychological Support, Presence of Chronic Diseases and Psychological Impact after Exposure according to the IES-R

This study analyzed the effects of selected COVID-19 pandemic-related variables (self-rated health status, having served in quarantine, psychological support, presence of chronic illnesses and post-exposure psychological impact according to IES-R) on nurses' psychological variables during the SARS-CoV-2 pandemic.

Based on the collected data, it was observed that the chance of insomnia increased with the increase in the severity of the trait "agitation" according to the IES-R (OR = 1.217, $p = 0.002$) (Table 2).

Table 2. The influence of the self-assessment of health, quarantine, psychological support, presence of chronic diseases and dimensions according to the Impact of Event Scale—Revised (IES-R) on the occurrence of insomnia according to the AIS.

Factor		b	OR	−95% CI	+95% CI	t	*p*
Intercept		−2.044	0.130	0.026	0.647	6.203	0.013
Quarantine	No (ref.)						
	Yes	0.266	1.305	0.570	2.985	0.396	0.529
Psychologist support	No (ref.)						
	Yes	0.261	1.298	0.662	2.545	0.577	0.448
Self-assessed health status	Poor/average (ref.)						
	Good	−0.607	0.545	0.154	1.934	0.882	0.348
	Very good	−0.755	0.470	0.115	1.918	1.108	0.293
Chronic disease	No (ref.)						
	Yes	−0.226	0.798	0.386	1.649	0.372	0.542
IES-R	Intrusion	0.066	1.068	0.985	1.157	2.553	0.110
	Stimulation	0.196	1.217	1.075	1.377	9.649	0.002
	Avoiding	−0.083	0.920	0.836	1.012	2.921	0.087

b—regression coefficient, OR—odds ratio, CI—confidence interval, ref.—reference level, IES-R—Impact of Event Scale—Revised.

Model IV explained approximately 40% of the variance in the anxiety variable according to the Generalized Anxiety Disorder (GAD-7) questionnaire ($F(8, 198) = 18.387$, $p < 0.001$). Those in quarantine had significantly higher levels of anxiety than those who did not have this experience ($\beta_{stand.} = 0.123$, $p = 0.026$). Study nurses who rated their health as very good had significantly lower levels of anxiety than those who rated their health as poor or average ($\beta_{stand.} = -0.132$, $p = 0.023$). As the level of intrusiveness according to the IES-R of the subjects increased, the level of anxiety according to GAD-7 increased significantly ($\beta_{stand.} = 0.340$, $p = 0.001$); furthermore, the increase in the level of agitation according to the IES-R caused a significant increase in the level of anxiety ($\beta_{stand.} = 0.366$, $p = 0.002$) (Table 3).

Table 3. Effect of the self-assessment of health, quarantine, psychological support, presence of chronic diseases and dimensions of the Impact of Event Scale—Revised (IES-R) on the level of anxiety according to GAD-7 (model IV).

Factor		b	$\beta_{stand.}$	−95% CI	+95% CI	t	*p*
Intercept		2.856				3.681	0.000
Quarantine	No (ref.)						
	Yes	0.841	0.123	0.015	0.231	2.242	0.026
Psychologist support	No (ref.)						
	Yes	−0.124	−0.023	−0.130	0.085	−0.416	0.678
Self-assessed health status	Poor/average (ref.)						
	Good	−0.851	−0.100	−0.208	0.009	−1.805	0.073
	Very good	−1.288	−0.132	−0.247	−0.018	−2.285	0.023
Chronic disease	No (ref.)						
	Yes	0.067	0.012	−0.098	0.121	0.207	0.836
IES-R	Intrusion	0.236	0.340	0.137	0.543	3.304	0.001
	Stimulation	0.316	0.366	0.132	0.600	3.085	0.002
	Avoiding	−0.087	−0.102	−0.276	0.072	−1.155	0.249

b—regression coefficient, $\beta_{stand.}$—standardized regression coefficient, CI—confidence interval, ref.—reference level, IES-R—Impact of Event Scale—Revised.

Model V explained approximately 41% of the variation in the variable of depression according to the Patient Health Questionnaire-9 (PHQ-9) ($F(8, 198) = 22.715$, $p < 0.001$). Study nurses who rated their health as very good had significantly lower levels of depression according to the PHQ-9 than those who rated their health as poor or average ($\beta_{stand.} = -0.147$, $p = 0.011$). Among the respondents, as the level of intrusiveness according to the IES-R increased, the level of depressiveness measured using the PHQ-9 increased significantly ($\beta_{stand.} = 0.387$, $p < 0.001$); furthermore, the increase in the level of arousal according to the IES-R caused a significant increase in depressiveness ($\beta_{stand.} = 0.347$, $p = 0.004$) (Table 4).

Table 4. Effect of self-rated health, quarantine, psychological support, presence of chronic diseases and the Impact of Event Scale—Revised (IES-R) dimensions on the level of depression according to the PHQ-9 (model V).

Factor		b	$\beta_{stand.}$	−95% CI	+95% CI	t	*p*
Intercept		2.908				3.287	0.001
Quarantine	No (ref.)						
	Yes	0.703	0.090	−0.018	0.198	1.643	0.102
Psychologist support	No (ref.)						
	Yes	−0.004	−0.001	−0.108	0.107	−0.011	0.991
Self-assessed health status	Poor/average (ref.)						
	Good	−1.009	−0.103	−0.211	0.005	−1.876	0.062
	Very good	−1.642	−0.147	−0.261	−0.034	−2.555	0.011

Table 4. *Cont.*

Factor		b	$\beta_{stand.}$	−95% CI	+95% CI	t	*p*
Chronic disease	No (ref.)						
	Yes	−0.579	−0.087	−0.196	0.022	−1.568	0.119
IES-R	Intrusion	0.308	0.387	0.185	0.589	3.781	0.000
	Stimulation	0.344	0.347	0.115	0.580	2.944	0.004
	Avoiding	−0.150	−0.153	−0.326	0.020	−1.740	0.083

b—regression coefficient, $\beta_{stand.}$—standardized regression coefficient, CI—confidence interval, ref.—reference level, IES-R—Impact of Event Scale—Revised.

Model VI explained approximately 24% of the variance in the stress variable according to The Perceived Stress Scale (PSS-10) ($F(8, 198) = 9.287$, $p < 0.001$). Individuals who rated their health as good had significantly lower levels of stress than those who rated their health as poor or average ($\beta_{stand.} = -0.149$, $p = 0.017$). As the intrusion level according to the IES-R of the subjects increased, the stress level according to the PSS-10 increased significantly ($\beta_{stand.} = 0.281$, $p = 0.016$) (Table 5).

Table 5. Effect of the self-assessment of health, quarantine, psychological support, presence of chronic diseases and dimensions of the Impact of Event Scale—Revised (IES-R) on stress level (model VI).

Factor		b	$\beta_{stand.}$	−95% CI	+95% CI	t	*p*
Intercept		6.039				24.030	0.000
Quarantine	No (ref.)						
	Yes	0.076	0.039	−0.083	0.161	0.627	0.531
Psychologist support	No (ref.)						
	Yes	0.049	0.031	−0.090	0.153	0.510	0.610
Self-assessed health status	Poor/average (ref.)						
	Good	−0.368	−0.149	−0.272	−0.027	−2.408	0.017
	Very good	−0.062	−0.022	−0.151	0.107	−0.338	0.735
Chronic disease	No (ref.)						
	Yes	0.016	0.009	−0.114	0.133	0.151	0.880
IES-R	Intrusion	0.056	0.281	0.053	0.510	2.430	0.016
	Stimulation	0.051	0.206	−0.057	0.470	1.545	0.124
	Avoiding	0.008	0.033	−0.163	0.229	0.330	0.742

b—regression coefficient, $\beta_{stand.}$—standardized regression coefficient, CI—confidence interval, ref.—reference level, IES-R—Impact of Event Scale—Revised.

4. Discussion

The years 2020 and 2021 in Poland became a challenging period due to the startling changes in social functioning that occurred with the announcement of the SARS-CoV-2 pandemic. As many as 8000 to 12,000 cases of coronavirus infection were reported daily between 1 and 4 January 2021. More than half of the beds designated for COVID-19 patients were occupied. During this period, a significant number of people struggled with symptoms of tension, anxiety, restlessness and sleep disturbances [12,13]. Healthcare workers were particularly vulnerable to stress symptoms. According to scientific analyses, mood and sleep disorders were most common in this occupational group during the pandemic period [14,15].

According to the results of our study, most of the nurses surveyed scored highly on the perceived stress scale. More than half of the respondents demonstrated moderate and mild levels of anxiety and almost 10% demonstrated severe anxiety symptoms. Almost half of the nurses surveyed suffered from sleep disorders. Almost one-third of the respondents showed full depressive symptoms and another one-third of the respondents showed mild depressive symptoms. An online survey of a group of physicians conducted in Turkey in March 2020 showed that more than half of the medics experienced symptoms of anxiety and depression [16]. Similar results were obtained by other researchers that examined the severity of stress of people working in hospitals during the COVID-19 pandemic [17–21]. Similar results were obtained by Nakhostin; however, in their scientific report, the analysis included a group of medical students [22].

According to the results of our study, more than half of the respondents indicated a lack of psychological support in the workplace. According to the study of Kang et al. [1], in terms of psychological support, 36.3% of the respondents received written psychoeducational materials (i.e., pamphlets, brochures and books), half of the respondents received psychological support through the media (which included online psychological support, as well as information obtained through television and online platforms) and 17.5% participated in group psychological counseling. It was noted that the higher the level of exposure to COVID-19 patients, the more severe the mental health disorders [23].

The nursing professionals of a COVID-19 team have significant levels of anxiety, depression and stress, and the factors associated with depression and stress were identified [24]. According to the study by Appel et al., the nursing professionals of the COVID-19 team studied had significant levels of anxiety, depression and stress, and the factors associated with depression and stress were identified [25].

According to a meta-analysis by Al Maqubali that estimated the combined prevalence of stress, anxiety, depression and sleep disturbance among nurses during the COVID-19 pandemic, the combined prevalences of stress, anxiety, depression and sleep disturbance (43%, 37%, 35% and 43%, respectively) among nurses during the COVID-19 outbreak suggested that at least one-third of nurses experienced stress, anxiety, depression and sleep disturbance. These findings are higher than those reported in the general population during the same period [26]. Shi et al. reported that, in the general population, 24% had stress, 32% had anxiety, 28% had depression and 29% had insomnia. This was because nurses were more likely to be patients with COVID-19 [27].

Lai et al. [28] conducted a cross-sectional, questionnaire-based study of the mental health of workers exposed to direct contact with COVID-19 patients. The results indicated that depressive and anxiety symptoms were present in half of the respondents, insomnia symptoms were present in over one-third of the respondents and distress as measured by the IES-R was present in nearly three-quarters of the respondents. Higher rates of anxiety symptoms were reported in women compared with men. Frontline workers, i.e., those involved in the direct diagnosis, treatment and care of patients with COVID-19, had a higher risk of depressive symptoms, insomnia and distress. The above results are consistent with those of Ten et al. [29] and Chew et al. [30].

The research work of Yin and Zeng [31] focused on the needs of nursing staff members. Qualitative analyses revealed the predominant needs for maintaining health and safety, needs for interpersonal relationships and warmth, concern from the community and needs for knowledge about COVID-19.

In Li's study [32], the most significant finding was that nursing staff who did not work directly with patients with COVID-19 had higher levels of vicarious traumatization compared with those who worked on the front line of medicine. According to Li et al. [33], this may have been due to their psychological preparation, the work experience of this group and they volunteered to work on the front line. The authors recommend that those medical workers who are not directly involved in the treatment of patients with COVID-19 should also be included in the support offered.

Our results indicated that men had significantly lower levels of depression compared with women. Similar results were obtained by Albert et al. The prevalence rate of anxiety and depressiveness was found to be higher in women, which probably reflects the gender difference in anxiety and depressive symptoms [34]. A study by Liu et al. found that nursing staff showed higher prevalence estimates for both anxiety and depressive symptoms compared with physicians. These findings may be partially challenged by the fact that nurses are predominantly female, but may also be attributed to the fact that they may be at higher risk of contracting infections from COVID-19 patients because they spend more time on the wards, provide direct patient care and are responsible for collecting sputum for viral detection [35]. Unfortunately, there have also been reports of suicide, as healthcare workers deal with accumulated psychological pressure and intense fear of death [36,37]. This is particularly worrisome given that healthcare personnel are already at an increased risk for suicide compared with the general population [38].

Initially, data from previous epidemics, most notably the SARS epidemic, were considered when organizing psychological support due to the lack of current research findings. Data on the negative consequences of isolation during SARS were also highlighted. The most common direct effects of the 9-day quarantine in medical services included experiencing emotions and conditions such as exhaustion, irritability, anxiety, withdrawal from relationships with others, insomnia, attention deficit disorder and impaired occupational functioning, including considering quitting work [39].

The results of our study showed that almost half of the subjects were in quarantine. People in quarantine showed higher levels of anxiety as measured by GAD-7 than those who did not have this experience. Significantly, the effects of quarantine were a predictor of symptoms of post-traumatic stress disorder within 3 years of the outbreak [40]. After the quarantine period, medical staff were reported to have persistent symptoms of avoidant, protective behaviors, such as avoiding crowded rooms, public places or contact with people with signs of infection [41]. The outreach organized for medical personnel during the COVID-19 pandemic was initially built on experiences and guidelines from the SARS outbreak. One recommendation was for screening for depression, anxiety and suicide risk for medical personnel, as for those infected or awaiting test results, especially since the experience of the SARS outbreak indicated significant stress among medical personnel, continuing even one year after the outbreak. Based on the experience of previous epidemics and extensive studies of various population groups, a mental health strategy was developed in China early in the COVID-19 epidemic [42,43].

Pappa et al. [44] conducted a systematic review and meta-analysis of the prevalence of anxiety, depression and insomnia among healthcare workers during the COVID-19 pandemic. Anxiety was assessed in 12 studies, with a prevalence of 23.2%; depression was assessed in 10 studies, with a prevalence of 22.8%. Labrague and De Los Santos [45] found that 37.8% of nurses surveyed had dysfunctional levels of anxiety. Labrague and De Los Santos indicated that COVID-19 anxiety was associated with social support, organizational support and personal resilience. These findings support the current study showing that frontline nurses were affected by anxiety during the COVID-19 pandemic. To help healthcare workers provide care in extremely challenging clinical settings, such as the COVID-19 pandemic, emotional and behavioral responses among workers should be recognized and enhanced through education and training to overcome fear and empathic distress [46].

A study by Alnazly et al. demonstrated the presence of fear, depression, anxiety and stress among healthcare workers during the COVID-19 pandemic. Workers surveyed identified social support from family and friends as important during the pandemic and demonstrated the need for increased social support to adjust to psychological stress. Factors found to be associated with psychological distress were male gender, aged 40 years or older and having a life partner or more clinical experience [47].

Published data strongly suggest that the health status of medical professionals is significantly impacted due to the ongoing COVID-19 pandemic. The clinical picture in this population shows an increase in depressive symptoms, anxiety and insomnia [41]. Psychological support, access to up-to-date data on new treatment options and adequate comfort by matching staff to patients has a positive impact on health care and will reduce errors that can have dramatic consequences [35]. It is essential to ensure the safety of workers through the availability of personal protective equipment, i.e., disinfectants, masks, goggles, visors, protective shoes and protective suits, that meet all required standards. These reports are very alarming. They indicate the need to build a strategy of mental health protection, undertake more intensive preventive actions toward medical workers and monitor the state of the mental health of this professional group after the end of the pandemic.

Limitations

Although the literature on this matter is scarce, a few studies that analyzed the nurses' psychological functioning (which assessed the frequency of depression, anxiety, insomnia, the level of perceived stress or the assessment of experienced traumatic events according to the Impact of Events Scale) have already been published during the COVID-19 pandemic. Unfortunately, our study had some limitations due to the extensive questionnaire administered to nurses. In Poland, there has been a shortage of nursing staff in hospitals for years, and due to the COVID-19 pandemic, nurses felt this shortage even more strongly; therefore, obtaining willing nurses to participate in the study was quite difficult. In addition, our study focused on employees of only one hospital in Szczecin, and it was a cross-sectional study, which means we cannot assess the long-term consequences of the COVID-19 pandemic on the mental health of healthcare workers. Despite the limitations of our study, it is worth mentioning that its advantage was the individual approach to the studied professional group. Therefore, it is advisable to conduct further research and take preventive measures to protect the mental health of nursing staff.

5. Conclusions

1. Education, gender and age were the variables that significantly affected the severity of anxiety, depression and insomnia of the studied nurses working with patients with COVID-19.
2. The form of employment was one of the factors that influenced the intensity of anxiety of the studied nurses.
3. Along with the intensity of intrusion in the studied nurses also increased the level of anxiety, depression and stress.
4. The positive self-assessment of the health of the surveyed nurses had a significant impact on the reduction of anxiety and depression during the implementation of care for patients with COVID-19.

Supplementary Materials: The following supporting information can be downloaded at: https://www.mdpi.com/article/10.3390/ijerph19031435/s1, Table S1. STROBE statement—Checklist of items that should be included in reports of case–control studies.; Table S2. Sociodemographic variables of respondents; Table S3. Outcome measures: insomnia according to the AIS, generalized anxiety according to GAD-7, Impact of Events Scale (IES-R), depression according to the PHQ-9 and stress according to the PSS-10 in the entire cohort; Table S4. Outcome measures: insomnia according to the AIS, generalized anxiety according to GAD-7, Impact of Events Scale (IES-R), depressiveness according to the PHQ-9 and stress according to the PSS-10 in the entire cohort by category; Table S5. The influence of sociodemographic variables on the level of anxiety; Table S6. Influence of sociodemographic variables on the level of depression according to the Patient Health Questionnaire-9 (PHQ-9) (model II); Table S7. The influence of sociodemographic variables on the level of stress according to The Perceived Stress Scale (PSS-10) (model III).

Author Contributions: Conceptualization, K.R. and A.M.C.; methodology, M.S.; software, M.S.; validation, M.P. and J.S.-P.; formal analysis, M.P.; investigation, P.U.; resources, J.S.-P.; data curation, J.S.-P.; writing—original draft preparation, K.R.; writing—review and editing, A.M.C.; visualization, E.G.; supervision, E.G.; project administration, P.U.; funding acquisition, E.G. All authors have read and agreed to the published version of the manuscript.

Funding: This research received no external funding.

Institutional Review Board Statement: The study was conducted according to the guidelines of the Declaration of Helsinki and approved by the Ethics Committee of the Pomeranian Medical University in Szczecin (KB-0012/25/04/2020/Z).

Informed Consent Statement: Informed consent was obtained from all subjects involved in the study.

Data Availability Statement: Data sharing not applicable.

Acknowledgments: We thank all participants for their participation and all the staff of the survey team for their efforts that made this study possible.

Conflicts of Interest: The authors declare no conflict of interest.

References

1. Gawrych, M. Mental Health of Medical Workers during COVID-19 Pandemic—Literature Review. Available online: http://www.psychiatriapolska.pl/uploads/onlinefirst/Gawrych_PsychiatrPolOnlineFirstNr213.pdf (accessed on 28 November 2021).
2. Badura-Brzoza, K.; Bułdak, R.; Dębski, P.; Kasperczyk, S.; Woźniak-Grygiel, E.; Konka, A.; Brzoza, Z. The Stress of the SARS-CoV-2 Virus Pandemic and Pro-Health Behaviors among Medical Personnel—Preliminary Report. Available online: https://www.researchgate.net/profile/Pawel-Debski/publication/353290956_The_stress_of_the_SARS-CoV-2_virus_pandemic_and_pro-health_behaviors_among_medical_personnel_-_preliminary_report/links/6109151b1e95fe241aa6423b/The-stress-of-the-SARS-CoV-2-virus-pandemic-and-pro-health-behaviors-among-medical-personnel-preliminary-report.pdf (accessed on 28 November 2021).
3. Perrotta, G. Anxiety disorders: Definitions, contexts, neural correlates and strategic therapy. *J. Neur. Neurosci.* **2019**, *6*, 42.
4. Święcicki, Ł. Depression—Definition, classification and causes. *Psychiatr. W Prakt. Ogólnolekarskiej* **2002**, *2*, 151–160.
5. Grygorczuk, A. The notion of stress in medicine and psychology. *Psychiatria* **2008**, *5*, 111–115.
6. Szambor, T.; Wasiak, J.; Urbańska, A.; Składanowski, M. Relationship between taking medical care of people infected with COVID-19 and mental health of healthcare professionals. *Pol. J. Public Health* **2019**, *129*, 4. [CrossRef]
7. Juczyński, Z.; Ogińska-Bulik, N. Measurement of post-traumatic stress disorder—Polish version of Impact Event Scale-Revised. *Psychiatria* **2009**, *6*, 15–25.
8. Spitzer, R.L.; Kroenke, K.; Williams, J.B.; Löwe, B. A brief measure for assessing generalized anxiety disorder. *Arch Intern. Med.* **2006**, *166*, 1092–1097. [CrossRef]
9. Tomaszewski, K.; Zarychta, M.; Bieńkowska, A.; Chmurowicz, E.; Nowak, W.; Skalska, A. Validation of the Patient Health Questionnaire-9 Polish version in the hospitalised elderly population. *Psychiatr. Pol.* **2011**, *45*, 2.
10. Fornal-Pawłowska, M.; Wołyńczyk-Gmaj, D.; Szelenberger, W. Validation of the Polish version of the Athens Insomnia Scale. *Psychiatr. Pol.* **2011**, *45*, 211–222.
11. Cohen, S.; Kamarck, T.; Mermelstein, R. The Perceived Stress Scale PSS-10. In *Stress Measurement and Stress Management Tools*; Juczyński, Z., Ogińska-Bulik, N., Eds.; Pracownia Testów Psychologicznych PTP: Warsaw, Poland, 2009.
12. Torales, J.; O'Higgins, M.; Castaldelli-Maia, J.M.; Ventriglio, A. The outbreak of COVID–19 coronavirus and its impact on global mental health. *Int. J. Soc. Psychiatry* **2020**, *66*, 317–320. [CrossRef]
13. Duszyński, J.; Afelt, A.; Ochab-Marcinek, A.; Owczuk, R.; Pyrć, K.; Rosińska, M. *Understanding COVID-19. Development of the COVID-19 Team at the President of the Polish Academy of Sciences*; PAN: Warsaw, Poland, 2020.
14. Wu, T. Prevalence of mental health problems during the COVID-19 pandemic: A systematic review and meta-analysis. *J. Affect. Disord.* **2021**, *281*, 91–98. [CrossRef]
15. Santabárbara, J.; Bueno-Notivol, J.; Lipnicki, D.M.; Olaya, B.; Pérez-Moreno, M.; Gracia-García, P.; Ozamiz-Etxebarria, N. Prevalence of anxiety in health care professionals during the COVID-19 pandemic: A rapid systematic review (on published articles in Medline) with meta-analysis. *Prog. Neuropsychopharmacol. Biol. Psychiatry* **2021**, *107*, 110244. [CrossRef] [PubMed]
16. Elbay, R.Y.; Kurtulmuş, A.; Arpacıoğlu, S.; Karadere, E. Depression, anxiety, stress levels of physicians and associated factors in COVID–19 pandemics. *Psychiatry Res.* **2020**, *290*, 113130. [CrossRef] [PubMed]
17. Du, J.; Dong, L.; Wang, T.; Yuan, C.; Fu, R.; Zhang, L. Psychological symptoms among frontline healthcare workers during COVID–19 outbreak in Wuhan. *Gen. Hosp. Psychiatry* **2020**, *67*, 144–145. [CrossRef] [PubMed]
18. Xing, L.Q.; Xu, M.L.; Sun, J.; Wang, Q.X.; Ge, D.D.; Jiang, M.M. Anxiety and depression in frontline health care workers during the outbreak of COVID–19. *Int. J. Soc. Psychiatry* **2020**, *24*, 20764020968119. [CrossRef]
19. Rossi, R.; Socci, V.; Pacitti, F.; Di Lorenzo, G.; Di Marco, A.; Siracusano, A. Mental Health Outcomes Among Frontline and Second-Line Health Care Workers During the Coronavirus Disease 2019 (COVID–19) Pandemic in Italy. *JAMA Netw. Open* **2020**, *3*, e2010185. [CrossRef]
20. Bohlken, J.; Schömig, F.; Lemke, M.R.; Pumberger, M.; Riedel-Heller, S.G. COVID-19 pandemic: Stress experience of healthcare workers—A short current review. *Psychiatr. Prax.* **2020**, *47*, 190–197.
21. Cheung, T.; Fong, T.K.H.; Bressington, D. COVID-19 under the SARS Cloud: Mental Health Nursing during the Pandemic in Hong Kong. *J. Psychiatr. Ment. Health Nurs.* **2021**, *28*, 115–117. [CrossRef]
22. Nakhostin-Ansari, A.; Sherafati, A.; Aghajani, F.; SaeidKhonji, M.; Aghajani, R.; Shahmansouri, N. Depression and Anxiety among Iranian Medical Students during COVID–19 Pandemic. *Iran. J. Psychiatry* **2020**, *15*, 228–235. [CrossRef]
23. Kang, L.; Ma, S.; Chen, M.; Yang, J.; Wang, Y.; Li, R. Impact on mental health and perceptions of psychological care among medical and nursing staff in Wuhan during the 2019 novel coronavirus disease outbreak: A cross-sectional study. *Brain Behav. Immun.* **2020**, *87*, 11–17. [CrossRef]

24. Nadeem, F.; Sadiq, A.; Raziq, A.; Iqbal, Q.; Haider, S.; Saleem, F.; Bashaar, M. Depression, Anxiety, and Stress Among Nurses During the COVID-19 Wave III: Results of a Cross-Sectional Assessment. *J. Multidiscip. Healthc.* **2021**, *14*, 3093–3101. [CrossRef]
25. Appel, A.P.; Carvalho, A.; Santos, R. Prevalence and factors associated with anxiety, depression and stress in a COVID-19 nursing team. *Rev. Gaúcha De Enferm.* **2021**, *42*, e20200403. [CrossRef] [PubMed]
26. Al Maqbali, M.; Al Sinani, M.; Al-Lenjawi, B. Prevalence of stress, depression, anxiety and sleep disturbance among nurses during the COVID-19 pandemic: A systematic review and meta-analysis. *J. Psychosom. Res.* **2020**, *141*, 110343. [CrossRef] [PubMed]
27. Shi, L.; Lu, Z.A.; Que, J.Y.; Huang, X.L.; Liu, L.; Ran, M.S.; Gong, Y.M.; Yuan, K.; Yan, W.; Sun, Y.K.; et al. Prevalence of and risk factors associated with mental health symptoms among the general population in China during the coronavirus disease 2019 pandemic. *JAMA Netw. Open* **2020**, *3*, e2014053. [CrossRef] [PubMed]
28. Lai, J.; Ma, S.; Wang, Y.; Cai, Z.; Hu, J.; Wei, N. Factors associated with mental health outcomes among health care workers exposed to coronavirus disease 2019. *JAMA Netw. Open* **2020**, *3*, e203976. [CrossRef]
29. Tan, B.Y.Q.; Chew, N.W.S.; Lee, G.K.H.; Jing, M.; Goh, Y.; Yeo, L.L.L. Psychological impact of the COVID-19 Pandemic on health care workers in Singapore. *Ann. Intern. Med.* **2020**, *173*, 317–320. [CrossRef]
30. Chew, N.W.S.; Lee, G.K.H.; Tan, B.Y.Q.; Jing, M.; Goh, Y.; Ngiam, N.J.H. A multinational, multicenter study on the psychological outcomes and associated physical symptoms amongst healthcare workers during COVID-19 outbreak. *Brain Behav. Immun.* **2020**, *88*, 559–565. [CrossRef]
31. Yin, X.; Zeng, L. A study on the psychological needs of nurses caring for patients with corona-virus disease 2019 from the perspective of the existence, relatedness, and growth theory. *Int. J. Nurs. Sci.* **2020**, *7*, 157–160.
32. Li, Z.; Ge, J.; Yang, M.; Feng, J.; Qiao, M.; Jiang, R. Vicarious traumatization in the general public, members, and non-members of medical teams aiding in COVID-19 control. *Brain Behav. Immun.* **2020**, *88*, 916–919. [CrossRef]
33. Li, Z.; Ge, J.; Yang, M.; Feng, J.; Liu, C.; Yang, C. Vicarious traumatization: A psychological problem that cannot be ignored during the COVID-19 pandemic. *Brain Behav. Immun.* **2020**, *87*, 74. [CrossRef]
34. Albert, P.W. Why is depression more prevalent in women? *J. Psychiatry Neurosci.* **2015**, *4*, 219–221. [CrossRef]
35. Liu, Q.; Luo, D.; Haase, J.E.; Guo, Q.; Wang, X.Q.; Liu, S.; Xia, L.; Liu, Z.; Yang, J.; Yang, B.X. The experiences of health-care providers during the COVID-19 crisis in China: A qualitative study. *Lancet Glob. Health* **2020**, *8*, e790–e798. [CrossRef]
36. Montemurro, N. The emotional impact of COVID-19: From medical staff to common people. *Brain Behav. Immun.* **2020**, *84*, 23–24. [CrossRef] [PubMed]
37. Papoutsi, E.; Giannakoulis, V.; Ntella, V.; Pappa, S.; Katsaounou, P. Global burden of COVID-19 pandemic on healthcare workers. *ERJ Open Res.* **2020**, *6*, 00195–2020. [CrossRef] [PubMed]
38. West, C.P.; Dyrbye, L.N.; Shanafelt, T.D. Physician burnout: Contributors, consequences and solutions. *J. Intern. Med.* **2018**, *283*, 516–529. [CrossRef] [PubMed]
39. Bai, Y.; Lin, C.C.; Lin, C.Y.; Chen, J.Y.; Chue, C.M.; Chou, P. Survey of stress reactions among health care workers involved with the SARS outbreak. *Psychiatr. Serv.* **2004**, *55*, 1055–1057. [CrossRef]
40. Wu, P.; Fang, Y.; Guan, Z.; Fan, B.; Kong, J.; Yao, Z. The psychological impact of the SARS epidemic on hospital employees in China: Exposure, risk perception, and altruistic acceptance of risk. *Can. J. Psychiatry* **2009**, *54*, 302–311. [CrossRef]
41. Reynolds, D.L.; Garay, J.R.; Deamond, S.L.; Moran, M.K.; Gold, W.; Styra, R. Understanding, compliance and psychological impact of the SARS quarantine experience. *Epidemiol. Infect.* **2008**, *136*, 997–1007. [CrossRef]
42. Wong, T.W.; Yau, J.K.Y.; Chan, C.L.W.; Kwong, R.S.Y.; Ho, S.M.Y.; Lau, C.C. The psychological impact of severe acute respiratory syndrome outbreak on healthcare workers in emergency departments and how they cope. *Europ. J. Emerg. Med.* **2005**, *12*, 13–18. [CrossRef]
43. Lee, A.M.; Wong, J.G.; McAlonan, G.M.; Cheung, V.; Cheung, C.; Sham, P.C. Stress and psychological distress among SARS survivors 1 year after the outbreak. *Can. J. Psychiatry* **2007**, *52*, 233–240. [CrossRef]
44. Pappa, S.; Ntella, V.; Giannakas, T.; Giannakoulis, V.G.; Papoutsi, E.; Katsaounou, P. Prevalence of depression, anxiety, and insomnia among healthcare workers during the COVID-19 pandemic: A systemic review and meta-analysis. *Brain Behav. Immun.* **2020**, *88*, 901–907. [CrossRef]
45. Labrague, L.J.; De Los Santos, J. COVID-19 anxiety among front-line nurses: Predictive role of organizational support, personal resilience and social support. *J. Nurs. Manag.* **2020**, *22*, 1653–1661. [CrossRef]
46. Hassannia, L.; Taghizadeh, F.; Moosazadeh, M.; Zarghami, M.; Taghizadeh, H.; Dooki, A.F.; Fathi, M.; Alizadeh-Navaei, R.; Hedayatizadeh-Omran, A.; Dehghan, N. Anxiety and Depression in Health Workers and General Population During COVID-19 in IRAN: A Cross-Sectional, S. *MedRxiv* **2020**, *1*, 40–49. [CrossRef] [PubMed]
47. Alnazly, E.; Khraisat, O.M.; Al-Bashaireh, A.M.; Bryant, C.L. Anxiety, depression, stress, fear and social support during COVID-19 pandemic among Jordanian healthcare workers. *PLoS ONE* **2021**, *16*, e0247679. [CrossRef] [PubMed]

International Journal of
Environmental Research and Public Health

MDPI

Systematic Review

Prevalence of Depression and Anxiety in Nurses during the First Eleven Months of the COVID-19 Pandemic: A Systematic Review and Meta-Analysis

Barbara Ślusarska, Grzegorz Józef Nowicki *, Barbara Niedorys-Karczmarczyk and Agnieszka Chrzan-Rodak

Department of Family and Geriatric Nursing, Medical University of Lublin, Staszica 6 Str., PL-20-081 Lublin, Poland; basiaslusarska@gmail.com (B.Ś.); baskaniedorys@gmail.com (B.N.-K.); agnieszkachrzan607@op.pl (A.C.-R.)

* Correspondence: gnowicki84@gmail.com; Tel.: +48-814-486-810

Abstract: The high risk of coronavirus (COVID-19) infection can increase the physical and psychological strain on nurses in professional practice, which can lead to mental health problems. The purpose of this systematic review and meta-analysis is to establish and estimate the combined incidence of depression and anxiety among nurses during the COVID-19 pandemic using standard measurement tools. A systematic search of the electronic databases PubMed, Web of Science, and SCOPUS was carried out to identify cross-sectional studies in the period from 3 March 2020 to 18 February 2021. Two reviewers independently and critically evaluated the studies which have been included, using the Agency for Healthcare Research and Quality checklist. We have identified twenty-three studies (n = 44,165) from nine countries. The combined incidence of depression among nurses was 22% (95% CI 0.15–0.30, I^2 = 99.71%), and anxiety symptoms 29% (95%CI 0.18–0.40, I^2 = 99.92%). No significant difference was observed in the percentage of depression and anxiety between the study subjects working on the frontlines vs. those in a mixed group (those working on the frontlines and behind the lines). This meta-analysis shows that over one-fifth of nurses in professional practice during the COVID-19 epidemic suffer from depression disorders, and almost one-third experience anxiety symptoms. This underscores the importance of providing comprehensive psychological support strategies for nurses working in pandemic conditions. Further longitudinal research is necessary to assess the severity of mental health symptoms related to the COVID-19 epidemic factor.

Keywords: symptoms; depression symptoms; COVID-19; frontlines; nurses; meta-analysis; systematic review

Citation: Ślusarska, B.; Nowicki, G.J.; Niedorys-Karczmarczyk, B.; Chrzan-Rodak, A. Prevalence of Depression and Anxiety in Nurses during the First Eleven Months of the COVID-19 Pandemic: A Systematic Review and Meta-Analysis. *Int. J. Environ. Res. Public Health* **2022**, *19*, 1154. https://doi.org/10.3390/ijerph19031154

Academic Editors: Richard Gray and Sonia Udod

Received: 12 December 2021
Accepted: 16 January 2022
Published: 20 January 2022

1. Introduction

The Severe Acute Respiratory Coronavirus-2 (SARS-CoV-2) pandemic has brought about many socio-economic changes in many countries; it has also triggered heavy burdens on health systems around the world, many of which had already been struggling with problems [1]. The World Health Organization (WHO) declared a global pandemic of SARS-CoV-2 on 11 March 2020 [2]. Since then, many countries have introduced limitations on social interaction and people have had to adapt to new restrictions at work and to the demands of social isolation. Nurses in their turn commenced working in the new reality of the pandemic, being on the frontlines of the fight against coronavirus, and their work plays a key role in the well-being and health of society as a whole [3,4].

Nurses have had to confront numerous problems which had, and continue to have, an effect on the quality of their work and their mental health [5–7]. The large number of cases increased the number of patients hospitalized with COVID-29, and often the state of health of these patients was very serious, requiring specialist care in intensive care units. Another problem is nurse staffing shortages all over the world, aggravated during the pandemic by sick leaves associated with SARS-CoV-2 infections. The already-existing nursing personnel shortage has dramatically worsened. One consequence of this has been increased workloads. There was also the problem of availability of equipment and personal protective gear. There have been situations where, due to the shortage of protective equipment, healthcare workers (HCW) faced the need to work without full epidemic protection [8,9]. Nurses worry both about the health of their loved ones, and about the risk of bringing the virus into their homes. The pandemic has caused thousands of deaths, which can be a source of existential stress [8,10].

The phenomenon of the COVID-19 pandemic and dynamic changes in the health care system have created difficult and even crisis situations in the lives of HCWs. Crisis situations as states of disorganization cause a person to experience a sense of fear, shock, emotional and psychological destabilization, and difficulties in getting through specific situations [11]. During the coronavirus pandemic, HCWs have faced crisis situations that increased the risk of physical and psychological suffering, conducive to the development of symptoms of anxiety, depression, and other emotional crises [12], as well as psychological disorders manifesting in states of anxiety, panic, or emotional disorders [13]. A review of the mental health literature related to the COVID-19 pandemic reveals preliminary evidence suggesting that symptoms of anxiety and depression and reports of stress are common psychological reactions to the COVID-19 pandemic [14]. In a systematic umbrella review of the global evidence of seven meta-analyses on the incidence of anxiety and depression among HCWs during the COVID-19 pandemic, it was shown that the overall incidence of states of anxiety or depression in HCWs during the COVID-19 epidemic were 24.94% and 24.83%, respectively [15]. In a systematic umbrella review of global evidence comprising ten systematic reviews, on the other hand, it was found that in the group of HCWs, the incidence of anxiety among nurses ranged from 22.8% to 27% while the incidence of depression among nurses was 28% [16].

The COVID-19 pandemic has put HCWs around the world in an unprecedented situation, but the risk of adverse psychological effects is particularly high among nurses. Healthcare workers, including large numbers of nurses, face difficult conditions and limited resources in caring for COVID-19 patients, putting them at an increased risk of depression and anxiety [14]. Therefore, it is essential to continue assessing the mental health of nurses and other high-risk groups at the forefront of this pandemic. The scale of this phenomenon changes over time, so it becomes increasingly important to understand the extent of nurses' mental health problems and needs, and to recognize the nature of these changes, in order to provide mental health services and implement effective psychological interventions [17].

The fast-paced and changeable nature of the mental health emergency during the COVID-19 pandemic and the numerous studies from various countries on the most common mental health problems among nurses that have been published in recent months are prerequisites for systematic reviews. For that reason, the goal of the present study is to update and refine the results of current systematic reviews and meta-analyses published by Olaya et al. [18], Al Maqbali et al. [19], Fernandez et al. [16], and Varghese et al. [20], and to carry out a systematic review and meta-analysis of published studies in the long term over the first eleven months of the COVID-19 pandemic that pertain to the prevalence of anxiety and depression among nurses only. Therefore, this systematic review and meta-analysis had the goal of determining any spread of mental health problems in terms of incidence of depression and anxiety among nurses during the COVID-19 pandemic, with respect to standard measurement tools and taking into account the results of long-term (eleven months) studies assessing the severity of mental health disorders.

We focused our review and meta-analysis on nurses only, the long duration of the pandemic (i.e., eleven months), the use of standardized measurement tools for anxiety and depression, and factors that could be selected relating to the incidence of depression and anxiety, such as gender, marital status, test sites (Asia vs. other continents), and places of employment during the COVID-19 pandemic (first line vs. mixed) of the respondents.

2. Materials and Methods

2.1. Study Design

This study was conducted in accordance with the recommendations of Preferred Reporting Items for Systematic Reviews and Meta-analyses (PRISMA) [21]. The systematic review protocol is not available in any databases and is available from the authors. The PRISMA checklist for this study is available in Table S1.

2.2. Search Strategy

Relevant articles from the moment the WHO announced the coronavirus pandemic, i.e., from 11 March 2020 to 18 February 2021, were searched for in the PubMed, Web of Science, and SCOPUS databases. Only English-language articles were sought. The article search was performed using an alternate combination of, and/or, the following terms: "COVID", "COVID-19", "Severe Acute Respiratory Syndrome Coronavirus 2", "SARS-CoV-2", "SARSCoV2", "SARS CoV2", "2019-nCov", "2019 Novel Corona virus", "Coronavirus Disease 2019", "Coronavirus Disease-19", "SARS Coronavirus 2", "nurses", "nursing personnel", "registered nurses", "nursing staff", "mental health", "mental health disorders", "stress", "stress disorder", "post-traumatic stress", "PSTD", "mental wellbeing", "psychological distress", "depression", and "anxiety". The search strategy used for each database is given in the Supplementary Materials, Table S2. After key articles were identified, manual document searches and tracking were performed for each reference on the list of key articles to increase the sensitivity of the literature search. In the case of a more comprehensive search, there would have been no limit to the results.

2.3. Selection Criteria

The selection criteria for relevant articles were the following: (1) the articles were cross-sectional, cohort, or case-control studies; (2) the participants were nurses working in various healthcare facilities during the coronavirus pandemic; (3) the articles were written in English; (4) the articles were published in peer-reviewed journals; (5) the degree of depression or anxiety was measured with a standardized questionnaire; and (6) the studies had sufficient data for calculating the degree of depression or anxiety in groups of practicing nurses.

Studies were excluded if (1) they were reviews, commentaries, editorials, or summaries of conferences; (2) they were not concerned with the goals of our review; (3) they were conducted on a small group of fewer than twenty respondents; (4) they included representatives of various medical professions without the possibility of extracting separate results for nurses; or (5) there were no clear cut-off points for standardized tools measuring the severity of depression and anxiety, and mean results were not taken into account.

Two independent reviewers reviewed the titles and abstracts and then the full text of potential articles, in accordance with the inclusion and exclusion criteria. Any discrepancies were established by consensus with a third reviewer.

2.4. Data Extraction

The data were extracted by one independent reviewer using predefined data extraction forms. The extracted data were then verified by a second reviewer. All disagreements were resolved by consensus with a third reviewer. The information extracted included characteristics of the study (author, year, and country of publication, study design, and sample size), characteristics of the samples (gender, age, marital status, place of work during the coronavirus pandemic), estimation of the dissemination of depression and anxiety, diagnostic criteria for depression and anxiety, and the research tool used to assess depression and anxiety.

2.5. Quality Assessment

Two independent authors assessed the risk of bias of the included studies. Discrepancies were resolved, by consensus, with a third author. In the analyzed cross-sectional studies, the evaluation form recommended by the Agency for Healthcare Research and Quality [22] was used. The checklist consisted of eleven items. Each item was rated as "yes", "no", or "unclear". One point was assigned for each item, if the research met the methodological standards. For ratings of "no" or "unclear", zero points were assigned. Results with a score of zero to three points indicated a low-quality study, four to seven points indicated a moderate quality study, and eight to eleven points indicated a high-quality study.

2.6. Ethical Approval

No ethical approval was obtained for the study because we used published data that had already been ethically validated.

2.7. Statistics Analysis

Pooled prevalence of depression and anxiety were calculated using meta-analytic methods. Modeling with random effects and the restricted maximum likelihood (REML) estimator was used to account for between-study heterogeneity. I^2 statistics were calculated to provide a measure of the proportion of overall variation attributable to between-study heterogeneity. Differences in response rate between categories of study definition, number of drugs, and number of types of malignancies were assessed using the Q test for heterogeneity in meta-regression. To examine the influence of several included characteristics on the prevalence of depression and anxiety, we performed a meta-regression. The following factors were studied: percentage of women, percentage of respondents who were married, the place where the study was conducted (Asia vs. other continents), and the place of work during the COVID-19 pandemic (front lines vs. mixed). The Egger test was used to assess the possibility of publication bias. Meta-analysis was conducted using meta for package (R version 3.3.3); $p < 0.05$ was considered statistically significant.

3. Results

3.1. Study Inclusion

The literature search process and the process for selecting studies are detailed in Figure 1. A total of 3367 studies were identified in the databases. After removing duplicates, 2569 were searched, 2417 of which were then excluded by study title and 112 of which were excluded on the basis of the abstract, leaving 40 studies for the eligibility phase. The full text of these articles was assessed by independent reviewers for eligibility. Fifteen articles were excluded at this stage because they did not meet eligibility requirements for the reasons listed in Figure 1. Following a critical evaluation of the full texts of the articles by consensus, two articles were excluded because it was not possible to define the incidence of depression and anxiety in the analyzed research. Moreover, the decision was made at this stage to include for further analysis only part of the results in an article that evaluated the level of anxiety and depression in nurses during the period of exacerbation and during the stable period of the COVID-19 pandemic [23]. As that article's research for both periods of the pandemic was conducted with the same group of nurses, it was decided to include only the results obtained during the exacerbation period of the pandemic. In the end, twenty-three studies were used in the qualitative analysis, eighteen of which analyzed the level of depression and twenty-two of which analyzed the level of anxiety.

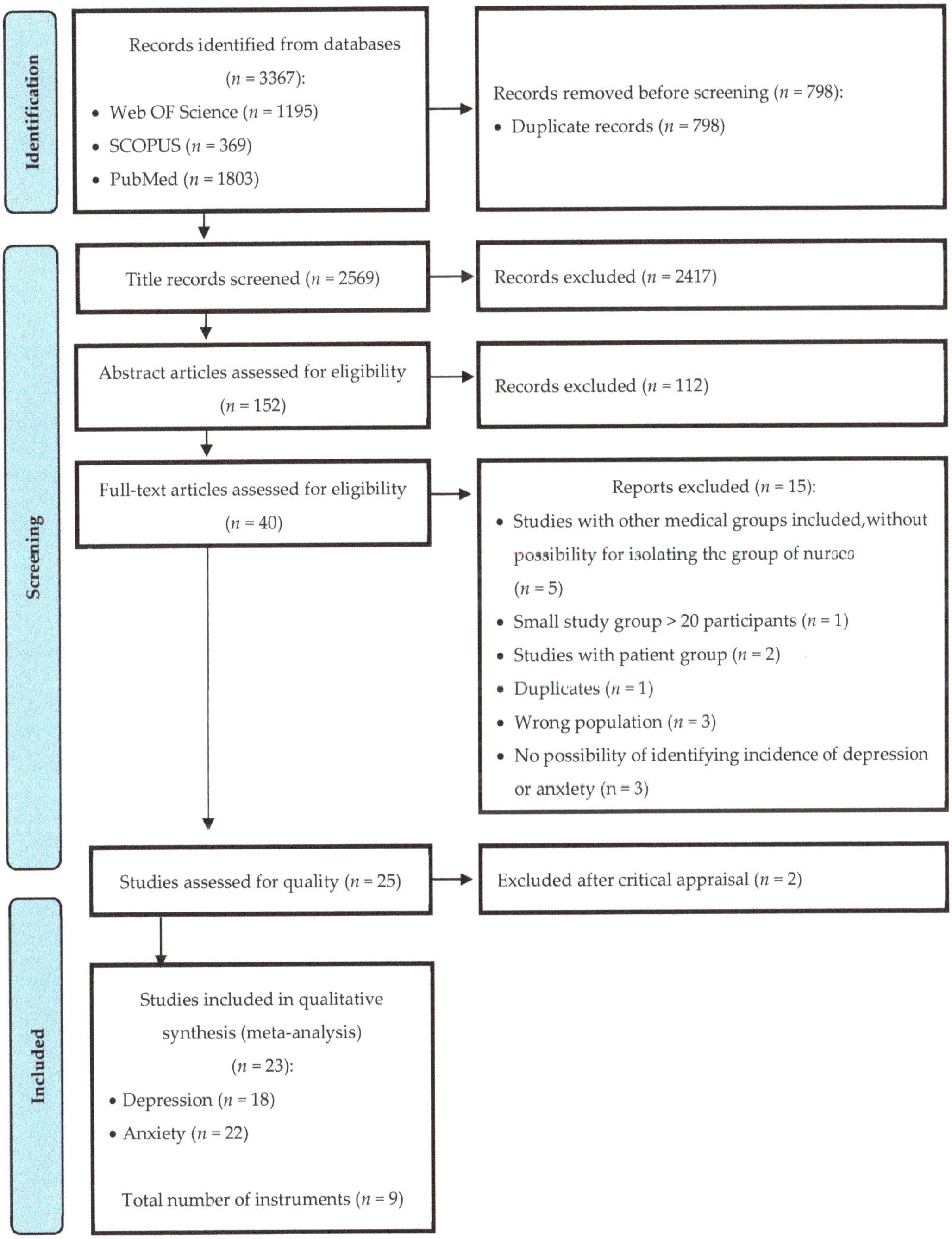

Figure 1. PRISMA flow diagram.

3.2. Description of Included Studies

A summary of the studies selected for our meta-analysis is presented in Table 1. The total sample size analyzed in the twenty-three studies that were included was 44,165 nurses, with sample sizes of each study ranging from 88 to 21,119 participants. With respect to the gender of the participants, one study did not give information on the gender of its participants [24]; this study included 3676 nurses. Of the 40,489 nurses in studies where the percentage of men and women was specified, 95.81% (n = 38,792) were women. In fifteen of the studies [6,25–38], the average age of respondents was determined by the mean, which ranged from 28.8 to 45.1 years; in the remaining studies [9,23,39–43], the age distribution was described by categories. In one study [24], neither average age nor age categories was given.

The research was conducted in nine countries: China (56.52%, n = 13) [23,26–29,32,34,35,38–42], the Philippines (8.7%, n = 2) [30,31], the United States (8.7%, n = 2) [6,9], Turkey (4.35%, n = 1) [36], Saudi Arabia (4.35%, n = 1) [25], Iran (4.35%, n = 1) [33], Great Britain (4.35%, n = 1) [37], Brazil (4.35%, n = 1) [43], and Canada (4.35%, n = 1) [24]. In eleven of the studies, nurses working on the front lines were surveyed [26,28,30–32,34,36,39–41,43], while in the other studies the nurses were working on the front lines as well as behind the lines in the fight against COVID-19, without distinct categories.

3.3. Quality Assessment

The studies were scored with the aid of the AHRQ checklist. In evaluating the quality of the analyzed studies according to AHRQ assessment criteria, as many as fifteen of the studies were characterized as being of moderate quality, while the remaining eight were characterized as being of low quality. None of the studies received scores indicative of high quality. Detailed results of the evaluation of the quality of the studies included in this meta-analysis are presented in the Supplementary Materials, Table S3.

3.4. Characteristics of Instruments Used to Assess Depression and Anxiety Levels

The characteristics of the nine tools used to assess the severity of depression and anxiety symptoms and the cut-off points for the scales adopted in this meta-analysis are presented in Table 2.

In thirteen of the studies [6,9,23–26,32–35,37,39,41] the Patient Health Questionnaire (PHQ-9) for evaluating the severity of depression symptoms was used. In four of the studies [27–29,42], the Self-Rating Depression Scale (SDS) was used to assess depression symptoms.

Six tools for assessing the severity of anxiety symptoms were systematically identified among the studies included in the review. In twelve studies [6,9,23–25,32–35,37,39,41] this tool was the Generalized Anxiety Disorder (GAD-7) assessment. In four studies [27–29,42] the Self-Rating Anxiety Scale (SAS) was used. In two of the studies [30,31], the Coronavirus Anxiety Scale (CAS) was used to assess the severity level of anxiety. In one study, [40] the Hamilton rating scale for anxiety (HAMA) was used, and one study [36] used the State-Trait Anxiety Inventory (STAI).

Two articles identified two tools consisting of two subscales that assessed both depression and anxiety symptoms at the same time. In one of these articles [38], this tool was the short version of the Depression Anxiety Stress Scale (DASS-21). In the other article, the Hospital Anxiety and Depression Scale (HAD) was used [43].

Table 1. Characteristics of the included studies.

No.	First Author (Year)/Country	Study Design	Study Size	Participants	Age, Years (Mean ± SD or n (%))	Female n (%)	Married n (%)	Position	Start Date	End Date	Depression Assessment Tool	n (%) with Depression	Anxiety Assessment Tool	n (%) with Anxiety	Survey Method	Quality Score
1.	Abu-Snieneh (2021)/Saudi Arabia [25]	cross-sectional study	1265	nurses from all regions of Saudi Arabia	28.83 ± 5.29	1101 (87)	783 (61.9)	Mixed	April 2020	June 2020	PHQ-9	329 (25.9)	GAD-7	234 (18.5)	Online survey	5
2.	An et al. (2020)/China [26]	cross-sectional study	1103	Emergency Department nurses from all regions of China	32.20 ± 7.61	1001 (90.8)	710 (64.4)	Frontline	15 March 2020	20 March 2020	PHQ-9	176 (16)	N/A	N/A	Online survey	4
3.	Cai et al. (2020)/China [23]	longitudinal study	709	nurses from Renmin Hospital of Wuhan University (outbreak period of the pandemic)	≥ 30 287 (40.4)	684 (96.5)	376 (53)	Mixed	29 January 2020	2 February 2020	PHQ-9	109 (15.4)	GAD-7	84 (11.8)	Online survey	7
4.	Han et al. (2020)/China [27]	cross-sectional survey	21,119	nurses from 14 prefecture and city hospitals in Gansu Province, located in northwest China	31.89 ± 7.08	20909 (98.6)	15499 (73.1)	Mixed	7 February 2020	10 February 2020	SDS	1738 (8.2)	SAS	996 (4.7)	Online survey	5
5.	Hong et al. (2021)/China [39]	cross-sectional study	4692	nurses from the Chongqing region	≥ 31 2043 (43.6)	4548 (96.9)	3013 (64.2)	Frontline	8 February 2020	14 February 2020	PHQ-9	442 (9.4)	GAD-7	379 (8.1)	Online survey	4
6.	Hu et al. (2020)/China [28]	cross-sectional study	2014	nurses from two hospitals in Wuhan	30.99 ± 6.17	1754 (87.1)	1230 (61.1)	Frontline	13 February 2020	24 February 2020	SDS	217 (10.7)	SAS	288 (14.3)	Online survey	5
7.	Jiang et al. (2020)/China [29]	cross-sectional study	1569	nurses from the Linxia Hui Autonomous Prefecture	30.93 ± 6.48	1550 (98.8)	1170 (74.6)	Mixed	6 February, 2020	10 February 2020	SDS	127 (8.1)	SAS	68 (4.3)	Online survey	3
8.	Labrague et al. (2021)/Philippines [31]	cross-sectional study	736	nurses from frontline hospital and public health nurses in Western Samar	31.9 ± 7.35	574 (78.1)	312 (42.45)	Frontline	1 September 2020	1 October 2020	N/A	N/A	CAS	130 (37.4)	Online survey	3
9.	Labrague et al. (2020)/Philippines [30]	cross-sectional study	325	nurses from frontline hospital in Region 8, Philippines	30.94 ± 6.67	243 (74.8)	108 (33.2)	Frontline	25 April 2020	25 May 2020	N/A	N/A	CAS	123 (37.8)	PAPI	4
10.	Li et al. (2020)/China [12]	cross-sectional study	176	nurses from tertiary hospitals in Wuhan city, Hubei province that were designated to receive new patients with COVID-19	≥30 72 (40.8)	136 (77.3)	88 (50)	Frontline	Unknown	Unknown	N/A	N/A	HAMA	136 (77.3)	Online survey	3
11.	Pang et al. (2021)/China [32]	cross-sectional study	282	nurses from three hospitals that received patients with COVID-19 in both Guangdong and Hubei Provinces	31.61 ± 7.60	250 (88.65)	169 (59.93)	Frontline	10 March 2020	20 March 2020	PHQ-9	160 (56.74)	GAD-7	134 (47.52)	Online survey	4
12.	Pouralizadeh et al. (2020)/Iran [33]	cross-sectional study	441	Nurses working in the province of Guilan at the University of Medical Sciences hospital	36.34 ± 8.74	420 (95.2)	335 (76)	Mixed	7 April 2020	12 April 2020	PHQ-9	165 (37.5)	GAD-7	171 (38.7)	Online survey	3
13.	Tu et al. (2020)/China [34]	cross-sectional study	100	nurses from Wuhan in "Huoshenshan" hospital	34.44 ± 5.85	100 (100)	70 (70)	Frontline	7 February 2020	24 February 2020	PHQ-9	10 (10)	GAD-7	2 (2)	Online survey	4

Table 1. *Cont.*

No.	First Author (Year)/Country	Study Design	Study Size	Participants	Age, Years (Mean ± SD or n (%))	Female n (%)	Married n (%)	Position	Start Date	End Date	Depression Assessment Tool	n (%) with Depression	Anxiety Assessment Tool	n (%) with Anxiety	Survey Method	Quality Score
14.	Wang et al. (2021)/China [35]	cross-sectional study	586	nurses working in Nanjing in the province of Jiangsu	31.07 ± 7.54	563 (96.08)	353 (60.24)	Unknown	14 February 2020	3 March 2020	PHQ-9	64 (11.09)	GAD-7	40 (6.83)	Online survey	6
15.	Xiong et al. (2020)/China [41]	cross-sectional study	223	nurses from one of the public tertiary hospitals in Xiamen, Fujian Province	≥36 77 (34.5)	217 (97.3)	Unknown	Frontline	16 February 2020	25 February 2020	PHQ-9	15 (6.7)	GAD-7	27 (12.1)	Online survey	5
16.	Yurtseven et al. (2021)/Turkey [36]	cross-sectional study	270	Nurses working in a university hospital operating as a pandemic hospital	36.83 ± 9.23	237 (87.77)	193 (71.48)	Frontline	Unknown	Unknown	N/A	N/A	SAI	249 (92.4)	Online survey	3
17.	Zheng et al. (2021)/China [42]	cross-sectional study	3 228	nurses from Sichuan Province and Wuhan City	≥30 1706 (52.9)	3121 (96.7)	Unknown	Mixed	27 January 2020	3 February 2020	SDS other cutoff points	N/A	SAS	122 (3.8)	Online survey	4
18.	Roberts et al. (2021)/United Kingdom [37]	cross-sectional study	255	nurses working in respiratory clinical areas	45.1 ± 9.77	226 (88.6)	Unknown	Mixed	1 May 2020	1 June 2020	PHQ-9	31 (17.2)	GAD-7	40 (20.9)	Online survey	3
19.	Dal'Bosco et al. (2020)/Brazil [43]	cross-sectional study	88	nurses working at a regional university hospital of reference for coping with COVID-19 in Paraná	≥ 31 51 (58)	79 (89.8)	32 (36.4)	Frontline	March 2020	April 2020	HAD-D	22 (25)	HAD-A	43 (48.9)	Online survey	5
20.	Arnetz et al. (2020)/USA [9]	cross-sectional study	695	nurses working in the state of Michigan	≥45 376 (54.7)	644 (93.6)	Unknown	Mixed	7 May 2020	29 May 2020	PHQ-9	167 (26.1)	GAD-7	144 (22.6)	Online survey	3
21.	Havaei et al. (2021)/Canada [24]	cross-sectional study	3 676	members of the provincial nurses' union	Unknown	Unknown	Unknown	Mixed	January 2020	July 2020	PHQ-9	1391 (41.4)	GAD-7	1273 (37.6)	Online survey	3
22.	Kim et al. (2021)/USA [6]	cross-sectional study	320	nurses who graduated from the nursing school at a private, 4-year liberal arts university in Southern California	33 (min-max: 21–67) BRAK SD	302 (94.4)	Unknown	Mixed	20 April 2020	10 May 2020	PHQ-9	83 (26)	GAD-7	138 (43)	Online survey	5
23.	Mekonen et al. (2021)/China [38]	cross-sectional study	293	nurses working in the northwest of Amhara Regional	29.6 ± 5.1	133 (45.4)	156 (53.2)	Mixed	25 September 2020	20 October 2020	DASS-21 Depression	162 (55.3)	DASS-21 Anxiety	204 (69.6)	PAPI	6

Abbreviations: PHQ-9: 9-item Patient Health Questionnaire; GAD-7: 7-item Generalized Anxiety Disorder; SDS: Self-Rating Depression Scale; SAS: Self-Rating Anxiety Scale; CAS: Coronavirus Anxiety Scale; PAPI: Paper and Pencil Interview; HAMA: the Hamilton rating scale for anxiety; BDI: Beck Depression Inventory; SAI: State Anxiety Inventory; DASS-21: Depression Anxiety Stress Scales (short version); HAD: Hospital Anxiety and Depression Scale; HAD-D: Hospital Anxiety and Depression Scale, subscales for identifying depression; HAD-A: Hospital Anxiety and Depression Scale, subscales for identifying anxiety;

Table 2. Characteristics of research tools used in assessing depression and anxiety levels.

Instrument	Name Abbreviation	Characteristic Being Assessed	Administration Method	Number of Items, (Sub)Scale(s) (Number of Items)	Response Options, Range of Score	The Cut-Off Point Adopted in the Meta-Analysis
Patient Health Questionnaire	PHQ-9	Depression	Self-reported	9 items	Dichotomous scoring system and 4-points Likert scale 0–27 - normal (0–4), - mild depression (5–9), - moderate depression (10–14), - severe depression (15–27)	≥10 points
Self-Rating Depression Scale	SDS	Depression	Self-reported	20 items	Dichotomous scoring system and 4-points Likert scale 25–100 - normal (25–52), - mild depression (53–62), - moderate depression (63–72), - severe depression (≥73)	≥63 points
Depression Anxiety Stress Scales	DASS-21	Depression/Anxiety	Self-reported	21 items, on 7 items for each subscale: - depression - anxiety - stress	Dichotomous scoring system and 4-points Likert scale 0–21 for each subscale	Depression ≥ 10 points Anxiety ≥ 8 points
Hospital Anxiety and Depression Scale	HAD	Depression/Anxiety	Self-reported	14 items, on 7 items for each subscale: - HAD-A-anxiety - HAD-D-depression	Dichotomous scoring system 0–21 for each subscale	≥8 points for each subscale:

Table 2. *Cont.*

Instrument	Name Abbreviation	Characteristic Being Assessed	Administration Method	Number of Items, (Sub)Scale(s) (Number of Items)	Response Options, Range of Score	The Cut-Off Point Adopted in the Meta-Analysis
Generalized Anxiety Disorder	GAD-7	Anxiety	Self-reported	7 items	Dichotomous scoring system and 4-points Likert scale 0–21 - normal (0–4), - mild anxiety (5–9), - moderate anxiety (10–14), - severe anxiety (15–27)	≥10 points
Self-Rating Anxiety Scale	SAS	Anxiety	Self-reported	20 items	Dichotomous scoring system and 4-points Likert scale 25–100 - normal (25–49), - mild anxiety (50–59), - moderate anxiety (60–69), - severe anxiety (70–100)	≥60 points
Coronavirus Anxiety Scale	CAS	Anxiety	Self-reported	5 items	Dichotomous scoring system and 5-points Likert scale 5–25	≥9 points
The Hamilton rating scale for anxiety	HAMA	Anxiety	Self-reported	14 items	Dichotomous scoring system 0–56	≥7 points
State Anxiety Inventory	SAI	Anxiety	Self-reported	20 items	Dichotomous scoring system and 4-points Likert scale 20–80 - normal (≤36), - moderate anxiety (37–42), - high anxiety (≥43)	≥37 points

3.5. Incidence of Depression among Nurses during the COVID-19 Pandemic

Figure 2 presents the percentage for occurrence of depression estimated by the analyzed studies. The incidence of depression among nurses during the COVID-19 pandemic was reported in eighteen of the studies, totaling 39,430 respondents. The combined overall rate of depression as assessed by all tools was 22% (95% CI 0.15–0.30, I^2 = 99.71%). The depression rate in thirteen of the studies (14,347 nurses), assessed with the PHQ-9 tool, was 23% (95% CI 0.15–0.31, I^2 = 99.27%). In the remaining five studies (n = 25,083 nurses), using other tools (SDS, HAD-D and DASS-21 Depression), the depression rate was 21% (95% CI 0.03–0.38, I^2 = 99.87%).

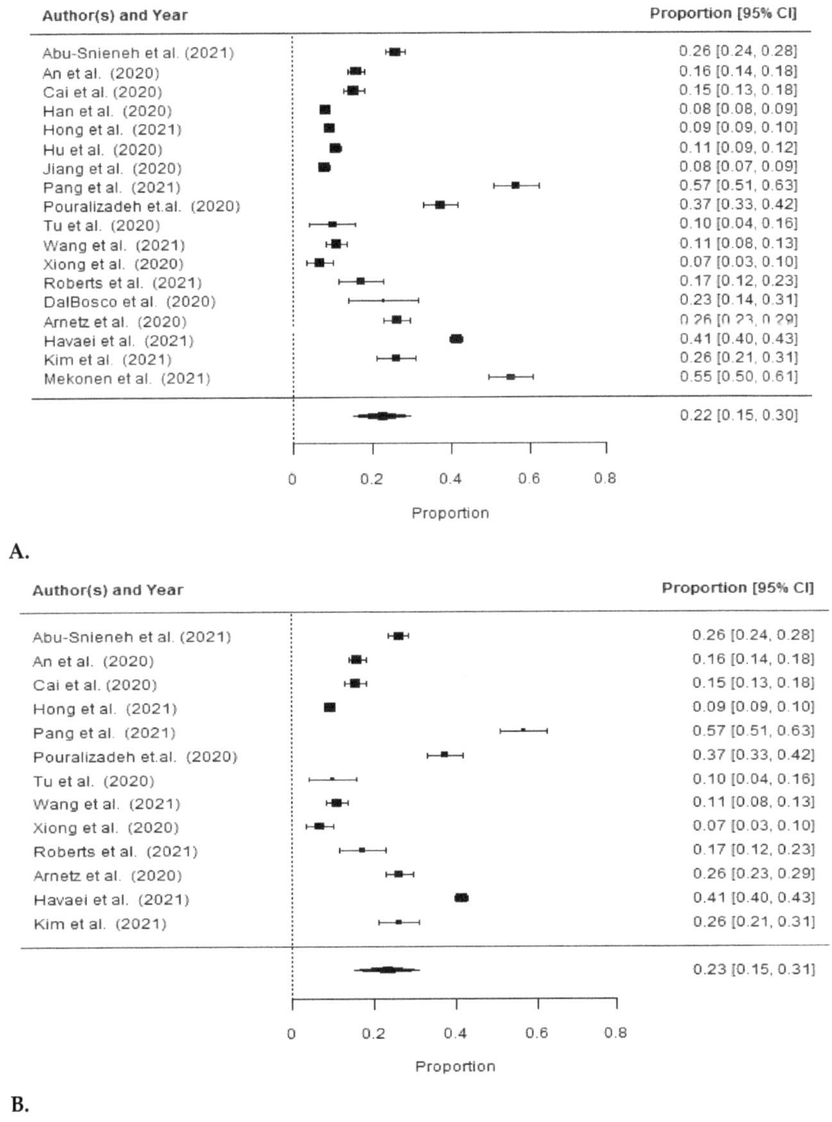

Figure 2. *Cont.*

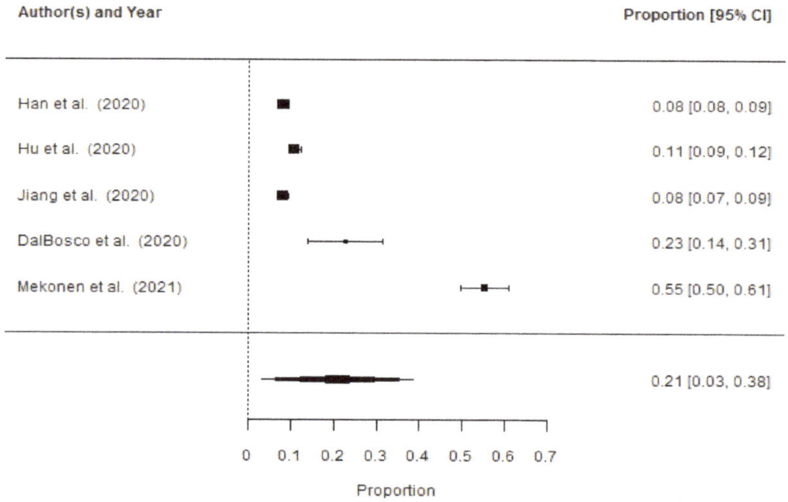

C.

Figure 2. Forest plot for the prevalence of depression among nurses: (**A**) overall result; (**B**) assessment scale PHQ-9; (**C**) remaining assessment scales, excluding PHQ-9.

3.6. Incidence of Anxiety among Nurses during the COVID-19 Pandemic

Figure 3 presents the percentage of the occurrence of anxiety estimated in the analyzed studies. Twenty-two of the studies assessed the intensity of anxiety during the COVID-19 pandemic among 43,062 nurses. The overall percentage of respondents with anxiety disorders was 29% (95% CI = 0.18–0.40, I^2 = 99.92%). In twelve of the studies (n = 13,244), the severity of anxiety was assessed on the GAD-7 scale, and the percentage of persons with anxiety was 22% (95% CI = 0.14–0.31, I^2 = 99.42%). In four of the studies, anxiety was assessed on the SAS scale (n = 27,930). The percentage of respondents with anxiety assessed by the SAS scale was 7% (95% CI = 0.02–0.12, I^2 = 99.49%). For the other 1888 nurses who were evaluated for anxiety by CAS, HAMA, SAI, HAD-A, and DASS-21, the incidence of anxiety was assessed at 57% (95% CI = 0.35–0.79, I^2 = 99.30%).

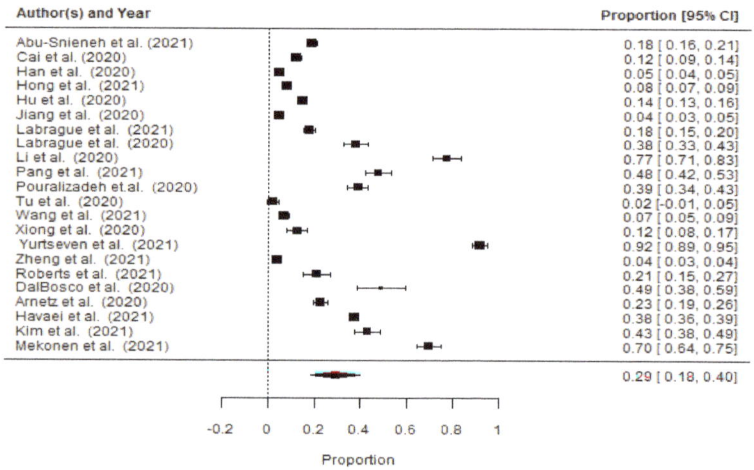

A.

Figure 3. *Cont.*

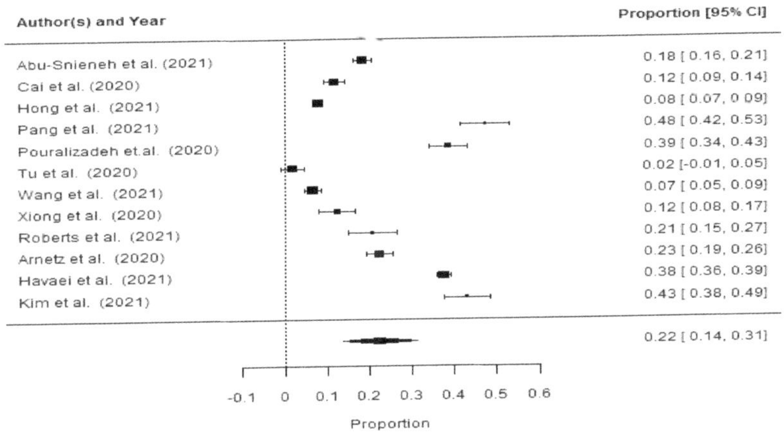

B.

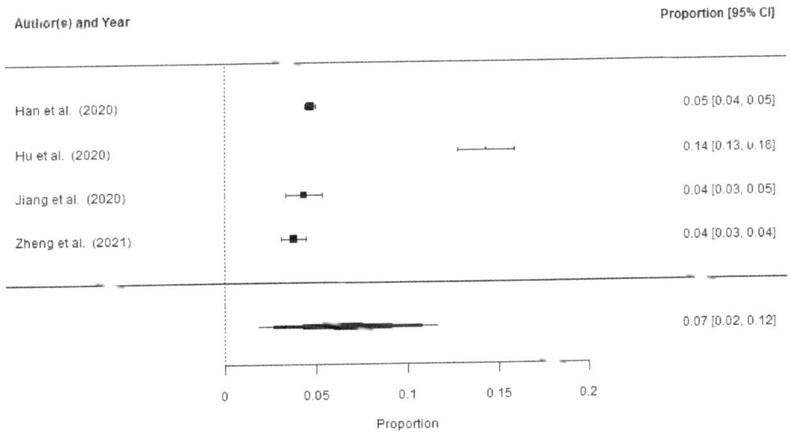

C.

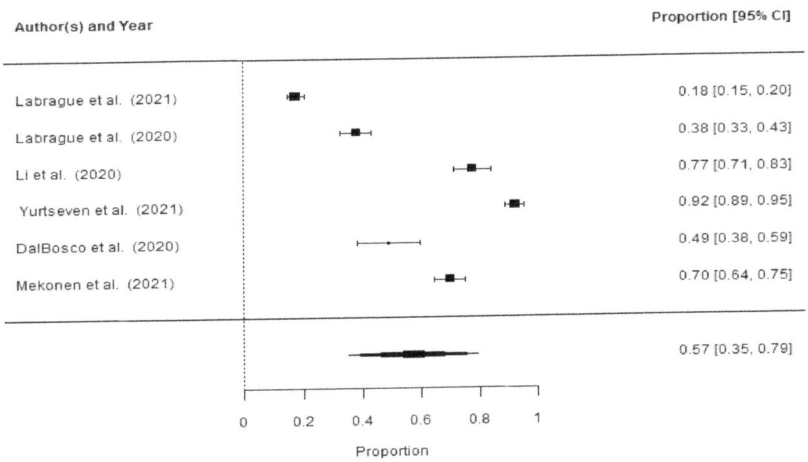

D.

Figure 3. Forest plot for the prevalence of anxiety among nurses: (**A**) overall result; (**B**) assessment scale GAD-7; (**C**) assessment scale SAS; (**D**) remaining assessment scales, excluding GAD-7 and SAS.

3.7. Factors Relating to the Incidence of Depression and Anxiety

A percentage of the women participating in this study was significantly and negatively associated with the incidence of depression (b = −0.008, 95% CI = −0.013–0.0036, p = 0.01) and anxiety (b = −0.012, 95% CI = −0.020–0.0047, p = 0.039) in the research reporting the incidence of both depression and anxiety. There was no significant relationship between the percentage of married respondents in the study and the incidence of depression (b = −0.004, 95% CI = −0.0133–0.0052, p = 0.39) or anxiety (b = −0.0049, 95% CI = −0.016–0.006, p = 0.38). A similar lack of relationships was observed when the studies were narrowed down, with depression and anxiety assessed only via PHQ-9 or GAD-7.

Table 3 presents a comparison of the percentage of depression and anxiety in relation to the location where the study was conducted (Asia vs. the other continents) and the respondents' places of work during the COVID-19 pandemic (frontlines vs. mixed). No significant percentage difference was observed in depression or anxiety between those working on the frontlines and those behind the lines. There was no significant correlation between the place where the research was carried out and the frequency of anxiety.

Table 3. Factors related to the incidence of depression and anxiety.

Variable	Depression			Anxiety		
	Proportion	95% CI	p	Proportion	95%CI	p
Place of research:						
	All instruments					
Asia	0.18	(0.09–0.26)	0.063	0.25	(0.11–0.38)	0.196
Other continents	0.31	(0.20–0.43)		0.40	(0.20–0.61)	
	Only PHQ-9			Only GAD-7		
Asia	0.21	(0.10–0.31)	0.44	0.18	(0.07–0.29)	0.15
Other continents	0.28	(0.13–0.42)		0.31	(0.17–0.45)	
Position:						
	All instruments					
Frontline	0.19	(0.07–0.31)	0.45	0.31	(0.15–0.46)	0.43
Mixed	0.25	(0.15–0.35)		0.23	(0.11–0.35)	
	Only PHQ-9			Only GAD-7		
Frontline	0.20	(0.06–0.33)	0.54	0.17	(0.02–0.32)	0.40
Mixed	0.25	(0.18–0.33)		0.26	(0.16–0.35)	

3.8. Publication Bias

The funnel plot demonstrated a mild asymmetry in prevalence of depression and anxiety (Supplementary Materials, Figures S1 and S2). However, the p-value for the Egger's test was 0.32 and 0.10 for depression and anxiety, respectively, indicating no, or undetected, publication bias.

4. Discussion

During the pandemic, the high risk of infection and the spread of COVID-19 increased the physical and mental burden of all healthcare workers, including nurses active in their profession [39]. With respect to psychological disorders, nurses are seen as a high-risk group even when working without the additional burden of a pandemic [44,45]. A state of poor mental health in nurses can be detrimental not only to nurses themselves but can also affect the quality of patient care [45]. Unfortunately, nursing shortages are an ongoing problem the world over. High turnover and absenteeism due to illness can cause staff overload and an inability to meet the expectations of patients and their families. An over-taxed team can put patients at risk of a greater error rate, longer hospitalization, and even mortality [46]. Thus, as the prevalence of mental health disorders among nurses increases, so will the economic, social, and individual effects of these disorders [45]. The SARS-CoV-2 pandemic has put a heavy burden on healthcare systems all around the world. To broaden our understanding of the experiences of nurses during the COVID-19 pandemic, we conducted a systematic literature review and meta-analysis of the prevalence of mental health problems in the areas of depression and anxiety disorders in the nursing population during the COVID-19 pandemic, based on the long period of time (eleven months) for which data on the topic has been collected.

The pooled analysis of the data consisted of cross-sectional studies in an overall group of 44,165 nurses. The goal of our systematic review and meta-analysis was to determine the prevalence of anxiety- and depression-related mental health problems among nurses during the COVID-19 pandemic. Severity levels of anxiety and depression were assessed in twenty-three studies [6,9,23–43], the results of which were analyzed. Four articles addressed the incidence of anxiety itself, as well as the factors intensifying it, among working nurses [30,31,36,40]. Meta-analysis indicates that the incidence of depression among nurses during the COVID-19 pandemic is 22% (95% CI = 0.15–0.30, I^2 = 99.71%), and the incidence of anxiety is 29% (95% CI = 0.18–0.40, I^2 = 99.92%). The considerable heterogeneity of these results should be emphasized. Our discoveries highlight an important issue regarding nurses and their mental health issues during the COVID-19 pandemic.

An extensive analysis of the literature showed that several systematic reviews and meta-analyses on the incidence of mental health disorders, among HCWs and in the general population, have already been published. Saragih et al. [47] conducted a systematic review and meta-analysis of studies on the spread of anxiety and depression among healthcare workers. In the studies they analyzed, 27.9% of the participants were doctors, 43.7% nurses, and 7% were other kinds of healthcare workers. They determined that the incidence of anxiety among healthcare workers was 39% and the incidence of depression was 36%. A similar systematic review and meta-analysis was carried out by Hao et al. [48]. Their results indicated an incidence of depression and anxiety in healthcare workers of 24.1% and 28.6%, respectively.

In contrast, the results of a large-scale meta-analysis of evidence summarizing seventy-one published articles on mental health problems during the COVID-19 pandemic, covering a group of 146,139 people from China, the United States, Japan, India, and Turkey, and including patients with confirmed COVID-19 infections, healthcare workers, and the general population, showed a frequency of anxiety symptoms at 32.6% and a frequency of depressive disorders at 27.6% during the COVID-19 pandemic. The authors of that meta-analysis also made the noteworthy observation that mental health problems (i.e., anxiety and depression) had the highest incidence in COVID-19 patients, and that lower levels of anxiety and depression, as well as sleep problems, were observed in healthcare professionals than in the general population. Another systematic review and meta-analysis found that the prevalence of depression among all healthcare workers was 24% (95% CI = 20–28%), while among nurses it was 25% (95% CI = 18–33%), among doctors it was 24% (95% CI = 16–31%), and for frontline healthcare workers it was 43% (95% CI = 28–59%) [18].

Al Maqbali et al. [19] conducted a systematic review and meta-analysis of the spread of stress, depression, anxiety, and sleep disorders among nurses during the COVID-19 pandemic. Their results indicated that the incidence of anxiety was 37% (95% CI = 32–41%), while the incidence of depression was 35% (95% CI = 31–39%). In another systematic review and meta-analysis that assessed the spread of mental health disorders among nurses, it was found that the incidence of anxiety symptoms among the surveyed nurses was 33% (95% CI = 24–43%) with significant heterogeneity (I^2 = 99.4%, $p < 0.01$), while the occurrence of depression was 32% (95% CI = 21–44%), with significant heterogeneity (I^2 = 99.4%, $p < 0.01$) [20].

In our meta-analysis, we found a lower incidence of anxiety and depression symptoms than in the studies cited above. The higher incidence of anxiety and depression in the meta-analyses conducted by Saragih et al. [47] and by Liu et al. [49], in comparison with our own results, may be related to distinctions in the work carried out in the various professions among the respondents. The duration of data collection in these studies also has significance. Higher rates of anxiety and depression, in comparison with our results, were also demonstrated in meta-analyses carried out on groups of nurses, i.e., in the meta-analyses of Al. Maqbali et al. [19] and Varghese et al. [20]. Our systematic review and meta-analysis summarize publications from both the onset of the pandemic and the period that followed (covering eleven months), compared to the cited systematic reviews and meta-analyses. It is therefore worthwhile to compare the results obtained in our meta-analysis with the results of meta-analyses published in this field before the COVID-19 pandemic. Unfortunately, there are not many such publications in the literature. Results of a systematic review and meta-analysis of the incidence of depression among nurses of various departments and hospitals in Iran indicated the prevalence of depression symptoms as being at a level of 26.88% (95% CI = 21.45–31.91%) [50]. A trend of change in the rate of incidence of depression can therefore be observed in this example, taking into account the time of publication of data from the various meta-analyses within the narrative analysis. However, a hypothesis that chronic effect factors related to the COVID-19 epidemic are a self-regulating restraint on the incidence of depressive and anxiety disorders among nurses cannot constitute a prerequisite for outreach and intervention studies for alleviating mental health problems among nurses and helping them cope with their burdens.

The prolonged duration of the COVID-19 pandemic also prompts a search for evidence of its long-term psychological effect on HCW. A replication cross-sectional study one year after the COVID-19 outbreak to assess the mental health outcomes of HCW (n = 1 033) at an academic hospital in Verona (Italy) found that the percentage of HCW above the cut-off point increased from 2020 to 2021 across all performance domains (anxiety, 50.1% vs. 55.7, $p < 0.05$; depression, 26.6% vs. 40.6%, $p < 0.001$). In turn, a multivariate analysis showed that one year after the COVID-19 outbreak, nurses were more likely to experience anxiety and depression than other HCWs [51].

The measurement tools used to assess the prevalence of anxiety and depression, namely their psychometric properties and the cut-off points that were adopted, may be important factors in the differences identified in meta-analyses. In our research, we sought to select studies on the basis of depression and anxiety being measured by the use of standardized questionnaires, and we made critical quality assessments of the studies that were included. In terms of moderation, analysis of a large-scale meta-analysis of the evidence [49] of the moderating role of measuring tools on the results in assessing mental health problems among research participants during a pandemic was confirmed, with results varying significantly depending on the scale used. Thus, the high prevalence of mental health problems during the COVID-19 pandemic, including anxiety symptoms and depressive disorders, may indicate (when analyzed in a fairly large sample) that heterogeneous results for these mental health problems may be caused by the use of non-standardized tools without reliable psychometric properties being maintained for the studied populations. Another possible reason for the differences in prevalence is the variation in the cut-off points for elevated symptoms for the same measurement instrument of the studied variable, which we took into account when qualifying studies for our analysis (for details, see Table 1).

In addition, research results published in scientific journals have provided very timely and significant evidence that the COVID-19 pandemic poses a threat to the mental health of individuals. However, it should be noted that most of these studies were conducted in the early and peak periods of the pandemic's development, which may indicate an overestimation of the frequency of these problems. Furthermore, in the interests of sharing new research results in a timely manner, articles that were not of high quality have been published in some journals. Our quality assessment using the AHRQ checklist showed that eight of the twenty-three articles included in the review were of low quality. It should be noted that all studies included in our meta-analysis used self-reported standardized questionnaires to assess symptomatology of depression and anxiety. Moreover, the use of a large variety of scales could lead to differences in the assessment of depression and anxiety occurrence. In fact, our results showed that studies using the SDS (Self-Rating Depression Scale) questionnaire indicated lower rates of depression, while studies using CAS, HAMA, SAI, HAD-A, and DASS-21 indicated a much higher prevalence of anxiety. Despite the convenience of using the same standardized measurement tools for an initial assessment of the characteristics of a diagnosis based on clinical interviews, it is not always possible for this usage to be fully reflected in epidemiological studies, because these are simply screening tools and require in-depth clinical diagnostic follow-up.

Study Limitations

When interpreting our results, it is necessary to take certain limitations into account. First, most of the studies included in the meta-analysis used convenient samples, so their representativeness of the nursing population may be unreliable. Second, depression and anxiety were evaluated mainly by using self-reported data from questionnaires that might also introduce other psychological and emotional manifestations, e.g., strongly expressing public approval of the medical profession during the pandemic. Such data may also be less accurate than data from full clinical interviews. Third, an assessment of the incidence of depression and anxiety among nurses in professional practice, based on their inclusion in cross-sectional studies in the meta-analysis, makes it difficult to establish a causal relationship between the pandemic and depression and anxiety. Depressive disorders and anxiety symptoms in the included studies had not been assessed before the pandemic. This has limited our ability to investigate additional psychological strains on nurses caused by the COVID-19 pandemic, as we do not have data on their prior mental state. For this reason, it is necessary to be careful when interpreting our results. In addition, our systematic review was conducted mainly in medical databases (PubMed, SCOPUS, and Web of Science); therefore, some articles, especially those related to psychology, may not be reflected. Further, our research did not take into account reports that concerned all health care professionals, among which a group of nurses was included as a subset.

Finally, we found certain sources of heterogeneity. In the articles we analyzed, various scales were used and various cut-off values were adopted. For example, the use of the SDS questionnaire was associated with lower rates of depression, and the use of the CAS, HAMA, SAI, HAD-A, and DASS-21 scales were associated with higher rates of anxiety. In addition, the studies we analyzed were carried out at various points of time; the feelings of nurses might differ as the COVID-19 pandemic runs its course from the moment when it first appeared. Many new scientific papers on COVID-19 are published each day, and as the pandemic continues, we have ever-increasing knowledge about it, which makes it difficult to conduct an up-to-date and in-depth review.

Another limitation is the fact that the vast majority of the studies analyzed in the present review came from Asia, mainly China, with only a small portion coming from other continents. This geographical and cultural context may have influenced various types of psychological responses to the same stressor among healthcare workers; therefore, the obtained results should not be generalized for all nurses. Yet another important limitation is the fact that due to the use of the selected inclusion and exclusion criteria, it is possible that relevant articles may have been omitted in the first stage of collecting the data for this review.

Future studies should strive to investigate the prevalence of depression and anxiety among nurses in other countries and, where possible, use random sampling as well as longitudinal designs for determining the evolution of mental health problems in this population. In addition, subsequent systematic reviews and meta-analyzes could consider the severity of depression and anxiety in nurses at different periods of the pandemic, taking into account milestones in the fight against the pandemic.

5. Conclusions

To summarize, our systematic review and meta-analysis provide a long-term and comprehensive synthesis of existing evidence confirming the incidence of depressive disorders in more than one-fifth of those studied, and anxiety symptoms among just under one-third of nurses, during the COVID-19 pandemic. These findings help quantify the emerging need for psychological support for nurses within the context of the COVID-19 pandemic. As new evidence continues to emerge, we will be able to continue updating this meta-analysis and carrying out further efforts in analyzing factors related to the epidemic, to facilitate planning at the national level, improve mental health security system interventions, and design prospective solutions for similar epidemic events involving those in the nursing profession in the future.

Supplementary Materials: The following are available online at https://www.mdpi.com/article/10.3390/ijerph19031154/s1, Table S1: PRISMA Checklist, Table S2: Search strategy and search terms; Table S3: Quality assessment result of observational studies (n = 23) using the questioner according The Agency for Healthcare Research and Quality (AHRQ); Figure S1: Funnel plot for meta-analysis of the prevalence of depression; Figure S2: Funnel plot for meta-analysis of the prevalence of depression (A: for all tools; B: only for GAD-7).

Author Contributions: Conceptualization, B.Ś. and G.J.N.; methodology, B.Ś. and G.J.N.; triage of the studies, B.N.-K. and A.C.-R.; data analysis, G.J.N. and B.Ś.; writing—original draft preparation, B.Ś., G.J.N., B.N.-K. and A.C.-R.; writing—review and editing, B.Ś. and G.J.N.; supervision, B.Ś. and G.J.N. All authors have read and agreed to the published version of the manuscript.

Funding: This research received no external funding.

Institutional Review Board Statement: Not applicable.

Informed Consent Statement: Not applicable.

Data Availability Statement: The datasets used and/or analyzed during the current study are available from the corresponding author on reasonable request.

Conflicts of Interest: The authors declare no conflict of interest.

References

1. Aiken, L.H.; Sloane, D.M.; Bruyneel, L.; Van den Heede, K.; Sermeus, W.; RN4CAST Consortium. Nurses' reports of working conditions and hospital quality of care in 12 countries in Europe. *Int. J. Nurs. Stud.* **2013**, *50*, 143–153. [CrossRef]
2. World Health Organization. Announces COVID-19 Outbreak a Pandemic Retrieved. Available online: http://www.euro.who.int/en/heps//:coronavirus.jhu.edu/map.alth-topics/health-emergencies/coronavirus-covid-19/news/news/2020/3/who-announces-covid-19-outbreak-a-pandemic (accessed on 10 March 2021).
3. Pfefferbaum, B.; North, C.S. Mental health and the COVID-19 pandemic. *N. Engl. J. Med.* **2020**, *383*, 510–512. [CrossRef]
4. Li, X.; Zhou, Y.; Xu, X. Factors associated with the psychological well-being among front-line nurses exposed to COVID-2019 in China: A predictive study. *J. Nurs. Manag.* **2021**, *29*, 240–249. [CrossRef]
5. Halcomb, E.; McInnes, S.; Williams, A.; Ashley, C.; James, S.; Fernandez, R.; Stephen, C.; Calma, K. The experiences of primary healthcare nurses during the COVID-19 pandemic in Australia. *J. Nurs. Scholarsh.* **2020**, *52*, 553–563. [CrossRef]
6. Kim, S.C.; Quiban, C.; Sloan, C.; Montejano, A. Predictors of poor mental health among nurses during COVID-19 pandemic. *Nurs. Open.* **2021**, *8*, 900–907. [CrossRef]
7. Di Tella, M.; Romeo, A.; Benfante, A.; Castelli, L. Mental health of healthcare workers during the COVID-19 pandemic in Italy. *J. Eval. Clin. Pract.* **2020**, *26*, 1583–1587. [CrossRef]
8. Shechter, A.; Diaz, F.; Moise, N.; Anstey, D.E.; Ye, S.; Agarwal, S.; Birk, J.L.; Brodie, D.; Cannone, D.E.; Chang, B.; et al. Psychological distress, coping behaviors, and preferences for support among New York healthcare workers during the COVID-19 pandemic. *Gen. Hosp. Psychiatry* **2020**, *66*, 1–8. [CrossRef]
9. Arnetz, J.E.; Goetz, C.M.; Sudan, S.; Arble, E.; Janisse, J.; Arnetz, B.B. Personal protective equipment and mental health symptoms among nurses during the COVID-19 pandemic. *J. Occup. Environ. Med.* **2020**, *62*, 892–897. [CrossRef] [PubMed]
10. Zaka, A.; Shamloo, S.E.; Fiorente, P.; Tafuri, A. COVID-19 pandemic as a watershed moment: A call for systematic psychological health care for frontline medical staff. *J. Health Psychol.* **2020**, *25*, 883–887. [CrossRef] [PubMed]
11. James, R.K.; Gilliland, B.E. *Crisis Intervention Strategies*; Cengage Learning: Belmont, MA, USA, 2017.
12. Li, X.; Li, S.; Xiang, M.; Fang, Y.; Qian, K.; Xu, J.; Li, J.; Zhang, Z.; Wang, B. The prevalence and risk factors of PTSD symptoms among medical assistance workers during the COVID-19 pandemic. *J. Psychosom. Res.* **2020**, *139*, 110270. [CrossRef] [PubMed]

13. Heitzman, J. Impact of COVID-19 pandemic on mental health. *Psychiatr. Pol.* **2020**, *54*, 187–198. [CrossRef]
14. Rajkumar, R.P. COVID-19 and mental health: A review of the existing literature. *Asian J. Psychiatr.* **2020**, *52*, 102066. [CrossRef]
15. Sahebi, A.; Nejati-Zarnaqi, B.; Moayedi, S.; Yousefi, K.; Torres, M.; Golitaleb, M. The prevalence of anxiety and depression among healthcare workers during the COVID-19 pandemic: An umbrella review of meta-analyses. *Prog. Neuropsychopharmacol. Biol. Psychiatry* **2021**, *107*, 110247. [CrossRef]
16. Fernandez, R.; Sikhosana, N.; Green, H.; Halcomb, E.J.; Middleton, R.; Alananzeh, I.; Trakis, S.; Moxham, L. Anxiety and depression among healthcare workers during the COVID-19 pandemic: A systematic umbrella review of the global evidence. *BMJ Open.* **2021**, *11*, e054528. [CrossRef]
17. Goldmann, E.; Galea, S. Mental health consequences of disasters. *Annu. Rev. Public Health* **2014**, *35*, 169–183. [CrossRef]
18. Olaya, B.; Pérez-Moreno, M.; Bueno-Notivol, J.; Gracia-García, P.; Lasheras, I.; Santabárbara, J. Prevalence of depression among healthcare workers during the COVID-19 outbreak: A systematic review and meta-analysis. *J. Clin. Med.* **2021**, *10*, 3406. [CrossRef] [PubMed]
19. Al Maqbali, M.; Al Sinani, M.; Al-Lenjawi, B. Prevalence of stress, depression, anxiety and sleep disturbance among nurses during the COVID-19 pandemic: A systematic review and meta-analysis. *J. Psychosom. Res.* **2021**, *141*, 110343. [CrossRef] [PubMed]
20. Varghese, A.; George, G.; Kondaguli, S.V.; Naser, A.Y.; Khakha, D.C.; Chatterji, R. Decline in the mental health of nurses across the globe during COVID-19: A systematic review and meta-analysis. *J. Glob. Health* **2021**, *11*, 05009. [CrossRef] [PubMed]
21. Page, M.J.; Moher, D.; Bossuyt, P.M.; Boutron, I.; Hoffmann, T.C.; Mulrow, C.D.; Shamseer, L.; Tetzlaff, J.M.; Akl, E.A.; Brennan, S.E.; et al. PRISMA 2020 explanation and elaboration: Updated guidance and exemplars for reporting systematic reviews. *BMJ* **2021**, *372*, n160. [CrossRef] [PubMed]
22. Rostom, A.; Dube, C.; Cranney, A.; Saloojee, N.; Sy, R.; Garritty, C.; Sampson, M.; Zhang, L.; Yazdi, F.; Mamaladze, V.; et al. Celiac disease. *Evid. Rep. Technol. Assess. (Summ.)* **2004**, *104*, 1–6.
23. Cai, Z.; Cui, Q.; Liu, Z.; Li, J.; Gong, X.; Liu, J.; Wan, Z.; Yuan, X.; Li, X.; Chen, C.; et al. Nurses endured high risks of psychological problems under the epidemic of COVID-19 in a longitudinal study in Wuhan China. *J. Psychiatr. Res.* **2020**, *131*, 132–137. [CrossRef] [PubMed]
24. Havaei, F.; Ma, A.; Staempfli, S.; MacPhee, M. Nurses' workplace conditions impacting their mental health during COVID-19: A cross-sectional survey study. *Healthcare* **2021**, *9*, 84. [CrossRef] [PubMed]
25. Abu-Snieneh, H.M. Psychological factors associated with the spread of Coronavirus disease 2019 (COVID-19) among nurses working in health sectors in Saudi Arabia. *Perspect. Psychiatr. Care.* **2021**, *57*, 1399–1408. [CrossRef] [PubMed]
26. An, Y.; Yang, Y.; Wang, A.; Li, Y.; Zhang, Q.; Cheung, T.; Ungvari, G.S.; Qin, M.Z.; An, F.R.; Xiang, Y.T. Prevalence of depression and its impact on quality of life among frontline nurses in emergency departments during the COVID-19 outbreak. *J. Affect Disord.* **2020**, *276*, 312–315. [CrossRef] [PubMed]
27. Han, L.; Wong, F.K.Y.; She, D.L.M.; Li, S.Y.; Yang, Y.F.; Jiang, M.Y.; Ruan, Y.; Su, Q.; Ma, Y.; Chung, L.Y.F. Anxiety and depression of nurses in a North West Province in China during the period of novel coronavirus pneumonia outbreak. *J. Nurs. Scholarsh.* **2020**, *52*, 564–573. [CrossRef]
28. Hu, D.; Kong, Y.; Li, W.; Han, Q.; Zhang, X.; Zhu, L.X.; Wan, S.W.; Liu, Z.; Shen, Q.; Yang, J.; et al. Frontline nurses' burnout, anxiety, depression, and fear statuses and their associated factors during the COVID-19 outbreak in Wuhan, China: A large-scale cross-sectional study. *EClinicalMedicine* **2020**, *24*, 100424. [CrossRef]
29. Jiang, M.; Li, S.; She, D.; Yan, F.; Chung, Y.F.; Han, L. The psychological effect of 2019 coronavirus disease outbreak on nurses living in Islamic culture dominant region, China. *Arch. Psychiatr. Nurs.* **2020**, *34*, 513–519. [CrossRef] [PubMed]
30. Labrague, L.J.; De Los Santos, J.A.A. COVID-19 anxiety among front-line nurses: Predictive role of organisational support, personal resilience and social support. *J. Nurs. Manag.* **2020**, *28*, 1653–1661. [CrossRef] [PubMed]
31. Labrague, L.J.; De Los Santos, J.A.A. Prevalence and predictors of coronaphobia among frontline hospital and public health nurses. *Public Health Nurs.* **2021**, *38*, 382–389. [CrossRef]
32. Pang, Y.; Fang, H.; Li, L.; Chen, M.; Chen, Y.; Chen, M. Predictive factors of anxiety and depression among nurses fighting coronavirus disease 2019 in China. *Int. J. Ment. Health Nurs.* **2021**, *30*, 524–532. [CrossRef]
33. Pouralizadeh, M.; Bostani, Z.; Maroufizadeh, S.; Ghanbari, A.; Khoshbakht, M.; Alavi, S.A.; Ashrafi, S. Anxiety and depression and the related factors in nurses of Guilan University of Medical Sciences hospitals during COVID-19: A web-based cross-sectional study. *Int. J. Afr. Nurs. Sci.* **2020**, *13*, 100233. [CrossRef] [PubMed]
34. Tu, Z.H.; He, J.W.; Zhou, N. Sleep quality and mood symptoms in conscripted frontline nurse in Wuhan, China during COVID-19 outbreak: A cross-sectional study. *Medicine* **2020**, *99*, e20769. [CrossRef] [PubMed]
35. Wang, Q.Q.; Fang, Y.Y.; Huang, H.L.; Lv, W.J.; Wang, X.X.; Yang, T.T.; Yuan, J.M.; Gao, Y.; Qian, R.L.; Zhang, Y.H. Anxiety, depression and cognitive emotion regulation strategies in Chinese nurses during the COVID-19 outbreak. *J. Nurs. Manag.* **2021**, *29*, 1263–1274. [CrossRef] [PubMed]
36. Yurtseven, Ş.; Arslan, S. Anxiety levels of university hospital nurses during the COVID-19 pandemic. *Perspect. Psychiatr. Care* **2021**, *57*, 1558–1565. [CrossRef] [PubMed]
37. Roberts, N.J.; McAloney-Kocaman, K.; Lippiett, K.; Ray, E.; Welch, L.; Kelly, C. Levels of resilience, anxiety and depression in nurses working in respiratory clinical areas during the COVID pandemic. *Respir. Med.* **2021**, *176*, 106219. [CrossRef] [PubMed]
38. Mekonen, E.; Shetie, B.; Muluneh, N. The Psychological impact of COVID-19 outbreak on nurses working in the Northwest of Amhara Regional State Referral Hospitals, Northwest Ethiopia. *Psychol. Res. Behav. Manag.* **2021**, *13*, 1353–1364. [CrossRef]

39. Hong, S.; Ai, M.; Xu, X.; Wang, W.; Chen, J.; Zhang, Q.; Wang, L.; Kuang, L. Immediate psychological impact on nurses working at 42 government-designated hospitals during COVID-19 outbreak in China: A cross-sectional study. *Nurs. Outlook* **2021**, *69*, 6–12. [CrossRef]
40. Li, R.; Chen, Y.; Lv, J.; Liu, L.; Zong, S.; Li, H.; Li, H. Anxiety and related factors in frontline clinical nurses fighting COVID-19 in Wuhan. *Medicine* **2020**, *99*, e21413. [CrossRef]
41. Xiong, H.; Yi, S.; Lin, Y. The psychological status and self-efficacy of nurses during COVID-19 outbreak: A cross-sectional survey. *Inquiry* **2020**, *57*, 46958020957114. [CrossRef]
42. Zheng, R.; Zhou, Y.; Fu, Y.; Xiang, Q.; Cheng, F.; Chen, H.; Xu, H.; Fu, L.; Wu, X.; Feng, M.; et al. Prevalence and associated factors of depression and anxiety among nurses during the outbreak of COVID-19 in China: A cross-sectional study. *Int. J. Nurs. Stud.* **2021**, *114*, 103809. [CrossRef]
43. Dal'Bosco, E.B.; Floriano, L.S.M.; Skupien, S.V.; Arcaro, G.; Martins, A.R.; Anselmo, A.C.C. Mental health of nursing in coping with COVID-19 at a regional university hospital. *Rev. Bras. Enferm.* **2020**, *73* (Suppl. 2), e20200434. [CrossRef]
44. Almazan, J.U.; Albougami, A.S.; Alamri, M.S. Exploring nurses' work-related stress in an acute care hospital in KSA. *J. Taibah Univ. Med. Sci.* **2019**, *14*, 376–382. [CrossRef] [PubMed]
45. Maharaj, S.; Lees, T.; Lal, S. Prevalence and risk factors of depression, anxiety, and stress in a cohort of Australian nurses. *Int. J. Environ. Res. Public Health* **2018**, *16*, 61. [CrossRef]
46. Tuckett, A.; Winters-Chang, P.; Bogossian, F.; Wood, M. 'Why nurses are leaving the profession . . . lack of support from managers': What nurses from an e-cohort study said. *Int. J. Nurs. Pract.* **2015**, *21*, 359–366. [CrossRef]
47. Saragih, I.D.; Tonapa, S.I.; Saragih, I.S.; Advani, S.; Batubara, S.O.; Suarilah, I.; Lin, C.J. Global prevalence of mental health problems among healthcare workers during the COVID-19 pandemic: A systematic review and meta-analysis. *Int. J. Nurs. Stud.* **2021**, *121*, 104002. [CrossRef]
48. Hao, Q.; Wang, D.; Xie, M.; Tang, Y.; Dou, Y.; Zhu, L.; Wu, Y.; Dai, M.; Wu, H.; Wang, Q. Prevalence and risk factors of mental health problems among healthcare workers during the COVID-19 pandemic: A systematic review and meta-analysis. *Front. Psychiatry* **2021**, *12*, 567381. [CrossRef]
49. Liu, X.; Zhu, M.; Zhang, R.; Zhang, J.; Zhang, C.; Liu, P.; Feng, Z.; Chen, Z. Public mental health problems during COVID-19 pandemic: A large-scale meta-analysis of the evidence. *Transl. Psychiatry* **2021**, *11*, 384. [CrossRef] [PubMed]
50. Fereidouni, Z.; Dehghan, A.; Najafi Kalyani, M. The prevalence of depression among nurses in Iran: A systematic review and meta-analysis. *Int. J. Med. Rev.* **2018**, *5*, 163–167. [CrossRef]
51. Lasalvia, A.; Bodini, L.; Amaddeo, F.; Porru, S.; Carta, A.; Poli, R.; Bonetto, C. The sustained psychological impact of the COVID-19 pandemic on health care workers one year after the outbreak—A repeated cross-sectional survey in a Tertiary Hospital of North-East Italy. *Int. J. Environ. Res. Public Health* **2021**, *18*, 13374. [CrossRef] [PubMed]

International Journal of
Environmental Research and Public Health

MDPI

Article

Spirituality in Patients at the End of Life—Is It Necessary? A Qualitative Approach to the Protagonists

E. Begoña García-Navarro [1,2,3,*], Alicia Medina-Ortega [1] and Sonia García Navarro [1,3,4]

1 Nursing Department, University of Huelva, 21007 Huelva, Spain; aliciadelosmaresaxo@gmail.com (A.M.-O.); soniagarcianavarro@gmail.com (S.G.N.)
2 Social Studies and Social Intervention Research Center (ESEIS), Contemporary Thinking and Innovation for Social Development Research Center (COIDESO), Faculty of Nursing, University of Huelva, 21007 Huelva, Spain
3 Coping In the End of Life Reseach Center (AFLV), INVESTIGA+, Junta de Andalucía, 41008 Sevilla, Spain
4 United Clinical Management (U.G.C. Los Rosales), Distrito Huelva-Costa-Condado-Campiña, 21007 Huelva, Spain
* Correspondence: bego.garcia@denf.uhu.es

Abstract: Spirituality is the most unknown aspect of palliative care despite being the need that is most altered in the last moments of life. Objective. To identify on the one hand the spiritual needs of patients who are at the end of life and on the other hand, the way in which nursing professionals can work to provide effective accompaniment in this process. Method. A qualitative study was conducted which applied different data collection techniques. This was done to describe the phenomenon from a holistic perspective in relation to experts' perceptions of the competencies required by health professionals and palliative patients' spiritual needs. Semi-structured interviews were conducted within both populations. In order to analyze the qualitative data collected through interviews, discourse was analyzed according to the Taylor–Bodgan model and processed using Atlas.ti software. Results. Three well-differentiated lines of argument are extracted from the discourse in each of the groups, on the one hand in the group of patients they define the concept of spirituality, system of values and beliefs, and the Factors that influence the spirituality of patients at the end of life (differentiating palliative care areas/other areas) and on the other, the professionals agree with the patients in the line of argument of concept of spirituality although they define more metaphysical categories and the other two lines of argument that result are the spiritual attention in this process and the need for formation in spirituality. Conclusions. The provision of spiritual care gives meaning to the actions of nursing professionals when it comes to providing end-of-life care, achieving holistic care, humanizing death, and promoting a dignified end.

Keywords: spirituality; palliative care; nursing skills; end-of-life

Citation: García-Navarro, E.B.; Medina-Ortega, A.; García Navarro, S. Spirituality in Patients at the End of Life—Is It Necessary? A Qualitative Approach to the Protagonists. *Int. J. Environ. Res. Public Health* **2022**, *19*, 227. https://doi.org/10.3390/ijerph19010227

Academic Editors: Richard Gray, Sonia Udod and Paul B. Tchounwou

Received: 11 November 2021
Accepted: 24 December 2021
Published: 26 December 2021

1. Introduction

In a first approach to the word Spirituality, it is necessary to mention that it comes from the Latin spirit, which means breathing, vitality. If this concept is related to the word Alma, in Latin anima, it means the capacity for transcendence [1]. A more contemporary definition is described by Mytko and Knight [2] as a set of feelings that lead the individual to connect with himself, with others, with the purpose of life or with nature in search of value and meaning, to find peace and harmony. These authors mention the difference between the constructs of Spirituality and Religiosity, indicating that they are not exclusive of each other, that they can overlap or exist separately, as long as, carefully, they are categorized and interpreted. Under this same conceptual line, Puchalski describes spirituality as the aspect of the human condition that refers to the way in which individuals seek and express meaning and purpose, as well as the way in which they express a state of connection with the moment, with oneself (self), with others, with nature and with the significant or Sacred [3].

The appreciation of the spiritual dimension and the inclusion of professionals trained in palliative and spiritual care capable of listening to fears and pain providing hope and recognition to terminally ill patients are the basis of spiritual care models. This model of care has its foundations in the biopsychosocial–spiritual model of care [4] and the patient-centered model of care [5].

Spirituality is the least understood aspect of end-of-life care despite, surprisingly, being the most altered need in this process. Spirituality is a priority in the fundamental objectives of palliative care work. Palliative care focuses on improving the patient's quality of life, and this cannot be favored as a whole if the spiritual dimension is not addressed [6]. In the words of Stanislav Grof: *"Spiritual development is an evolutionary capacity that is innate to all human beings"*. It describes an impulse towards totality and the discovery of one's true potential [7]. It is as common and natural as birth, physical growth, and death, being an integral part of our existence. It is a classic concept, in the same way as the concept of human beings and their fear of facing death and the search for vital meaning. This means that, at the end-of-life, this fear and anguish grows exponentially making spiritual care hugely important for terminally ill patients [8]. For patients in palliative circumstances, spirituality is considered as a driving force to provide an optimal response to the circumstances of these individuals in relation to their own existence. "The practice of spirituality is also seen as an agent for the transformation and regulation of emotions, with this representing an effective tool for reducing levels of depression and anxiety in those who find themselves in the final stages of life" [9].

A high percentage of hospitalized patients are faced with emotions such as anguish, fear, depression, anger, dissatisfaction, etc., which are emotions with a high emotional and spiritual load. Nursing must care for these emotions [6]. According to studies conducted by Silvia Caldeira, *"spiritual anguish is defined as a state of suffering which is related with a lack of meaning in life"* [10]. In order to tackle this diagnostic, spiritual care must be provided by nursing professionals. This care should consider the way in which professionals are and act with both patients and their families. It should, therefore, be perceived as a holistic dimension of palliative care which preserves dignity and facilitates patients in their search for vital meaning and the relief of suffering [8].

It should be recognized that this sphere is a competence which must come, not only from psychology professionals belonging to the palliative care team but, also, from within the entire multidisciplinary team [11]. Different studies show that the nursing plays an important role at the time of facing death. Facing death appropriately poses the need to know the best way to act when faced with situations which generate great suffering and anxiety. This is the case as much for the individual living the end-of-life process, as for the professionals accompanying them and conditions their approach to providing care fitted to patient needs. An appropriate approach helps patients have a good death [10–12].

At its heart, all nursing care provision is based on spirituality as it is guided by hope, compassion and the conviction that an individual's life remains full of possibilities, even though it is limited in certain aspects [12,13]. Nonetheless, some challenges are encountered in real life. Indeed, despite spiritual care being an integral part of nursing care, it's provision is highly diverse and can be influenced by the individual, cultural, and educational background of each nurse [13]. In the same way, a number of prejudices with regards to nursing are found in the healthcare system. Nurses have been judged to have underestimated the spiritual dimension in care and various factors have been proposed to explain this limitation. These factors include a lack of awareness of its importance and a lack of preparation, incorrect interpretation of the term spirituality, lack of desire to provide spiritual care. However, different systematic reviews have served to demonstrate [8–14] that in the nursing setting, nurses demonstrate an understanding of spiritual and religious care that is in tune with the construct that is advocated in the present day as much in the current Spanish setting as in Europe and the United States. Professionals have also indicated that patients serve as a mirror of their own mortality and, when health workers are open to listening and sharing anguish, they are able to understand the process gone through by patients and facilitate the search for making sense of the illness itself. Nevertheless, professionals who are not able to face up to their own problems with regards to death will find it even more difficult to face up to the death of another person and with seek to distance themselves from it [15]. The attitudes of nurses towards this type of care is favorable, although a need to raise awareness of specific related care responsibilities is detected. Training relating to some aspects of intervention needs to be completed [16].

With the development of the study we propose on the one hand to identify the spiritual needs of patients in a situation of terminality through their discourse and on the other, by the hand of experts in palliative care, to know what professional skills are decisive to respond to the needs of patients at the end of life. In this way, the foundations would be laid for future lines of research aimed at establishing proposals for improvement based on evidence.

2. Materials and Methods

A qualitative design and phenomenological approach was followed through content analysis as described by Taylor and Bodgan [17]. We have used this methodology since it allows us to know the emic of the participants, that is, to understand the perception of people, as well as feelings and thoughts, from their testimonies, full of meanings, symbols, intentions, motives, and beliefs. Esta investigación se adhiere a las directrices del COREQ [18].

In order to respond to the proposed objectives, we address two populations. On the one hand, we selected palliative patients belonging to care support groups in the municipality and on the other hand we selected expert professionals that worked in in end-of-life processes in the same geographical setting. The sampling strategy was theoretical sampling, a technique that was developed by Glaser and Strauss [19] and where the sample is selected through the use of a successive strategy, progressive incorporation of informants, and evidence of similar studies, coinciding in a total of 10 expert professionals. However, in the group of patients, given the difficulties of accessibility to palliative patients voluntarily reported to be informants, the snowball sampling technique was used [20], we were able to reach 7 patients who behaved in a heterogeneous sample, and given their generosity and need for expression we managed to saturate in each of the dimensions found.

Intentional sampling was carried out during the months from May to November 2020. The sample size was determined progressively during the course of the research incorporating informants until the saturation of the information was reached [21]. In other words, research activities were continued until no new data pertaining to thematic categories could be extracted. In order to be considered for inclusion, this patient group had to comply with the criteria of belonging to the municipality under study, being of adult age, having been informed of their diagnosis and prognosis, having been informed about the process to be undergone, and, finally, having signed an informed consent form. In the case of expert professionals in end-of-life processes, once relevant individuals agreed to participate, the only criterion was that they provided written informed consent.

In order to analyze the discourse obtained in the interviews, the model described by Taylor–Bodgan [17] (Table 1).

The research team meets to obtain the script of the interviews and we carried out a pilot test with a professor and a collaborating student. Subsequently, the principal investigator conducted in-depth interviews with the aim of further exploring some of the dimensions that had emerged in the first interviews and thus obtaining more data.

Interviews were recorded and transcribed. The research team listened to and read the interviews in order to make an initial superficial interpretation. This provided a general idea which supported a more in-depth analysis (identification of relevant recurring themes, search for similarities and differences between themes in order to develop codes-dimensions and, with these, thematic categories. The repetition of codes—dimensions—on behalf of researchers—blind analysis—indicated that the analysis got to the essence and exposed the meaning of the studied phenomenon).

Table 1. In-process analysis approach in qualitative research (Talor–Bogdan).

Stage	Action
Discovery (search for topics by browsing the data in every possible way)	1. Read the data repeatedly 2. Keep track of themes, insights, interpretations and ideas 3. Look for emerging topics 4. Build topologies 5. Develop concepts and theoretical propositions 6. Read the bibliographic material 7. Develop a history guide
Coding (meeting and analysis of all the data that refer to themes, ideas, concepts, interpretations and propositions)	• Develop coding categories • Encode all data • Separate the data belonging to the various coding categories • See what data has been left • Refine your analysis
Data revitalization (interpret them in the context in which/where they were collected)	1. Requested o unsolicited data 2. Observer influence on stage 3. Who was there? (differences between what people say and do when are alone and when there are others in the place) 4. Direct and indirect data 5. Source (distinguishing between the perspective of a single person and that of a larger group 6. Our own assumption (critical self reflection)

The two study populations were made up of patients and expert professionals in end-of-life processes. In order to ensure validity and reliability, the entire process of coding and analyzing discourse was conducted independently by three members of the research team. Discrepancies were discussed until consensus was reached.

The study was conducted according to the guidelines of the Declaration of Helsinki, and approved by the Ethics Committee PPEIBA, government of Andalusia, Spain (protocol code 01/2020 CEPP and date of approval 18 January 2020).

3. Results

3.1. Participant Characteristics

Seventeen informants were interviewed. This included seven patients, of both sexes and with different illness progression states, undergoing palliative processes. This also included ten end-of-life expert professionals, these were representative in terms of age, gender, and years of experience in the field (Table 2).

The coding of discourse from interview transcripts produced 27 different codes. Of these, 17 were generated in the patient group and 10 in the expert population. This basis was developed using the data management program Atlas.ti. In consideration of the repetition of utterances in relation to each code, six lines of argument emerged which were equally distributed within both population groups, suggesting that the concept of spiritually coincided in each population (Table 3).

3.2. Lines of Argument

Line of argument 1 (patient group), coincides with line of argument 4 (professional expert group) with regards to the concept of spirituality. This agreement is not so much seen in the content overall, which is understandable given existing differences between both populations, but in reference to the search for the meaning of life as a cornerstone of spirituality (Table 4).

Considering further the idea of individual projection used by the palliative patient group to discuss spirituality relative to end-of-life processes, a code emerges which reached saturation very quickly. This code referred to connecting with others in order to give meaning to the processes. Selected patients also added accompaniment and communication to this concept.

Table 2. Sociodemographic characteristics of those interviewed.

Participant	Patient/Professional	Age	Disease Evolution Palliative Care Experience (Years)	Sex
Participant 1	Palliative Patient	74	4	Female
Participant 2	Palliative Patient	78	2	Male
Participant 3	Palliative Patient	45	0	Male
Participant 4	Palliative Patient	64	6	Female
Participant 5	Palliative Patient	69	3	Female
Participant 6	Palliative Patient	51	4	Female
Participant 7	Palliative Patient	60	3	Female
Participant 8	Nursing Professional	53	17	Female
Participant 9	Academic Professional	47	17	Female
Participant 10	Nursing Professional	60	28	Female
Participant 11	Nursing Professional	49	24	Female
Participant 12	Nursing Professional	56	28	Female
Participant 13	Nursing Professional	55	24	Male
Participant 14	Academic Professional	34	10	Female
Participant 15	Nursing Professional	41	16	Female
Participant 16	Nursing Professional	48	22	Female
Participant 17	Nursing Professional	56	26	Male

"I am really well attended to by all of my family. My sister-in-law comes every other day to see me and asks me many questions. I am grateful to my wife for all of the help and love that she is giving me, and of course for caring for me completely. I feel really loved by the people who are around me, they really go out of their way".

(Patient Palliative 02)

"I tell my daughter not to suffer because of me, that she has to live he r life. My daughter gets scared a lot because she thinks that I am going to bleed out and I have to cheer her up".

(Patient Palliative 04)

Table 3. Origin of study categories and subcategories according to population group.

Study Population	Line of Argument	Categories	Work Experience	Scientific Evidence	Emerging Discourse
Palliative care patient	Concept of spirituality	Meaning of life	*	*	
		Connection with others	*	*	
		Hope			*
	System of values and beliefs	Patient's system of values and beliefs	*	*	
		System of values and beliefs linked with religion and metaphysical phenomenon			*
		Spirituality in end-of-life care	*	*	
		Spirituality in society			*
	Factors that influence the spirituality of patients at the end of life	Worries/concerns	*	*	
		Conflict			*
		Coping strategies			*
		Social support	*	*	
		Sense of security	*	*	
		Proximity to death	*		
		Feelings of despair			*
		Pain	*	*	
		Fear of suffering	*	*	
		Body image			*
		Family background			*
End-of-life processes: Professional	Concept of spirituality	Spirituality	*	*	
		Evolution of spirituality			*
	Spiritual care	Spirituality in clinical care	*	*	
		Spirituality in palliative care units			*
	Training needs pertaining to spirituality	Need for spirituality training	*	*	
		Degree training			*
		Postgraduate training			*
		Personal experience			*
		Tools to evaluate patients' spiritual needs			*

The * symbol indicates that each category described has been generated in the different techniques shown in the column headings: Work Experience, Scientific Evidence y Emerging Discourse.

Turning attention back to the patient group, a second line of argument is found which was called as system of values and beliefs, and was deemed to be fundamental for understanding the spiritual end-of-life component. As with the other arguments generated by this population, the intensity of this component meant that it was tightly linked with the moment being lived at the time of data collection. Further, this line of argument defined codes that were highly relevant to end-of-life accompaniment. On the one hand, the system of values and beliefs emerged at a general level. On the other hand, something more metaphysical was coded. It is important to highlight that all of the discourse transcripts were coded as highlighting this component, with saturation occurring prematurely following discussion of faith and religion.

> *"I believe so, the idea that there is someone and that I turn to them at certain times. I believe in a higher being, accompaniment exists at certain moments. Yes at times when I need them, when it gives me stability. But I am not practicing at all".*
>
> *(Patient Palliative 02)*

Another dimension, linked with one's belief system and, at the same time, spirituality, that was generated by informants was hope.

> *"I when I lead a normal and acceptable life I feel super satisfied, I have learned to enjoy the small things. Get up and do three things in my house, it's the most wonderful thing in the world to me, because maybe in the future I won't be able to. I have hope again. I am able to cling onto anything. With really small things, share time with others. I think that that is really positive and it helps me a lot in these moments".*
>
> *(Patient Palliative 01)*

The palliative patient population also coincided with the expert professional population with regards to the need for palliative care to include attention to spirituality. Differences emerged in patient discourse which pertained to the approach taken in palliative units and in other units.

> *"In palliative patient they do it really well, because they approach that facet, they treat your symptoms, but also your concerns".*
>
> *(Patient palliative 03)*

The last line of argument generated from patient discourse, Line of argument 3, pertains to the factors that influence patient spirituality at the end of life. This argument is characterized by a large volume of emergent dimensions, with all being born out of service user perceptions. Saturation was reached with regards to the need to address conflict (Table 5).

With regards to the expert professional group, we previously described a line of argument that is in sync with another given by patients, however, another two arguments stand out for revealing idiosyncrasies of this group. Namely, these are spiritual care and training needs for effectively providing this care.

One of the subcategories underlying this first argument is spirituality in clinical and spiritual care. Utterances gathered together in relation to this dimension came from discourse that focused on a need that is currently not catered for, not even in palliative care.

> *"I'll sum it up in a really simple way, if when the moment comes you are not capable of standing 25 minutes of hugs and grief with a person in your arms, you're not qualified. We are used to working with the pain ladder and when one approaches on an existential level the reality of a person who is dying they must be able to open up, to tremble with the other and above all to look with them into the abyss, I think that it isn't done well because I think that we live with little awareness us professionals".*
>
> *(Professional expert 08)*

> *"Because there isn't the custom of talking about this, and less in those moments at the end of life. For me it was much more difficult to do it at other services where there was a lot of need because it wasn't expected of me, in the palliative context it is. But there isn't any assessment of the life project, religious dimension, celebrations, last rites; rites are really important to the spiritual dimension. It isn't integrated as a part of the job. Because there is a need to respond to what is expected of the nurse"*
>
> *(Professional expert 02)*

Table 4. Line of argument 1 patients: Concept of spirituality vs. line argument 4 Professional expert: Concept of spirituality.

	Role		
Line of Argument 1 Vs. Line of Argument 4	Professional expert	EXP02	*"It is the need that men and women have to transcend daily life, giving it meaning. The same with passions, that can be related with the image of some type of God or specific ideas ... that people can demonstrate solidarity with each other is nothing more than the most beautiful or wonderful branches of spirituality. It is a dimension that is within all human beings, and not only in each human being, but also in every town"*
		EXP07	*"Spirituality, which does not identify with a single unique divinity, is the expression of the essence of a person from where everything is governed and finds value. A person who does not have spirituality bears a higher burden of internal defeat. They lack the foundations and nutrients that help to interpret life ... A society without spirituality is dead, it gets manipulated by whatever ideology regardless of where it comes from. For this, mature spirituality leads individuals and society to be critical"*
	Palliative Patients	PPAL01	*"I am very satisfied with the life I have led before the illness, and with the life I lead now. I go out, I don't hide myself away at home. I don't ask for things I can't do. I don't have that feeling of "I could have done that and I didn't do it"*
		PPAL03	*"I know everything I have, I don't stop asking because I want to know how long I have left to live and how I am going to be up until I die"*
		PPAL07	*"But I want to be awake up until the end if I don't have strong pains. Until the end I want to see my children, my grandchildren, my neighbors, my daughters-in-law. I wouldn't like to lose my mind or say silly things"*

Table 5. Line of argument 3, palliative patient group. Factors that influence patient spirituality at the end of life.

Line Argument: Concept of Spirituality	Role			
Line Argument: Concept of Spirituality	Palliative Patients	need to address conflict	PPAL3	*"People are not really used to expressing anything that is not exactly physical, for this reason I try to resolve conflict both talking and without talking"*
		coping strategies	PPAL6	*"I am dealing with it 100% well, don't consider it, I move forward, I keep going. I am great, I always say that I am good, it is better to not dwell"*
		social support	PPAL3	*"My husband is my main support, because my children support me, they call me every day, but they live in Madrid. They really do care for me a lot. But without him I wouldn't have had the strength to go on"*
		sense security	PPAL7	*"It makes me feel good being able to lead the most normal life possible. To be able to have a beer someday with friends, any little thing will do for me"*
		closeness to death	PPAL2	*"I know I'm in a very advanced stage of metastasis but then... how it's going to be, what I'm going to feel...... I think everything will be fine and that relaxes"*
		feelings of despair	PPAL4	*"But yesterday got me a bit despairing, and I said "now whatever has to happen". Plus I really wanted to cry and I said "now I can't stand this anymore"*
		pain	PPAL2	*My legs I can hardly move them for the pain. And for this I take a lot of painkillers every day, that has morphine. up until now they haven't given me a single day without pain. They tell me that my pain is very difficult because it is in the bones and the nerves"*
		fear of suffering	PPAL1	*"Ay goodness me, that I don't have to suffer much when I am dying, that my loved ones don't see me suffer so that they don't suffer, that I fall asleep one night, but the suffering . . . "*
		body image	PPAL7	*"7 years ago now I had an operation for breast cancer, they gave me a prosthetic and it looks awful, looking at it, it's the difference between the two that you notice even with clothes, but it doesn't bother me as much now because I have other concerns"*
		family background	PPAL5	*"Four siblings have died of the same thing. And my mum, I think it is hereditary. There's more to come . . . I had a really bad time when they went, with my twin, we always used to go out together . . . . It is obvious that my destiny is what it is, the same as my family"*

Other experts, in this same category, had already pointed to training as the answer to integrating the spiritual component into end-of-life care. The absence of this care is linked with the scarcity of competencies in this area.

> *"If it isn't taught or if no experience is given of spirituality in the teaching of medicine or nursing, well we run the big risk of putting ourselves in front of a sick person without criteria that help us to understand beyond what is presented in their illness. It is never our job to judge anybody, but to be the doctor to whom the person can flow what they really want to express from inside of them. And all of this in a climate of confidence and serenity. Embodied spirituality is also this expression of support in daily things that make life more dignified".*
>
> *(Professional expert 10)*

Finally, the presentation of results is ended with the sixth line of argument, which was alluded to in all of the aforementioned categories and for which a code emerged following specialization of discourse. This code refers to the training needs of professionals to approach the spirituality of patients who find themselves undergoing end-of-life processes. Some utterances agreed on the need to know oneself and undergo introspection in order to be able to attend to another.

> *"The patients open up the path to this search and I study. A lot of things come out of your own free will, but, are you doing it right or not? It isn't easy to bring serenity to someone who is dying, that this process that they go through is a process of personal and family growth, if you yourself don't believe it. First you have to wake up within yourself, then you have to train yourself to not do things wrong, because without wanting to you can do harm".*
>
> *(Professional expert 04)*

Other utterances refer to the need to conduct team training in an interdisciplinary way in order to be able to provide holistic patient care.

> *"From our daily experience in hospitals at no time is a formal meeting space found where it is possible to work on teamwork in all of the required areas. And this is a mistake because it limits a lot the reach of care to patients and to those around them. Medical care and nursing slip into healthcare, but the spiritual is not integrated".*
>
> *(Professional expert 07)*

4. Discussion

The two populations under study in this research coincide in defining spirituality, in describing it as a way to connect with others and give meaning to the final process they are experiencing—in the case of palliative patients—or to give meaning to their existence and contact with life in the case of expert professionals. Authors, like Torralba [22], define spiritual intelligence as a form of existential or transcendent intelligence which enables human beings to question the meaning of their existence. It allows them to step away from reality, favors the elaboration of a life project, and permits them to transcend materiality, interpret symbols and understand the wisdom of life.

Another of the dimensions described in the results where both groups, coincide is the need to addressing the spiritual component in end-of-life care. Various authors [3,4,6] agree that treatment that strives to provide integral and dignified care must attend to all dimensions of the human being and tackle all patient and family needs. It should converge to include "dying well", the absence of suffering (in terms of the physical, emotional and spiritual) and the absence of pain for both the inflicted individual and their family. The present study, in accordance with a previous study [3], verified that these spiritual needs are present during the final moments, even when the patient is not aware of it. This is exemplified by the comment: *"I have learned to enjoy the small things. Get up and do three things in my house, it's the most marvelous thing in the world for me, because maybe in the future I won't be able to"* (Patient Palliative 01). Other previous research studies have also revealed similar outcomes [11,12]. Torralba [22,23] named needs of a spiritual nature that were conceived by the philosopher Simone Weils [24], in which the need to find meaning during these moments of life and reconciliation with oneself require spiritual intelligence. These can also be extrapolated from the discourse provided by unwell individuals in response to the situation in which they find themselves as a means to overcome it.

Delving deeper into the narrative of interviewed patients undergoing end-of-life processes, two main worries or concerns emerged with arise at these moments [22]. Specifically, these were concern around what death would be like or what would take place at the moment of death (Patient palliative 01) and fear of suffering (Patient Palliative 04). At the same time, references to spirituality emerged in all aspects of life as a method of help and support. This is demonstrated in the quote: "*A lot of pain, but always positive, wanting to better myself, wanting to be strong and smiling for my husband, for my son, for my parents and my sister . . .* " (Patient Palliative 03). Similar outcomes have also been described in works conducted in the clinical setting [3,25].

Based on the discourse resulting from the content analysis of expert professionals, the physical and emotional vulnerability developed to end-of-life processes causes an increase in the spiritual needs of patients and their families. These needs must be satisfied by health professionals in the end-of-life care setting. These results coincide with previous studies [3,4], that spiritual needs permeate the discourse of informants along with the importance of addressing them in order to provide comprehensive and exemplary care to patients and families involved in palliative care.

Besides, outcomes of the present study demonstrate the importance of spirituality at these moments and the huge impact of the quality of care, in the same way as reflected in other research [3]. It can be concluded that, based on the discourse of participating informants, the spiritual dimension is a felt need pertaining to the population of palliative patients in Huelva.

According to the palliative patients interviewed, nursing professionals must attend to the spiritual needs of patients at the end of life. There are authors [26] who agree on this idea, and conclude the need to include it in the academic world. An idea that in turn coincides with the speeches provided by the expert professionals interviewed. For instance, "*I have the feeling that this dimension is not touched upon not even when covering other material. The spiritual dimension is not integrated in the curriculum anywhere, therefore, nobody has to give it*" (Professional expert 02). The study confirms that spirituality is forgotten about. Nonetheless, it is true that students present high indices of knowledge and positive attitudes towards spirituality [8], although deficiencies are observed in knowledge and the delivery of nursing interventions related with spirituality [11]. New generations of students will be the future of the nursing profession. If these students are not trained to meet this need, spirituality will once again become an empty space in "integral" care plans.

With regards to discourse provided by professionals, it was revealed that positive attitudes exist along with a predisposition towards spiritual care. Such spiritual care is not only for religious individuals but also includes atheists and agnostics. This is in accordance with the concept of holistic health care proposed by the World Health Organization, which includes the integration of spirituality in nurses' care plans in line with previously conducted studies [12].

According to various studies [3,11] and two of the interviewed experts (Professionals Experts 01, 05), the act itself of working at a palliative care unit, where professionals continuously come into contact with death, should help them develop skills to provide spiritual care. In this sense, the compassion satisfaction shown by the care provider to the sick person connects with that individual and, at the same time, helps the professional manage their own feelings and compassion satisfaction [27].

The concept of spirituality defined by the panel overall agrees with current understanding of the construct, not only in the Spanish context but, also in Europe [7,13,22,28]. "Spirituality, which does not identify with a single unique divinity, is the expression of the essence of a person from where everything is governed and finds value" (EXP05). Spiritual care is understood as being basic to nursing care, as indicated by: "Each one is how they are, this generates suffering at the time of death and if you as a professional don't mitigate that, death is not as dignified as it should be" (Professional expert 01); "Spirituality is the capacity to tremble with the other person" (Professional expert 04). The importance of training in this environment was emphasized, in both nursing degrees and postgraduate training, and of the use of therapeutic tools and tools to detect spiritual suffering. This was outlined in the quote: "But we realized that it wasn't just an exploratory tool but a therapeutic tool. Those who use it must be really aware, be in control, know how far to go, when they have to interrupt, when is the right moment and when no, for this you have to be trained" (Professional expert 03). Similar outcomes have been reflected in various articles [3,4,6,24,29].

Strengths and Limitations

This study is innovative as it describes the need for spiritual accompaniment in the final process of life from the perspective not only of the professional who performs it, but of the protagonists themselves, the patients who are in this process. More studies and research, both quantitative and qualitative, are needed that contemplate the spiritual need, as well as the competences of nursing professionals for their development both in our field of study—palliative care—and outside it. Therefore, this research should be extended to different health professionals, doctors, nurses and psychologists, as well as to different areas where addressing the end of life is a priority.

Social awareness, and specifically of health professionals, in the spiritual field is fundamental, so this content should be included in the most initial stages of individual education. "A society without spirituality is dead, breathless, without criteria, it allows itself to be manipulated by whatever ideology it comes from. That is why a mature spirituality makes the person and society critical, open, non-manipulable, constructive: free".

5. Conclusions

The provision of spiritual care gives meaning to the actions performed by nursing professionals and the end of life, achieving holistic care, humanizing death, and promoting a dignified end. In the present work, it is true that spiritual accompaniment was seen to be challenged by its very nature given that the experimental paradigm did not achieve complete understanding or exploration. This being said, obtained outcomes verify that the spiritual dimension is understood by professionals on hand to accompany as a human universal and, with that, approaching it correctly will help other needs to be addressed. For this reason, following elaboration of the present study, it can be concluded that better training is required in this setting. Such training should be transversal, and be included within the Nursing degree, as well as in postgraduate training. This would promote the lifelong learning of nursing professionals in the city. In this way, social awareness could be strengthened within the nursing context in a way that encourages professionals working in the field to contemplate spiritual accompaniment as an indispensable aspect of care plans.

In the run up to the end of life, a lack of spiritual care becomes even more tangible for patients. Through the present study it can be confirmed that not only palliative patients are impacted by this dimension and, instead, spiritual conflict take occur at any vital stage and generate suffering. Nursing must be on hand to meet this need and mitigate its potential consequences through the route of integral and personalized care.

Author Contributions: Conceptualization, E.B.G.-N.; Formal analysis, A.M.-O. and E.B.G.-N. Research and analysis S.G.N., A.M.-O., and E.B.G.-N. Writing and preparation of the first draft E.B.G.-N. Drafting A.M.-O., S.G.N., and E.B.G.-N. All authors have read and agreed to the published version of the manuscript.

Funding: This research received no external funding.

Institutional Review Board Statement: The study was conducted according to the guidelines of the Declaration of Helsinki, and approved by Ethics Committee PPEIBA, government of Andalusia, Spain (protocol code 01/2020 CEPP and date of approval 18 January 2020).

Informed Consent Statement: Informed consent was obtained from all subjects involved in the study.

Conflicts of Interest: The authors declare no conflict of interest.

References

1. Volker, G. *Filosofía de la Psicología*; Herder: Barcelona, Spain, 2006.
2. Mytko, J.J.; Knight, S.J. Body, mind and spirit: Towards the integration of religiosity and spirituality in cancer quality of life research. *Psychooncology* **1999**, *8*, 439–450. [CrossRef]
3. Puchalski, C.; Ferrell, B.; Virani, R.; Otis-Green, S.; Baird, P.; Bull, J.; Chorchinov, H.; Handzo, G.; Nelson-Becker, H.; Prince-Paul, M.; et al. La mejora de la calidad de los cuidados espirituales como una dimensión de los cuidados paliativos: El informe de la Conferencia de Consenso. *Med. Paliativa* **2011**, *1*, 20–40. [CrossRef]
4. Benito, E.; Barbero, J.; Dones, M. *Espiritualidad en Clinica. Una Propuesta de Evaluación y Acompañamiento Espiritual en Cuidados Paliativos*; Sociedad Española de Cuidados Paliativos: Madrid, Spain, 2014; ISBN 978-84-940224-3-2.
5. Vincensi, B.B. Interconnections: Spirituality, spiritual care, and patient-centered care. *Asia-Pac. J. Oncol. Nurs.* **2019**, *6*, 104. [CrossRef]
6. Arrieira, I.C.D.O.; Thofehrn, M.B.; Porto, A.R.; Moura, P.M.M.; Martins, C.L.; Jacondino, M.B. Espiritualidade nos cuidados paliativos: Experiência vivida de uma equipe interdisciplinar. *Rev. da Esc. Enferm. da USP* **2018**, *52*, 3312. [CrossRef]
7. Reich, K.H. Spiritual development: Han F. de Wit's and Stanislav Grof's differing approaches. *Zygon®* **2001**, *6*, 509–520. [CrossRef]
8. Pinedo, M.T.; Jiménez, J.C. Cuidados del personal de enfermería en la dimensión espiritual del paciente. Revisión sistemática. *Cult. Cuid. Rev. Enfermería Humanid* **2017**, *48*, 110–118. [CrossRef]
9. Velosa, T.; Caldeira, S.; Capelas, M. Depression and Spiritual Distress in Adult Palliative Patients: A Cross-Sectional Study. *Religions* **2017**, *19*, 156. [CrossRef]
10. Caldeira, S.; Pinto, S.; Capelas, M. Spiritual care at the end of life. *Nurs Stand.* **2013**, *28*, 41–45. [CrossRef]
11. Codorniu, N.; Guanter, L.; Molins, A.; Utor, L. *Competencias Enfermeras en Cuidados Paliativos*; Sociedad Española de Cuidados Paliativos: Madrid, Spain, 2013; ISBN 978-84-940224-0-7.
12. Ortega, Á.M.; Ruiz-Fernández, M.D.; Ortiz-Amo, R.; Cabrera-Troya, J.; Carmona-Rega, I.M.; Ibáñez-Masero, O. Atención recibida al final de la vida en los servicios de urgencias desde la perspectiva de los cuidadores: Estudio cualitativo. *Enferm. Clin.* **2019**, *29*, 10–17. [CrossRef] [PubMed]
13. Rudilla, D.; Soto-Rubio, A.; Pérez, M.A.; Galiana, L.; Fombuena, M.; Oliver, A. Intervenciones psicológicas en espiritualidad en cuidados paliativos: Una revisión sistemática. *Med. Paliativa* **2018**, *25*, 203–212. [CrossRef]
14. Morillo-Martín, M.; Galán, J.M.; Llanos, F. Actitudes de las Enfermeras ante los Cuidados Espirituales y Religiosos en un Hospital General. *Index Enferm.* **2017**, *26*, 152–156.
15. Martins, H.; Caldeira, S. Spiritual Distress in Cancer Patients: A Synthesis of Qualitative Studies. *Religions* **2018**, *20*, 285. [CrossRef]
16. Rogers, M.; Wattis, J.; Khan, W.; Curran, S. A questionnaire-based study of attitudes to spirituality in mental health practitioners and the relevance of the concept of spiritually competent care. *J. Psychiatr. Ment. Health Nurs.* **2019**, *28*, 1165–1175. [CrossRef]
17. Taylor, S.J.; Bogdan, R. *Introducción a los Métodos Cualitativos de Investigación*; Paidós: Barcelona, Spain, 1987; ISBN 84-7509-816-9.
18. Tong, A.; Sand, P.; Craig, J. Consolidated criteria for reporting qualitative research (COREQ): A 32-item checklist for interviews and focus groups. *Inter. J. Qual. Health Care* **2007**, *19*, 349–357. [CrossRef]
19. Glaser, B.; Strauss, A. *The Discovery of Grounded Theory: Strategies for Qualitative Research*; Aldine: Chicago, IL, USA, 1967.
20. Ghaljaie, F.; Naderifar, M.; Goli, H. Snowball sampling: A purposeful method of sampling in qualitative research. *Strides Dev. Med. Educ.* **2017**, *14*, e67670. [CrossRef]
21. Fusch, P.I.; Ness, L.R. Are we there yet? Data saturation in qualitative research. *Qual. Rep.* **2015**, *20*, 1408–1416. [CrossRef]
22. Torralba, F. *Inteligencia Espiritual*; Plataforma: Barcelona, Spain, 2010; ISBN 978-84-96981-74-4.
23. Torralba, F. Necesidades espirituales del ser humano, Cuestiones preliminares. *Labor Hosp.* **2004**, *271*, 7–16.
24. Rozelle-Stone, A.R.; Stone, L. *Simone Weil and Theology*; Bloomsbury: New York, NY, USA, 2013; ISBN 9780567424303.
25. Kruizinga, R.; Scherer-Rath, M.; Schilderman, J.B.A.M.; Weterman, M.; Young, T.; van Laarhoven, H.W.M. Images of God and attitudes towards death in relation to spiritual wellbeing: An exploratory side study of the EORTC QLQ-SWB32 validation study in palliative cancer patients. *BMC Palliat Care* **2017**, *8*, 56–67. [CrossRef] [PubMed]
26. Benito, E. Los cuidados espirituales, entraña de los cuidados paliativos. *Med. Paliativa* **2011**, *18*, 1–3. [CrossRef]
27. Oliver, A.; Benito, E.; Sansó, N.; Galiana, L. Cuestionarios de atención espiritual en cuidados paliativos: Revisión de la evidencia para su aplicación clínica. *Psicooncología* **2007**, *13*, 385–397. [CrossRef]
28. Buceta, M.; Bermejo, J.C.; Villacieros, M. Elementos potenciadores de la satisfacción por compasión en profesionales sociosanitarios. *An. Psicol.* **2019**, *35*, 323–331. [CrossRef]
29. Miqueletto, M.; Silva, L.; Figueira, C.B.; Dos Santos, M.R.; Szylit, R.; de Faria, C.R. Espiritualidade de famílias com um ente querido em situação de final de vida. *Rev. Cuid.* **2017**, *8*, 1616–1627. [CrossRef]

International Journal of
Environmental Research and Public Health

Article

Nursing Home's Measures during the COVID-19 Pandemic: A Critical Reflection

Hongli Sam Goh [1,*], Vivian Tan [2], Chen-Na Lee [3], Hui Zhang [4] and M Kamala Devi [4]

1 Nursing Administration, Kwong Wai Shiu Hospital, Singapore 328127, Singapore
2 Lee Ah Mooi Nursing Home, Singapore 168871, Singapore; vuivui.tan@gmail.com
3 Department of Internal Medicine, Singapore General Hospital, Singapore 168753, Singapore; chenna_lee@hotmail.com
4 Alice Lee Centre for Nursing Studies, Yong Loo Lin School of Medicine, National University of Singapore, Singapore 117597, Singapore; nurzh@nus.edu.sg (H.Z.); nurmkd@nus.edu.sg (M.K.D.)
* Correspondence: nurghs@gmail.com

Abstract: This study examined the pandemic measures taken by nursing leaders to cope with COVID-19 at a nursing home in Singapore. The pandemic has affected over 215 countries, sparking a series of containment and pandemic measures by governments and healthcare organizations worldwide. Long-term care facilities are especially vulnerable to the pandemic, but little has been reported about the nursing homes' measures in handling the pandemic. The present study used Morley's (2014) three-stage critical reflection method to review meeting minutes, organizational emails, and government advisories on the COVID-19 pandemic measures undertaken by nursing leaders at a nursing home in Singapore between January and June 2020. The pandemic measures were broadly classified into four groups: (1) infection surveillance and containment measures; (2) ensuring continuity in clinical care and operational support; (3) resource and administrative coordination; and (4) staff training and development. Nurses have played a vital role in the fight against COVID-19 by ensuring continuity in patient care and demonstrating clinical leadership in pandemic efforts. This study proposes a useful nursing pandemic structure that outlines a set of functions and measures required for handling a pandemic and that can be applied to various medical emergencies and contingencies.

Keywords: long-term care; community nursing; COVID-19; coronavirus; workforce; SARS-CoV-2; pandemic

Citation: Goh, H.S.; Tan, V.; Lee, C.-N.; Zhang, H.; Devi, M.K. Nursing Home's Measures during the COVID-19 Pandemic: A Critical Reflection. *Int. J. Environ. Res. Public Health* **2022**, *19*, 75. https://doi.org/10.3390/ijerph19010075

Academic Editors: Richard Gray and Sonia Udod

Received: 21 November 2021
Accepted: 20 December 2021
Published: 22 December 2021

1. Introduction

In December 2019, a novel coronavirus, COVID-19, emerged and has resulted in a pandemic affecting over 215 countries worldwide within a short span of five months. As of 30 June 2021, 181,521,067 people have been infected globally, with 3,937,437 deaths [1]. Singapore reported its first COVID-19 case on 23 January 2020. Due to rapid local community transmission, the country raised its Disease Outbreak Response System Condition (DORSCON) alert level to orange on 7 February 2020. On 7 April 2020, the country introduced "circuit breaker" measures to stamp the sharp rise in COVID-19 cases within the community [2]. Due to the unknown pathology of the disease, its high transmission rate, and asymptomatic infections, this pandemic sparked a flurry of clinical guidelines put forth by governments and healthcare organizations worldwide to contain its spread and impact [3].

Long-term care facilities are especially vulnerable to infectious diseases due to their residents' profile, infrastructure constraints, manpower and resource shortages, and limited government funding [4]. These systemic challenges have contributed to reports of COVID-19 transmission within nursing homes in the United States, the United Kingdom, and Singapore [5–7]. In Singapore, the majority of the nursing homes resemble dormitory-style residential conditions with shared communal facilities and close proximity among residents [8]. The physical layout, coupled with the systemic challenges nursing homes face, could provide the impetus for the COVID-19 outbreak. Tan and Seetharaman reported high rates of acute respiratory symptoms among nursing home residents, making it difficult for clinicians to differentiate COVID-19 cases from non-COVID-19 ones [9].

Management guidelines for the COVID-19 outbreak can be more complex for nursing homes than those of acute hospitals due to differences in physical layout, resources, and residents' disease profiles [9]. In a local news report, a nursing home operator had to resort to seeking assistance and additional manpower from the Ministry of Health (MOH) to support its daily operations when several of its staff and residents were infected with COVID-19 and required to quarantine. Staff shortages and lean resources have been identified as contributory causes [10]. Although governmental bodies have been swift in introducing pandemic guidelines, success is contingent on the extent and pace of implementation by nursing homes. While there have been several published reports on COVID-19 pandemic measures taken by acute hospitals and primary and tertiary care centers [11–13], little has been reported about measures taken in the long-term care sector. Therefore, there is a need to shed light on the efforts and measures taken by nursing leaders to manage COVID-19 within nursing home settings.

2. Materials and Methods

This study examined the pandemic measures taken by nursing leaders to cope with COVID-19 at a charitable home in the long-term care sector in Singapore. The study employed Morley's three-stage critical reflection method involving data immersion, deconstruction, and reconstruction to generate recommendations for practice [14,15]. The method is based on several theoretical traditions, including Schon's reflective practice, critical post-modernism theory, and discourse analysis. The researchers chose this method as it was helpful in exploring assumptions and actions within the social context and re-interpreting their meaning for renewed options for societal action [15].

The study was conducted at a 624-bedded charitable nursing home in central Singapore. In Singapore, there are a total of 16,221 beds across 77 nursing homes, which fall into three categories: public (n = 24, 31.1%), private (n = 31, 40.3%), and charitable/not-for-profit (n = 22, 28.6%) [16]. Most public and charitable nursing homes receive substantial government subsidies, operate under donor funding, and require co-payment from clients. On the contrary, as private nursing homes are not under the MOH subsidy scheme, clients are required to make direct out-of-pocket payments [17]. The majority of the public and charitable nursing homes' layout resembles dormitory-style living conditions shared between 6 and 12 residents, who are mostly elderly and require a moderate to high level of care assistance [17]. However, private nursing homes vary widely in living conditions, from single- or double-bedded private rooms to a dormitory with as many as 30 residents [17].

According to Morley's (2014) three-stage critical reflection approach, the first stage involved two researchers (G.H.S. and V.T.) collating documents, making field notes about the pandemic measures at the nursing home, and immersing themselves in the data from January to June 2020 [14]. The second stage involved deconstruction, with the two researchers discussing and generating evolving concepts [14]. They analyzed various data sources, such as meeting minutes, organizational emails, and government advisories. Finally, the third stage involved reconstruction, with the researchers grouping the final concepts into categories with critical incidents as supporting examples and proposing a set of actions for change [14]. The study's trustworthiness was ensured by prolonged data immersion and member checking of notes [15].

The study was reviewed by the institutional management and exempted from ethics approval, as it did not involve any human subjects. Permission was given by the management team to report and publish the findings of the study.

3. Results

The pandemic measures adopted by the nurse leaders at the nursing home are classified into four groups: (1) infection surveillance and containment measures; (2) ensuring continuity in clinical care and operational support; (3) resource and administrative coordination; and (4) staff training and development. These measures, which have continually evolved in response to the MOH's national directives and the DORSCON alert level, are discussed in the following section.

3.1. Infection Surveillance and Containment Measures

In January 2020, when news of the COVID-19 outbreak was reported in China, the nursing home set up a command center and a nursing taskforce committee to monitor the situation. The Nursing Director and the Infection Control Nurse (ICN) chaired the nursing taskforce committee and sat in the command center to oversee the nursing home's pandemic response and coordination efforts. They managed the setup of the screening counter and the surveillance system for staff/visitor traffic movement and served as the subject matter expert for the command center. The ICN was also responsible for reviewing national pandemic guidelines; consulting other experts; and liaising with the MOH, other government agencies, and healthcare organizations. *"The ICN would provide a daily update and submission of data to MOH* via *AIC [Agency for Integrated Care]. She would work with the Clinical Director to collate the information from other non-nursing departments. They will disseminate any information to the rest of the nursing home"* (MM1, Infection Control Nurse).

The ICN's role proved pivotal to the nursing home's capability to cope with the pandemic measures. She mobilized the necessary resources and support from the nursing workforce at short notice. For example, the ICN had to review and contextualize government guidelines into organizational directives for each department. *"We [ICN and Nursing Director] need to translate the MOH DORSCON alert level into organization-specific directives on infection prevention measures for frontline and admin staff"* (JN1, Infection Control Nurse).

The ICN also worked with the nurse clinician to coordinate mask-fitting exercises for over 400 staff within three weeks to ensure that they were prepared for the COVID-19 pandemic measures. As a result, when the COVID-19 cases spiked in May 2020 with widespread community transmission in Singapore, the nursing home had already instituted organizational guidelines on pandemic measures and established vital infrastructures to cope with the pandemic per the MOH directives.

3.2. Ensuring Continuity in Clinical Care and Operational Support

When Singapore implemented the DORSCON Orange alert level in February 2020 to contain small clusters of COVID-19 transmission within the community, the nursing home intensified manpower and resource planning efforts to ensure continuity in clinical practice care and operational support. To ensure sufficient manpower, the nurse managers informed all frontline staff to defer non-essential overseas trips. In addition, they explored alternative staffing arrangements, such as spilt-team/spilt-site arrangement, a 12 h shift rotation, and an extension of work hours. *"The nursing home will be implementing the "split-team; split-site" arrangement for all non-essential staff"* (OE1, Nursing Director). A ward-specific staffing threshold was also set for the possible activation of additional staffing in the event of high work absenteeism. To sustain adequate resources for clinical operations, nurse managers projected ward utilization rates for essential resources, such as personal protective equipment (PPE). Areas for the consolidation of services were also identified, resulting in the delegation of non-essential tasks to non-clinical staff and the suspension of certain services. The Nursing Director mentioned, "Non-clinical staff will be deployed and assigned to man certain areas such as registration counter or visitor escort" (OE1).

The nurse managers played a crucial role in ensuring continuity of care for the residents. They had to increase ward round frequencies and provide constant communication with staff and oversee their compliance with the prevailing infection control directives, which were continuously changing at a rapid pace. They also assessed vulnerable residents with acute respiratory symptoms for medical referral, screened residents' outpatient appointments, and rescheduled non-essential ones to minimize residents' movement out of the nursing home. Nurse Manager 4 said: *"We are doing more frequent ward rounds to comb the wards to make sure that there are no sick residents with ARI [acute respiratory infection]"* (JN2). The constant presence of the nurse managers at the frontline also helped to ensure rapid information dissemination, staff compliance to pandemic directives, and the monitoring of staff safety and welfare during this trying period.

The nursing team also relied on information and communication technology to substitute face-to-face family visits with remote visitation and important meetings with web-based conferencing. During a meeting, the Nursing Director reported: *"The Admission team has used Zoom to facilitate tele-visitation between our residents and family members"* (MM5). These measures assisted the nursing home in maintaining communication with residents' next of kin and friends during the pandemic.

3.3. Resources and Administrative Coordination

Two non-nursing administrative staff members assisted the nursing taskforce committee in logistics and administrative and manpower support functions, which centered on inventory management, organizational and documentation support, and data collation required for government reporting. The administrative staff assisted the Nursing Director in conducting business continuity planning for the entire nursing home, such as spilt-site and spilt-team work arrangements and identifying areas for service consolidation. They also assisted the ICN in data collation for mandatory reporting to the MOH. As data were primarily in hardcopy format, collating such information can be challenging and time-wasting. The Infection Control Nurse commented: *"J and M [pseudonyms] continue to support me ICN in gathering information based on the MOH's demand as collating such information from different departments at short notice at the behest of the MOH can be technically draining for me"* (MM2). The administrative staff proved valuable in helping the clinicians with mundane tasks, thus freeing them to focus on coordination and communication efforts with various governmental agencies.

Other than operational and administrative support, the administrative staff also supported the nurse managers in overseeing human resource matters, such as staff welfare and lodging. Nurse Manager 2 said during a meeting: *"We must be physically present to make sure our staff are okay, and they know we are there for them. If they are stressed, we can always activate H.R. to support them, whether it is finance or emotional issue."* (MM2). When workplace segregation was instituted to minimize staff movement within the 624-bedded facility, the administrative staff coordinated with the human resource personnel to ensure similar living arrangements within the nursing home dormitory for the foreign staff to minimize risks for cross-cluster transmission. Temporary accommodations were also arranged if foreign staff were issued quarantine orders or evicted from rental housing by their landlords. Other resources, such as a helpline for psychological support and food catering, were also arranged to ensure staff welfare and mental well-being. Nursing Director: *"Management and H.R. should pay more attention to staff welfare. The following measures may be considered: Provide recognition for staff in small tangible ways, e.g., words of encouragement, surprise pack, subscribe to entertainment channels on T.V. for stay-in staff to watch in-house"* (GA1).

3.4. Staff Training and Development

The last function pertains to the specific training needs of nursing staff to handle the pandemic. This function was assigned to the nurse educator to coordinate and conduct essential training, such as upskilling the long-term care nurses' competencies in pandemic management. At the behest of the Agency for Integrated Care, the nurse educator was tasked with helping to organize mask-fitting train-the-trainer courses for the long-term care sector, including the general practitioners, clinic staff, and other nursing homes that might not have the capabilities to support such efforts.

When Singapore introduced the "circuit breaker" measures, a tighter set of safe distancing measures, in April 2020 to stem the spike in COVID-19 cases, many training providers were restricted from conducting face-to-face training, forcing many essential training programs, such as cardiopulmonary resuscitation and the use of personal protective equipment, to cease temporarily. These measures prompted the training department to revamp their courseware for online delivery, such as recording procedural skills and teleconferencing platforms to enable continuous learning. Nurse Educator: *"The education team has no choice but to stop [classroom] training and convert them into online learning. This will allow us to continue to train our staff"* (OE5). At the same time, the nurse educator also worked with the training team to rapidly build its training infrastructure, such as the learning management system. The nurse educator commented on how the COVID-19 pandemic had a positive aspect in regard to expediting the nursing home's use of technology to continue operations and training. As a result, the nurse educator converted her training materials to electronic format and utilized web-based communication technologies to deliver her staff training to more staff.

4. Discussion

The creation of the nursing taskforce committee, which consists of nurse leaders and the ICN, proved valuable in the early establishment of communication channels and the coordination of infection surveillance and containment efforts at the nursing home. As the government continues to roll out new directives during the COVID-19 situation, the structure and functions of the nursing taskforce committee have evolved, resulting in its existing framework. In this framework, the nursing taskforce committee plays a crucial role in reviewing the latest pandemic guidelines and advising the command center on clinical operations and resource management as subject matter experts. In addition, the Nursing Director coordinates internal communication to keep all stakeholders updated on government advisories on the COVID-19 situation. At the same time, the ICN serves as the primary contact point for external communication with the MOH, other government agencies, and healthcare organizations.

The current nursing pandemic framework has provided the nurse leaders with a highly efficient approach to handle the COVID-19 situation at the nursing home (Figure 1). The Nursing Director and ICN assume the infection surveillance and containment measures function and direct the nursing taskforce committee in collaboration with the command center to set the overall direction and efforts for the pandemic. The ICN oversees the surveillance and containment measures, such as staff/visitor's movement, infrastructures, and security points. During the pandemic, two key issues emerged for the nursing taskforce committee: (1) the exigency of data collation for the real-time monitoring of suspected/confirmed cases and (2) the review of multiple COVID-19 reports of pandemic responses. In our experience, the establishment of a dynamic pandemic response system is lacking in the long-term care sector due to heterogeneity in organizational systems and processes, limited funding and governmental support in infrastructure development. Paterson et al. highlighted the daunting task of reviewing the overwhelming number of COVID-19 reports published almost daily, much less developing effective pandemic strategies accordingly [18]. This laborious but necessary process has resulted in the nursing home dedicating two nurse leaders to assist the ICN in the data collation and review of the latest COVID-19 directives from the government [18].

	Structure of Nursing Taskforce Committee
Lines of Command	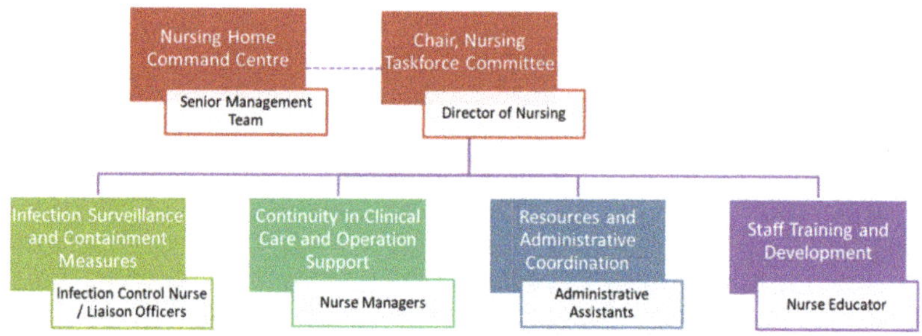

Measures	Functions of Nurse Leaders During a Pandemic			
	Infection Surveillance and Containment Measures	**Ensuring Continuity in Clinical Care and Operational Support**	**Resources and Administrative Coordination**	**Staff Training and Development**
Procedural Measures	1. Provide on-site support for non-nursing services. 2. Oversee compliance to infection control practices for non-ward areas. 3. Handling contingencies e.g., suspect and confirmed cases.	1. Teleconferencing for essential meetings with staff, management and external stakeholders. 2. Review of high-risk and vulnerable residents for medical referral. 3. Screening and rescheduling of essential follow-up appointments for residents. 4. Ensure staff compliance to infection control practices. 5. Ensure continual support from operations, e.g., environmental services, food, and linen.	1. Data collation and reporting to ICN.	1. Revamp existing courseware and convert it to online delivery. 2. Conduct essential training: ▪ PPE retraining and training for administrative staff and vendors. ▪ Conducting mass swab testing for COVID. ▪ Performing high-risk procedures, e.g., Aerosol-generating procedures.
Administrative Measures	4. Liaison and subject matter expert for infection disease matters. 5. Review and synthesis of international and national guidelines and translation of evidences into organizational directives. 6. Data collation, analysis and reporting to senior management and ministry.	6. Resource planning and control: ▪ Project and plan enough resources, especially PPE, during the next 2–3 months. ▪ Ration of controlled items. 7. Manpower planning: ▪ Handling staff leave. ▪ Alternative manning hours. ▪ Deployment of manpower pool.	2. Review business continuing plans for essential services. 3. Resource management, especially PPE. 4. Manpower support coordination: ▪ Split-site arrangement-ward and staff segregation. ▪ Split-work arrangement. 5. Supply of food for staff staying in the dormitories. 6. Staff welfare and support.	3. Develop a guide on how to utilize the ICT system to support in-house training.
Structural Measures	7. Oversee the establishment of pandemic infrastructures and areas: ▪ Triage and screening counter for visitors and vendors. ▪ Access control points and security management. ▪ Surveillance system for staff and visitors' movement.	8. Set up and facilitate teleconsultation with locum physicians. 9. Set up and facilitate remote visitation via teleconferencing platforms. 10. Ward segregation and bed management.	7. Identification and designation of empty spaces for mass cohort for suspected cases/staff accommodation.	4. Establishment of ICT support to support online delivery.

Figure 1. *Cont.*

	▪ Identification and demarcation of containment/holding areas. ▪ Identification and placement of pandemic information within the organization. ▪ Identification and placement of hand sanitizer within the organization.			

Figure 1. Pandemic nursing framework at the nursing home.

The nurse managers assumed the function of ensuring continuity in clinical care and operational support, such as manpower and resource planning, clinical care coordination, documentation, and environmental control. The two non-nursing administrative staff members assisted the nursing taskforce committee with resources and administrative coordination by focusing on inventory management, organizational support, and data collation. These concerted efforts allowed the nursing taskforce committee to implement government-issued directives in a timely and effective manner and the nursing home to ensure sufficient resources for daily operations despite a supply crunch. For example, there were reports of healthcare organizations facing shortages in PPE, disinfectants, and other essential items worldwide, prompting the World Health Organization to issue advisories on the prudent use of PPEs during the COVID-19 pandemic [19,20].

The nurse educator assumed the staff training and development function by conducting essential training and upskilling the long-term care nurses' competencies in pandemic management. She also contributed to the development of the online training infrastructures to ensure continuity in essential staff training. Several studies have highlighted the importance of staff upskilling and cross-training to enable their competencies to handle the pandemic and deployment to critical work areas when needed [9,21,22]. At the time of this writing, the nursing home has generated sufficient training infrastructure and resources to offer their in-house long-term care training courses to other nursing homes using online delivery.

This study reports the current framework to provide nurse leaders with pandemic management strategies. Although some have considered pandemics a natural disaster and considered the use of disaster nursing models to inform disaster risk reduction strategies, the pandemic presents a different set of challenges, involving a less hazardous but more dynamic situation than other natural disasters [21]. There are currently limited studies to guide nursing functions and measures during a pandemic. In several studies on pandemic measures within nursing homes, Stall et al. detailed the different phases of pandemic measures outlining the various responses implemented to stabilize an outbreak situation in Toronto, Canada. At the same time, Yen et al. described the use of environmental scanning and control to mitigate COVID-19 risks in Taiwan [23,24]. In the U.S. and Europe, several studies outlined the challenges long-term care facilities faced and proposed a series of measures to be taken to protect these organizations during the COVID-19 pandemic [25,26]. Our study contributed to the literature by providing nursing home leaders with a better understanding of the structures, functions, and measures required for handling future pandemic situations, particularly in data collation, communication, and resource management.

5. Conclusions

Being the largest workforce in healthcare, nurses have played a vital frontline role in the fight against COVID-19. They have demonstrated clinical leadership by maintaining care continuity, directing pandemic efforts, and building organizational capabilities to handle the crisis. This study highlighted several challenges nurse leaders faced in the long-term care sector during a pandemic, requiring a multi-prong, collaborative, and coordinated approach involving various stakeholders. As the long-term care setting presents unique challenges, international and national guidelines need to be contextualized into the sector-specific and organizational directives before they can be implemented successfully.

The present study proposes a useful nursing pandemic structure that outlines a set of functions and measures required for handling a pandemic and that can be applied to various medical emergencies and contingencies. The structure can also be used to guide the curriculum and develop core competencies in pandemic management for nurses in the long-term care sector. Nurse educators can also utilize the framework to develop training materials to improve the staff's capability in handling pandemics in the future.

Author Contributions: Conceptualization, H.S.G. and V.T.; methodology, H.S.G. and H.Z.; validation, M.K.D. and C.-N.L.; formal analysis, H.S.G. and V.T.; writing—original draft preparation, H.S.G. and H.Z.; writing—review and editing, M.K.D. and C.-N.L. All authors have read and agreed to the published version of the manuscript.

Funding: This research received no external funding.

Institutional Review Board Statement: Not applicable.

Informed Consent Statement: Not applicable.

Data Availability Statement: The data presented in this study are available on request from the corresponding author. The data are not publicly available due to privacy restrictions.

Acknowledgments: The authors would like to thank the senior management team of the nursing home for their permission to share and publish the report.

Conflicts of Interest: The authors declare no conflict of interest.

References

1. World Health Organization (WHO). *Standard Precautions in Health Care*; World Health Organization: Geneva, Switzerland, 2021.
2. Chen, P.; Yap, J.C.-H.; Hsu, L.Y.; Teo, Y.Y. COVID-19 and Singapore: From early response to circuit breaker. *Ann. Acad. Med. Singap.* **2020**, *49*, 561–572. [CrossRef]
3. Peeri, N.C.; Shrestha, N.; Rahman, M.S.; Zaki, R.; Tan, Z.; Bibi, S.; Baghbanzadeh, M.; Aghamohammadi, N.; Zhang, W.; Haque, U. The SARS, MERS and novel coronavirus (COVID-19) epidemics, the newest and biggest global health threats: What lessons have we learned? *Int. J. Epidemiol.* **2020**, *49*, 717–726. [CrossRef]
4. Davidson, P.M.; Szanton, S.L. Nursing homes and COVID 19: We can and should do better. *J. Clin. Nurs.* **2020**, *29*, 2758–2759. [CrossRef]
5. Barnett, M.L.; Grabowski, D.C. Nursing Homes Are Ground Zero for COVID-19 Pandemic. *JAMA Heal. Forum* **2020**, *1*, e200369. [CrossRef]
6. Morciano, M.; Stokes, J.; Kontopantelis, E.; Hall, I.; Turner, A.J. Excess mortality for care home residents during the first 23 weeks of the COVID-19 pandemic in England: A national cohort study. *BMC Med.* **2021**, *19*, 71. [CrossRef] [PubMed]
7. Tan, L.F.; Seetharaman, S.K. COVID-19 outbreak in nursing homes in Singapore. *J. Microbiol. Immunol. Infect.* **2021**, *54*, 123–124. [CrossRef]
8. Wong, G.H.Z.; Pang, W.S.; Yap, P. A paradigm shift in regulating and running nursing homes in Singapore. *J. Am. Med. Dir. Assoc.* **2014**, *15*, 440–444. [CrossRef] [PubMed]
9. Tan, L.F.; Seetharaman, S. Preventing the spread of COVID 19 to nursing homes: Experience from a Singapore Geriatric Centre. *J. Am. Geriatr. Soc.* **2020**, *68*, 942. [CrossRef]
10. Lai, L. All Staff, Residents at Homes for the Elderly to be Tested for Covid-19. *The Straits Times*, 8 May 2020. Available online: https://www.straitstimes.com/singapore/all-staff-and-residents-at-nursing-homes-to-be-tested-for-covid-19-starting-with-those-who(accessed on 1 November 2021).
11. Lee, C.C.M.; Thampi, S.; Lewin, B.; Lim, T.J.D.; Rippin, B.; Wong, W.H.; Agrawal, R.V. Battling COVID-19: Critical care and peri-operative healthcare resource management strategies in a tertiary academic medical centre in Singapore. *Anaesthesia* **2020**, *75*, 861–871. [CrossRef] [PubMed]
12. Lim, W.H.; Wong, W.M. COVID-19: Notes From the Front Line, Singapore's Primary Health Care Perspective. *Ann. Fam. Med.* **2020**, *18*, 259–261. [CrossRef] [PubMed]
13. Mason, D.J.; Friese, C.R. Protecting Health Care Workers Against COVID-19—and Being Prepared for Future Pandemics. *JAMA Health Forum* **2020**, *1*, e200353. [CrossRef]
14. Morley, C. Using critical reflection to research possibilities for change. *Br. J. Soc. Work* **2014**, *44*, 1419–1435. [CrossRef]
15. Morley, C. *Critical Reflection as a Research Methodology*; Nova Publishers: New York, NY, USA, 2008.
16. Ministry of Health Singapore. Beds in Inpatient Facilities and Places in Non-Residential Long-Term Care Facilities. Available online: https://www.moh.gov.sg/resources-statistics/singapore-health-facts/beds-in-inpatient-facilities-and-places-in-non-residential-long-term-care-facilities (accessed on 13 December 2021).

17. Ho, E.; Huang, S. *Care Where You Are: Enabling Singaporeans to Age Well in the Community*; Lien Foundation: Singapore, 2018.
18. Paterson, C.; Gobel, B.; Gosselin, T.; Haylock, P.J.; Papadopoulou, C.; Slusser, K.; Rodriguez, A.; Pituskin, E. Oncology Nursing During a Pandemic: Critical Reflections in the Context of COVID-19. *Semin. Oncol. Nurs.* **2020**, *36*, 151028. [CrossRef] [PubMed]
19. Feng, S.; Shen, C.; Xia, N.; Song, W.; Fan, M.; Cowling, B.J. Rational use of face masks in the COVID-19 pandemic. *Lancet Respir. Med.* **2020**, *8*, 434–436. [CrossRef]
20. Livingston, E.; Desai, A.; Berkwits, M. Sourcing Personal Protective Equipment During the COVID-19 Pandemic. *JAMA* **2020**, *323*, 1912–1914. [CrossRef]
21. Huang, L.; Lin, G.; Tang, L.; Yu, L.; Zhou, Z. Special attention to nurses' protection during the COVID-19 epidemic. *Crit. Care* **2020**, *24*, 120. [CrossRef]
22. Jackson, D.; Bradbury-Jones, C.; Baptiste, D.; Gelling, L.; Morin, K.; Neville, S.; Smith, G.D. Life in the pandemic: Some reflections on nursing in the context of COVID-19. *J. Clin. Nurs.* **2020**, *29*, 2041–2043. [CrossRef]
23. Yen, M.-Y.; Schwartz, J.; King, C.-C.; Lee, C.-M.; Hsueh, P.-R. Recommendations for protecting against and mitigating the COVID-19 pandemic in long-term care facilities. *J. Microbiol. Immunol. Infect.* **2020**, *53*, 447–453. [CrossRef]
24. Stall, N.M.; Farquharson, C.; Fan Lun, C.; Wiesenfeld, L.; Loftus, C.A.; Kain, D.; Johnstone, J.; McCreight, L.; Goldman, R.D.; Mahtani, R. A hospital partnership with a nursing home experiencing a COVID 19 outbreak: Description of a multiphase emergency response in Toronto, Canada. *J. Am. Geriatr. Soc.* **2020**, *68*, 1376–1381. [CrossRef] [PubMed]
25. Heckman, G.A.; Kay, K.; Morrison, A.; Grabowski, D.C.; Hirdes, J.P.; Mor, V.; Shaw, G.; Benjamin, S.; Boscart, V.M.; Costa, A.P. Proceedings from an International Virtual Townhall: Reflecting on the COVID-19 Pandemic: Themes from Long-Term Care. *J. Am. Med. Dir. Assoc.* **2021**, *22*, 1128–1132. [CrossRef]
26. Langins, M.; Curry, N.; Lorenz-Dant, K.; Comas-Herrera, A.; Rajan, S.; World Health Organization. The COVID-19 pandemic and long-term care: What can we learn from the first wave about how to protect care homes? *Eurohealth* **2020**, *26*, 77–82.

International Journal of
Environmental Research and Public Health

MDPI

Article

The Impact of COVID-19 on Levels of Adherence to the Completion of Nursing Records for Inpatients in Isolation

Mercedes Fernández-Castro [1], José-María Jiménez [1,*], Belén Martín-Gil [1], María-Fé Muñoz-Moreno [1], María-José Castro [2], María-José Cao [2] and María López [2]

1 Hospital Clínico Universitario de Valladolid, 47002 Valladolid, Spain; mefernandezc@saludcastillayleon.es (M.F.-C.); bmartingi@saludcastillayleon.es (B.M.-G.); mfmunozm@saludcastillayleon.es (M.-F.M.-M.)
2 Nursing Faculty, University of Valladolid, 47005 Valladolid, Spain; mariajose.castro@uva.es (M.-J.C.); mjcao@enf.uva.es (M.-J.C.); maria.lopez.vallecillo@uva.es (M.L.)
* Correspondence: josejimenez@enf.uva.es; Tel.: +34-983-183025

Abstract: The COVID-19 pandemic has led to an increased workload for nurses and organisational and structural changes, which have been necessary to meet the needs of inpatients in isolation. Aim: To describe the impact of the COVID-19 pandemic on levels of adherence to the completion of nursing records that document the risk of developing pressure ulcers, falling, and social vulnerability among hospitalised patients in isolation. Methods: Observational pre-post comparison study. Comparison between nursing records (the Braden, Downton, and Gijón scales) belonging to 1205 inpatients took place in two phases. Phase 1: 568 patients admitted in February 2020, prior to the COVID-19 pandemic, vs. phase 2: 637 patients hospitalised with COVID-19 in March–April 2020, during the peak of the first wave of the pandemic. This research adheres to the STROBE guidelines for the reporting of observational studies. Results: The degree of completion of the Braden, Downton, and Gijón scales decreased significantly in phase 2 vs. phase 1 ($p < 0.001$). The mean Downton and Gijón scale scores for patients admitted in phase 1 were higher compared to those of patients admitted in phase 2 ($p < 0.001$). The mean Braden scale score in phase 2 was higher than in phase 1 ($p < 0.05$). Conclusion: During the COVID-19 pandemic, there was a decrease in the completion of nursing records in the clinical records of patients in isolation. The levels of risk of developing PUs, falling, and social vulnerability of patients admitted to hospital were lower during the first wave of the pandemic.

Keywords: nursing records; patient isolation; COVID-19; nursing care; nurses

Citation: Fernández-Castro, M.; Jiménez, J.-M.; Martín-Gil, B.; Muñoz-Moreno, M.-F.; Castro, M.-J.; Cao, M.-J.; López, M. The Impact of COVID-19 on Levels of Adherence to the Completion of Nursing Records for Inpatients in Isolation. *Int. J. Environ. Res. Public Health* **2021**, *18*, 11262. https://doi.org/10.3390/ijerph182111262

Academic Editors: Richard Gray and Sonia Udod

Received: 21 September 2021
Accepted: 25 October 2021
Published: 27 October 2021

1. Introduction

On 12 March 2020, the World Health Organisation declared the spread of the severe acute respiratory syndrome coronavirus 2 (SARS-CoV-2) to be a pandemic [1]. The number of confirmed cases worldwide has exceeded 49.7 million, while the number of deaths has risen to more than 1.2 million. In March 2020, during the first wave of the pandemic, the number of confirmed cases of COVID-19 (coronavirus disease 2019) in Spain was 78,797 compared to 693,282 worldwide. The number of new cases and deaths reported in Europe increased exponentially in November 2020. Spain emerged as the country with the sixth highest number of COVID-19 cases worldwide, with more than 2000 new cases per million inhabitants [1].

In this context, hospital managers were required to make considerable organisational and structural changes to meet the needs arising from isolating inpatients and to protect healthcare workers [2]. Isolation is the priority course of action in these cases. However, the negative repercussions of isolation on patients must be taken into account, as they are associated with negative psychological effects, such as risk of developing anxiety and depression; the occurrence of a greater number of adverse events, such as falls; and reduced contact with healthcare workers [3,4]. Isolation inevitably entails limited contact with other patients, disruption of daily life, no visitors, and less interaction with hospital staff. These restrictions may lead to feelings of loneliness, neglect, social exclusion, and stigmatisation [5].

Given the rapid rise in the numbers of infected patients requiring hospitalisation, units admitting patients with suspected or confirmed COVID-19 have had to make a great effort to adapt to emerging needs in terms of material resources, newly hired personnel, and new protocols and procedures required to tackle the pandemic. COVID-19 has led to changes in nurse staffing and increased workload for nurses, which may have negatively affected the quality of nursing records [6]. The work environment is a conditioning factor in the implementation and use of electronic records, which means it may influence their quality and levels of completion [7].

If properly documented in the patient's clinical record, the following measures are possible: provision of pressure ulcer (PU) care through early identification of patients at risk of developing ulcers; recording of the number of PUs, if any; fall prevention by assessing the risk of falling during hospitalisation; analysis of the causes of a patient's fall; and identification of socially at-risk patients. Records intended to assess and identify risks among inpatients are essential for developing evidence-based initiatives capable of preventing such risks. Patient assessments using scales and interventions must be conducted regardless of the clinical environment and should be the same for all patients, whether or not they are in isolation. When a patient's condition is critical or complex, further nursing care is needed [8], and it is essential that this care is recorded.

A unified approach could help frontline healthcare professionals to standardise data collection and increase the efficiency and performance of their work. Documentation is crucial for the communication of healthcare teams and patient outcome measurement and monitoring [9]. This will require continuous training, regular updates, feedback, support from staff, and regular monitoring of records [10].

A number of studies have shown that nurses' workload is significantly associated with the quality of care provided [11] and that nurses' workload and patient deaths are positively correlated [12]. The time required to keep electronic records in their daily work can be a source of frustration and exhaustion for nurses, who experience it as additional workload [13]. Nursing records are an important clinical resource, as they are necessary for assessing the delivery of care, enhancing the quality of nursing care, and improving nurses' work environment and workload [14].

Previous experiments have shown that improving training and implementing best clinical practices is helpful in increasing the completion of nursing records in clinical records and in integrating said completion into nurses' routine work procedures [15].

Further studies and comprehensive tools are needed to analyse this phenomenon in greater depth. There is a need for studies assessing the impact of isolation on safety indicators, in addition to psychological aspects, while taking into account potential collateral damage caused by isolation.

The objective of this study is to describe the impact of the first wave of the COVID-19 pandemic on levels of adherence to the completion of nursing records that document the risk of developing PUs, falling, and risk of social vulnerability among hospitalised patients in isolation.

2. Materials and Methods

2.1. Study Design

This is an observational pre–post comparison study on the nursing records of patients hospitalised in a tertiary care hospital in the public healthcare system before and during the first phase of the COVID-19 pandemic.

2.2. Sampling and Participants

The study population consisted of the records of 1205 inpatients: 568 patients admitted to the Internal Medicine, Vascular Surgery, Otorhinolaryngology, and Cardiology inpatient units at a University Clinical Hospital between 1 and 29 February 2020 (prior to the pandemic) and 637 patients admitted to these same units between 15 March and 15 April 2020 with COVID-19 diagnoses (during the peak of the first wave of the pandemic). These units were repurposed to treat patients with COVID-19 from the second half of March.

2.3. Data Collection

Data collection took place in two phases (pre- and post-COVID-19 at the same units), which assessed the completion of electronic records, including the Braden, Downton, and Gijón scales.

Risk of developing PUs was measured using the Braden scale. Scores range from 6 to 26. Scores below 12 points indicate a high risk of developing PUs; scores between 13 and 14 indicate a moderate risk; and scores between 15 and 18 indicate a low risk [16]. The risk of falling was measured using J.H. Downton's scale. Scores range from 0 to 14, with scores $\geq$ 3 indicating risk of falling [17]. Socio-familial risk among patients aged 75 or older was measured using the socio-familial Gijón scale. Scores range from 5 to 25. Scores $\leq$ 8 indicate a low risk; scores from 8 to 9 indicate a moderate risk; and scores $\geq$ 10 indicate a high risk [18].

Phase 1 took place between 1 and 29 February 2020. The electronic records of patients hospitalised before the pandemic were collected. Phase 2 took place between 15 March and 15 April 2020 (during the first wave of the pandemic). The electronic records of patients admitted for COVID-19 were collected.

In both phases, the following variables were also analysed: sex, age, mean length of stay, falls, number of PUs, and places where the PUs originated.

2.4. Data Analysis

All statistical analyses were performed using IBM SPSS v. 24.0 software (IBM, Armonk, New York, NY, USA). Quantitative variables were described using means, standard deviations, and minimum and maximum scores. Qualitative variables were described by their distribution of frequencies. Associations between qualitative variables were analysed using Pearson's chi-squared test. Quantitative values were compared using Student's *t*-test for paired samples or using ANOVA for more than two samples. The statistical significance threshold for all tests was set at $p < 0.05$.

3. Results

The records of 1205 patients were analysed, 54.8% of whom were men and 45.2% women, with a mean age of 70.46 (SD = 16.1) years. In total, 47% of patients were admitted in February 2020 with a mean stay of 9.42 (SD = 2.1) days, and 53% of patients were admitted between 15 March 2020 and 15 April 2020 with a mean stay of 9.18 (SD = 2.8) days. There were no differences between the two periods by sex. By age group, 32.7% were $\leq$65 and 67.3% > 65 years. However, differences in age were identified. In phase 1, the number of women was 252 and that of men was 316. In phase 2, there were 293 women and 344 men. Regarding the age group, the group $\leq$ 65 years in phase 1 consisted of 166 patients and 228 patients in phase 2. The group > 65 years in phase 1 consisted of 402 patients and 409 patients in phase 2. The mean age decreased considerably, from 72 (SD = 17) years to 69 (SD = 15) years among patients who had tested positive for COVID-19 ($p = 0.02$).

The degree of completion of the Braden, Downton, and Gijón scales decreased significantly in phase 2 with respect to phase 1 ($p < 0.001$). See Table 1.

Table 1. The degree of completion of the Braden, Downton, and Gijón scales recorded between study phases 1 and 2.

	Study Periods						
	Phase 1		Phase 2		Total		
Number of Patients Assessed	n = 568		n = 637		n = 1205		
Nursing Records Completed	n	%	n	%	n	%	p-Value
Braden scale	498	87.7	350	54.9	848	100	<0.001
Downton scale	338	59.5	231	36.3	569	100	<0.001
Gijón scale	224	62.7	133	37.3	357	100	<0.001

The level of adherence to the completion of the records did not show statistically significant differences between the two phases in terms of sex.

The completion of the Braden and Downton scales was significantly higher in the first phase for the group over 65 years (0.012 and $p = 0.003$); see Table 2.

Table 2. Analyses of completion of scales for age group and sex.

	Phase	Sex				p-Value	Age				p-Value
		Man		Woman			≤65		>65		
		n	%	n	%		n	%	n	%	
Braden scale	1	274	58.9%	224	58.5%	0.897	144	52.6%	354	61.7%	0.012
	2	191	41.1%	159	41.5%		130	47.4%	220	38.3%	
Downton scale	1	184	59.5%	154	59.2%	0.939	73	49.0%	265	63.1%	0.003
	2	125	40.5%	106	40.8%		76	51.0%	155	36.9%	
Gijón scale	1	114	62.3%	110	63.2%	0.857	18	54.5%	206	63.6%	0.306
	2	69	37.7%	64	36.8%		15	45.5%	118	36.4%	

Assessment records using the Downton and Gijón scales revealed scores consistent with a higher risk of falling and social vulnerability in phase 1 compared to phase 2. However, the risk of developing PUs during hospital stay increased in phase 2; see Table 3.

Table 3. Mean scores for the Braden, Downton, and Gijón scales between study phases 1 and 2.

	Phase 1 Mean (SD †)	Phase 2 Mean (SD †)	t-Test for Independent Samples			p-Value
			Differences in Means	95% CI		
				Lower Bound	Upper Bound	
Braden scale	17.83 (4.47)	18.45 (4.41)	−0.62	−1.23	−0.01	0.04
Downton scale	2.78 (1.67)	1.87 (1.50)	0.91	0.65	1.17	<0.001
Gijón scale	6.88 (2.44)	3.68 (1.79)	3.20	2.76	3.64	<0.001

† Standard deviation.

The number of PUs recorded decreased in phase 2 (phase 1: $n = 60$; 76% vs. phase 2: $n = 21$; 26%; $p < 0.001$). However, an increase in the number of patients who developed PUs during their hospital stay was also observed in phase 2 compared to phase 1 (phase 1: $n = 7$; 33.3% vs. phase 2: $n = 15$; 25%; $p = 0.033$).

Regarding the number of falls, six falls were recorded in each of the study periods, with a total of 12 (phase 1: $n = 6$; 1.05% vs. phase 2: $n = 6$; 0.94%; $p > 0.005$). No statistical significance was observed given the small sample size of patients who experienced a fall during these periods.

Regarding the analyses of demographics (age group and sex), completion level of scale records, and scores, the completion of the Braden and Downton scales was significantly higher in the first phase for the group over 65 years (0.012 and $p = 0.003$). No statistically significant differences were observed when comparing risks between phase 1 and phase 2 in terms of sex or age; see Table 4.

Table 4. Analyses of risk scale scores for age group and sex.

	Phase	Sex	Mean (SD)	p-Value	Age	Mean (SD)	p-Value
Braden scale	1	Man	18.21 (4.35)	0.278	≤65	20.47 (3.21)	0.960
		Woman	17.37 (4.57)		>65	16.76 (4.46)	
	2	Man	18.53 (4.09)	0.221	≤65	20.76 (3.28)	
		Woman	18.36 (4.78)		>65	17.09 (4.43)	
Downton scale	1	Man	2.57 (1.6)	0.221	≤65	1.71 (1.29)	0.825
		Woman	3.05 (1.73)		>65	3.08 (1.65)	
	2	Man	1.81 (1.52)	0.221	≤65	1 (0.99)	
		Woman	1.95 (1.48)		>65	2.3 (1.52)	
Gijón scale	1	Man	6.82 (2.68)	0.470	≤65	6.5 (3.19)	0.947
		Woman	6.94 (2.18)		>65	6.91 (2.37)	
	2	Man	3.45 (1.49)	0.470	≤65	3.27 (0.59)	
		Woman	3.92 (2.05)		>65	3.73 (1.88)	

4. Discussion

This study reports a decrease in the completion of nursing records assessing the risk of developing PUs, experiencing falls, and social vulnerability among inpatients with COVID-19 in isolation.

The COVID-19 pandemic has resulted in a clear decrease in adherence to the completion of the Braden, Downton, and Gijón scales. Nurses' failure to record their work does not necessarily mean that they do not complete this work. When nurses have greater workloads, they prioritise their interventions by attaching greater importance to patient care than to recording activities [19]. This may explain why the number of records decreased during the pandemic. This is especially relevant considering that we are comparing the same units and the same staff between two periods, pre- and post-COVID-19. The literature has discussed the unintended effects that can result from the need for strict isolation during the pandemic, which may include incomplete patient documentation [20].

The risk of developing PUs during hospital stays increased in phase 2, as did the number of patients who developed PUs during their hospital stay. Nursing records are a necessary clinical source of relevant information for assessing nursing care, so incomplete or missing records hinder health decision making [14] and, as in this case, hinder health decision making regarding COVID-19 patients. A decrease in the frequency of assessment of the risk of developing PUs using the Braden scale may represent a barrier to early detection and regular risk assessment [21].

The levels of risk of falling and risk of social vulnerability of patients admitted to hospital during phase 2 were lower than during phase 1. The occurrence of adverse events in hospitals depends, to a great extent, on the mean length of stay. In this case, the mean lengths of hospital stays were similar in the two study periods, meaning that this factor could not have influenced the analysis. However, the mean age of patients admitted to hospital during the first wave of the COVID-19 pandemic was lower than it was prior to the pandemic. This may be linked to the Downton and Gijón scale scores showing a greater risk of falling and experiencing social vulnerability prior to the pandemic than during the first wave of the pandemic, which may suggest that age, rather than isolation, is the risk factor in this case. The availability of assessment tools that include age as a predictor of risk will help to identify at-risk patients more accurately [22]. The decrease in mean age in phase 2 could be explained by the fact that the samples may have changed markedly as the units were used for unplanned care of COVID-19 patients and may not represent the types of patients in each unit prior to COVID-19.

Nurses have been deeply involved in the prevention and management of the COVID-19 pandemic in a health system capable of dealing with public health emergencies. Assessment records of the risk of developing PUs must be included in the standardisation of care in new hospital departments and in ongoing improvements to contingency plans [23]. A number of studies associate the risk of developing PUs with severe patient distress in the form of vomiting, shortness of breath, severe pain at rest, urinary problems, and low albumin levels in laboratory tests [21]. This is a clinical scenario similar to that of patients with COVID-19, which justifies the use of the Braden scale in all cases. The decrease in the number of PUs recorded may also be explained or influenced by the decrease in the mean age of the patients admitted to the study units during the pandemic, since age is considered to be a risk factor in developing PUs [21]. However, the number of PUs that occurred while in strict isolation in hospital is particularly worrying, since frequent patient repositioning and mobilisation avoid skin exposure to friction and are vital in PU prevention [24]. The study findings suggest that patient isolation may be associated with a decrease in the frequency of risk assessment and patient mobilisation, leading to decreased PU prevention.

The number of records on the risk of falls among inpatients decreased during the pandemic, which, together with the individual's risk assessment and personal profile, serves as a risk indicator. The occurrence of falls causing injuries and the risk of falling are related [25]. Fall risk assessments provide information necessary for determining the risk of serious clinical outcomes. Therefore, conducting them enables nurses to identify individuals at high risk of falling and put preventative measures in place [26]. Some studies have found a statistically significant relationship between isolation and the occurrence of falls causing injury [27], which means that risk assessment should be a priority in patient safety. Management of the risk of falling is closely related to recording of this risk, and the correct recording of falls enables the factors contributing to them to be identified [28].

A decrease in the number of records on the risk of social vulnerability was also observed. Hospitals have been overwhelmed and professionals have become exhausted during the pandemic, but it must be borne in mind that unfavourable social and family circumstances can result in prolonged hospital stays, readmissions, reduced quality of life, and lower life expectancy among patients. Therefore, early identification of patients at risk and referral to social services facilitates the integration of patients into the social and family spheres, as health problems in the elderly may result in social and family problems and vice versa [29,30].

Analysing the reasons for the decline in the number of nursing records is essential for making care management decisions that prevent these situations from recurring in the event of health system overloads. Quality indicators must be enhanced by improving a number of care-related processes, such as documentation, risk assessments, and reports, which enable nurses to promptly identify at-risk patients and implement specific interventions [31]. Measures that may contribute to preventing a lack of completion of nursing records during the COVID-19 pandemic may include training staff in the use of electronic records systems [15,32] through continued professional development and having nurse managers monitor records to quickly identify any deficiencies [20]. Most importantly, management strategies are needed to allow sufficient time and resources to ensure that nurses are able to effectively perform all important aspects of care, setting staffing levels at the necessary average. Employing low numbers of permanent staff and relying on temporary staff and redeployments jeopardise quality of care and patient safety [33]. It may be necessary to rearrange shift patterns and allocate new nursing staff to reduce nurses' workload and improve the quality of nursing care [34]. Further studies are needed to identify the impact of these measures on nursing records in terms of quantity and quality and to assess the effects of work overload on the quality of nursing records and care provided [12].

The main limitations of this study may be that the sample is limited to a single hospital at a particular moment in time and the unmeasured differences in patient population between phases. Other limitations include the biases inherent to a retrospective study based on past records, although these records are standardised using validated scales to minimise variability.

5. Conclusions

Adherence to the completion of nursing records decreased during the first wave of the pandemic. The quality of care is reflected to a great extent in the clinical records that nurses keep for their patients.

The decrease in the number of nursing records in cases of isolation should prompt the directors of healthcare facilities and healthcare workers to reflect on the need to take measures to encourage recording of risk assessments.

There is a need for further studies on potential solutions to these situations.

Author Contributions: Conceptualisation, M.F.-C., B.M.-G., J.-M.J. and M.L.; formal analysis, M.F.-C., B.M.-G., J.-M.J. and M.L.; validation, M.F.-C., B.M.-G., M.-F.M.-M., J.-M.J., M.-J.C. (María-José Castro), M.-J.C. (María-José Cao) and M.L.; investigation, M.F.-C., B.M.-G., J.-M.J. and M.L.; data curation, M.F.-C., B.M.-G., M.-J.C. (María-José Castro) and M.-J.C. (María-José Cao); statistical analysis, M.-F.M.-M.; writing—original draft preparation and visualisation, M.F.-C., B.M.-G., M.-F.M.-M., J.-M.J., M.-J.C. (María-José Castro), M.-J.C. (María-José Cao) and M.L.; supervision, M.F.-C., B.M.-G., J.-M.J. and M.L. All authors have read and agreed to the published version of the manuscript.

Funding: This research received no external funding.

Institutional Review Board Statement: The study was conducted according to the guidelines of the Declaration of Helsinki and approved by the East Valladolid Health Area's Clinical Research Ethics Committee (protocol code: PI-GR-COVID-20-1861).

Informed Consent Statement: Informed consent was obtained from all subjects involved in the study.

Data Availability Statement: The data presented in this study are available on request from the corresponding author.

Conflicts of Interest: The authors declare no conflict of interest.

References

1. World Health Organization (WHO). Coronavirus Disease (COVID-2019) Weekly Epidemiological Update and Weekly Operational Update. 2020. Available online: https://www.who.int/emergencies/diseases/novel-coronavirus-2019/situation-reports (accessed on 8 March 2021).
2. Cao, Y.; Li, Q.; Chen, J.; Guo, X.; Miao, C.; Yang, H.; Chen, Z.; Li, C.; Li, L. Hospital Emergency Management Plan during the COVID-19 Epidemic. *Acad. Emerg. Med.* **2020**, *27*, 309–311. [CrossRef]
3. Purssell, E.; Gould, D.; Chudleigh, J. Impact of isolation on hospitalised patients who are infectious: Systematic review with meta-analysis. *BMJ Open* **2020**, *10*, e030371. [CrossRef]
4. Tran, K.; Bell, C.; Stall, N.; Tomlinson, G.; McGeer, A.; Morris, A.; Gardam, M.; Abrams, H.B. The Effect of Hospital Isolation Precautions on Patient Outcomes and Cost of Care: A Multi-Site, Retrospective, Propensity Score-Matched Cohort Study. *J. Gen. Intern. Med.* **2017**, *32*, 262–268. [CrossRef]
5. Gammon, J.; Hunt, J. Source isolation and patient wellbeing in healthcare settings. *Br. J. Nurs.* **2018**, *27*, 88–91. [CrossRef]
6. Bei-Lei, L.; Yong-Xia, M.; Fa-Yang, M.; Zhen-Xiang, Z.; Qin, C.; Ming-Ming, S.; Yuan-Yuan, F. Current status and nurses' perceptions of the electronic tabular nursing records in Henan, China. *J. Nurs. Manag.* **2019**, *27*, 616–624. [CrossRef] [PubMed]
7. Kutney-Lee, A.; Sloane, D.M.; Bowles, K.H.; Burns, L.R.; Aiken, L.H. Electronic Health Record Adoption and Nurse Reports of Usability and Quality of Care: The Role of Work Environment. *Appl. Clin. Inform.* **2019**, *10*, 129–139. [CrossRef]
8. Yu, H.Y.; Ahn, E.K.; Seo, E.J. Relationship between the frequency of nursing activities and adverse outcomes in patients with acute coronary syndrome: A retrospective cohort study. *Nurs. Health Sci.* **2019**, *21*, 531–537. [CrossRef]
9. Sprague, E.; Reynolds, S.; Brindley, P. Patient Isolation Precautions: Are They Worth It? *Can. Respir. J.* **2016**, *2016*, 5352625. [CrossRef] [PubMed]
10. McCarthy, B.; Fitzgerald, S.; O'Shea, M.; Condon, C.; Hartnett-Collins, G.; Clancy, M.; Sheehy, A.; Denieffe, S.; Bergin, M.; Savage, E. Electronic nursing documentation interventions to promote or improve patient safety and quality care: A systematic review. *J. Nurs. Manag.* **2019**, *27*, 491–501. [CrossRef]
11. Chang, L.Y.; Yu, H.H.; Chao, Y.C. The Relationship between Nursing Workload, Quality of Care, and Nursing Payment in Intensive Care Units. *J. Nurs. Res.* **2019**, *27*, 1–9. [CrossRef] [PubMed]
12. Fasoi, G.; Patsiou, E.C.; Stavropoulou, A.; Kaba, E.; Papageorgiou, D.; Toylia, G.; Goula, A.; Kelesi, M. Assessment of Nursing Workload as a Mortality Predictor in Intensive Care Units (ICU) Using the Nursing Activities Score (NAS) Scale. *Int. J. Environ. Res. Public Health* **2020**, *18*, 79. [CrossRef] [PubMed]
13. Harris, D.A.; Haskell, J.; Cooper, E.; Crouse, N.; Gardner, R. Estimating the association between burnout and electronic health record-related stress among advanced practice registered nurses. *Appl. Nurs. Res.* **2018**, *43*, 36–41. [CrossRef] [PubMed]

14. Akhu-Zaheya, L.; Al-Maaitah, R.; Bany Hani, S. Quality of nursing documentation: Paper-based health records versus electronic-based health records. *J. Clin. Nurs.* **2018**, *27*, e578–e589. [CrossRef] [PubMed]
15. Ting, J.; Garnett, A.; Donelle, L. Nursing education and training on electronic health record systems: An integrative review. *Nurse Educ. Pract.* **2021**, *55*, 103168. [CrossRef]
16. Cho, I.; Noh, M. Braden Scale: Evaluation of clinical usefulness in an intensive care unit. *J. Adv. Nurs.* **2010**, *66*, 293–302. [CrossRef]
17. Bueno-García, M.J.; Roldán-Chicano, M.T.; Rodríguez-Tello, J.; Meroño-Rivera, M.D.; Dávila-Martínez, R.; Berenguer-García, N. Characteristics of the Downton fall risk assessment scale in hospitalised patients. *Enferm. Clin.* **2017**, *27*, 227–234. [CrossRef] [PubMed]
18. Alarcón, M.T.; González-Montalvo, J.I. La escala sociofamiliar de Gijón, instrumento útil en el hospital general. *Rev. Esp. Geriatr. Gerontol.* **1998**, *33*, 178–179.
19. De Marinis, M.G.; Piredda, M.; Pascarella, M.C.; Vincenzi, B.; Spiga, F.; Tartaglini, D.; Alvaro, R.; Matarese, M. 'If it is not recorded, it has not been done!'? Consistency between nursing records and observed nursing care in an Italian hospital. *J. Clin. Nurs.* **2010**, *19*, 1544–1552. [CrossRef]
20. Karki, S.; Leder, K.; Cheng, A.C. Patients under contact precautions have an increased risk of injuries and medication errors: A retrospective cohort study. *Infect. Control Hosp. Epidemiol.* **2013**, *34*, 1118–1120. [CrossRef]
21. Skogestad, I.J.; Martinsen, L.; Børsting, T.E.; Granheim, T.I.; Ludvigsen, E.S.; Gay, C.L.; Lerdal, A. Supplementing the Braden scale for pressure ulcer risk among medical inpatients: The contribution of self-reported symptoms and standard laboratory tests. *J. Clin. Nurs.* **2017**, *26*, 202–214. [CrossRef]
22. Børsting, T.E.; Tvedt, C.R.; Skogestad, I.J.; Granheim, T.I.; Gay, C.L.; Lerdal, A. Prevalence of pressure ulcer and associated risk factors in middle- and older-aged medical inpatients in Norway. *J. Clin. Nurs.* **2018**, *27*, e535–e543. [CrossRef]
23. Wang, H.; Feng, J.; Shao, L.; Wei, J.; Wang, X.; Xu, X.; Shao, R.; Zhang, M.; He, J.; Zhao, X.; et al. Contingency management strategies of the Nursing Department in centralized rescue of patients with coronavirus disease 2019. *Int. J. Nurs. Sci.* **2020**, *7*, 139–142. [CrossRef]
24. Manderlier, B.; Van Damme, N.; Verhaeghe, S.; Van Hecke, A.; Everink, I.; Halfens, R.; Beeckman, D. Modifiable patient-related factors associated with pressure ulcers on the sacrum and heels: Secondary data analyses. *J. Adv. Nurs.* **2019**, *75*, 2773–2785. [CrossRef] [PubMed]
25. Mojtaba, M.; Alinaghizadeh, H.; Rydwik, E. Downton Fall Risk Index during hospitalisation is associated with fall-related injuries after discharge: A longitudinal observational study. *J. Physiother.* **2018**, *64*, 172–177. [CrossRef] [PubMed]
26. Nilsson, M.; Eriksson, J.; Larsson, B.; Odén, A.; Johansson, H.; Lorentzon, M. Fall Risk Assessment Predicts Fall-Related Injury, Hip Fracture, and Head Injury in Older Adults. *J. Am. Geriatr. Soc.* **2016**, *64*, 2242–2250. [CrossRef]
27. Gandra, S.; Barysauskas, C.M.; Mack, D.A.; Barton, B.; Finberg, R.; Ellison, R.T., 3rd. Impact of contact precautions on falls, pressure ulcers and transmission of MRSA and VRE in hospitalized patients. *J. Hosp. Infect.* **2014**, *88*, 170–176. [CrossRef]
28. Registered Nurses' Association of Ontario. *Preventing Falls and Reducing Injury from Falls*, 4th ed.; RNAO: Toronto, ON, Canada, 2017; pp. 25–60.
29. Calvillo-King, L.; Arnold, D.; Eubank, K.J.; Lo, M.; Yunyongying, P.; Stieglitz, H.; Halm, E.A. Impact of social factors on risk of readmission or mortality in pneumonia and heart failure: Systematic review. *J. Gen. Intern. Med.* **2013**, *28*, 269–282. [CrossRef]
30. Chan, B.; Goldman, L.E.; Sarkar, U.; Guzman, D.; Critchfield, J.; Saha, S.; Kushel, M. High perceived social support and hospital readmissions in an older multi-ethnic, limited English proficiency, safety-net population. *BMC Health Serv. Res.* **2019**, *19*, 334. [CrossRef] [PubMed]
31. Bjarnadottir, R.I.; Herzig, C.T.A.; Travers, J.L.; Castle, N.G.; Stone, P.W. Implementation of Electronic Health Records in US Nursing Homes. *Comput. Inform. Nurs.* **2017**, *35*, 417–424. [CrossRef]
32. Gossen, A.; Mehring, B.; Gunnell, B.S.; Rheuban, K.S.; Cattell-Gordon, D.C.; Enfield, K.B.; Sifri, C.D. The Isolation Communication Management System. A Telemedicine Platform to Care for Patients in a Biocontainment Unit. *Ann. Am. Thorac. Soc.* **2020**, *17*, 673–678. [CrossRef]
33. Saville, C.; Monks, T.; Griffiths, P.; Ball, J.E. Costs and consequences of using average demand to plan baseline nurse staffing levels: A computer simulation study. *BMJ Qual. Saf.* **2021**, *30*, 7–16. [CrossRef] [PubMed]
34. Gao, X.; Jiang, L.; Hu, Y.; Li, L.; Hou, L. Nurses' experiences regarding shift patterns in isolation wards during the COVID-19 pandemic in China: A qualitative study. *J. Clin. Nurs.* **2020**, *29*, 4270–4280. [CrossRef] [PubMed]

International Journal of
Environmental Research and Public Health

MDPI

Article

Gender Bias and the Lack of Equity in Pandemic Nursing in China: A Qualitative Study

Pingting Zhu [1,2,*], Qiwei Wu [1], Xinyi Liu [1], Ericka Waidley [3,*], Qiaoying Ji [1] and Ting Xu [1]

1 School of Nursing, Yangzhou University, Yangzhou 225009, China; MZ120201760@yzu.edu.cn (Q.W.); MX120190879@yzu.edu.cn (X.L.); MZ120201761@yzu.edu.cn (Q.J.); MX120201102@yzu.edu.cn (T.X.)
2 Jiangsu Key Laboratory of Zoonosis, 136 Jiangyang Middle Road, Yangzhou 225009, China
3 School of Nursing, Linfield University, 2900 NE 132nd Ave, Portland, OR 97230, USA
* Correspondence: ptzhu@yzu.edu.cn (P.Z.); ewaidley@linfield.edu (E.W.)

Abstract: There has long been a gender bias in medicine. This qualitative study aims to identify the experience of sexism among frontline female nurses and further explore their expectations and possible strategies to get rid of gender bias. This is a descriptive phenomenological study of 23 female nurses with 11 ± 3.98 years of experience who spent 36 ± 6.50 days at the frontline during the initial COVID-19 outbreak. We employed Colaizzi's phenomenological analysis method to understand the subjective experiences, revealing the following themes: (a) materialization of gender identity; (b) incoordinate relationships; (c) future voice of female nurses. The gender bias experienced by female frontline nurses further challenges their emotional identity and self-identity. Therefore, it is important to require extensive consciousness-raising and policy support to defend female nurses' rights.

Keywords: COVID-19; sexism; female nurses; gender equity; gender bias; female stereotype; pandemic

Citation: Zhu, P.; Wu, Q.; Liu, X.; Waidley, E.; Ji, Q.; Xu, T. Gender Bias and the Lack of Equity in Pandemic Nursing in China: A Qualitative Study. *Int. J. Environ. Res. Public Health* 2021, 18, 10273. https://doi.org/10.3390/ijerph181910273

Academic Editors: Richard Gray and Sonia Udod

Received: 28 August 2021
Accepted: 28 September 2021
Published: 29 September 2021

1. Introduction

The eye of the COVID-19 storm caused deadly destruction in Wuhan that was visible throughout the world. Doctors and nurses from all over the country joined the efforts to fight against the epidemic [1]. Female nurses accounted for two-thirds of the total number of the medical support team [2]. These female nurses were efficient in delivering care to the COVID-19 patients and assisted in stabilizing the pandemic in Wuhan [3,4]. One year has passed since the beginning of the pandemic in Wuhan, and the recognition of the female nurses appears to have gradually disappeared. However, while watching the pandemic unfold, it increased the awareness of the issue of women's interests post-disaster. An example of this awareness is the Beijing Declaration and Platform for Action in 2020 which highlighted that equality between women and men is a fundamental condition for social justice and sustainable development. It is regarded as a milestone all over the world for gender equality and the holistic development of women. However, even with these developments, which are regarded as benchmarks for change, women's rights issues are being ignored [5].

Medicine is traditionally regarded as a male-dominated field, which may be a universal consensus worldwide [6]. This conception is not about gender ratios, as in fact, there are far more women than men in the medical field, but refers to a dominant cultural form based on a particular kind of logic that embraces heroism and rationalism [7]. Previous research pointed to "the Matilda effect" to describe a bias denying recognition within the medical field [8,9]. Even with the female-dominated response to the pandemic, the traditional gender gap issues in healthcare continue to exist [10,11]. During the epidemic, in numerous reports praising frontline female nurses, we would have thought that the performance of women would be the recognition needed to boost the culmination and long-term benefits of feminism. However, the peak that occurred during the pandemic was just that, a single occurrence. Then, it fell off a cliff, below the original level, and got stuck in stigmatization [12].

There are still many people who believe that compassion and caring for patients is driven by the cogs of femininity [13]. Such unconscious, nonmalicious biases and gender expectations also existed behind the widespread coverage of Wuhan. Most frontline real-time professional spokespersons tend to be men, which to a certain extent conceals women's professional and leadership abilities and also suppresses women's voices. Statistically, more than four out of five of the COVID-19 decision-makers were identified as men [14]. In contrast, when the photo lens cut to the picture of women, it tended to show facial blisters and bloodstains squeezed out by masks, rather than expressions of expertise and confidence in providing care. Therefore, in such an ultra-high-risk environment, men, who are a minority of nurses, appear to have a higher authority than women, which seems to be a declaration of frontline sovereignty and public conviction [15]. In this research, female nurses who had volunteered to go to Wuhan were interviewed. The aim of this study is to investigate the gender bias experienced by female nurses during and after COVID-19 supporting assignments.

2. Materials and Methods

2.1. Research Design

This research adopted interpretative phenomenological analysis to understand the subjective experiences and the reasons for these experiences amongst female nurses [16,17]. Critical qualitative content analysis was reported according to the COREQ checklist.

2.2. Participants and Recruitment

Participants who had work experience in the COVID-19 outbreak in Wuhan were recruited using a purposive snowball strategy through the Jiangsu Commission of Health. The inclusion criteria for participants consisted of the following: (1) was a volunteer participant when the epidemic broke out in Wuhan, (2) female, and (3) over the age of 18 years. The exclusion criteria were male nurses and an inability to complete the interview. To determine the number of the sample in qualitative research, and considering the determination of the number of the sample, data saturation (no more new information emerging) was found to be achievable with 16 female nurses (n = 23) [18].

2.3. Data Collection

The study data were collected from September to November 2020. The data collection used a semistructured interview methodology with participants from three hospitals in Yangzhou, Jiangsu province. We used it to guide interviews after a literature review of a large number of feminist theories. Nevertheless, there is no single feminist theory or singular understanding of feminism. However, there is certainly a starting point of feminist theory: "feminism is a movement to end sexism, sexist exploitation, and oppression" [6,19–22]. A semistructured interview is a common mode in phenomenological research that helps to remove gender bias in research by allowing women to express their ideas, opinions, or experiences in their own language, while capturing women's voices, especially those in line with feminist ideals [6,23]. It consisted of open-ended questions (Table 1). Field testing for potential participants was conducted, and the questions were modified prior to the formal application of the interview questions [24]. Researchers strive to establish trust and a comfortable atmosphere before entering the topic and starting the interview with a regular conversation (e.g., "How is your day?"). Participants enter a relaxed state where rapport is developed over time. Each interview was conducted for approximately 60–90 min in the meeting room of the participants' hospital.

Table 1. Interview questions.

	Open-Ended Questions
1.	Can you talk about your experience of supporting Wuhan?
2.	During your support period, have you ever been subjected to gender bias? Could you please specify.
3.	What does gender equality mean to you?
4.	How do you feel about your career?
5.	What barriers/difficulties related to your gender if any have you faced during your carrier advancement?
6.	How did you feel when you were confronted with the barriers?
7.	What do you think of the phenomenon of gender bias?

2.4. Data Analysis

Transcribed interview data were imported into qualitative analysis software Nvivo Version 12. Data were analyzed using Colaizzi's phenomenological analysis method [25,26]. The transcripts were read carefully several times by researchers, and then initial codes, categories, and subcategories were identified. Three main themes were formed by describing the categories in detail. Several strategies were used to ensure trustworthiness and credibility. The transcripts were sent to the participants to confirm the accuracy of the transcribed content. The coding and categorization processes were performed independently by the two researchers. The researchers had regular and continuing discussions to verify the appropriateness of the conceptual meanings and terminology. The audit trail was maintained to ensure all analysis steps could be traced back to original interviews. All research results were presented through the consensus reached by the whole team after discussion.

2.5. Ethical Considerations

The Ethics Committee of the School of Nursing of Yangzhou University approved the study (IR code: YZUHL2020002). Prior to data collection, the researchers provided a self-introduction to the participants and explained the study objectives and methodology. Verbal (on WeChat) and/or written (face to face) informed consent was obtained from all participants. All principles of confidentiality and anonymity were maintained during the study. The participants were told they had the freedom to withdraw from the study at any time without consequences.

3. Results

The study cohort included 23 female nurses who had worked as frontline nurses in Wuhan during the COVID-19 epidemic in 2019. The mean age of participants was 32 years old with a mean work experience of 11 years. All participants were registered nurses. The demographic characteristics of the participants are presented in Table 2.

Table 2. Demographic characteristics of the study participants.

	Mean ± SD or n (%)
Age (years)	32 ± 3.80
Clinical work experience (years)	11 ± 3.98
Length of time in Wuhan (days)	36 ± 6.50
Marital status	
Married	17 (73.9)
Single	6 (26.1)

Three themes were extracted from the content of the interviews: materialization of gender identity, incoordinate correlations, and future voice of female nurses.

3.1. *Theme 1—Materialization of Gender Identity*

Two-thirds of the interviewees expressed experiences of suffering materialization of gender identity. Various examples were given by the participants. We divided this theme into three subthemes: salutation should not be gendered, symbolization of "head shaving", and substitution of identity.

3.1.1. Salutation Should Not Be Gendered

Participants felt that media professionals often create attention-grabbing words for high exposure and that these words were often offensive because they were the product of the combination with gender, such as "female frontline soldier". For participants with the same frontline experience, gendered salutations were infuriating.

> "It's really uncomfortable to be particularly emphasized on gender issues, and there is no need to emphasize gender in the same experience." (Participant 15)

> "Women do need to overcome more difficulties at the emotional and physical level compared with men in the special environment at the frontline of the epidemic. These combined word collocations seem to praise a woman, but the excessive emphasis on gender is a misunderstanding of these praise words." (Participant 11)

3.1.2. Symbolization of "Head Shaving"

Participants explained that head shaving was done in the beginning of the epidemic to reduce the chance of becoming infected when little was known about COVID-19. Because they were also afraid of unknown viruses, head shaving was easier to accept compared to the risk of infection. Some participants said that the use of "head shaving" to highlight their contributions to the frontline was a gender bias stemming from a male perspective in portraying female nurses.

> "The media showed the photos of female nurses with shaved hair in public view. It was shocking at first, and it was a subversion of the image of women. But it's been reposted over and over again and it's not just visual fatigue, and I started wondering is that all we can do?" (Participant 8)

Others say that "shaving and supporting" was a sense of ritual in their heart and that the sense of the ritual was not to care about whether or not to shave their beautiful hair but that afterward they were ready to fight the unknown virus.

> "Everyone else had their head shaving, so I did the same. It seemed that the mission to join the frontline has begun at that time." (Participant 2)

3.1.3. Substitution of Social Identity

As the epidemic in China unfolded, the focus on the female nurses tended to paint a picture of these professionals as wives and mothers versus one of experienced healthcare professionals willing to be deployed on a moment's notice to care for COVID patients. Some participants felt it was "ignoring their expertise" because they clearly knew that some of their original social roles would not be fulfilled if they chose to go to the frontline.

> "It is a personal choice to go to the frontline for support, and the media likes to use special headlines related to family roles to exaggerate the atmosphere." (Participant 4)

One participant said that these headlines related to social roles were involuntarily touching, but the growing number of reports made her feel guilty about her family because media coverage of the role of a mother or wife was a stimulus, a source of empathy.

> "There is no need to use females' other social roles to exaggerate the situation. It would be a handicap." (Participant 12)

3.2. Theme 2—Incoordinate Correlations

Female stereotypes often lead to preconceptions that lead to incoordinate correlations. We divided this theme into two subthemes: professionalism is not the same as gender characteristics, arbitrary definitions using female stereotypes.

3.2.1. Professionalism Is Not the Same as Gender Characteristics

Some participants said that in caring for COVID-19 patients, being humane and talking softly was perceived by patients as feminine rather than as a nurse. Even if this understanding is encountered in the day-to-day work, in the frontline, they wanted to be seen as a nurse who was willing to take risks to care for them, rather than as a woman, because defining them by their gender inevitably accentuates their feminine characteristics.

> "In the consensus of the public, women represent gentleness, but it does not mean that I will choose a career because of my gender." (Participant 7)

Participants were exposed to the popular belief that men were equal to doctors and women to nurses. Because everyone in the shelter was wearing the same personal protective clothing, patients identified gender by height and voice. The gender was determined only to confirm whether the medical staff should be addressed as doctor or nurse. People's subconscious perception of doctors and nurses was mentioned.

> "Even in the subconscious of the nation, the difference between men and women among medical staff is mainly the difference between doctors and nurses, thinking that we are secondary." (Participant 6)

> "When it's a man, patients call him doctor, but he's a male nurse." (Participant 21)

3.2.2. Arbitrary Definitions Using Female Stereotypes

In describing the experience, one participant said that if a male nurse was administering an infusion to a patient and the patient felt pain, the patient would just say "forget it". As for the female nurse, she would be accused of not being gentle enough.

> "Why should we emphasize the distinction between men and women? This is a very strange phenomenon. After all, we do all the same things." (Participant 1)

Family stereotypes of the female even influence their career choices.

> "Nursing was the career my family chosen for me because they thought it was a suitable job for a girl. I think that's probably because of 'inherently feminine trait'." (Participant 3)

3.3. Theme 3—Future Voice of Female Nurses

Reality often shows the circumstances of female nurses in a cruel way [27]. However, as more female nurses receive the recognition they deserve, their voices are becoming stronger, and they are beginning to voice their dissatisfaction and demands [28].

3.3.1. The Need to Remove Gender-Colored Spectacles

Not being trusted and not feeling involved at work was described as an "invisible barrier" by participants, especially when they mentioned that the patient's symptoms and discomfort could be related to psychological causes, which was perceived as a lack of expertise because it has been assumed that only females talk about psychological issues.

> "Raising questions or comments at work were not being acknowledged. But I think compared with men, women have no shortage of knowledge." (Participant 16)

3.3.2. Career Development

Consideration for career advancement would not be a priority if women were not involved in specific tasks, such as frontline supporting.

> "In the past, leaders would give male colleagues more opportunities for continuing education. Since returning from Wuhan, I seem to be the first in line to get some chances to learn, such as the training of specialist nurses." (Participant 2)

Participants mentioned that a female's fertility could be a career uncertainty and that pregnant nurses were treated like "ball players" by various departments because they were unable to have night shifts and were taken on a heavy workload.

> "The head nurse will propose to the human resources department that male nurses are needed, after all, they do not need maternity leave." (Participant 3)

Men still hold essential positions on temporary assignments (frontline working in Wuhan).

> "The spokesmen and team leaders are all men." (Participant 19)

3.3.3. Creating a Gender-Friendly Working Environment

In the early phase of COVID-19, feminine products were deficient. It was difficult for female workers to have access to feminine napkins, tampons, and other comfort measures during deployment. Even though China had a "green channel" for emergency supplies, these feminine products were not available at first.

> "I heard that those who have just arrived in Wuhan to support were not provided with enough female products because all material deliveries are based on protective equipment. But women make up the majority of nurses population, and women's supplies should also be given priority." (Participant 5)

As for supporting dangerous areas like Wuhan, the medical condition of female nurses should be checked before they go.

> "One team member went to Wuhan and found out that she was pregnant, so we did not let her into the quarantine area. Other medical teams had similar situations and all of them were (flown) ... back to Yangzhou." (Participant 14)

4. Discussion

The purpose of this study was to investigate the gender bias and inequality experienced by female nurses during and after supporting the Wuhan assignments.

Gender inequality is a major challenge to global health, and the existence of gender inequalities and prejudices impedes the delivery of effective and efficient healthcare services by health systems [29,30]. The foundation of the health system includes achieving goals of universal health and sustainable development, and if gender equality is not achieved, then building on a shaky foundation is not sustainable. Embedding a series of gender biases in the health system can greatly undermine female's enthusiasm and work ability and chips away at the foundation of patient care services [31]. Similarly, in a traditional hierarchical medical environment, there is concern that a culture of bullying is acceptable at the lower levels of the pyramid. In addition, female nurses who have just started work are subject not only to gender bias, but also to vertical workplace bullying [32–34]. If allowed to continue, these behaviors create a culture of distrust and fear of retribution and contribute to high turnover rates in many institutions. High turnover can shake up the healthcare industry, especially in the event of a pandemic. It was, therefore, important to know whether female nurses who render care in Wuhan experienced gender bias and their feelings, as this will have implications for future recruitment rates of female nurses in the medical profession and support rates after the outbreak.

Whether gender bias occurs at the frontline or after the supporting mission is over (e.g., deployment to the front lines of the pandemic), the contradictions in roles and recognition are unavoidable. From a macro level, it is closely related to cultural background, social process, and social ideology. Although the status of Chinese women is consistently being scrutinized throughout the world, there continues to be an intermittent influence of traditional values that affect the evolution of their role. The mainstream traditional belief in China is Confucianism, which evolved after the washing of history and the subsequent ideological revolution. Many Chinese are trying to abandon the ideological dregs of "men are superior to women" and "men farming and women weaving" [35]. However, Confucianism has an unshakable position in the long history of China, and the side effects of Confucianism are still detrimental to women [36].

Female nurses experienced a gender bias in vocabulary that could be found in this study. The media reports, which emphasized gender symbols, were seen as a sign of disrespect. Female nurses were portrayed as an expectant ideology using the materialization of gender identity. Previous studies have shown that high rates of materialization of women are commonly used in the media, for example, by highlighting women's bodies in advertising [37]. The materialization of women in media has long been argued to affect men's attitudes in ways that could lower the social value of women [37,38]. Clearly, media reports are not correct for frontline nurses, who are expected to demonstrate professional medical skills during their frontline experiences rather than rely on their appearance and identities to be considered heroes of the moment. Such stereotyped female power roles are the embodiment of the ideology of patriarchal society [39]. The media tends to commoditize this gendered power, but in fact, women need to be seen as individuals who can speak and be heard.

"Femininity" and "nurse" always seem to be matching words. Previous studies have shown that patients experience a lot of confusion when presented with male nurses [40,41]. Moreover, male nurses can gain more tolerance, which is a new difference in this study. A systematic review and narrative synthesis study reported that the public's impression of nursing is uneven [42]. Some people believe that nurse specialists are more knowledgeable than general practitioners and that they are also medical staff who can be contacted first, while others believe that nurses are followers of doctors and have not received higher education [42]. Research in the United Kingdom shows that parents are less likely to encourage nursing as a career choice [43], and a survey of public perceptions of nursing conducted in the United States reported that nursing was highly respected as a career [44]. In this study, nursing was found to be an occupation with feminine characteristics recommended by parents to their daughters. Thus, gender bias has been linked with preferences supportive of traditional gender roles.

The so-called "gender equality paradox" is the fact that gender segregation occurs across occupations. In a field often thought to be dominated by men, the medical domain, women are often seen as playing only a supporting role. It will take 99.5 years to close the global gender gap, even though the majority of the world's healthcare professionals are female [5]. Female nurses present a pyramidal position distribution that indicates that only a small number of women are at the decision-making level at the top of the pyramid, while the larger base group is at the bottom of the pyramid and accounts for most grassroots workers [13,45]. Due to this distribution, healthcare leaders may prioritize male nurses for professional development opportunities and job promotion. The deployment of female nurses during the pandemic may indicate that changes in gender equality in China remain unclear; this is because participants were unsure whether increased opportunities were due to awareness of gender equality or to being on the front lines.

The passive gender schema is integrated into the entire external environment that is unfavorable to women. Studies have shown that the reasons for women's career barriers in the workplace are believed to be psychological factors such as dependency and obedience [32]. Therefore, women are also labeled as sensitive and fragile, not strong enough, lacking the spirit of hardship, and generally unable to withstand high pressure in management positions [46]. On the contrary, it is these labels that make people think that caring for patients is a bounden duty commensurate with the female character. Women's career development is often referred to as the "glass ceiling" to indicate invisible obstacles [47]. Previous studies have shown that this phenomenon is caused by the linkage of many factors [48,49]. These factors can include stereotypes, maternal stress (e.g., child-rearing and undertaking housework), and lack of role models for high-ranking women. As the accumulation effect of disadvantages increases, the ceiling continues to be a realistic barrier that cannot be broken through. In order to make small cracks in this barrier, it is important to create a work environment suitable for women.

There were some limitations in this study. First, it was conducted only for healthcare professionals in Yangzhou city, limiting the representativeness of the sample and the generalizability of the results. Second, quantitative approaches, which can be employed to measure perceived gender bias in female nurses, were not components of this study.

5. Conclusions

Current research on gender bias has focused chiefly on surgery departments, with few studies focusing on the experience of female nurses during the pandemic. This study adds to new evidence of gender bias and inequities in medicine. Using this new evidence to speak out for female power and using tension and contradiction as a driving force will facilitate further thought about these issues. Continuing research on women's roles and rights in society, specifically in healthcare environments, provides an inexhaustible driving force for narrowing the distance in gender equality.

Author Contributions: Conceptualization, P.Z. and Q.W.; methodology, P.Z. and Q.W.; software, X.L.; validation, P.Z. and Q.W.; formal analysis, X.L. and Q.J.; investigation, Q.W., X.L., Q.J. and T.X.; writing—original draft preparation, Q.W.; writing—review and editing, P.Z. and E.W.; supervision, P.Z. and E.W. All authors have read and agreed to the published version of the manuscript.

Funding: This research was funded by Science Foundation of Nursing Research of Yangzhou University, grant number HX2002, and Postgraduate Research & Practice Innovation Program of Jiangsu Province, grant number SJCX21_1653.

Institutional Review Board Statement: The study was conducted according to the guidelines of the Declaration of Helsinki and approved by the Ethics Committee of Yangzhou University (No. YZUHL2020002).

Informed Consent Statement: Informed consent was obtained from all subjects involved in the study.

Data Availability Statement: The data presented in this study are available on request from the corresponding author.

Acknowledgments: Thanks to all those who participated in this study and Yangzhou University for providing funding.

Conflicts of Interest: The funders had no role in the design of the study. The authors declare no conflict of interest.

References

1. Liu, Q.; Luo, D.; Haase, J.E.; Guo, Q.; Wang, X.Q.; Liu, S.; Xia, L.; Liu, Z.; Yang, J.; Yang, B.X. The experiences of health-care providers during the covid-19 crisis in china: A qualitative study. *Lancet Glob. Health* **2020**, *8*, e790–e798. [CrossRef]
2. Daily, C.P.S. Xi Expressed Sincere Condolences to Women on the Front Line and on All Fronts of the Epidemic. 2020. Available online: http://paper.people.com.cn/rmrb/html/2020-03/09/nw.D110000renmrb_20200309_2-01.htm (accessed on 17 May 2021).
3. Health Commission of Hubei Province. The Control of Leaving Hubei Outside Wuhan Was Lifted on 8 April 2020. Available online: http://wjw.hubei.gov.cn/bmdt/ztzl/fkxxgzbdgrfyyq/fkdt/202003/t20200325_2189939.shtml (accessed on 17 May 2021).
4. Xiong, Y.; Peng, L. Focusing on health-care providers' experiences in the covid-19 crisis. *Lancet Glob. Health* **2020**, *8*, e740–e741. [CrossRef]
5. The Lancet. 2020: A critical year for women, gender equity, and health. *Lancet* **2020**, *395*, 1. [CrossRef]
6. Sharma, M. Applying feminist theory to medical education. *Lancet* **2019**, *393*, 570–578. [CrossRef]
7. Bleakley, A. Gender matters in medical education. *Med. Educ.* **2013**, *47*, 59–70. [CrossRef] [PubMed]
8. Patel, S.R.; St Pierre, F.; Velazquez, A.I.; Ananth, S.; Durani, U.; Anampa-Guzmán, A.; Castillo, K.; Dhawan, N.; Oxentenko, A.S.; Duma, N. The matilda effect: Underrecognition of women in hematology and oncology awards. *Oncologist* **2021**, *26*, 779–786. [CrossRef]
9. Woitowich, N.C.; Jain, S.; Arora, V.M.; Joffe, H. Covid-19 threatens progress toward gender equity within academic medicine. *Acad. Med.* **2021**, *96*, 813–816. [CrossRef]
10. Stewart-Brown, S. Gender diversity in academic medicine. *BMJ* **2020**, *371*, m4076. [CrossRef]

11. Vijayasingham, L.; Govender, V.; Witter, S.; Remme, M. Employment based health financing does not support gender equity in universal health coverage. *BMJ* **2020**, *371*, m3384. [CrossRef]
12. Mostafa, A.; Sabry, W.; Mostafa, N.S. Covid-19-related stigmatization among a sample of egyptian healthcare workers. *PLoS ONE* **2020**, *15*, e0244172. [CrossRef]
13. Carlsson, M. Self-reported competence in female and male nursing students in the light of theories of hegemonic masculinity and femininity. *J. Adv. Nurs.* **2020**, *76*, 191–198. [CrossRef] [PubMed]
14. van Daalen, K.R.; Bajnoczki, C.; Chowdhury, M.; Dada, S.; Khorsand, P.; Socha, A.; Lal, A.; Jung, L.; Alqodmani, L.; Torres, I.; et al. Symptoms of a broken system: The gender gaps in covid-19 decision-making. *BMJ Glob. Health* **2020**, *5*, e003549. [CrossRef] [PubMed]
15. Asr, F.T.; Mazraeh, M.; Lopes, A.; Gautam, V.; Gonzales, J.; Rao, P.; Taboada, M. The gender gap tracker: Using natural language processing to measure gender bias in media. *PLoS ONE* **2021**, *16*, e0245533. [CrossRef] [PubMed]
16. Byatt, K. The bmj should be adventurous and lead the way on qualitative research. *BMJ* **2016**, *352*, i1471. [CrossRef] [PubMed]
17. Bergdahl, E.; Berterö, C.M. The myth of induction in qualitative nursing research. *Nurs. Philos.* **2015**, *16*, 110–120. [CrossRef]
18. Saunders, B.; Sim, J.; Kingstone, T.; Baker, S.; Waterfield, J.; Bartlam, B.; Burroughs, H.; Jinks, C. Saturation in qualitative research: Exploring its conceptualization and operationalization. *Qual. Quant.* **2018**, *52*, 1893–1907. [CrossRef] [PubMed]
19. Steen, M. Historical perspectives on women and mental illness and prevention of depression in women, using a feminist framework. *Issues Ment. Health Nurs.* **1991**, *12*, 359–374. [CrossRef]
20. Lauve-Moon, K.R.; Enman, S.; Hentz, V. Mainstreaming gender: An examination of feminist methodology in social work research. *Soc. Work* **2020**, *65*, 317–324. [CrossRef] [PubMed]
21. Im, E.O. Current trends in feminist nursing research. *Nurs. Outlook* **2010**, *58*, 87–96. [CrossRef]
22. Webb, C. Feminist research: Definitions, methodology, methods and evaluation. *J. Adv. Nurs.* **1993**, *18*, 416–423. [CrossRef]
23. de Witt, L.; Ploeg, J. Critical appraisal of rigour in interpretive phenomenological nursing research. *J. Adv. Nurs.* **2006**, *55*, 215–229. [CrossRef]
24. Kallio, H.; Pietilä, A.M.; Johnson, M.; Kangasniemi, M. Systematic methodological review: Developing a framework for a qualitative semi-structured interview guide. *J. Adv. Nurs.* **2016**, *72*, 2954–2965. [CrossRef]
25. Haase, J.E. Components of courage in chronically ill adolescents: A phenomenological study. *Adv. Nurs. Sci.* **1987**, *9*, 64–80. [CrossRef]
26. Thomas, J.; Harden, A. Methods for the thematic synthesis of qualitative research in systematic reviews. *BMC Med. Res. Methodol.* **2008**, *8*, 45. [CrossRef]
27. Hay, K.; McDougal, L.; Percival, V.; Henry, S.; Klugman, J.; Wurie, H.; Raven, J.; Shabalala, F.; Fielding-Miller, R.; Dey, A.; et al. Disrupting gender norms in health systems: Making the case for change. *Lancet* **2019**, *393*, 2535–2549. [CrossRef]
28. Gill, J.; Baker, C. The power of mass media and feminism in the evolution of nursing's image: A critical review of the literature and implications for nursing practice. *J. Med. Humanit.* **2019**, *42*, 371–386. [CrossRef] [PubMed]
29. Liang, R.; Dornan, T.; Nestel, D. Why do women leave surgical training? A qualitative and feminist study. *Lancet* **2019**, *393*, 541–549. [CrossRef]
30. El Arnaout, N.; Chehab, R.F.; Rafii, B.; Alameddine, M. Gender equity in planning, development and management of human resources for health: A scoping review. *Hum. Resour. Health* **2019**, *17*, 52. [CrossRef] [PubMed]
31. Krieger, N. Discrimination and health inequities. *Int. J. Health Serv.* **2014**, *44*, 643–710. [CrossRef]
32. Hauw-Berlemont, C.; Aubron, C.; Aissaoui, N.; Bodet-Contentin, L.; Boissier, F.; Fartoukh, M.S.; Jourdain, M.; Le Marec, J.; Pestel, J.; Salmon Gandonnière, C.; et al. Perceived inequity, professional and personal fulfillment by women intensivists in france. *Ann. Intensive Care* **2021**, *11*, 72. [CrossRef]
33. Trépanier, S.G.; Peterson, C.; Fernet, C.; Austin, S.; Desrumaux, P. When workload predicts exposure to bullying behaviours in nurses: The protective role of social support and job recognition. *J. Adv. Nurs.* **2021**, *77*, 3093–3103. [CrossRef]
34. Mahase, E. Gender pay gap in general practice is 35%, report finds-owing to age, working hours, and partnerships. *BMJ* **2020**, *368*, m112. [CrossRef]
35. Li, Y.; Chen, H. Gender convergence or divergence in the relationship between late-life depression and multiple stressors: Evidence from a national survey in china. *J. Women Aging* **2021**, 1–14. [CrossRef]
36. Xiao, L.; Wang, F. Examining the links between beauty ideals internalization, the objectification of women, and ambivalent sexism among chinese women: The effects of sexual orientation. *Arch. Sex Behav.* **2021**, *50*, 553–562. [CrossRef]
37. Carrotte, E.R.; Prichard, I.; Lim, M.S. "Fitspiration" on social media: A content analysis of gendered images. *J. Med. Internet Res.* **2017**, *19*, e95. [CrossRef]
38. Wright, P.J.; Tokunaga, R.S. Men's objectifying media consumption, objectification of women, and attitudes supportive of violence against women. *Arch. Sex. Behav.* **2016**, *45*, 955–964. [CrossRef] [PubMed]
39. Meier, T.; Boyd, R.L.; Mehl, M.R.; Milek, A.; Pennebaker, J.W.; Martin, M.; Wolf, M.; Horn, A.B. Stereotyping in the digital age: Male language is "ingenious", female language is "beautiful"—And popular. *PLoS ONE* **2020**, *15*, e0243637. [CrossRef] [PubMed]
40. Sasa, R.I. Male nurse: A concept analysis. *Nurs. Forum* **2019**, *54*, 593–600. [CrossRef] [PubMed]
41. Tollison, A.C. Stereotype threat in male nurse-patient interactions. *J. Nurs. Educ.* **2018**, *57*, 614–619. [CrossRef]
42. Girvin, J.; Jackson, D.; Hutchinson, M. Contemporary public perceptions of nursing: A systematic review and narrative synthesis of the international research evidence. *J. Nurs. Manag.* **2016**, *24*, 994–1006. [CrossRef]

43. Neilson, G.R.; McNally, J. The negative influence of significant others on high academic achieving school pupils' choice of nursing as a career. *Nurse Educ. Today* **2013**, *33*, 205–209. [CrossRef]
44. Donelan, K.; Buerhaus, P.; Desroches, C.; Dittus, R.; Dutwin, D. Public perceptions of nursing careers: The influence of the media and nursing shortages. *Nurs. Econ.* **2008**, *26*, 143–150. [PubMed]
45. Onumah, C.; Wikstrom, S.; Valencia, V.; Cioletti, A. What women need: A study of institutional factors and women faculty's intent to remain in academic medicine. *J. Gen. Intern. Med.* **2021**, *36*, 2039–2047. [CrossRef] [PubMed]
46. Kardashian, A.; May, F.P. Empowering early career female gastroenterologists and hepatologists. *Nat. Rev. Gastroenterol. Hepatol.* **2019**, *16*, 644–645. [CrossRef]
47. Morgenroth, T.; Kirby, T.A.; Ryan, M.K.; Sudkämper, A. The who, when, and why of the glass cliff phenomenon: A meta-analysis of appointments to precarious leadership positions. *Psychol. Bull.* **2020**, *146*, 797–829. [CrossRef] [PubMed]
48. Manzi, F.; Heilman, M.E. Breaking the glass ceiling: For one and all? *J. Pers. Soc. Psychol.* **2021**, *120*, 257–277. [CrossRef]
49. Krishnan, N.; Biggerstaff, D.; Szczepura, A.; Dolton, M.; Livingston, S.; Hattersley, J.; Eris, J.; Ascher, N.; Higgins, R.; Braun, H.; et al. Glass slippers and glass cliffs: Fitting in and falling off. *Transplantation* **2019**, *103*, 1486–1493. [CrossRef] [PubMed]

International Journal of
Environmental Research and Public Health

MDPI

Article

Analyzing the Impact of COVID-19 Trauma on Developing Post-Traumatic Stress Disorder among Emergency Medical Workers in Spain

Carmen M. Martínez-Caballero [1,†], Rosa M. Cárdaba-García [1,2,3,†], Rocío Varas-Manovel [1], Laura M. García-Sanz [1], Jorge Martínez-Piedra [4], Juan J. Fernández-Carbajo [1], Lucía Pérez-Pérez [2,3,5], Miguel A. Madrigal-Fernández [2,3,6], M. Ángeles Barba-Pérez [2,3,6], Elena Olea [2,3,7], Carlos Durantez-Fernández [8] and M. Teresa Herrero-Frutos [1,*]

1 Emergencies Management (SACYL), 40002 Segovia, Spain; cmmartinez@saludcastillayleon.es (C.M.M.-C.); rcardaba@saludcastillayleon.es (R.M.C.-G.); mvarasma@saludcastillayleon.es (R.V.-M.); lmgarcias@saludcastillayleon.es (L.M.G.-S.); jjfernandez@saludcastillayleon.es (J.J.F.-C.)
2 Nursing Department, Faculty of Nursing, University of Valladolid, 47005 Valladolid, Spain; lucia.perez@uva.es or luperper2@hotmail.com (L.P.-P.); miguelangel.madrigal@uva.es or miguelanmad@gmail.com (M.A.M.-F.); mariaangeles.barba@uva.es (M.Á.B.-P.); elena.olea@uva.es (E.O.)
3 Nursing Care Research (GICE), Faculty of Nursing, University of Valladolid, 47005 Valladolid, Spain
4 Health Transportation Group, 40195 Segovia, Spain; jorgemp29@gmail.com
5 Primary Care Management Valladolid West (SACYL), 47012 Valladolid, Spain
6 University Clinical Hospital of Valladolid, 47003 Valladolid, Spain
7 Instituto de Biología y Genética Molecular (IBGM), Universidad de Valladolid-CSIC, 47005 Valladolid, Spain
8 Faculty of Health Sciences, University of Castilla-La Mancha, 45600 Talavera de la Reina, Spain; carlos.durantez@uclm.es
* Correspondence: rosamaria.cardaba@uva.es or therrerof@saludcastillayleon.es
† Mrs. Carmen M. Martínez-Caballero and Dra. Rosa M. Cárdaba-García have contributed as IP in the research.

Citation: Martínez-Caballero, C.M.; Cárdaba-García, R.M.; Varas-Manovel, R.; García-Sanz, L.M.; Martínez-Piedra, J.; Fernández-Carbajo, J.J.; Pérez-Pérez, L.; Madrigal-Fernández, M.A.; Barba-Pérez, M.Á.; Olea, E.; et al. Analyzing the Impact of COVID-19 Trauma on Developing Post-Traumatic Stress Disorder among Emergency Medical Workers in Spain. *Int. J. Environ. Res. Public Health* **2021**, *18*, 9132. https://doi.org/10.3390/ijerph18179132

Academic Editors: Richard Gray, Sonia Udod and Marcello Covino

Received: 6 July 2021
Accepted: 26 August 2021
Published: 30 August 2021

Abstract: The early stages of the COVID-19 pandemic presented the characteristics of a traumatic event that could trigger post-traumatic stress disorder. Emergency Medical Services workers are already a high-risk group due to their professional development. The research project aimed to analyse the impact of the COVID-19 pandemic on EMS professionals in terms of their mental health. For this purpose, we present a descriptive crosssectional study with survey methodology. A total of 317 EMS workers (doctors, nurses, and emergency medical technicians) were recruited voluntarily. Psychological distress, post-traumatic stress disorder, and insomnia were assessed. The instruments were the General Health Questionnaire-12 (GHQ-12), the Davidson Trauma Scale (DTS-8), and the Athens Insomnia Scale (AIS-8). We found that 36% of respondents had psychological distress, 30.9% potentially had PTSD, and 60.9% experienced insomnia. Years of work experience were found to be positively correlated, albeit with low effect, with the PTSD score ($r = 0.133$). Finally, it can be stated that the COVID-19 pandemic has been a traumatic event for EMS workers. The number of professionals presenting psychological distress, possible PTSD, or insomnia increased dramatically during the early phases of the pandemic. This study highlights the need for mental health disorder prevention programmes for EMS workers in the face of a pandemic.

Keywords: emergency medical services; post-traumatic stress disorder; mental status; sleep disorders; COVID-19 pandemic

1. Introduction

In Spain, the SARS-CoV-2 pandemic started on 31 January 2020, when the first case was diagnosed on the island of La Gomera, and the first death from Coronavirus Disease 2019 (COVID-19) occurred on 13 February 2020 in Valencia. Since the first confirmed case was reported on 31 January 2020, more than 405,000 cases and 28,000 deaths have been reported in Spain [1]. According to the ENE–COVID seroprevalence study, one in ten Spaniards had been infected with the virus by November 2020 [2]. It was not until 14

March 2020 that the Spanish state decreed a state of alarm and limited the movement of people throughout the territory [3]. On 28 March, all nonessential onsite work activities were suspended for 15 days [4]. Spain has suffered four waves of the COVID-19 pandemic, with the first wave being the most aggressive in terms of morbidity and mortality, with the highest number of deaths in March and April. The highest number of coronavirus deaths in one day (950) was recorded on 2 April [5,6]. We are currently in the fifth wave of the pandemic, although, as of 26 June 2021, it is not mandatory to wear masks outdoors if safe distances of at least 1.5 m are maintained between individuals [7].

Post-traumatic stress disorder (PTSD) is defined in the DSM-V in section B as the "presence of one or more of the following intrusive symptoms associated with the traumatic event, beginning after the traumatic event" [8]. The symptoms referred to are: recurrent, involuntary, intrusive, or distressing memories of the traumatic event; recurrent distressing dreams in which the content of the dream is related to the traumatic event; dissociative reactions such as flashbacks in which the subject feels or acts as if the traumatic event is being replayed; intense or prolonged psychological distress on exposure to internal or external factors resembling the traumatic event; and intense physiological reactions to internal or external factors resembling the traumatic event. This definition is specified with other characteristics that do not exactly fit the object of study of this research. It should be noted that the current definition of PTSD does not state that a specific time must have passed since the traumatic event in order for an individual to suffer from this syndrome only that the associated symptoms must remain for at least one month and negatively affect the individual's life [8].

The scientific literature indicates that traumatic symptoms may appear immediately, after weeks, or even months after exposure, and, in most cases, they appear in the first six months after the triggering event. Unlike an acute stress reaction, PTSD symptoms do not disappear after a few weeks and tend to persist over time [9].

PTSD was originally described in wartime contexts, and shortly thereafter, it was also seen in survivors of death camps and sexual assaults. Natural disasters and terrorist attacks are also documented as triggers for PTSD [10]. PTSD has also been associated with previous epidemics, such as the one generated by the Ebola virus [11].

Individuals working in the emergency medical services experience direct contact with death and with events that can be considered traumatic. Although their academic training should be adequate to deal with these situations, the reality is that this is not the case [12], and, in hostile situations such as wars, natural disasters, and terrorist attacks, it is not uncommon for PTSD to develop in health personnel on the front line. [13]. Despite this, professionals often do not readily accept that they suffer from symptoms associated with PTSD, as it is often understood to be a weakness at work [14]. It is assumed that health personnel who work in EMS have the capacity to cope with events that can be traumatic, which is not always the case—it should not be forgotten that the most frequently attended incidents in these services are not emergent but urgent and that the actual and practical experience in catastrophic situations such as a pandemic may only be theoretical [15]. In fact, these professionals should be trained to face situations similar to those experienced during the COVID-19 pandemic, but the reality is quite different; as a result, such individuals are at risk of developing PTSD [16]. Despite several studies on the mental health of EMS workers in recent years, there is not enough previous data prior to the last two decades, as there was previously not much interest in assessing the mental health of frontline EMS workers [17].

It is widely known that since the beginning of the COVID-19 pandemic, an increase in mental illness has been observed [18]. A decrease in psychological wellbeing associated with higher values of anxiety and depression has been observed in the general population, in COVID-19 patients, and, above all, in healthcare workers, especially among those on the front line [19–21]. One of the most common symptoms in healthcare personnel has been insomnia [22,23]. Some studies relate these consequences to occupational factors such as professional category, workplace, and the means available to protect against possible COVID-19 infection, among others [24,25].

We are aware that previous studies have been published on the impact of the pandemic on healthcare workers [26,27], highlighting the deterioration in mental health and problems related to sleep and rest, but, to our knowledge, no studies have yet been published with data on the negative impact on mental health and PTSD symptoms focusing on emergency medical services (EMS) workers. Moreover, the scientific literature offers few examples that include all professional categories involved in Spanish EMS (physicians, nurses, and emergency medical technicians (EMTs)) who have worked during the pandemic [28]. EMS workers are considered to be a group at particular risk of developing PTSD in general terms [9], since, while the prevalence of PTSD in the general population ranges between 1% and 3% [13], in EMS in particular, it is estimated to be 11% during catastrophic events [29].

The initial hypothesis of the study was that the COVID-19 pandemic was associated with poor mental health status, insomnia, and an increased risk of developing PTSD in prehospital emergency professionals. The overall objective was to determine the impact of the early stages of the COVID-19 pandemic on the mental health of workers of the "Gerencia de Emergencias Sanitarias de Castilla y León" (GESACYL) and the "Servicio de Urgencias Médicas de Madrid 112" (SUMMA 112). Specifically, validated instruments were used to quantify the mental health of the first responders, to measure the presence of insomnia, to assess the frequency of PTSD, and to describe the variables most frequently related to the three previous aspects.

In this paper, readers will find a descriptive study methodology based on survey data collection. Next, a descriptive analysis of the main variables is presented to further the search for correlations between variables that have significance in the development of mental health problems, insomnia, and PTSD. In this way, a discussion is established with the findings of other authors, accepting the limitations of this research, and assessing the implications that the results have for clinical practice.

2. Materials and Methods

2.1. Design

A descriptive crosssectional study with survey methodology is presented.

2.2. Study Sample

The study population was EMS workers (physicians, nurses, and EMTs) from two different regions of Central Spain: Castile and León "Gerencia de Emergencias Sanitarias de Castilla y León" (GESACYL) and Madrid "Servicio de Urgencias Médicas de Madrid 112" (SUMMA 112).

A total of 317 workers were recruited, and the response rate was 37.6%. A volunteer sampling method was adopted, via corporate email.

The inclusion criteria established were as follows: over 18 years of age, working in GESACYL or SUMMA112, being a physician, nurse, or EMT, being active during the COVID-19 pandemic, having worked almost exclusively in prehospital care (at least 90% of the total number of working days), agreeing to participate in the investigation, having basic computer skills, and being Spanish-speaking. Those who did not meet the aforementioned inclusion criteria and those who ticked the box on the questionnaire stating that they did not consent to participate in this study were excluded.

2.3. Ethical Aspects

The study was approved by the Ethics Committee for Drug Research of the Valladolid East Health Area, with registration code PI 139-20 NO HRHV, on 6 June 2020. This study conformed to the STROBE Initiative (Strengthening the Reporting of Observational Studies in Epidemiology) for observational studies of the EQUATOR Initiative [30].

2.4. Recruitment of the Sample

The sample was recruited by contacting the participants through the corporate email service of the emergency institutions of Castile and Leon and Madrid, sending them a link to the self-administered survey developed using the online Google Forms® tool, in which the participants declared that they met the requirements to be part of the study sample. The recruitment strategy was carried out by sending an email reminder one and three weeks after the initial referral. In no case were participants offered any incentive to be part of the sample. The data collection period was from 20 May 2020 to 26 July 2020, a period early on during the first wave of the pandemic; according to the DSM-V definition of PTSD, this was appropriate, as symptomatology may appear immediately after a traumatic event [8].

2.5. Study Variables

The variables considered were sociodemographic (age, sex, number of people living together during the pandemic, and change in body weight during the pandemic); work-related (professional category, place of work, type of unit, experience in the service, and change of function during the pandemic); occupational safety aspects (previous practical training in the use of protective equipment, availability of sufficient protective equipment in the unit, removal of protective equipment that did not comply with regulations, information on the pandemic and its evolution, testing for COVID-19, need for home isolation, presence of COVID-19 symptoms, and hospitalization for COVID-19); and variables associated with psychological health (concern about the possibility of contracting the disease, concern about harming loved ones, anxiety symptoms before the pandemic, anxiety symptoms during the pandemic, treatment of anxiety before the pandemic, treatment of anxiety during the pandemic, need for psychological support before the pandemic and during the pandemic, knowledge of the existence or not of a psychological support unit for employees, work environment of the unit, and existence of specific training courses for anxiety control for workers).

2.6. Instruments

The instruments used were the General Health Questionnaire-12 (GHQ-12), the Davidson Trauma Scale (DTS-8), and the Athens Insomnia Scale (AIS-8).

2.6.1. General Health Questionnaire-12

The General Health Questionnaire-12 (GHQ-12) is a 12 item self-administered questionnaire that detects psychological distress. There are six positive items (e.g., "Have you been able to concentrate?") and six negative items (e.g., "Have you lost confidence?"). Each item has four possible responses—according to a four-level Likert scale—aimed at capturing the intensity of the respondents' feelings for the given item. The possible responses for the six positive items in the questionnaire, together with the score assigned to them, were 0 = more than usual; 0 = same as usual; 1 = less than usual; and 1 = much less than usual. For the negative items, possible responses were 0 = absolutely not; 0 = no more than usual; 1 = somewhat more than usual; and 1 = much more than usual. Thus, the possible total score on the questionnaire ranged from 0 to 12. The interpretation of the total score is as follows: from 0 to 4: no psychological distress; from 5 to 6: probable psychological distress; and from 7 to 12: psychological morbidity. The GHQ-12 has a reliability according to different studies with Cronbach's alpha ranging from 0.82 to 0.86 [31,32]. In the sample of this study, a result of 0.85 was obtained for the mentioned test.

2.6.2. Davidson Trauma Scale

The Davidson Trauma Scale (DTS-8) is a questionnaire that can be self-administered or interviewed and consists of eight items. This scale is used to detect suspicion of a potential diagnosis of post-traumatic stress syndrome. The questions refer to the last week and are measured by a five-level Likert scale, with possible values (0,1,2,3,4). Value 0 corresponds to the least stressful response. The total score of the questionnaire is obtained by adding the scores of the eight items, and it therefore ranges from 0 to 32. Higher scores on the scale are related to a higher possibility of suspected PTSD. The interpretation established by the authors of the original test is by means of ranges as follows: from 0 to 7: no suspicion of PTSD; from 8 to 11: it cannot be determined whether or not PTSD exists; 12 or more: suspicion of PTSD [33]. The scale presents adequate internal consistency, with a Cronbach's alpha of 0.71–0.91 [34]. The value of Cronbach's alpha obtained in the study sample was 0.87.

2.6.3. Athens Insomnia Scale

The Athens Insomnia Scale (AIS-8) is a self-assessment survey consisting of eight items. Its purpose is to detect insomnia-type sleep disorders. The first four items assess possible insomnia problems from a quantitative point of view, the fifth item asks about sleep quality, while the last three items assess the daytime impact of insomnia. The evaluation questions refer to the last week and are measured on a four-level Likert scale, which translates into values (0,1,2,3), with 0 being the absence of a problem and 3 the maximum severity. The total score of the questionnaire is obtained by adding the scores of the eight items, and it therefore ranges from 0 to 24. Higher scores on the questionnaire are associated with more insomnia. Authors who have evaluated the scale based on the diagnosis of insomnia of the International Classification of Diseases in its 10th revision (ICD-10) establish that a score equal to or higher than six points determines a diagnosis of insomnia. The internal consistency of the test measured by Cronbach's alpha is around 0.90 [35]. The AIS-8 showed a high degree of internal homogeneity, obtaining a Cronbach's alpha of 0.91 for the whole sample.

2.7. Data Analysis

The statistical procedure and data analysis were performed by means of a descriptive analysis of frequencies and response percentages, centrality (mean), and dispersion (standard deviation) in quantitative variables. Quantitative variables were analyzed by normality test (Kolmogorov–Smirnov) prior to the inferential analysis, looking for significant relationships between variables by means of Pearson's r test, ANOVA, and Student's t test. The statistical significance level used was $p = 0.05$ or lower. The statistical program used was SPSS® v.24.

3. Results

3.1. Sample Description

The sample consisted of 317 health professionals from the Health Emergency Services of Castile and Leon (80.4%) and Madrid (19.6%), who voluntarily agreed to participate in the study. In relation to the sociodemographic variables of the sample, 52.7% were men, 46.4% women, and 0.9% replied "Other". The most frequent age range was between 40 and 49 years (42.9%). Only 16.1% lived alone during the pandemic, while households of four or more constituted 41.3% of the total. Overall, 120 respondents (37.9%) gained weight during the pandemic. Of those who gained weight, 61.2% declared having gained less than 1 kg.

3.2. Occupational Considerations

The following is a description of the variables related to the health profession and work setting. By professional category, 61 respondents were physicians (19.2%), 78 nurses (24.6%), and 178 emergency health technicians (56.2%). Half of the respondents worked in advanced life support units (50.5%). The most common time period for which respondents had worked in the service was between 10 and 20 years (54.9%), followed by less than 10 years (25.6%). Overall, 223 respondents (70.3%) changed their care functions during the pandemic, but only 41 persons (12.9%) were reassigned to a specific contingency hospital for patients diagnosed with COVID-19.

3.3. Job Security in the Pandemic

Working in healthcare during the pandemic has entailed a number of risks, which are described below.

A large number of people (94.3%) felt worried about the possibility of contracting the disease at work and about the possibility of passing it on to their family members (96.8%).

Overall, 202 respondents (63.7%) stated that they had received prior theoretical training in their service on the use of personal protective equipment (PPE) necessary in case of biological risk, and 60.6% stated that they had received practical training regarding the use of personal protective equipment.

In total, 205 respondents (64.7%) had adequate means of protection in their work during the pandemic, but in 78.9% of cases, it was necessary to remove the protective equipment provided by their service as it did not comply with the protection regulations.

In total, 238 respondents (75.1%) affirmed that they had not been informed by their service of the possibility of a COVID-19 pandemic occurring prior to the state of confinement, while 48.3% (153) had been informed by the public health administration of the evolution of the pandemic.

Most of the workers (93.4%) had been tested for SARS-CoV-2 infection; in 35.3% of cases, they had been tested with both a PCR test and an antibody screening test.

A total of 19.2% (61) required home isolation because they had had a high-risk encounter in their work environment. A total of 33.8% had experienced symptoms associated with COVID-19 infection, but only six persons (1.9%) required hospital admission.

3.4. Mental Health Considerations

The respondents reported their mental health in terms of its pre- and postpandemic status as follows.

Twelve percent had experienced symptoms of anxiety prior to the pandemic, compared to 65.6% who stated that they had experienced anxiety-related symptoms during the pandemic. Overall, 20.5% had taken anxiolytics prior to the pandemic, a figure that decreased to 18.9% during the pandemic. Similarly, the need for psychological support was reported by 24.0% before the pandemic and by 9.8% during the pandemic.

In total, 37.2% of the respondents stated that their service had a psychological support unit, but a similar number, 36.0%, did not know if they had access to such a support unit. Training courses aimed at anxiety control were given within the unit in which they worked in 26.2% of the cases, and in 46.7% of the cases, the psychological health of the workers could be dealt with normally.

3.5. Questionnaire Results

Regarding the mental health of the participants, in the GHQ-12, the mean score of the sample in the questionnaire was 5.26 (SD = 3.18). The GHQ-12 scores of the participants indicate that 37.5% showed no pathology, 26.5% showed possible psychological pathology, and 36% showed signs of psychological pathology, according to the cutoff points of the scale.

In relation to PTSD, assessed by the DTS-8 questionnaire, the mean score was 9.26 (SD = 6.04). According to the cutoff point of this scale ($\geq$12 points), 30.9% of the people in the sample present suspected post-traumatic stress syndrome.

Regarding the perception of sleeping difficulties, which was measured by the AIS-8 scale, the mean score of the participants on the instrument was 7.39 (SD = 4.94). Regarding the cutoff point of the scale ($\geq$6 points), 60.9% experienced sleeping difficulties.

The most significant items in each of the three instruments (GHQ-12, DTS-8, and AIS-8) are shown in Table 1. If we take into account those variables that offer responses other than the YES/NO dichotomy, we can observe that the groups with the greatest number of individuals suffering from sleep difficulties were: the age group between 40 and 49 years, women, EMTs, EMS workers in Castilla y León, EMS workers in advanced units, those who had been working for between 10 and 20 years, those who lived with four or more people, those who had undergone serological tests, and those who had gained less than 1 kg in weight. In general, these groups also demonstrated the greatest prevalence of signs of suspected psychological pathology, suspected PTSD, and insomnia (Table 2).

Table 1. Items from the GHQ-12, DTS-8, and AIS-8 instruments with the greatest significance (n = 317).

GHQ-12	
Items with the highest scores in the scale	Percentage (%)
Thinking of self as worthless	88.3
Losing confidence	75.7
DTS-8	
Items with the highest scores in the scale	Percentage (%)
Experiencing less interest in things previously enjoyed	4.7
Imagining or remembering painful, recurring images that cannot be put out of mind	3.8
AIS-8	
Items with the highest scores in the scale	Percentage (%)
Sleep induction	4.4
Final awakening	3.2
Total sleep duration	3.2
Sleep quality	3.2

Table 2. Sociodemographic distribution of polytomous variables according to the results of GHQ-12: suspected psychological pathology (GHQ-12 = 5–6), DTS-8: suspicion of post-traumatic stress disorder (DTS-8 $\geq$ 12), and AIS-8: insomnia (AIS-8 $\geq$ 6) (n = 317).

Variables	**GHQ-12 Psychological Pathology**		**DTS-8 PTSD**		**AIS-8 Insomnia**	
	n	%	n	%	n	%
Age (years)						
≤29	19	4.1	29	9.1	29	9.1
30–39	31	9.8	26	8.2	42	13.2
40–49	41	12.9	39	12.3	78	24.6
50–59	26	8.2	22	6.9	40	12.6
≥60	3	0.9	2	0.6	4	1.3
Gender						
Female	68	21.5	52	16.4	108	34.1
Male	46	14.5	43	13.6	82	25.9
Professional category						
Physician	19	6	15	4.7	36	11.4
Nurse	31	9.8	22	6.9	54	17
Emergency medical technician	64	20.2	61	19.2	103	32.5
Emergency Service						
SACYL	90	28.4	74	23.3	148	46.7
SUMMA 112	24	7.6	24	7.6	45	14.2

Table 2. *Cont.*

Variables	GHQ-12 Psychological Pathology		DTS-8 PTSD		AIS-8 Insomnia	
	n	%	*n*	%	*n*	%
Type of EMS						
ALS	56	17.7	39	12.3	99	31.2
BLS	40	12.6	41	12.9	70	22.1
Work experience (years)						
<10	29	9.1	18	5.7	52	16.4
10 to 20	63	19.9	56	17.7	106	33.4
21 to 30	18	5.7	18	5.7	27	8.5
>30	4	1.3	6	1.9	8	2.5
Number of people per household						
1	21	6.6	18	5.7	33	10.4
2	21	6.6	20	6.3	39	12.3
3	21	6.6	15	4.7	34	10.7
>4	51	16.1	45	14.2	87	27.4
Tests						
PCR	14	4.4	14	4.4	18	5.7
Ig M/Ig G	43	13.6	79	24.9	90	28.4
Both	50	15.8	39	12.3	70	22.1
Weight gained (Kg)						
<1	64	20.2	58	18.3	113	35.6
1 to 2	4	1.3	4	1.3	5	1.6
2 to 3	10	3.2	3	0.9	12	3.8
3 to 4	19	6	18	5.7	28	8.8
>4	28	8.8	9	2.8	10	3.2

Abbreviations: PTSD, post-traumatic stress disorder; SACYL, Sanidad de Castilla y León; SUMMA 112, Servicio de Urgencias Médicas de Madrid; EMS, emergency medical services; ALS, advanced life support; BLS, basic life support.

3.6. Comparison of Means and Correlations

Subsequently, an inferential analysis was carried out between variables, with the intention of searching for relationships between the general variables and the results of the total scores of the GHQ-12, DTS-8, and AIS-8, which, in all cases, approximately followed a normal distribution.

Depending on the type of variable, Student's t tests were used for dichotomous variables, ANOVA for variables with more than two possible answers, and Pearson's r correlation coefficient for quantitative variables.

Relationships were found between the GHQ-12 total score indicating the psychological health of the person and the following variables: gender, changes in job functions, having undergone previous theoretical and practical training on the use of PPE, the type of SARS-CoV-2 test, having required isolation, having experienced symptoms of the disease, having had adequate PPE during the pandemic, having had PPE removed from the service because it was not adequate, having been worried about contracting the disease and about transmitting it to family, anxiety symptoms prior to and during the pandemic, use of anxiolytics during the pandemic, requiring psychological support prior to and during the pandemic, and dealing with mental health issues normally in the work unit.

In addition, relationships were found between the DTS-8 total score, showing the risk of post-traumatic stress, and the following variables: gender, changes in job duties, having had prior theoretical and practical training on the use of PPE, the type of SARS-CoV-2 testing, having had appropriate PPE during the pandemic, having been worried about contracting the disease, anxiety symptoms prior to and during the pandemic, use of anxiolytics prior to and during the pandemic, requiring psychological support prior to and during the pandemic, and dealing with mental health issues normally in the work unit.

Relationships were also found between the AIS-8 total score indicating the presence of insomnia and the following variables: gender, service in which they work, having undergone previous theoretical and practical training on the use of PPE, having been worried about contracting the disease, weight gain during confinement, anxiety symptoms before and during the pandemic, use of anxiolytics before and during the pandemic, requiring psychological support before and during the pandemic, and dealing with mental health issues normally in the work unit (Tables 3 and 4).

Table 3. Inferential analysis: Student *t* test means comparison.

Variables	Instrument (Total Score)	Levene Test	*t* Value	Level of Significance *p*	IC 95%	
					Min	Max
Emergency service	AIS-8	0.554	−1.964	0.050 *	−2.743	0.002
Functions	GHQ-12	0.696	−2.449	0.015 *	−1.716	−0.187
	DTS-8	0.846	−2.540	0.012 *	−3.248	−0.408
Theoretical training	GHQ-12	0.340	2.422	0.016 *	0.168	1.620
	DTS-8	0.005	2.213	0.028 *	0.178	3.084
	AIS-8	0.055	3.389	0.001 *	0.809	3.047
Practical training	GHQ-12	0.295	2.693	0.007 *	0.263	1.689
	DTS-8	0.000	2.755	0.006 *	0.571	3.441
	AIS-8	0.250	2.608	0.010 *	0.361	2.579
Need for quarantine	GHQ-12	0.929	−2.428	0.016 *	−1.979	−0.207
COVID-19 symptoms	GHQ-12	0.645	−2.392	0.017 *	−1.637	−0.159
Adequate personal equipment	GHQ-12	0.000	4.145	0.000 *	0.742	2.084
	DTS-8	0.021	4.946	0.000 *	2.040	4.735
	AIS-8	0.160	4.800	0.000 *	1.593	3.805
Contagion concern	GHQ-12	0.337	−4.790	0.000 *	−5.050	−2.109
	DTS-8	0.023	−3.978	0.000 *	−8.519	−2.881
	AIS-8	0.090	−2.884	0.004 *	−5.762	−1.089
Transmission concern	GHQ-12	0.012	−3.775	0.000 *	−5.757	−1.812
Weight gained	AIS-8	0.222	−2.604	0.010 *	−2.597	−0.362
Anxiety prepandemic	GHQ-12	0.629	−3.135	0.002 *	−2.771	−0.634
	DTS-8	0.651	−2.362	0.019 *	−4.490	−0.409
	AIS-8	0.449	−3.003	0.003 *	−4.201	−0.875
Anxiety during pandemic	GHQ-12	0.356	−11.104	0.000 *	−4.179	−2.921
	DTS-8	0.001	−8.946	0.000 *	−6.566	−4.197
	AIS-8	0.960	−7.188	0.000 *	−4.975	−2.836
Anxiety treatment prepandemic	DTS-8	0.254	−2.645	0.009 *	−3.840	−0.564
	AIS-8	0.027	−4.491	0.000 *	−4.318	−1.687
Anxiety treatment during pandemic	GHQ-12	0.837	−7.468	0.000 *	−3.977	−2.318
	DTS-8	0.080	−6.147	0.000 *	−6.652	−3.426
	AIS-8	0.838	−5.717	0.000 *	−5.199	−2.537
Need for psychological support prepandemic	GHQ-12	0.855	−2.197	0.029 *	−1.734	−0.096
	DTS-8	0.071	−3.338	0.001 *	−4.150	−1.072
	AIS-8	0.001	−4.170	0.000 *	−4.515	−1.604

Table 3. *Cont.*

Variables	Instrument (Total Score)	Levene Test	*t* Value	Level of Significance *p*	IC 95%	
					Min	Max
Need for psychological support during pandemic	GHQ-12 DTS-8 AIS-8	0.876 0.090 0.309	−6.489 −6.293 −4.305	0.000 * 0.000 * 0.000 *	−4.789 −8.907 −5.714	−2.561 −4.664 −2.129
Positive behavior in the service	GHQ-12 DTS-8 AIS-8	0.965 0.206 0.179	2.394 2.522 2.636	0.017 * 0.012 * 0.009 *	0.152 0.374 0.369	1.552 3.028 2.541

* Statistical significance bilateral level 0.05; Abbreviation: IC, interval level of significance.

Table 4. Inferential analysis: analysis of variance (ANOVA).

Variables	Instrument Total Score	Level of Significance *p*
Gender	GHQ-12 DTS-8 AIS-8	0.000 * 0.000 * 0.000 *
Professional category	GHQ-12 DTS-8 AIS-8	0.107 0.613 0.310
Type of Service	GHQ-12 DTS-8 AIS-8	0.564 0.244 0.414
SARS-COV-2 test	GHQ-12 DTS-8 AIS-8	0.011 * 0.001 * 0.159
Withdrawn personal equipment	GHQ-12 DTS-8 AIS-8	0.026 * 0.972 0.993
Psychological support unit	GHQ-12 DTS-8 AIS-8	0.154 0.868 0.658

* Statistical significance at level 0.05.

In addition, a positive, although weak, relationship was found between time worked in the service and DTS-8 ($r = 0.133$, with a significance level $p = 0.050$), so that as the time worked in the service increased, so did the DTS-8 scale score, resulting in a greater risk of developing PTSD (Table 5).

Table 5. Inferential analysis: Pearson's *r* correlation coefficient.

Variables	GHQ-12 Total Score	DTS-8 Total Score	AIS-8 Total Score
Age	−0.068	−0.032	−0.088
Year of work experience	−0.049	0.133 *	0.091
Number of people per household	−0.015	0.043	0.041
Weight gained	0.024	0.024	0.081

* Statistical significance at level 0.05.

Considering the total scores on the instruments used (GHQ-12, DTS-8, and AIS-8), we sought to identify relationships between them and determined that there was a significant correlation according to the Pearson's r coefficient for a bilateral level 0.01 of a moderate positive type between the total GHQ-12 score and the total DTS-8 score (r = 0.622), and between the total GHQ-12 score and the total AIS-8 score ($r = 0.556$). There was also a strong positive correlation between the DTS-8 total score and the AIS-8 total score ($r = 0.724$). Accordingly, higher GHQ-12 scores (poorer mental health) were related to higher DTS-8 scores (greater likelihood of PTSD) and vice versa. Higher GHQ-12 scores (poorer mental health) were related to higher AIS-8 scores (greater insomnia) and vice versa. Finally, higher DTS-8 scores (greater likelihood of PTSD) were related to higher AIS-8 scores (more insomnia) and vice versa.

4. Discussion

In light of the results obtained in this study, our working hypothesis, which proposed that the mental health of EMS workers in Castile y León and Madrid has worsened during the outbreak of the COVID-19 pandemic, seemed to hold. The potential presence of PTSD was found in 30.9% of the sample, which is significantly higher than values obtained before the pandemic in workers in other EMS, which had a prevalence of PTSD of 11% [28].

Outside the out-of-hospital emergency group, the data on the presence of PTSD in health professionals are lower than those found in our sample. During the epidemics of other coronavirus prior to the COVID-19 pandemic, PTSD symptoms were recorded in Canadian healthcare workers with a prevalence of 14.6% (Instrument: Revised Event Scale IES-R) [36], and among emergency personnel in Taiwan, the prevalence was 19.8% (Instrument: Davidson Trauma Scale-Chinese version (DTS-C) and Chinese Health Questionnaire-12 (CHQ-12)) [36]. In the meta-analysis conducted by Salehi et al. [37], two out of ten healthcare workers would have presented PTSD symptoms after epidemics of other coronavirus, and including the COVID-19 pandemic. This increases the percentages previously found but the values are still below those obtained in our sample. A review of the effects of work on health professionals during the pandemic shows that it is common for healthcare workers to recall images that have caused them distress, as was also the case in this study [38]. It is also common to find, in China, a lack of interest in activities that were previously of interest to doctors and nurses, as in our case [39].

The evaluation of the psychological impact on EMS workers in our study found psychological pathology in 36% of the sample. In addition, the greater the loss of psychological wellbeing, reflected by a higher GHQ-12 score, the higher the DTS-8 score. A negative relationship between decreased psychological wellbeing and PTSD diagnosis was found in this study, in line with previous findings in healthcare workers [40,41].

A total of 65.6% of the EMS workers surveyed in this study referred to anxiety symptoms during the early stages of the pandemic. These results are consistent with those observed both in the general population and among healthcare workers at the height of the pandemic. In China, elevated levels of fear, anxiety (30–70%) (Instrument: IES-R and Depression Anxiety and Stress Scale (DASS-21) [42–44], and depression (20.1%) have been described [45].

A study conducted in Denver, Colorado shows that, during the pandemic, frontline physicians suffered from a lack of confidence in their actions, as with the health professionals in our research, as well as a sense of helplessness and a feeling of uselessness in saving patients' lives [46].

In our study, concerns about the quality of PPE, which had to be removed because it did not meet current protection regulations, affected 78.9% of the respondents. Similarly, 75% of the sample reported being affected by the lack of initial information. The perception of insecurity and the fear of contagion caused an increase in anxiety, according to published works on the subject [47]. Although there was some research on PPE as early as May 2020 [48], in our case, the respondents accepted that, in some cases, protective equipment had to be recalled, possibly due to the shortages experienced during the first wave of the pandemic [49]. A study in China showed that training and coaching in the process of using personal protective equipment reduced stress among healthcare workers when they had to use it. It would therefore be necessary for such training to be carried out but the required frequency has not been specified [50].

In some cases, the surveyed EMS workers admitted to having redacted information prior to the pandemic, although it was more common for such information to have been provided during the pandemic. Studies have shown that both too little and too much information can be detrimental to the mental health of the general population [51,52].

Insomnia levels reflect pathological sleep impairment in 60% of EMS workers. The prevalence in the general population is estimated at around 3.9 to 22% [48,49], and among healthcare workers in general during the COVID-19 outbreak, the prevalence of insomnia reached 36% (Instrument: Insomnia Severity Index (ISS7)) [50], which shows that in the sample of EMS professionals analyzed, the presence of sleep problems was quite high compared to the general population and other healthcare workers. The most frequent psychological response in a group of Irish healthcare workers was difficulty initiating sleep [53]. A sleep study conducted in Bahrain on healthcare workers during the pandemic found that the sleep quality of the participants was poor, the number of hours for which they stayed asleep was reduced, and awakenings were frequent [54], consistent with the results found in the present study sample.

The proportional and positive relationships found in this study in the results between the GHQ-12 and AIS-8 instruments reinforce the relationship established in the literature between a loss of psychological wellbeing and insomnia [55].

In Wuhan, according to Lai et al. [56], increased exposure in toilets led to more frequent symptoms of anxiety, depression, and insomnia. In our study, concerns about contagion, stemming from occupational exposure, were apparent in 94.3% of the respondents. In addition, the results of the study showed a positive relationship between the results obtained in the measurement of psychological health, PTSD, and insomnia and the concern regarding self-contagion. The score on the three instruments used was higher in the concerned sample.

Concern about transmitting the disease to family members was also present in the sample in more than 90% of the cases, most frequently among respondents living with four or more people. Concerns about contracting the disease and about transmitting it to close relatives have already been reflected in other published studies [56,57].

With regard to testing for SARS-CoV-2 infection in EMS professionals in Castilla y León and Madrid, the volume of tests carried out was similar to that found in other investigations [58,59]. The same was true for the presence of symptoms, highlighting that, in many cases, healthcare workers have been asymptomatic carriers [60]. The figures for isolation and hospital admission did not differ from those found by other authors among healthcare professionals in hospital emergency departments, who were also frontline staff [61].

A study that recruited participants through social media found that the general population during the pandemic gained between 5 and 10 pounds in body weight, equivalent to between 2.2 and 4.4 kg. In our sample, the average weight gain was 1 K, which is half the lower limit of weight gain found in the general population study [62]. This may be because the healthcare workers had not been confined to the same extent because they were working, but studies are needed to demonstrate this.

In the sample collected, 16% of EMS workers did not live with others during the pandemic. In the literature, it remains unclear whether living alone increases risk among healthcare workers. However, in the United Kingdom, women in the general population who lived alone and were confined were considered at risk. Being female, a nurse, and belonging to the younger subgroup of workers are factors associated with an increased risk in several studies [63]. Consistent with these findings, women in our study showed a greater loss of psychological wellbeing, PTSD symptoms, and insomnia, which leads us to affirm that gender is a predisposing factor for PTSD risk in our sample.

Nonetheless, the most affected professional category in our sample was emergency health technicians. The studies cited above do not specifically mention the involvement of emergency medical technicians. However, emergency health technicians have previously shown worrying results in other surveys worldwide [64,65], and their situation may have worsened in the current context probably due to physical strain and increased workload, as may also have happened in other professional categories [66,67]. All these factors may contribute to the appearance of negative effects, in the short or long term, in a population already at risk [68,69].

There are no known previous studies of this type in the SEMs studied in this research, nor have we found any studies that take into account the modality of work (BLS and ALS), so it has not been possible to carry out comparisons with other authors' studies.

The most frequent demographic in our study was middle-aged individuals (40–49 years) with between 10 and 20 years of experience. In this study, the more experience that the healthcare workers (>20 years) had the less affected they were. Years of work experience has previously been related to resilience and identified as a protective factor [69].

Given the overwhelming presence of signs and, in some cases, clear alterations in the psychological health of out-of-hospital emergency workers in the communities studied, the need for support and prevention programs during crises such as the COVID-19 pandemic seems reasonable, as confirmed by other research [70–73].

The importance of identifying the underlying factors to prevent and treat before the onset of traumatic symptoms and to reduce the future consequences of PTSD is highlighted [74]. Likewise, scientific recommendations from mental health experts to maintain contact with family and friends, share information with colleagues in a positive way, schedule routines outside of work, be aware of one's feelings and emotions, maintain healthy lifestyle habits, and allow oneself to ask for help are suitable [75,76].

This research has a number of limitations. The first is due to the use of a descriptive crosssectional design that only provides a static picture of the problem but can serve as a basis for longitudinal studies. Therefore, it does not allow causality to be established between the factors and the risk of PTSD; it is consequently not possible to extrapolate the results to other populations. The second lies in the fact that the study sample was nonrandomly selected, mainly due to the epidemiological situation at the time, which precluded any other form of sampling, although it must be accepted that the sample may be biased. Despite this, it was a moderately large sample taking into account the small number of EMS workers compared to other levels of care, which tends to limit the biases that could arise from the selection and recall of participants. Finally, although information on previous mental health status was collected, this aspect was not taken into account when determining the correlations between the variables. In future research, it would be advisable to evaluate PTSD with a random sample that includes more professionals from other EMS to ensure the veracity of the results, using a random sample and a design that allows us to establish causal relationships, considering the previous mental health of the workers.

This study confirms that the COVID-19 pandemic has been a traumatic event for EMS workers having an impact on their wellbeing. One-third of them have manifested a potential diagnosis of PTSD in the early phases of the pandemic. In addition, stress, signs of psychological distress, and insomnia have been shown to be common among out-of-hospital healthcare workers.

Respondents most affected by PTSD were women, those aged 40 to 49 years, emergency health technicians, those with 10 to 20 years of experience, and those living with four or more people.

Both gender and concern about becoming infected are related to the risk of suffering from psychological pathology, PTSD, and insomnia.

In relation to the implications of the study for clinical practice, the authors defend the need to followup with those individuals who report a deterioration in their psychological health due to their professional work in the pandemic. We propose the creation of specific mental health programs for events similar to COVID 19 in the future, prioritizing mental health. This also requires an increase in public health human resources to cover the mental health care of out-of-hospital emergency health professionals. Given that the training of professionals to prepare them to face these situations is not adequate, it could be suggested that health training programs include this topic. In addition, coping strategies should be promoted for this group in order to better enable them to respond to traumatic events similar to those experienced during the pandemic. To achieve this, it would be necessary to establish a support unit for workers' mental health and to establish training courses within the working day that allow them to acquire these skills.

The paper adds a novel topic to the scientific literature, as the mental health of healthcare workers during the COVID-19 pandemic has been studied previously but not in out-of-hospital emergency personnel. Moreover, studies are usually limited to samples composed of doctors and nurses, without taking into account other healthcare professionals such as emergency health technicians. In addition, the timing of data collection is noteworthy as it took place relatively close to the end of the first wave of the pandemic, which gave an idea of how these staff were coping at that time and allows comparison with later stages.

A future line of research for the research team would be to reassess the same variables in the sample after the current fifth wave and thus obtain an idea of the evolution of the mental health of these out-of-hospital emergency healthcare professionals. In addition, we aim to carry out a qualitative study that will provide in-depth knowledge of the experiences of healthcare workers in their work during the SARS-CoV-2 pandemic.

5. Conclusions

This study confirms that the COVID-19 pandemic may have been a traumatic event for emergency workers. One-third of them reported a possible diagnosis of PTSD in emergency health workers who performed their professional work in the early phases of the pandemic. PTSD needs to be confirmed by further assessment, as the number may have increased or decreased after months of exposure to such a traumatic situation. In addition, stress, signs of psychological pathology, and insomnia have been shown to be common among out-of-hospital healthcare workers at the time of the research.

Respondents most affected by possible PTSD were women, those aged 40–49, emergency health technicians, those with 10–20 years of experience, and those living with four or more people. Both gender and preoccupation with illness were associated with the risk of psychological distress, the likelihood of PTSD, and insomnia.

The authors argue for the need to followup with those individuals who report a deterioration of their psychological health due to their professional work in the pandemic through specific health programs, as well as the prevention of such deterioration during future traumatic events similar to the COVID-19 pandemic.

Author Contributions: Conceptualization, C.M.M.-C. and R.M.C.-G.; methodology, R.V.-M., M.T.H.-F.; software, R.M.C.-G.; validation, L.M.G.-S., J.M.-P., L.P.-P. and M.A.M.-F.; formal analysis, R.M.C.-G.; investigation, C.M.M.-C., M.Á.B.-P. and E.O.; resources, C.D.-F. and M.T.H.-F.; data curation, L.P.-P. and C.D.-F.; writing—original draft preparation, C.M.M.-C., R.M.C.-G. and M.T.H.-F.; writing—review and editing, R.M.C.-G., J.M.-P. and J.J.F.-C.; visualization, C.D.-F.; supervision, R.M.C.-G. All authors have read and agreed to the published version of the manuscript.

Funding: This research received no external funding.

Institutional Review Board Statement: The study was conducted according to the guidelines of the Declaration of Helsinki and approved by the Ethics Committee for Drug Research of the Valladolid West Health Area (PI 139-20 NO HRHV on 6 June 2020).

Informed Consent Statement: Informed consent was obtained from all subjects involved in the study.

Data Availability Statement: The data presented in this study are available on request from the corresponding author.

Conflicts of Interest: The authors declare no conflict of interest. The funders had no role in the design of the study; in the collection, analyses, or interpretation of data; in the writing of the manuscript, or in the decision to publish the results.

References

1. Oliver, N.; Barber, X.; Roomp, K.; Roomp, K. Assessing the impact of the COVID-19 pandemic in Spain: Large-scale, online, self-reported population survey. *J. Med. Internet Res.* **2020**, *22*, e21319. [CrossRef] [PubMed]
2. Pollán, M.; Pérez-Gómez, B.; Pastor-Barriuso, R.; Oteo, J.; Hernán, M.A.; Pérez-Olmeda, M.; Sanmartín, J.L.; Fernández-García, A.; Cruz, I.; de Larrea, N.F.; et al. Prevalence of SARS-CoV-2 in Spain (ENE-COVID): A nationwide, population-based seroepidemiological study. *Lancet* **2020**, *396*, 535–544. [CrossRef]
3. Boletín Oficial del Estado. Real Decreto 463/2020, de 14 de Marzo, por el que se Declara el Estado de Alarma para la Gestión de la Situación de Crisis Sanitaria Ocasionada por el COVID-19. Available online: https://www.boe.es/eli/es/rd/2020/03/14/463 (accessed on 24 June 2021).
4. The Lancet Public Health. COVID-19 in Spain: A predictable storm? *Lancet* **2020**, *5*, e568.
5. World Health Organization. Coronavirus Disease (COVID-2019) Situation Reports. Available online: https://www.who.int/emergencies/diseases/novel-coronavirus-2019/situation-reports (accessed on 26 June 2021).
6. Mitjà, O.; Arenas, A.; Rodó, X.; Tobias, A.; Brew, J.; Benlloch, J.M. Experts' request to the Spanish Government: Move Spain towards complete lockdown. *Lancet* **2020**, *395*, 1193–1194. [CrossRef]
7. Boletín Oficial del Estado. Available online: https://boe.es/boe/dias/2021/06/25/ (accessed on 26 June 2021).
8. American Psychiatric Association. *DSM-5. Guía de Consulta de los Criterios Diagnosticos*, 5th ed.; Panamericana: Madrid, Spain, 2018.
9. Vance, M.C.; Kovachy, B.; Dong, M.; Bui, E. Peritraumatic distress: A review and synthesis of 15 years of research. *J. Clin. Psychol.* **2018**, *74*, 1457–1484. [CrossRef] [PubMed]
10. Berger, W.; Coutinho, E.S.F.; Figueira, I.; Marques-Portella, C.; Luz, M.P.; Neylan, T.C.; Marmar, C.R.; Mendlowicz, M.V. Rescuers at risk: A systematic review and meta-regression analysis of the worldwide current prevalence and correlates of PTSD in rescue workers. *Soc. Psychiatry Psychiatr. Epidemiol* **2012**, *47*, 1001–1011. [CrossRef] [PubMed]
11. Preti, E.; Di Mattei, V.; Perego, G.; Ferrari, F.; Mazzetti, M.; Taranto, P.; Di Pierro, R.; Madeddu, F.; Calati, R. The Psychological Impact of Epidemic and Pandemic Outbreaks on Healthcare Workers: Rapid Review of the Evidence. *Curr. Psychiatry Rep.* **2020**, *22*, 1–22. [CrossRef]
12. Ramírez-Santana, M.; Aguirre, J., Carvajal, N. Formación médica para afrontar emergencias y desastres: Experiencia de enseñanza-aprendizaje con trabajo colaborativo, uso de tecnologías de información y comunicación, y simulación. *FEM* **2020**, *23*, 243–249. [CrossRef]
13. Ward, C.L.; Lombard, C.J.; Gwebushe, N. Critical incident exposure in South African emergency services personnel: Prevalence and associated mental health issues. *Emerg. Med. J.* **2006**, *23*, 226–231. [CrossRef] [PubMed]
14. Carmassi, C.; Foghi, C.; Dell'Oste, V.; Cordone, A.; Bertelloni, C.A.; Bui, E.; Dell'Osso, L. PTSD symptoms in healthcare workers facing the three coronavirus outbreaks: What can we expect after the COVID-19 pandemic. *Psychiatry Res.* **2020**, *292*, 113312. [CrossRef]
15. Mojica-Crespo, R.; Morales-Crespo, M.M. Pandemic COVID-19, the new health emergency of international concern: A review. *Semergen* **2020**, *46*, 65–77. [CrossRef] [PubMed]
16. Iglesias Vázquez, J.A.; Echarri-Sucunza, A.; Ruíz-Azpiazu, J.I.; Pastrana-Blanco, J.L.; Guirao-Salinas, F.A.; Escriche-López, C.; Jiménez-Fábregas, X. Análisis de la organización y preparación para la respuesta ante la pandemia de COVID-19 por los ser-vicios médicos de emergencias extrahospitalarias en España. *Emergencias* **2021**, *33*, 151–153. [PubMed]
17. Gracía-Iglesias, J.J.; Gómez-Salgado, J.; Martín-Pereira, J.; Fagundo-Rivera, J.; Ayuso-Murillo, D.; Martínez-Riera, J.R.; Ruiz-Frutos, C. Impact of SARS-CoV-2 (Covid-19) on the mental health of healthcare professionals: A systematic review. *Rev. Esp. Salud Publica* **2020**, *94*, e202007088.
18. Fan, F.C.; Zhang, S.Y.; Cheng, Y. Incidence of psychological illness after coronavirus outbreak: A meta-analysis study. *J. Epidemiol. Community Health* **2021**, *75*, 836–842. [CrossRef] [PubMed]
19. Matalon, N.; Dorman-Ilan, S.; Hasson-Ohayon, I.; Hertz-Palmor, N.; Shani, S.; Basel, D.; Gross, R.; Chen, W.; Abramovich, A.; Afek, A.; et al. Trajectories of post-traumatic stress symptoms, anxiety, and depression in hospitalized COVID-19 patients: A one-month follow-up. *J. Psychosom. Res.* **2021**, *143*, 110399. [CrossRef] [PubMed]
20. Taquet, M.; Luciano, S.; Geddes, J.R.; Harrison, P.J. Bidirectional associations between COVID-19 and psychiatric disorder: Retrospective cohort studies of 62,354 COVID-19 cases in the USA. *Lancet Psychiatry* **2020**, *8*, 130–140. [CrossRef]
21. Vindegaard, N.; Benros, M.E. COVID-19 pandemic and mental health consequences: Systematic review of the current evidence. *Brain Behav. Immun.* **2020**, *89*, 531–542. [CrossRef]
22. Pappa, S.; Ntella, V.; Giannakas, T.; Giannakoulis, V.; Papoutsi, E.; Katsaounou, P. Prevalence of depression, anxiety, and insomnia among healthcare workers during the COVID-19 pandemic: A systematic review and meta-analysis. *Brain Behav. Immun.* **2020**, *88*, 901–907. [CrossRef] [PubMed]

23. Chew, N.W.; Lee, G.K.; Tan, B.Y.; Jing, M.; Goh, Y.; Ngiam, N.J.; Yeo, L.; Ahmad, A.; Khan, F.A.; Shanmugam, G.N.; et al. A multinational, multicentre study on the psychological outcomes and associated physical symptoms amongst healthcare workers during COVID-19 outbreak. *Brain Behav. Immun.* **2020**, *88*, 559–565. [CrossRef] [PubMed]
24. Danet, A.D. Psychological impact of COVID-19 pandemic in Western frontline healthcare professionals. A systematic review. *Med. Clin.* **2021**, *156*, 449–458. [CrossRef]
25. El-Hage, W.; Hingray, C.; Lemogne, C.; Yrondi, A.; Brunault, P.; Bienvenu, T.; Etain, B.; Paquet, C.; Gohier, B.; Bennabi, D.; et al. Health professionals facing the coronavirus disease 2019 (COVID-19) pandemic: What are the mental health risks? *Encephale* **2020**, *46*, S73–S80. [CrossRef]
26. Burillo-Putze, G.; Espinosa-Ramírez, S.; Lecuona-Fernández, M. Personal protection against COVID-19 in the emergency department: Neither heroes nor cowards. *Emergencias* **2020**, *32*, 223–224. [PubMed]
27. Calvo-Bonacho, E.; Catalina-Romero, C.; Fernández-Labandera, C.; Fernández-Meseguer, A.; González-Quintela, A.; Martínez-Muñoz, P.; Quevedo, L.; Valdivielso, P.; Sánchez-Chaparro, M.A. COVID-19 and Sick Leave: An Analysis of the Ibermutua Cohort of Over 1,651,305 Spanish Workers in the First Trimester of 2020. *Front. Public Health* **2020**, *8*, 580546. [CrossRef]
28. Eiche, C.; Birkholz, T.; Jobst, E.; Gall, C.; Prottengeier, J. Well-being and PTSD in German emergency medical services—A nationwide cross-sectional survey. *PLoS ONE* **2019**, *14*, e0220154. [CrossRef] [PubMed]
29. Petrie, K.; Milligan-Saville, J.; Gayed, A.; Deady, M.; Phelps, A.; Dell, L.; Forbes, D.; Bryant, R.A.; Calvo, R.A.; Glozier, N.; et al. Prevalence of PTSD and common mental disorders amongst ambulance personnel: A systematic review and meta-analysis. *Soc. Psychiatry Psychiatr. Epidemiol.* **2018**, *53*, 897–909. [CrossRef] [PubMed]
30. Vandenbroucke, J.P.; Von Elm, E.; Altman, D.G.; Gøtzsche, P.C.; Mulrow, C.D.; Pocock, S.J.; Poole, C.; Schlesselman, J.J.; Egger, M. Fortalecimiento de la presentación de informes de estudios observacionales en epidemiología (STROBE): Explicación y elaboración. *Gac. Sanit.* **2009**, *23*, 158.e1–158.e28. [CrossRef] [PubMed]
31. Goldberg, D. *Manual of the General Health Questionnaire*; NFER Publishing Company: Windsor, UK, 1978.
32. Sánchez-López, M.P.; Dresch, V. The 12-Item General Health Questionnaire (GHQ-12): Reliability, external validity and factor structure in the Spanish population. *Psicothema* **2008**, *20*, 839–843.
33. Davidson, J.R.T.; Colket, J.T. The eight-item treatment-outcome post-traumatic stress disorder scale: A brief measure to assess treatment outcome in post-traumatic stress disorder. *Int. Clin. Psychopharmacol.* **1997**, *12*, 41–46. [CrossRef] [PubMed]
34. Bobes, J.; Calcedo-Barba, A.; García, M.; François, M.; Rico-Villademoros, F.; González, M.P.; Bascarán, M.T.; Bousoño, M. Evaluación de las propiedades psicométricas de la versión española de cinco cuestionarios para la evaluación del trastorno de estrés postraumático. *Actas Esp. Psiquiatr.* **2000**, *28*, 207–218.
35. Soldatos, C.R.; Dikeos, D.G.; Paparrigopoulos, T.J. Athens Insomnia Scale: Validation of an instrument based on ICD-10 criteria. *J. Psychosom. Res.* **2020**, *48*, 555–560. [CrossRef]
36. Reynolds, D.L.; Garay, J.R.; Deamond, S.L.; Moran, M.K.; Gold, W.; Styra, R. Understanding, compliance and psychological impact of the SARS quarantine experience. *Epidemiol. Infect.* **2007**, *136*, 997–1007. [CrossRef] [PubMed]
37. Lin, C.-Y.; Peng, Y.-C.; Wu, Y.-H.; Chang, J.; Chan, C.-H.; Yang, D.-Y. The psychological effect of severe acute respiratory syndrome on emergency department staff. *Emerg. Med. J.* **2007**, *24*, 12–17. [CrossRef] [PubMed]
38. Salehi, M.; Amanat, M.; Mohammadi, M.; Salmanian, M.; Rezaei, N.; Saghazadeh, A.; Garakani, A. The prevalence of post-traumatic stress disorder related symptoms in Coronavirus outbreaks: A systematic-review and meta-analysis. *J. Affect. Disord.* **2021**, *282*, 527–538. [CrossRef] [PubMed]
39. Giorgi, G.; Lecca, L.I.; Alessio, F.; Finstad, G.L.; Bondanini, G.; Lulli, L.G.; Arcangeli, G.; Mucci, N. COVID-19-Related Mental Health Effects in the Workplace: A Narrative Review. *Int. J. Environ. Res. Public Health* **2020**, *17*, 7857. [CrossRef] [PubMed]
40. Kang, L.; Ma, S.; Chen, M.; Yang, J.; Wang, Y.; Li, R.; Yao, L.; Bai, H.; Cai, Z.; Yang, B.X.; et al. Impact on mental health and perceptions of psychological care among medical and nursing staff in Wuhan during the 2019 novel coronavirus disease outbreak: A cross-sectional study. *Brain Behav. Immun.* **2020**, *87*, 11–17. [CrossRef] [PubMed]
41. Castillo, D.; Ovalle, L.; Oyola, P.; Garavito, C. La resiliencia como estrategia de afrontamiento ante el estrés postraumático en combatientes. *Rev. Enfoques* **2016**, *2*, 83–90. [CrossRef]
42. Braquehais, M.D.; Vargas-Cáceres, S.; Gómez-Durán, E.; Nieva, G.; Valero, S.; Casas, M.; Bruguera, E. The impact of the COVID-19 pandemic on the mental health of healthcare professionals. *QJM* **2020**, *113*, 613–617. [CrossRef] [PubMed]
43. Song, X.; Fu, W.; Liu, X.; Luo, Z.; Wang, R.; Zhou, N.; Yan, S.; Lv, C. Mental health status of medical staff in emergency departments during the Coronavirus disease 2019 epidemic in China. *Brain Behav. Immun.* **2020**, *88*, 60–65. [CrossRef]
44. Wu, D.; Jiang, C.; He, C.; Li, C.; Yang, L.; Yue, Y. Stressors of nurses in psychiatric hospitals during the COVID-19 outbreak. *Psychiatry Res.* **2020**, *288*, 112956. [CrossRef]
45. Huang, Y.; Zhao, N. Generalized anxiety disorder, depressive symptoms and sleep quality during COVID-19 outbreak in China: A web-based cross-sectional survey. *Psychiatry Res.* **2020**, *288*, 112954. [CrossRef]
46. Rao, H.; Mancini, D.; Tong, A.; Khan, H.; Gutierrez, B.S.; Mundo, W.; Collings, A.; Cervantes, L. Frontline interdisciplinary clinician perspectives on caring for patients with COVID-19: A qualitative study. *BMJ Open* **2021**, *11*, e048712. [CrossRef] [PubMed]
47. Shahzad, F.; Du, J.; Khan, I.; Fateh, A.; Shahbaz, M.; Abbas, A.; Wattoo, M.U. Perceived Threat of COVID-19 Contagion and Frontline Paramedics' Agonistic Behaviour: Employing a Stressor–Strain–Outcome Perspective. *Int. J. Environ. Res. Public Health* **2020**, *17*, 5102. [CrossRef] [PubMed]

48. Vico-Romero, J.; Cabré-Roure, M.; Monteis-Cahis, R.; Palomera-Faneges, E.; Serra-Prat, M. Prevalencia de trastornos del sueño y factores asociados en pacientes hospitalizados. *Enferm. Clin.* **2014**, *24*, 276–282. [CrossRef] [PubMed]
49. Li, Y.; Qin, Q.; Sun, Q.; Sanford, L.D.; Vgontzas, A.N.; Tang, X. Insomnia and psychological reactions during the COVID-19 outbreak in China. *J. Clin. Sleep Med.* **2020**, *16*, 1417–1418. [CrossRef]
50. Buchholz, Y. COVID-19: Insomnio, depresión y ansiedad en el personal sanitario. *Mente Cereb.* **2020**, *120*, 30–31.
51. Farooq, A.R.; Fareeha, F. Information Overload and Infodemic in the COVID-19 Pandemic. *J. Pak. Med. Assoc.* **2020**, *70*, S162–S165.
52. Rovetta, A.; Bhagavathula, A.S. Global Infodemiology of COVID-19: Analysis of Google Web Searches and Instagram Hashtags. *J. Med. Internet Res.* **2020**, *22*, e20673. [CrossRef]
53. Fortune, D.G.; Richards, H.L.; Wormald, A.; Connor, K.O.; McKiernan, M.; Najt, P.; Dwyer, A.O.; Dea, E.O.; Burke, P.; Eustace, J. An investigation of psychological responses to COVID-19 in Irish healthcare workers: Longitudinal quantitative and nested qualitative study. *HRB Open Res.* **2021**, *4*, 15. [CrossRef] [PubMed]
54. Jahrami, H.; BaHammam, A.S.; AlGahtani, H.; Ebrahim, A.; Faris, M.; AlEid, K.; Saif, Z.; Haji, E.; Dhahi, A.; Marzooq, H.; et al. The examination of sleep quality for frontline healthcare workers during the outbreak of COVID-19. *Sleep Breath.* **2020**, *25*, 503–511. [CrossRef]
55. Lai, J.; Ma, S.; Wang, Y.; Cai, Z.; Hu, J.; Wei, N.; Wu, J.; Du, H.; Chen, T.; Li, R.; et al. Factors Associated with Mental Health Outcomes among Health Care Workers Exposed to Coronavirus Disease 2019. *JAMA Netw. Open* **2020**, *3*, e203976. [CrossRef] [PubMed]
56. Sandín, B.; Valiente, R.M.; García-Escalera, J.; Chorot, P. Impacto psicológico de la pandemia de COVID-19: Efectos negativos y positivos en población española asociados al periodo de confinamiento nacional. *Rev. Psicopatol. Psicol. Clin.* **2020**, *25*, 1–22. [CrossRef]
57. Lumley, S.F.; O'Donnell, D.; Stoesser, N.E.; Matthews, P.C.; Howarth, A.; Stephanie, B.H.; Marsden, B.D.; Cox, S.; James, T.; Warren, F.; et al. Antibody Status and Incidence of SARS-CoV-2 Infection in Health Care Workers. *N. Engl. J. Med.* **2021**, *384*, 533–540. [CrossRef] [PubMed]
58. Martin, C.; Montesinos, I. Dynamics of SARS-CoV-2 RT-PCR positivity and seroprevalence among high-risk healthcare workers and hospital staff. *J. Hosp. Infect.* **2020**, *106*, 102–106. [CrossRef] [PubMed]
59. Rivett, L.; Sridhar, S.; Sparkes, D.; Routledge, M.; Jones, N.K.; Forrest, S.; Young, J.; Pereira-Dias, J.; Hamilton, W.L.; Ferris, M.; et al. Screening of healthcare workers for SARS-CoV-2 highlights the role of asymptomatic carriage in COVID-19 transmission. *Epidemiol. Glob. Health* **2020**, *9*, e58728.
60. Gómez-Ochoa, S.A.; Franco, O.H.; Rojas, L.Z.; Raguindin, P.F.; Roa-Díaz, Z.M.; Wyssmann, B.M.; Guevara, S.L.R.; Echeverría, L.E.; Glisic, M.; Muka, T. COVID-19 in Health-Care Workers: A Living Systematic Review and Meta Analysis of Prevalence, Risk Factors, Clinical Characteristics, and Outcomes. *Am. J. Epidemiol.* **2020**, *190*, 161–175. [CrossRef] [PubMed]
61. Chico-Sánchez, P.; Gras-Valentí, P.; Mora-Muriel, J.G.; Algado-Sellés, N.; Sánchez-Payá, J.; Llorens, P. Impact of the COVID-19 pandemic on health care workers in a tertiary care hospital emergency department. *Emergencias* **2020**, *32*, 227–232. [PubMed]
62. Zachary, Z.; Brianna, F.; Brianna, L.; Garrett, P.; Jade, W.; Alyssa, D.; Mikayla, K. Self-quarantine and weight gain related risk factors during the COVID-19 pandemic. *Obes. Res. Clin. Pract.* **2020**, *14*, 210–216. [CrossRef]
63. Silva, D.F.O.; Cobucci, R.N. Prevalência de ansiedade em profissionais da saúde em tempos de COVID-19: Revisão sistemática com metanálise. *Cienc. Saude Coletiva* **2021**, *26*, 693–710. [CrossRef] [PubMed]
64. Almutairi, I.; Al-Rashdi, M.; Almutairi, A. Prevalence and predictors of depression, anxiety and stress symptoms in paramedics at saudi red crescent authority. *Saudi J. Med. Med. Sci.* **2020**, *8*, 105–111. [CrossRef]
65. Bentley, M.A.; Mac Crawford, J.; Wilkins, J.R.; Fernandez, A.R.; Studnek, J.R. An Assessment of Depression, Anxiety, and Stress among Nationally Certified EMS Professionals. *Prehospital Emerg. Care* **2013**, *17*, 330–338. [CrossRef]
66. Dutheil, F.; Mondillon, L.; Navel, V. PTSD as the second tsunami of the SARS-Cov-2 pandemic. *Psychol. Med.* **2020**, 1–2. [CrossRef] [PubMed]
67. Hannigan, B.; Nolan, F.; Chambers, M.; Turner, J. Mental health nursing at a time of crisis. *J. Psychiatr. Ment. Health Nurs.* **2021**, *28*, 123–125. [CrossRef] [PubMed]
68. Jakovljevic, M.; Bjedov, S.; Jaksic, N.; Jakovljevic, I. COVID-19 pandemia and public and global mental health from the per-spective of global health security. *Psychiatr. Danub.* **2020**, *32*, 6–14. [CrossRef] [PubMed]
69. Musso, M.; Tatum, D.; Hamer, D.; Hammarlund, R.; Son, L.; McMahon, P. The Relationship between Grit and Resilience in Emergency Medical Service Personnel. *Ochsner J.* **2019**, *19*, 199–203. [CrossRef] [PubMed]
70. Cheung, T.; Fong, T.K.; Bressington, D. COVID-19 under the SARS Cloud: Mental Health Nursing during the Pandemic in Hong Kong. *J. Psychiatr. Ment. Health Nurs.* **2020**, *28*, 115–117. [CrossRef]
71. Cuidando a los Profesionales. Available online: https://www.semes.org/informacion-para-profesionales-sobre-covid-19/cuidando-a-los-profesionales/ (accessed on 28 June 2021).
72. Cuidemos Nuestra Salud Mental. Available online: https://www.saludcastillayleon.es/HRHortega/es/actualidad/servicio-psiquiatria-salud-mental-elaborado-guia-ayudar-san (accessed on 24 June 2021).
73. Cuidando la Salud Mental del Personal Sanitario. Available online: http://www.sepsiq.org/file/InformacionSM/SEP%20COVID19-Salud%20Mental%20personal%20sanitario.pdf (accessed on 28 June 2021).
74. Blake, H.; Bermingham, F.; Johnson, G.; Tabner, A. Mitigating the Psychological Impact of COVID-19 on Healthcare Workers: A Digital Learning Package. *Int. J. Environ. Res. Public Health* **2020**, *17*, 2997. [CrossRef]

75. Bendau, A.; Ströhle, A.; Petzold, M.B. Salud mental en profesionales de la salud en la pandemia COVID-19. *Adv. Exp. Med. Biol.* **2021**, *1318*, 737–757.
76. López-Bueno, R.; Calatayud, J.; Ezzatvar, Y.; Casajús, J.A.; Smith, L.; Andersen, L.L.; Sánchez, G.F.L. Association between Current Physical Activity and Current Perceived Anxiety and Mood in the Initial Phase of COVID-19 Confinement. *Front. Psychiatry* **2020**, *11*, 729. [CrossRef] [PubMed]

International Journal of *Environmental Research and Public Health*

MDPI

Article

Investigating the Effective Factors of Using Personal Protective Equipment from the Perspective of Nurses Caring for COVID-19 Patients: A Cross-Sectional Study

Razieh Mokhtari [1], Ali Safdari [2], Davood Hekmatpou [1], Ali Sahebi [3], Siamak Moayedi [4], Mercedes Torres [4] and Mohamad Golitaleb [1,*]

1 Department of Nursing, School of Nursing, Arak University of Medical Sciences, Arak 3819693345, Iran; razieh.mokhtari91@gmail.com (R.M.); dr_hekmat@arakmu.ac.ir (D.H.)
2 Student Research Committee, Arak University of Medical Sciences, Arak 3819693345, Iran; asafdari.nu@gmail.com
3 Non-Communicable Diseases Research Center, Ilam University of Medical Sciences, Ilam 6931851147, Iran; ali.sahebi.phd@gmail.com
4 Department of Emergency Medicine, School of Medicine, University of Maryland, Baltimore, MD 21201, USA; mak.moayedi@som.umaryland.edu (S.M.); mtorres@som.umaryland.edu (M.T.)
* Correspondence: m.golitaleb@arakmu.ac.ir or mohamadgolitaleb@gmail.com; Tel.: +98-93-7936-6279

Abstract: Considering the importance of appropriate personal protective equipment (PPE) for preventing COVID-19 transmission, the aim of this study was to investigate the factors affecting the use of PPE from the perspective of the nurses caring for COVID-19 patients. This descriptive cross-sectional study surveyed 240 nurses working in the central COVID-19 hospitals of Arak, Iran. Nurses were enrolled in the study by a convenience sampling method. The data collection tool was a validated questionnaire. Data were analyzed by SPSS 16 software using descriptive statistics, analysis of variance (ANOVA), and independent sample *t*-test. Environmental (4.24 ± 0.45), personal (4.16 ± 0.42), and organizational (4.04 ± 0.50) factors all contribute significantly to nursing attitudes about PPE use ($p < 0.05$). The average score, combining all identified factors, was 4.15 ± 0.31. The most influential factor contributing to appropriate use of PPE was environmental, while the least impactful parameters were related to rules and regulations. Environmental factors have the greatest impact on the use of PPE from the perspective of the nurses caring for patients with COVID-19. Managers and healthcare organizations should provide appropriate and adequate PPE to nurses, educate them on proper use, and monitor the process to resolve barriers.

Keywords: COVID-19; personal protection equipment (PPE); nurse; protective equipment

Citation: Mokhtari, R.; Safdari, A.; Hekmatpou, D.; Sahebi, A.; Moayedi, S.; Torres, M.; Golitaleb, M. Investigating the Effective Factors of Using Personal Protective Equipment from the Perspective of Nurses Caring for COVID-19 Patients: A Cross-Sectional Study. *Int. J. Environ. Res. Public Health* **2021**, *18*, 7882. https://doi.org/10.3390/ijerph18157882

Academic Editors: Richard Gray and Sonia Udod

Received: 5 May 2021
Accepted: 13 July 2021
Published: 26 July 2021

Publisher's Note: MDPI stays neutral with regard to jurisdictional claims in published maps and institutional affiliations.

1. Introduction

The Association of Infection Control and Epidemiology Specialists supports measures to prevent the transmission of the novel coronavirus from patients to healthcare workers (HCWs) [1,2]. Strict adherence to infection prevention guidelines is a critical component of efforts to stop the spread of infectious and contagious diseases such as SARS-CoV-2 to healthcare personnel [2,3]. A study conducted in China showed that approximately one-third of those infected with COVID-19 were HCWs [4]. In Italy, 10% of healthcare providers contracted the virus, 3% of whom died [1]. This highlights the importance of providing appropriate personal protective equipment (PPE) for HCWs in order to prevent transmission in the healthcare environment [5,6].

Nurses are an essential component of the frontline team caring for COVID-19 patients. Their service is vital to the care of the sick and further efforts to end the pandemic [2,7]. The International Council of Nurses has recognized the key role of nurses in the treatment and care of patients with COVID-19 [8]. Considering the highly infectious nature of the disease and the dire consequences of HCW infections for healthcare infrastructure, it is important to pay close attention to the use of PPE [5,8].

The provision of adequate PPE to nurses has been a significant challenge throughout this pandemic. High cost, limited supply, and high rates of consumption have all contributed to PPE shortages experienced by HCWs worldwide. Shortages in PPE have caused great concern among HCWs regarding their safety and protection [8,9].

In a recent review, factors such as low skill, lack of training, insufficient access to PPE, and environmental factors were noted as barriers to the use of PPE by nurses [10]. In addition, personal characteristics including beliefs, attitudes, and values and organizational factors such as communication, training, performance feedback, and acceptance among colleagues or managers have been shown to influence nurses' rates of compliance with self-protection behaviors [8,10].

Previous studies have demonstrated that nurses who care for patients with a novel infectious disease (such as severe acute respiratory syndrome (SARS) or H1N1) may be unaware of the most up-to-date information regarding safe patient care and are ill-equipped with PPE [11,12]. The experience of Saudi nurses caring for Middle East respiratory syndrome (MERS) patients also showed that the nurses lacked adequate knowledge about the disease and were more vulnerable to contracting the virus [12]. Prior to the current COVID-19 pandemic, most recent studies regarding best practices for infection control of HCWs were based on lessons learned during the MERS, SARS, and H1N1 outbreaks [13–15]. Nursing compliance with preventive behaviors against respiratory infectious diseases such as SARS and H1N1 has been shown to be influenced by their level of knowledge [16,17], attitudes toward the disease [18], and risk perception [19]. To the best of our knowledge, no study has assessed the impact of individual, organizational, and environmental factors on the use of PPE by nurses caring for patients with COVID-19. We aimed to investigate factors affecting the use of PPE with a focus on nursing perspectives.

2. Methods

This was a descriptive cross-sectional study. The study population consisted of nurses caring for COVID-19 patients in the hospitals affiliated with Arak University of Medical Sciences. All nurses working in the COVID-19 care centers of Valiasr (n = 110) and Ayatollah Khansari (n = 130) hospitals were enrolled via the census sampling method (Figure 1). The study was approved by the Ethics Committee of the university and researchers obtained the permission of hospital directors and head nurses. The research team visited the target wards, spoke to the nurses individually and in groups, and asked eligible nurses to complete this anonymous questionnaire. This occurred during three working shifts (morning, evening, and night). Participants were assured about the confidentiality of their responses and the voluntary nature of the study. Inclusion criteria were having at least a bachelor's degree in nursing and at least six months of work experience. The exclusion criterion was an unwillingness to participate. The data collection tool, a paper-based questionnaire, was handed to eligible nurses and placed by the researcher into a folder after completion. The time needed to complete the questionnaire was 10 min. The data were collected from 5 October to 15 November 2020. For confidentiality, the questionnaires were filled out anonymously without any identifying data. The content validity of the questionnaire was confirmed by 10 nursing research experts. The content validity ratio (CVR) and the content validity index (CVI) of the checklist were calculated as 0.71 and 0.94, respectively. Moreover, the total reliability of its items was approved by a Cronbach's alpha of 0.88 (0.79 for environmental factors, 0.96 for organizational factors, and 0.90 for individual factors). The reliability was also confirmed based on calculating the correlation coefficient index (0.81) through a test–retest method in a pilot study of 15 nurses with an interval of 10 days.

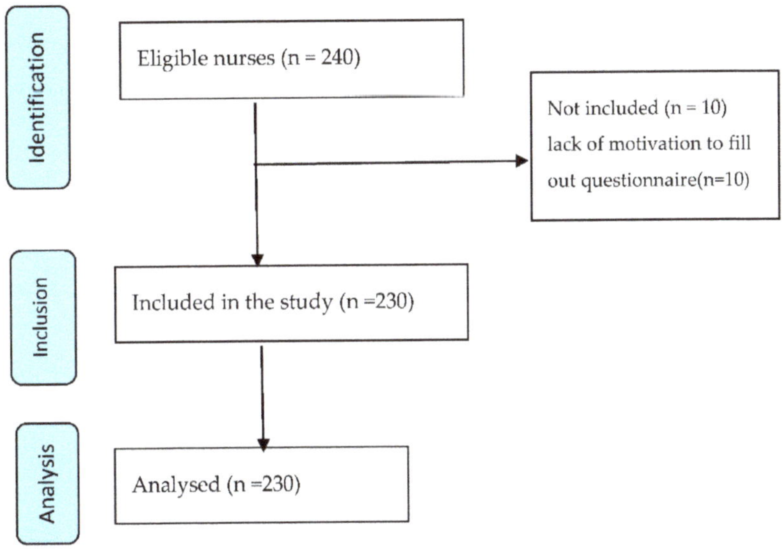

Figure 1. Flow diagram of the selection of study based on STROBE.

The questionnaire consisted of two parts. The first part included demographic information (gender, age, marital status, education, position, work experience, and previous attendance at any PPE training workshop). The second part consisted of 26 statements about the environmental (4 questions), organizational (9 questions), and individual (13 questions) factors affecting the respondent's use of PPE. The statements were scored based on a 5-point Likert scale (strongly agree = 5, agree = 4, no opinion = 3, disagree = 2, and strongly disagree = 1). Using this 5-point scale, the hypothetical average score of the population was assumed to be 3 (i.e., the middle point = the option of "no opinion") during data analysis. The mean score of each item and dimension was determined separately and compared with the hypothetical mean. A mean score of higher than 3 was regarded as above the average, while a mean score of less than 3 was considered below the average. To calculate the average score of each category, the scores of all questions were summed up and then divided by the total number of questions in that domain.

The data were analyzed by SPSS software (version 16) using descriptive statistics. The one-way ANOVA test was used to determine any significant differences when comparing the scores of more than two groups, and the independent sample Student *t*-test was used to examine the mean score differences between two-state variables.

3. Results

Out of 240 distributed questionnaires, 230 were returned, for a response rate of 95.8%. Table 1 shows that 195 nurses (84.4%) were female and 35 (15.2%) were male. Overall, 219 nurses (95.2%) had a bachelor's degree, and 11 (4.8%) had a master's degree. Regarding position, the majority of participants (187, 81.3%) were clinical nurses, while only two (0.9%) were supervisors. Most respondents were married (152, 66.1%). The mean duration of work experience was 12.38 $\pm$ 6.22 years, and the mean age was 37.23 $\pm$ 7.13 years. More than half of the nurses (126, 54.8%) had participated in PPE training workshops.

Table 1. Demographic characteristics of study participants.

Variables		*N* (%)
Gender	Female	195 (84.8%)
	Male	35 (15.2%)
Education	Bachelor's degree	219 (95.2%)
	Master's degree	11 (4.8%)
Marital status	Single	78 (33.9%)
	Married	152 (66.1%)
Previous participation in PPE training workshops	Yes	126 (54.8%)
	No	104 (45.2%)
Position	Nurse	187 (81.3%)
	Shift's chief	32 (13.9%)
	Head nurse	9 (3.9%)
	Supervisor	2 (0.9%)
Age in years (mean ± SD)		37.23 ± 7.13
Work experience in years (mean ± SD)		12.38 ± 6.22

The factors affecting the use of PPE by nurses participating in this survey were environmental (4.24 ± 0.45), individual (4.16 ± 0.42), and organizational (4.04 ± 0.50), listed in order of expressed importance. The average score for all categories was 4.15 ± 0.31. Considering homogeneous variances and normal distribution based on the Kolmogorov–Smirnov test ($p < 0.05$), the univariate *t*-test rendered significant results for all of the environmental, organizational, and individual factors ($p < 0.05$). Therefore, as the observed averages were significantly greater than the hypothetical mean (i.e., 3), these factors were found to have a substantial impact on decision making (Table 2).

Table 2. Univariate *t*-test for the mean score of the factors affecting nursing compliance with the use of PPE (cut off point = 3).

Dimensions	Mean	SD	*p*	T	df	Deviation from Hypothetical Mean
Environmental factors	4.24	0.45	0.001	41.48	229	1.24
Organizational factors	4.04	0.50	0.001	31.38	229	1.04
Personal factors	4.16	0.42	0.001	41.07	229	1.16
All Categories	4.15	0.31	0.001	56.18	229	1.15

After examining the homogeneity of variances using Levene's test ($p < 0.05$), a *t*-test was used to compare the mean scores obtained based on gender, education, marital status, and previous participation in a PPE training workshop (Table 3). Nurses with a bachelor's degree placed more importance on personal factors contributing to their decisions regarding PPE use when compared with nurses who held a master's degree, although this difference was not found to be highly significant ($p = 0.08$). The results of the *t*-test show that nursing compliance with the use of PPE was significantly associated with female gender ($p = 0.05$). An increased importance of environmental factors was significantly associated with being married ($p < 0.05$).

The results of the analysis of variance of the total score after confirming the homogeneity of variances based on Levene's test ($p < 0.05$) show that the highest and lowest total mean scores were related to the charge nurse and nurse supervisor positions, with mean scores of 129.80 and 65.50, respectively (Table 4).

Table 3. Comparison of the mean scores of the factors affecting nurses' compliance with using PPE based on gender, marital status, education, and previous participation in a PPE workshop.

Variables		Environmental Factors	Organizational Factors	Personal Factors	Average of All Factors
Gender	Female	4.24 ± 0.44	4.04 ± 0.48	4.17 ± 0.42	4.15 ± 0.30
	Male	4.24 ± 0.53	4.08 ± 0.60	4.06 ± 0.42	4.13 ± 0.35
p *		0.13	0.26	0.18	0.05
Education	Bachelor	4.23 ± 0.45	4.04 ± 0.50	4.17 ± 0.42	4.14 ± 0.31
	Master	4.56 ± 0.31	4.18 ± 0.62	3.94 ± 0.48	4.23 ± 0.32
p *		0.16	0.37	0.08	0.38
Marital Status	Single	4.15 ± 0.47	4.07 ± 0.48	4.20 ± 0.39	4.14 ± 0.30
	Married	4.29 ± 0.43	4.03 ± 0.51	4.13 ± 0.44	4.15 ± 0.31
p *		0.02	0.55	0.22	0.84
Participation in PPE workshop	Yes	4.28 ± 0.44	4.08 ± 0.47	4.19 ± 0.41	4.18 ± 0.29
	No	4.19 ± 0.46	4.00 ± 0.53	4.10 ± 0.32	4.10 ± 0.32
p *		0.95	0.60	0.16	0.70

* Independent t-test.

Table 4. The mean scores of the factors affecting the compliance of nurses with using PPE according to the nurses' positions.

Position	Mean	SD	Mean of Degree	p
Nurse	4.14	0.29	113.77	0.59
Shift's chief	4.22	0.40	129.80	
Head nurse	4.14	0.21	111.67	
Supervisor	3.98	0.18	65.50	
p = 0.13	Df1 = 3		Df2 = 226	F = 1.88

4. Discussion

HCWs are at the frontline of fighting COVID-19 and should use PPE to protect themselves against the disease. Conversely, wearing PPE increases their stress and workload [20]. Our results show that environmental factors were the most impactful on nurses' decisions regarding the use of PPE, while individual preferences carried less weight. A study from Pakistan showed that a lack of availability and inappropriate use of PPE were among the most notable factors contributing to the transmission of COVID-19 disease to HCWs [21]. Furthermore, an Italian study showed that proper education regarding the use of PPE was just as important as providing adequate supplies [22]. Adequate and appropriate access to PPE reduces the incidence of mental health disorders such as depression and anxiety in nurses [23]. Therefore, in addition to access to PPE, HCWs should receive the necessary and appropriate education to use this equipment safely. Our results show a relatively low importance of personal factors, such as knowledge, attitudes, and beliefs, on the use of PPE by nurses. A study in Nepal showed that it is possible to improve attitudes and safety performances by disseminating accurate information about COVID-19 transmission and infection [24,25]. It is likely that increased efforts aimed at educating nurses regarding COVID-19 transmissibility and infection could improve their attitudes toward, and compliance with, recommended PPE use.

Organizational factors also affected nurses' attitudes toward PPE to some degree. Healthcare organizations should consider continuously training their personnel to use PPE as a part of their COVID-19 pandemic response programs [26]. Furthermore, Delgado et al. showed that supporting HCWs should be among the strategic priorities of healthcare systems during this pandemic [27]. Ahmed et al. also showed that providing HCWs with

PPE is essential, and hospital managers and governments should implement measures to guarantee their access [28]. Overall, our study showed that the factors that had the greatest impact on the views of the nurses caring for patients with COVID-19 regarding the use of personal protective equipment were as follows: environmental factors such as availability of PPE, lack of barriers to safe work practices, and cleanliness and order of the workplace; organizational factors such as feedback from supervisors and safety officers regarding the use of PPE, providing constructive and continuous education to nurses on the use of PPE, addressing staff shortages, implementing quarantine and isolation policies, limiting time for patient care, and high work pressure and workload; personal factors such as believing in the effectiveness of PPE, perception of the organization's safety requirements, the impact of mental norms on the use of PPE, knowledge of coronavirus transmission routes, knowing how to use PPE, understanding the risk of contracting the COVID-19, and setting an example for colleagues by using PPE.(Table 5).

Table 5. Frequency, percentage, mean, and standard deviation of nurses' responses to the factors affecting the use of personal protective equipment.

Number	Factor Impacting the Use of PPE	High and Very High	Moderate	Low and Very Low	Mean	SD
1	The availability of PPE	215 (93.5%)	15 (6.5%)	0	4.53	0.61
2	The lack of barriers to safe work practices	210 (91.3%)	17 (7.4%)	3 (1.3%)	4.31	0.66
3	The cleanliness and order of the workplace	204 (88.8%)	21 (9.1%)	5 (2.1%)	4.33	0.75
4	The patient's clinical course deterioration	146 (63.7%)	72 (31.1%)	12 (5.2%)	3.79	0.86
5	The support of managers about the implementation of safety procedures	152 (66.1%)	63 (27.4%)	15 (6.5%)	3.76	0.88
6	Feedback from supervisors and safety officers regarding the use of PPE	168 (73%)	48 (20.9%)	14 (6.1%)	3.90	0.90
7	Providing constructive and continuous education to nurses on the use of PPE	190 (82.6%)	36 (15.7%)	4 (1.7%)	4.20	0.76
8	Staff shortage for patient care	188 (81.7%)	36 (15.7%)	6 (2.6%)	4.10	0.77
9	Managers' expectations on the use of PPE	178 (77.4%)	34 (14.8%)	18 (7.8%)	4.00	1.04
10	The impact of the workplace prevailing safety practices on using PPE	189 (82.2%)	34 (14.8%)	7 (3%)	4.09	0.80
11	Implementing quarantine and isolation policies	194 (84.7%)	30 (12.7%)	6 (2.6%)	4.12	0.76
12	Limited time for patient care	192 (83.4%)	29 (12.7%)	9 (3.9%)	4.13	0.80
13	High work pressure and workload	191 (83.1%)	27 (11.7%)	12 (5.2%)	4.09	0.85
14	Believing in the effectiveness of PPE to prevent infectious disease, such as COVID-19 transmission	208 (90.5%)	16 (6.9%)	6 (2.6%)	4.26	0.72
15	Perception of the organization's safety requirements	209 (91%)	17 (7.3%)	4 (1.7%)	4.22	0.69
16	The impact of mental norms on the use of PPE	215 (93.5%)	12 (5.2%)	3 (1.3%)	4.32	0.65
17	Having knowledge of coronavirus transmission routes	212 (92.3)	11 (4.7%)	7(3%)	4.29	0.71
18	Knowing how to use PPE	211 (91.8%)	15(6.5%)	4 (1.7%)	4.27	0.66
19	Understanding the risk of contracting the COVID-19	208 (90.5%)	22 (9.5%)	0	4.29	0.63
20	Believing in a reduction in the quality of patient–nurse communication when using PPE	165 (71.7%)	42 (18.3%)	23 (10%)	3.89	0.97

Table 5. *Cont.*

Number	Factor Impacting the Use of PPE	High and Very High	Moderate	Low and Very Low	Mean	SD
21	Believing in a reduction of agility in patient care when using PPE	183 (79.6%)	38 (16.5%)	9 (3.9%)	4.06	0.79
22	Previous infection of self, or colleague, with the coronavirus or other infectious diseases	207 (11.8%)	20 (86.9%)	3 (1.3%)	4.23	0.65
23	Setting an example for colleagues by using PPE	208 (90.5%)	21 (9.1%)	1 (0.4%)	4.28	0.64
24	Patients' expectations about nurses using PPE	172 (74.9%)	45 (19.5%)	13 (5.6%)	4.02	0.87
25	A positive attitude toward the protective effect of PPE	206 (89.6%)	24 (10.4%)	0	4.21	0.61
26	Valuing personal judgment over organizational policies	138 (60.1%)	67 (29.1%)	25 (10.8%)	3.68	0.94

Ultimately, healthcare systems have an important role in maintaining an adequate supply of PPE for nurses during the COVID-19 pandemic. If this role is neglected, organizations face declining quality of care, increased risk to staff, worsening levels of burnout, and an overall compromise in their efficiency and performance.

5. Limitations

A limitation of our study was the relatively low sample size. This can potentially reduce the generalizability of the results. One way to address this would be to pursue larger, multicenter studies in the future. In addition, if respondents were concerned regarding the confidentiality of their answers, they may have provided answers that were less critical of their workplace or organization. This may have altered the results to show a greater support for the use of PPE than in actual practice. This may also have resulted in less critique of the provision and organizational support for PPE than truly experienced. Counteracting this effect, however, may also be a concern for stigma against personal beliefs that conflict with hospital policy, therefore making participants less likely to express their personal beliefs if at odds with those of the organization. Finally, the cross-sectional design of the study may limit our results.

6. Conclusions

Environmental factors had the greatest impact on the use of PPE from the perspective of the nurses caring for COVID-19 patients. Managers and healthcare organizations should provide appropriate and adequate PPE to nurses, educate them on proper use, and monitor the process to resolve barriers.

Author Contributions: R.M. conceptualized the study with support from M.G., A.S. (Ali Safdari), D.H., S.M., M.T. and A.S. (Ali Sahebi). R.M., A.S. (Ali Safdari) and M.G. extracted the data for this study. R.M. cleaned and analyzed the data with support from A.S. (Ali Sahebi). And M.G., S.M., M.T. and D.H. wrote the first draft of the manuscript. All authors contributed to writing and finalizing the manuscript. All authors have read and agreed to the published version of the manuscript.

Funding: This research received no external funding.

Institutional Review Board Statement: The study was conducted according to the guidelines of the Declaration of Helsinki and approved by the COVID-19 Research Center (3627) and the Research Ethics Committee (IR.ARAKMU.REC.1399.092) of Arak University of Medical Sciences.

Informed Consent Statement: Informed consent was obtained from all subjects involved in the study.

Data Availability Statement: The dataset analyzed during the current study is available from the corresponding author upon reasonable request.

Acknowledgments: We would like to offer our special thanks to the nurses for their cooperation in this study during the harsh conditions under the COVID-19 pandemic.

Conflicts of Interest: The authors declare no conflict of interest.

References

1. Cao, Y.; Li, Q.; Chen, J.; Guo, X.; Miao, C.; Yang, H.; Chen, Z.; Li, C.; Li, L. Hospital Emergency Management Plan During the COVID-19 Epidemic. *Acad. Emerg. Med.* **2020**, *27*, 309–311. [CrossRef]
2. Choi, J.S.; Kim, K.M. Crisis Prevention and Management by Infection Control Nurses During the Middle East Respiratory Coro-Navirus Outbreak in Korea. *Am. J. Infect. Control.* **2016**, *44*, 480–481. [CrossRef]
3. Jenkins, E.K.; McAuliffe, C.; Hirani, S.; Richardson, C.; Thomson, K.C.; McGuinness, L.; Morris, J.; Kousoulis, A.; Gadermann, A. A Portrait of the Early and Differential Mental Health Impacts of the COVID-19 Pandemic in Canada: Findings from the First Wave of a Nationally Representative Cross-Sectional Survey. *Prev. Med.* **2021**, *145*, 106333. [CrossRef] [PubMed]
4. Saha, S.; Dutta, D. A Study on the Psychological Crisis During the Lockdown Caused Due to Covid-19 Pandemic. *Afr. J. Biol. Sci.* **2020**, *3*, 41–49.
5. Mokhtari, R.; Moayedi, S.; Golitaleb, M. COVID-19 Pandemic and Health Anxiety Among Nurses of Intensive Care Units. *Int. J. Ment. Health Nurs.* **2020**, *29*, 1275–1277. [CrossRef] [PubMed]
6. Greene, J.; Gibson, D.M. Workers at Long-Term Care Facilities and Their Risk for Severe COVID-19 Illness. *Prev. Med.* **2021**, *143*, 106328. [CrossRef]
7. Guo, Y.; Qin, W.; Wang, Z.; Yang, F. Factors Influencing Social Distancing to Prevent the Community Spread of COVID-19 Among Chinese Adults. *Prev. Med.* **2021**, *143*, 106385. [CrossRef]
8. Millar, R.C. Nursing a Patient With Covid-19 Infection. *Tasman. Med. J.* **2020**, *1*, 4–8.
9. Choi, J.-S.; Kim, J.-S. Factors Influencing Preventive Behavior Against Middle East Respiratory Syndrome-Coronavirus Among Nursing Students in South Korea. *Nurse Educ. Today* **2016**, *40*, 168–172. [CrossRef]
10. Moore, D.; Gamage, B.; Bryce, E.; Copes, R.; Yassi, A. Protecting Health Care Workers from SARS and Other Respiratory Pathogens: Organizational and Individual Factors That Affect Adherence to Infection Control Guidelines. *Am. J. Infect. Control* **2005**, *33*, 88–96. [CrossRef]
11. Kim, K.; Lee, O. Knowledge, Attitudes and Perceptions of Nurses on Personal Protective Equipment: Response to the Middle East Respiratory Syndrome Coronavirus. *J. Korean Acad. Fundam. Nurs.* **2016**, *23*, 402–410. [CrossRef]
12. Khalid, I.; Khalid, T.J.; Qabajah, M.R.; Barnard, A.G.; Qushmaq, I.A. Healthcare Workers Emotions, Perceived Stressors and Coping Strategies During a MERS-CoV Outbreak. *Clin. Med. Res.* **2016**, *14*, 7–14. [CrossRef]
13. Cowling, B.J.; Park, M.; Fang, V.J.; Wu, P.; Leung, G.M.; Wu, J.T. Preliminary Epidemiological Assessment of MERS-CoV Outbreak in South Korea, May to June 2015. *Eurosurveillance* **2015**, *20*, 21163. [CrossRef]
14. Hall, A.J.; Tokars, J.I.; Badreddine, S.A.; Bin Saad, Z.; Furukawa, E.; Al Masri, M.; Haynes, L.M.; Gerber, S.I.; Kuhar, D.T.; Miao, C.; et al. Health Care Worker Contact With MERS Patient, Saudi Arabia. *Emerg. Infect. Dis.* **2014**, *20*, 2148–2151. [CrossRef]
15. Park, H.; Lee, E.; Ryu, Y.; Kim, Y.; Kim, H.; Lee, H.; Yi, S.J. Epidemiological Investigation of MERS-CoV Spread in a Single Hospital in South Korea, May to June 2015. *Eurosurveillance* **2015**, *20*, 21169. [CrossRef]
16. Gautret, P.; Benkouiten, S.; Salaheddine, I.; Belhouchat, K.; Drali, T.; Parola, P.; Brouqui, P. Hajj pilgrims' Knowledge about Middle East Respiratory Syndrome Coronavirus, August to September 2013. *Eurosurveillance* **2013**, *18*, 20604. [CrossRef] [PubMed]
17. Khan, M.U.; Shah, S.; Ahmad, A.; Fatokun, O. Knowledge and Attitude of Healthcare Workers about Middle East Respiratory Syn-Drome in Multispecialty Hospitals of Qassim, Saudi Arabia. *BMC Public Health* **2014**, *14*, 1–7. [CrossRef]
18. Choi, J.-S.; Yang, N.-Y. Perceived Knowledge, Attitude, and Compliance With Preventive Behavior on Influenza A (H1N1) by University Students. *Korean J. Adult Nurs.* **2010**, *22*, 250–259.
19. Brug, J.; Aro, A.R.; Oenema, A.; De Zwart, O.; Richardus, J.H.; Bishop, G.D. SARS Risk Perception, Knowledge, Precautions, and in-Formation Sources, The Netherlands. *Emerg. Infect. Dis.* **2004**, *10*, 1486. [CrossRef]
20. Choudhury, A.; Singh, M.; Khurana, D.K.; Mustafi, S.M.; Sharma, S. Physiological Effects of N95 FFP and PPE in Healthcare Workers in COVID Intensive Care Unit: A Prospective Cohort Study. *Indian J. Crit. Care Med.* **2020**, *24*, 1169–1173. [CrossRef] [PubMed]
21. Ali, S.; Noreen, S.; Farooq, I.; Bugshan, A.; Vohra, F. Risk Assessment of Healthcare Workers at the Frontline Against COVID-19. *Pak. J. Med. Sci.* **2020**, *36* (COVID19-S4), S99–S103. [CrossRef]
22. Savoia, E.; Argentini, G.; Gori, D.; Neri, E.; Piltch-Loeb, R.; Fantini, M.P. Factors Associated With Access and Use of PPE During COVID-19: A Cross-Sectional Study of Italian Physicians. *PLoS ONE* **2020**, *15*, e0239024. [CrossRef] [PubMed]
23. Arnetz, J.E.; Goetz, C.M.; Sudan, S.; Arble, E.; Janisse, J.; Arnetz, B.B. Personal Protective Equipment and Mental Health Symptoms Among Nurses During the COVID-19 Pandemic. *J. Occup. Environ. Med.* **2020**, *62*, 892–897. [CrossRef]
24. Alao, M.A.; Durodola, A.O.; Ibrahim, O.; Asinobi, O.A. Assessment of Health Workers' Knowledge, Beliefs, Attitudes, and Use of Personal Protective Equipment for Prevention of COVID-19 Infection in Low-Resource Settings. *Adv. Public Health* **2020**, *2020*, 1–10. [CrossRef]
25. Nepal, R.; Sapkota, K.; Adhikari, K.; Paudel, P.; Adhikari, B.; Paudyal, N.; Sapkota, K.; Nepal, R. Knowledge, Attitude and Practice Regarding COVID-19 Among Healthcare Workers in Chitwan, Nepal. *J. Chitwan Med. Coll.* **2020**, *10*. [CrossRef]

26. Piché-Renaud, P.-P.; Groves, H.E.; Kitano, T.; Arnold, C.; Thomas, A.; Streitenberger, L.; Alexander, L.; Morris, S.K.; Science, M. Healthcare Worker Perception of a Global Outbreak of Novel Coronavirus (COVID-19) and Personal Protective Equipment: Survey of a Pediatric Tertiary-Care Hospital. *Infect. Control Hosp. Epidemiol.* **2021**, *42*, 261–267. [CrossRef]
27. Delgado, D.; Quintana, F.W.; Perez, G.; Liprandi, A.S.; Ponte-Negretti, C.; Mendoza, I.; Baranchuk, A. Personal Safety During the COVID-19 Pandemic: Realities and Perspectives of Healthcare Workers in Latin America. *Int. J. Environ. Res. Public Health* **2020**, *17*, 2798. [CrossRef] [PubMed]
28. Ahmed, J.; Malik, F.; Bin Arif, T.; Majid, Z.; A Chaudhary, M.; Ahmad, J.; Malik, M.; Khan, T.M.; Khalid, M. Availability of Personal Protective Equipment (PPE) Among US and Pakistani Doctors in COVID-19 Pandemic. *Cureus* **2020**, *12*, e8550.

International Journal of
Environmental Research and Public Health

MDPI

Article

The Transformational Experience of Junior Nurses Resulting from Providing Care to COVID-19 Patients: From Facing Hurdles to Achieving Psychological Growth

Yuk-Chiu Yip *, Ka-Huen Yip and Wai-King Tsui

School of Health Sciences, Caritas Institute of Higher Education, Hong Kong, China; khyip@cihe.edu.hk (K.-H.Y.); ztsui@cihe.edu.hk (W.-K.T.)
* Correspondence: jyip@cihe.edu.hk

Abstract: The rapid spread of coronavirus disease 2019 (COVID-19) has put significant pressure on junior nursing staff. The objective of this study was to examine the in-depth experiences of junior nurses in providing care for COVID-19 patients within an acute care setting. This study employed a phenomenological method to understand the situation from a first-person perspective. Purposive sampling was used. Interviews were performed with 40 junior nurses (<4 years of clinical experience) who provided direct care to COVID-19 patients in isolation wards in acute care settings in Hong Kong. The interviews were conducted from 1 January 2021 to 24 May 2021 via virtual conferencing software (Zoom) to maintain social distancing, and the responses were analysed using Colaizzi's seven-step method. Junior nurses' psychological experiences of providing direct care to COVID-19 patients were categorised into four main themes. First, there were hurdles in the early stages, in which participants experienced negative emotions, such as fear, anxiety, helplessness, and fatigue. Somatic symptoms, such as headaches and sleep disturbance, were reported. Second, the adoption of self-care coping strategies enabled nurses to confront the hurdles, signifying the start of self-transformation. Third, junior nurses maintained positivity under pressure by appreciating their sources of support (including their families and other important relationships in their lives). Professionalism was also found to reinforce positivity. Fourth, self-transformation resulted in psychological growth, which prepared junior nurses to be resilient and confident in their clinical practice to take up future challenges in the ongoing battle against the pandemic. The hurdles experienced by junior nurses at the early stage of their work in isolation wards provided the foundation upon which self-transformation took place. Being able to employ self-care coping strategies and further sustain positivity characterised the self-transformation process. Eventually, junior nurses became resilient and more capable of understanding both the negativity and positivity of their experiences. The self-transformation process also enabled junior nurses to recognise and appreciate the wider support system from various parties in society.

Keywords: coronavirus disease 2019 (COVID-19); junior nurses; transformational experience

Citation: Yip, Y.-C.; Yip, K.-H.; Tsui, W.-K. The Transformational Experience of Junior Nurses Resulting from Providing Care to COVID-19 Patients: From Facing Hurdles to Achieving Psychological Growth. *Int. J. Environ. Res. Public Health* **2021**, *18*, 7383. https://doi.org/10.3390/ijerph18147383

Academic Editors: Richard Gray and Sonia Udod

Received: 7 June 2021
Accepted: 6 July 2021
Published: 10 July 2021

1. Introduction

Coronavirus disease 2019 (COVID-19) is caused by a novel variant of the infectious coronavirus that was initially recognised in Wuhan, China, on 31 December 2019 [1]. The disease was classified as a pandemic by the World Health Organisation (WHO) on 11 March 2020, because of the rapid global spread of the virus [2]. Approximately 20% of COVID-19 patients suffer serious complications that require oxygen therapy or other forms of in-hospital intervention, and 5% of patients need to be admitted to intensive care [3].

Nurses have an important role to play in the support and assistance of patients during in-patient care. However, the nurses themselves are at considerable risk of contracting the virus, and it is virtually impossible to eliminate this threat [4]. The virus is highly contagious and can threaten the lives of nurses, and as it is a novel variant, the information related to standards of care and infection control is continually evolving. The influx of infected patients has led to significant alterations to the care settings in which nurses work, thus creating considerable challenges for nurses. Nurses are instrumental and highly involved in efforts to combat the virus. Providing 24/7 nursing care means that nurses are in proximity to COVID-19 patients from their admission to their discharge. Among healthcare professionals, nurses are most exposed to psychologically distressing situations during these difficult times [5,6].

Previous research has shown that, when unexpected natural disasters or pandemics arise, nurses frequently disregard their own health and safety to address the situation in front of them, working selflessly due to their strong ethics and professionalism [7]. Simultaneously, nurses may feel physically and mentally stressed, experiencing isolation and helplessness when faced with dangers to their health and the high-pressure continuous work required when public health emergency situations arise [8]. Research has demonstrated that while working closely with patients suffering from novel infectious diseases, nurses frequently experience fatigue, fear, anxiety, sleep disorders, loneliness and other challenges to both their physical and mental health [9–14]. One study showed that nurses attending to SARS patients experienced insomnia (37%), depression (38.5%), and posttraumatic stress (33%) [14]. However, some studies have also shown that working on a collective initiative to combat an epidemic requires nurses to grow professionally in the process and develop resilience to overcome the challenges posed by the outbreak [10,15].

Given that the COVID-19 pandemic is caused by a novel virus, many nurses are thus called to the frontline to provide care to patients, and these nurses may not be familiar with the disease. At the time this research was undertaken, junior nurses with fewer than 4 years of clinical practice were recruited on a voluntary basis to offer their professional help in acute care settings. This group of nurses has been under-researched in terms of their unique experiences on the frontline of the battle against the disease. Current research has noted that physicians experienced severe psychological distress [16,17]; however, there is little research regarding the psychological experiences faced by junior nurses who have been practicing for a certain period "in the field"—providing care to patients with confirmed COVID-19 in acute care settings. To fill this knowledge gap, this qualitative research investigated the in-depth and subjective experiences of junior nurses who provided direct care to patients with confirmed COVID-19 for at least six months using semi-structured interviews and employing a phenomenological methodology [18].

This research has practical implications in that the psychological conditions potentially affecting junior nurses, including fear, anxiety, and burnout, could be shown with empirical evidence so that timely and appropriate support could be provided by healthcare management who are responsible for developing policies to safeguard the mental health of nursing staff [19,20].

2. Methods

2.1. Research Design

In this qualitative study, junior nurses were comprehensively interviewed about their psychological experiences providing direct hospitalised care for patients with confirmed COVID-19. The data were analysed based on the phenomenological methodology suggested by Colaizzi [18]. With this method, the researchers attempted to understand the participants' subjective feelings and experiences by mentally returning to the situation itself.

2.2. Participants

The participants in this study were 40 junior nurses attending to patients with confirmed COVID-19 at public hospitals in Hong Kong, and purposive sampling was used. To recruit these participants, our research team approached four hospital clusters where isolation wards were established to admit patients with confirmed COVID-19 for hospitalised care. The research team members informed the department operation managers of these clusters information about the study and expressed our interests in interviewing their junior nursing staff. The research team members then individually followed up with junior nurses who obtained our research team contact information (email and/or phone) through their supervisors and showed interest in participating in this study. The inclusion criteria included the following: (1) being a nurse with at least 6 months (continuous or intermittent) of clinical experience in providing direct care to patients with confirmed COVID-19 in an isolation ward, (2) volunteering to participate in the study, and (3) being a nurse with fewer than 4 years of practical experience after graduation from pre-licensure academic studies. In this study, isolation wards were defined as wards in acute care settings that were equipped with multiple airborne infection isolation rooms (AIIRs) for in-patients with confirmed COVID-19. Each AIIR was a single-occupancy negative-pressure room with at least 12 air changes per hour. In addition, the exhaust of air from each AIIR within the isolation wards had to pass through a high-efficiency particulate air filter. Within each AIIR, an en-suite toilet facility was provided for infection-control purposes, such that individually isolated patients within an isolation ward did not share a toilet. Individual interviews continued until data saturation was reached at the 37th interview, after which no new information arose in the next three individual interviews (with two female participants and one male participant). The participants' characteristics can be found in Table 1. We enrolled six male and 34 female nurses between the ages of 21 and 35, with an average age of 28. The participants had an average of 7.5 months of experience in providing care to patients with confirmed COVID-19. At the time of the interview, the participants were 24–48 months (mean, 39 months) post-graduation. Among the participants, 38 nurses possessed a bachelor's degree, and two nurses had graduated with a higher diploma. Regarding marriage and children, one nurse was married with children, one was married without children and 38 were unmarried and without children.

Table 1. Participant characteristics.

Characteristic	All		Male		Female	
	n = 40		n = 6		n = 34	
	n	%	n	%	n	%
Age						
21–25	1	2.5	0	0	1	3
26–30	37	92.5	5	83	32	94
31–35	2	5	1	17	1	3
Education level						
Higher diploma	2	5	0	0	2	6
Bachelor's degree	38	95	6	100	32	94
Marriage and children						
Unmarried without children	38	95	6	100	32	94
Married without children	1	2.5	0	0	1	3
Married with children	1	2.5	0	0	1	3
Number of year(s) of post-licensure practical experience at time of interview						
1	0	0	0	0	0	0
2	6	15	0	0	6	18
3	18	45	4	67	14	41
4	16	40	2	33	14	41
Number of months providing direct care to hospitalised patients confirmed with COVID-19 at time of interview						
6	8	20	0	0	8	24
7	12	30	2	33	10	29
8	10	25	1	17	9	26
9	10	25	3	50	7	21

Table 1. *Cont.*

Characteristic	All		Male		Female	
	n = 40		*n* = 6		*n* = 34	
	n	%	*n*	%	*n*	%
Religious beliefs						
None	7	17.5	3	50	4	12
Christian	10	25	2	33	8	23.5
Buddhist	23	57.5	1	17	22	64.5
Other	0	0	0	0	0	0

2.3. Data Collection

All interviews were conducted by the researcher (Y.C.) at the participant's preferred time in a private password-protected Zoom (Nasdaq, San Jose, California, U.S.) meeting room from 1 January 2021 to 24 May 2021. Each interview took about 60–120 min, and the same interview guide was always used to reduce variation in the data-collection process. A panel of two experts—an academic qualitative scholar and a psychological consulting specialist—was formed to review and affirm the validity of the interview questions. All interviews were audio-recorded with the participants' written permission. Field notes were taken during the interviews to facilitate the collection of contextual information and thus, the data analysis. The interview guide questions are listed in Table 2. If the participant exhibited emotional distress during the interview, adequate psychological support was provided to prevent further psychological harm. The participants were also informed that they could withdraw consent at any time.

Table 2. Interview guide.

No.	Probing Questions
1.	How do you feel when you are called upon to provide direct nursing care to patients with confirmed COVID-19?
2.	How did your feelings change over time when you practiced as a junior nurse in an isolation ward to take care of these patients day and night?
3.	Can you describe some of your self-care coping strategies to meet your own psychological needs?
4.	In what ways do you think your self-care coping strategies help you on a psychological level?
5.	How do you stay positive when you feel distressed at work?
6.	Reflecting on your months of efforts in caring for patients with COVID-19, how do you perceive the negativity and positivity along the journey?

2.4. Data Analysis and Rigor

Data analysis was performed immediately after data collection using NVivo software (NVivo Version 12, QSR International). For individual interviews, the interview tapes were transcribed verbatim by two researchers (Y.C. and K.H.). Colaizzi's [18] phenomenological analysis method was used for systematically organising the data and field notes. This method includes a seven-step process to reveal emergent themes through (1) familiarisation with the collected data, (2) identification of the significant statements, (3) formulation of meanings alongside the use of the researcher's reflective bracketing, (4) clustering of themes, (5) formation of an exhaustion description, (6) development of the fundamental structure of the phenomenon, and (7) verification of the exhaustive description and fundamental structure [18].

Specifically, the recorded data of each interview were transcribed word for word and analysed by Colaizzi's [18] phenomenological analysis method throughout the data-analysis process. Two members of the research team (Y.C. and K.H.) independently reviewed the interview materials, summarised and extracted meaningful statements, and formulated different themes. The researchers compared the subthemes and identified the differences and similarities between them by looking at the picture holistically. The study's authors (Y.C., K.H., W.K.) discussed the results of their analyses to reach a consensus. To ensure a high level of rigor in this study, the study referenced the stringent criteria established by Lincoln and Guba [21]. The summary table provided below (see Table 3) illustrates how each of the criteria, in relation to credibility, dependability, confirmability, and transferability, was fulfilled. Member checking was also performed.

Table 3. Summary of strategies applied to achieve rigor.

Rigor Criteria	Purpose	Strategies to Achieve Rigor	Notes of Application
Credibility	To establish confidence that the results are true, credible, and believable	- Prolonged and varied engagement with each setting	- Engagement through participant observation in the field was infeasible at the time of this research. There was a strict "no third-party visit" policy (as imposed by the Hospital Authority) for the isolation wards admitting patients with confirmed COVID-19. This policy was to prevent the spread of the virus to the community. - However, a range of participants from different acute-care venues were approached through the nursing administration departments that have regular communications about clinical research with the authors' affiliated institution.
		- Interviewing process and techniques	- The interview guide was tested at two induction meetings after the ethics approval was granted. Two pilot interviews via Zoom were conducted, and the data from these two interviews were also included in the final data analysis.
		- Establishing investigators' authority	- All members of the research team had the required knowledge, data management skills, and practical experience of no less than 5 years in qualitative research to perform their roles.
		- Collection of referential adequacy materials	- Field notes were used to aid the documentation of the contextual information mentioned by the participants for accurate data analysis. Field notes were also analysed with the transcripts.
		- Peer debriefing	- Debriefing sessions were held regularly at 3-week intervals with the Fellows from the Hong Kong Academy of Nursing to ensure that there were no taken-for-granted biases, perspectives, or assumptions on the researchers' part.
Dependability	To ensure the findings of this qualitative inquiry would be repeatable if the inquiry occurred within the same cohort	- Rich description of study methods	- The study methods were described in detail and clearly in the research papers.
		- Establishing an audit trail	- All researchers formed a detailed track record of the data-collection process. - Member checking was performed to ensure the clarity of the meanings derived from the participants, thereby enhancing the validity of the accounts from the participants.
		- Stepwise replication of data	- All researchers assessed coding accuracy and inter-coder reliability throughout the data-analysis process.

Table 3. *Cont.*

Rigor Criteria	Purpose	Strategies to Achieve Rigor	Notes of Application
Confirmability	To extend the confidence that the results would be confirmed/corroborated by other researchers	- Reflexivity	- Measures such as reflexive journals and weekly investigator meetings were adopted.
Transferability	To extend the degree to which the results can be generalised/transferred to other contexts/settings	- Data saturation - Thick description	- Data saturation was reached when no new themes emerged from the participants. All three researchers reached a consensus on the attainment of data saturation. - Lengthy description was provided in the quotes of the participants, such that the meanings of the statements from the participants could be interpreted in context.

2.5. Ethical Review

All participants were informed of the details of the study. Informed consent was obtained from all participants. All methods were carried out in accordance with the relevant guidelines and regulations of the authors' affiliated institution. Participation was voluntary, and all participants were informed that they could withdraw from the study without any consequences. The confidentiality and anonymity of the participants were strictly ensured with encryption. Only the researchers had access to the study data. Ethical approval was obtained from the Research and Ethics Committee of the Caritas Institute of Higher Education in Hong Kong (HRE200133).

3. Results

Using phenomenological methods, we explored the psychological experiences of junior nurses providing direct care to patients with confirmed COVID-19. Four themes were identified from the observations, and they are summarised below:

3.1. Theme 1: Hurdles in the Early Stage

When participants experienced their first working week in isolation wards, they all demonstrated high stress and negative emotions.

3.1.1. Suffering Due to Overwork and Burnout

The increasing intake of confirmed cases of COVID-19 patients came with an increase in workload that was substantially greater than the normal workload experienced in nursing care services. They all complained that they were feeling unwell and tired. They felt exhausted both physiologically and psychologically.

> "After working non-stop for 8 h a day and wearing personal protective equipment all day, I often suffered from headaches and chest tightness. At the same time, the band of the surgical mask on my ears made me uncomfortable. Every time I finished my shift and took off my PPE, I was sweaty and my entire body ached. I felt very tired as if I was about to collapse, and I could fall asleep easily at any time. I often wished there was a bed right in front of me so I could jump onto it and fall asleep right away."

> "I was under a lot of pressure [said in a slightly raised tone while leaning towards the interviewer] ... I was mentally exhausted from keeping abreast of the updates on the admission situation in the various isolation wards ... The rapidly increasing number of protocols relating to isolation and disinfection and the overwhelming number of updates on nursing and medical interventions

simply wore me down ... I could not afford the time to have a psychological consultation, as I did not even have enough sleep."

Participants also expressed feelings of stress and helplessness in the face of a limited supply of personal protective equipment (PPE). They felt frustrated trying to perform nursing procedures when resources were tight. Meanwhile, the inadequate stock of PPE posed huge challenges to the nursing staff because they had to strike a delicate balance between meeting patients' needs and controlling the consumption of PPE in their daily practice within the boundaries set by the hospital infection-control protocols. Most participants adopted radical measures to minimise the usage of PPE as much as they could.

> "I felt drained and somewhat less capable to deliver care when resources were unprecedentedly and extremely tight ... I decided to drink less water and eat much less to reduce both the frequency of going to the toilet and, hence, the need to change my PPE."

3.1.2. Fear and Anxiety

Participants expressed fear and anxiety when they were asked by their department if they were willing to work voluntarily in isolation wards, because most of them had been practicing mainly in general adult medical and/or surgical wards in the past few years. Specifically, participants doubted if they could cooperate well at a professional level with the physicians and nursing staff in isolation wards because some of them were unfamiliar with the nursing care workflow and the operational logistics of isolation wards, both of which were different from those of general adult wards.

> "I worried that my nursing colleagues would feel unhappy with me because I worked slower than them ... I was afraid of potential criticism during my adaptation period [said with a frown] ... I worried that the doctors would blame me because I was considered not as competent as others who were used to working in an isolation ward setting ... I could not sleep very well and I had an upset stomach once I knew I would soon be relocated."

> "I used to work in paediatric units and adult medical wards ... The nursing and treatment items there (isolation wards) were all placed in different locations from the general ward settings ... The operating procedures and daily routines of nursing care in an isolation ward were different ... I felt very anxious and had difficulty falling asleep ... I pushed myself to the limit to adapt to the ward practices as quickly as I could."

Participants also expressed that their fear and anxiety stemmed from their limited knowledge of the disease and the relevant strategies of nursing management (for example, the mechanisms of pathogenesis, possible routes of transmission, treatment algorithms, and nursing interventions). They considered the above-mentioned knowledge important for them to accurately evaluate a patient's condition and treatment progress and to plan their nursing care accordingly.

> "Honestly, the feeling of fear drove me to put extra effort into learning ... My colleagues and I did not want to appear petrified when patients' inquiries and needs arose ... I would have felt uneasy if I were less knowledgeable than my co-workers and senior nurses who worked diligently to serve the patients with professionalism."

> "I was particularly concerned about possible sudden complications, like shortness of breath or unknown psychological conditions ... I am very concerned about the mental well-being of patients who need to receive treatment in an isolation ward. I need more knowledge from both research and updated nursing guidelines to support my practice. I felt dreadful for my lack of preparedness [sighed deeply]."

> "I always worried about what I should do if the patient's condition deteriorated in a split second ... I wondered whether the resuscitation effort would be uncoordinated because the nursing team was newly formed."

Social media (for example, disease updates forwarded through Twitter) may also have increased the fear and anxiety of junior nurses, as social-media messages may have suggested a seemingly "real" and particularly high risk of mortality for the individuals who contracted the novel virus.

> "I was academically trained to appraise scientific evidence ... I believe in science ... Yet I could not distance myself from the news that naturally came up on my Facebook and Twitter pages ... These newsfeeds about patients with confirmed COVID-19 terrified me because they focused on reporting the death rates and how critical the patients were."

3.1.3. Two-Way Relationships between Family Members

All participants came from families with spouses or aged parents. They cared greatly about the health of their family members and were worried about transmitting the virus to them if they got infected. Some participants had not informed their families that they had begun working in an isolation ward. Because of the nature of the disease (i.e., infected individuals may be clinically asymptomatic), many of the participants decided to stay away from their parents and spouses to protect their health and, in the meantime, to prevent any transmission of the virus from the hospital to the community.

> "I did not want to emotionally burden my husband during the pandemic. I did not let him know that I was working in an isolation ward ... I applied for a subsidy from my hospital so that I could rent an apartment ... My husband always cares about me, and I believe I have a duty as a responsible wife to protect him."

> "I dared not tell my parents that I was working in an isolation ward. Every day, I called my parents after work and told them I would stay and rest in the dormitory instead of returning home. I mostly stayed in a hotel when I was off duty ... I did not want to spread the virus to my family or the community ... Still, I was very worried about my dad, mom and grandma during the pandemic [tears up], and I knew they were worried about me too."

While participants demonstrated commitment to their professional duties in isolation wards, they were cognizant of the concern and worries from their families. The fact that their nursing work involved physical care and a risk of contracting the novel virus was a major disquieting factor for their family members. This reciprocal pattern of concern (both from the families to the participants and vice versa) was evident, as shown by the following quotes.

> "My mother was very worried that I would get infected by performing suction for patients ... She texted me a lot to check if I was okay at work. She had never been so anxious, even though she knew all about my profession and my current working environment (in an isolation ward) ... Yet I did not want my mother to be so uptight about my health; it was not good for her mentally."

> "My mum kept an eye out for news of any healthcare workers contracting the novel coronavirus. She looked so worried that I might get infected. That is why I was equally worried about her ... I knew she was mindful (more than ever) of the relevant news because I worked so closely with patients."

3.2. *Theme 2: Self-Care Coping Strategies*

Participants relied on their own self-care coping methods to manage the unprecedented work challenges that arose frequently in their clinical environment, as well as their emotions (including ups and downs) during the pandemic.

3.2.1. Continual Adjustment in Life

All participants engaged in their own psychological self-defence mechanisms, including distraction, humour, and rationalisation. Many participants channelled their emotions by confiding in trusted colleagues and companions. They relieved their stress and addressed their grievances either directly or indirectly through psychological tactics, online media, or other activities (for example, diary-writing, rhythmic breathing, meditation, and listening to music).

> "I rationalised things so I felt better while stressed. It was easy. When I got stressed for all sorts of things like criticism from colleagues, I told myself I was not that bad ... I may have been junior (in terms of practicing experience), and I had inadequate knowledge ... But I could improve by some self-learning and things would be fine."

> "I wrote a diary on Instagram to share my excitement and sadness ... Sometimes, I liked having video calls with my boyfriend to seek consolation. He is good at telling me humorous stories ... I also felt less anxious when I practiced rhythmic breathing or distracted myself by listening to music."

Some participants increased their sleeping time by going to bed earlier when they were under immense pressure. Some changed their diet and began exercising regularly to maintain their mental health.

> "I thought sleeping more is the best way to reduce stress. It temporarily took the emotional burden and stress off my shoulders ... I also liked doing some simple exercises like stretching and yoga regularly. Exercise brings me relaxation."

> "I was more aware of the importance of self-care to my well-being during this pandemic. For example, to strengthen my immune system, I was more selective in my diet choices. I ate more healthy food for breakfast, lunch and dinner."

3.2.2. Feelings of Unity

Participants pointed out that there could be various sources of stress and anxiety in one's practice in an isolation ward. Nonetheless, having a feeling of unity with the nursing team represented an effective coping strategy for many participants. Participants further elaborated that, because they felt the solidarity and unity of a nursing team, they were more active in seeking help for their negative emotions and difficulties. On many occasions, these negative emotions and difficulties could be mitigated through mutual support and motivation from colleagues.

> "Although I was new to the (isolation) ward, my feeling of unity drove me to seek clarification when I was in doubt ... When miscommunication was largely prevented by my active efforts, my anxiety decreased with time."

> "I thought my adaptation time was shorter than others because, at the start of my work in this unfamiliar ward, I regarded myself as an integral part of the team ... I supported others, and others did the same for me ... You must actively unite with your colleagues to manage the psychological hurdles arising from this rapidly changing pandemic situation [said in a firm tone of voice]."

3.2.3. Anchoring and Holding On

Participants felt uncertain about how to manage the hurdles and negative emotions, such as fear and anxiety, that arose from their practice. The volatility of the pandemic and the unclear implications of the nursing practice increased the participants' desire to search for an anchor point. The anchor point provided participants with psychological comfort and reassurance for them to cope with the hurdles. Participants identified this anchor point by actively reviewing the literature, international reports and any useful information on the Internet to compare what they encountered with the experiences around the world.

> "I needed a reference point psychologically. I was eager to know how the hardships I encountered in clinical settings were managed in other countries ... I felt more assured of my nursing practice if I knew other (developed countries) did similarly."

> "I looked over international materials to make sure I was not alone. I thought finding an anchor point in my mind was a self-care method in this difficult time."

Participants were able to hold on, continuing their hard work in clinical areas, when they derived a certain level of mental calmness from the psychological anchor point. They expressed that identifying an anchor point represented a rational way to manage the hurdles.

> "When I felt distressed, I looked around at what was happening throughout the world. I motivated myself by thinking up some reasons that helped me make sense of the clinical impacts of this pandemic."

3.3. Theme 3: Staying Positive under Pressure

Participants stayed positive under pressure by appreciating their sources of support, including their families, colleagues, friends, and other important relationships in their lives. Professionalism was found to play a role in reinforcing positivity. Participants were eventually able to sustain the positivity and, through self-transformation, summon the courage to face the stress and future challenges in their practice.

3.3.1. Appreciation for the People You Love and Live with

Participants expressed that working in an isolation ward and providing direct care to patients with COVID-19 represented a unique (albeit stressful) experience in their nursing practice. Participants admitted that they had not "lived through" any pandemic as they had at this time, because most of them were children during historical pandemics. For example, participants recalled that they were still in primary education when the severe acute respiratory syndrome—commonly known as SARS—pandemic struck Hong Kong in 2003. As the participants suggested, the uniqueness of the experience was characterised by being at the frontline in the battle against this pandemic, being a member of a nursing team to provide professional care, and being grown up and thus, accountable to their families. By reflecting upon the gain from this unique experience, participants were able to stay positive under stress.

> "My lovely parents supported and encouraged me to contribute in an isolation ward ... I was so thankful for all my loved ones because they rekindled my inner spirit as a nurse ... I am blessed and indebted to them for their care, love, motivation and support."

Participants also derived positive energy by reflecting upon the valuable relationships in their lives. They appreciated the essential affection, love, and friendship in their lives. They felt more positive because of an increasing awareness of the established rapport between the persons they knew and worked with and the emotional attachment to their families.

> "The working experience in this pandemic made me feel that nothing (people and relationships) should be taken for granted in life ... My mum always motivated me and gave me confidence ... I felt I am living in an enabling living and working space ... my helpful colleagues gave me a lot of strength when I was stressed."

3.3.2. Professional Identity and Sense of Responsibility

Participants believed that their professionalism kept them motivated to engage in the fight against the COVID-19 pandemic. Most of them lifted their spirits by reminding themselves of the fundamental nature of their nursing duty and their invaluable role in this fight. Their professionalism strengthened their positive belief regarding the need to perform and undertake duties of the nursing profession.

> "I kept reminding myself that this is my duty as a nurse ... I was involved in lifesaving work every day ... I was trained to provide high-quality and holistic care that aims to alleviate patients' suffering."

> "Although I was scared about the pandemic, I did not back off . . . I considered it my responsibility to take good care of the patients. This is what I believe, and I must go on . . . I think I was internally driven to work based on my philosophy of nursing."

3.3.3. Self-Transformation: From Fear to Courage

The participants achieved self-transformation when they went through the process of initially being stressed, afraid, and anxious to then staying strong through psychological adjustment. They eventually moved towards positivity by building courage with the adoption of self-care coping strategies, sustained their psychological growth, and became more prepared for the tasks ahead in their clinical practice.

> "At that moment, I felt that there was nothing I could not overcome . . . I had become one of the essential members of the nursing team [laughing out loud] . . . I was not scared anymore. What else could put me off now that I was not even afraid of death?"

> "After all these days, I never thought that I could be so strong [said with a sense of pride and a bright smile] and determined to take up the challenge."

3.4. Theme 4: Perceived Negativity and Positivity: Two Sides of Emotions

Although participants had negative feelings, like fear, anxiety, and worries, at the start of their work in isolation wards, being able to confront the hurdles signified the beginning of their self-transformation to become a resilient nurse in the battle against the pandemic. Through the self-care coping processes, they stayed positive and were more prepared for the future stressful situations in their practice. Ultimately, they were more capable of understanding both the negativity and positivity of their experiences. Participants emphasised that gaining confidence from practicing "in the field" is an essential factor in achieving self-transformation and subsequently recognised and appreciated the wider support system from various parties in society.

3.4.1. Gaining Confidence

All participants gained confidence with time by working in the field and resolving the emerging difficulties with courage. In taking up challenges, they were forced to learn and adapt to the changes brought about by the pandemic. Although they experienced anxiety and fear initially, these feelings decreased with an increasing level of confidence. The confidence gained from practice contributed to the resilience of the participants, signifying an important outcome of self-transformation. While participants began to gain confidence to play an active role in dealing with the effects of the pandemic at their workplace, they acquired a greater awareness of and increased appreciation for the effects of the wider policies relating to the control of the pandemic. They also demonstrated more determination to continue contributing in their professional roles.

> "I knew the government had been working hard, but at the beginning, I did not realise the effects . . . I tended to perceive their work negatively . . . But now, I think I have grown a lot in the past half year . . . Lately, I was so excited to hear that Lei Yue Mun Holiday Camp and Asia World-Expo had been converted into provisional hospitals to cope with the increasing number of patients with COVID-19. This played a significant triage function in our battle."

> "Being in the field was a vital learning process, even though the psychological growth I attained did not come easy . . . After all, a resilient nurse cannot be nurtured by learning within the school's environment. To me, building confidence in myself and persevering in a time of stress made me succeed in this journey."

3.4.2. Sources of Support from Various Parties in Society

As opposed to what they perceived at the beginning of their work in isolation wards, participants who had undergone self-transformation understood that, without concerted efforts from society, a single profession could not succeed in winning the battle against this pandemic. Following the self-transformation, they demonstrated maturity in terms of how they perceived the roles of their profession and the stakeholders in society. For example, they were grateful for the cooperation and respect from the patients.

> "Those outside the hospitals claimed that nurses were afraid of being infected with COVID-19, but it was not like that. I had never thought about quitting the job. I felt safe with the (infection control) protocols and felt supported by the hospital… I felt cheerful when the patients thanked us for our care."

Participants also appreciated the support from the hospital management, particularly the welfare provisions that were encouraging and supporting the nursing staff. The support from senior colleagues gave the participants hope. Other forms of support from society were equally valuable to the participants.

> "The hospital provided us (nurses) with extra cash allowances and hotel accommodation allowances. After 2 weeks of nursing work, we (nurses) were given an extra day of paid leave so that we could have ample rest… From time to time, some companies donated small gifts and supplies to support us in this fight against the pandemic. I am very moved [smiles]! Even our professional nursing bodies (i.e., the Association of Hong Kong Nursing Staff and the Hong Kong Academy of Nursing) have sent us gifts to show their support. Many video clips with supportive and encouraging messages to the nursing staff have also been uploaded online."

4. Discussion

This research employed phenomenological methods to examine the experiences of junior nurses who provided direct care for patients with confirmed COVID-19. The outcomes of the interviews could be broadly categorised into four themes: (1) hurdles in the early stage, (2) self-care coping strategies, (3) staying positive under pressure, and (4) perceived negativity and positivity: two sides of emotions.

The interviews revealed that the participants experienced significant discomfort and exhaustion as a result of their heavy workload, the scale of the outbreak, the large number of patients who required care and treatment, and the insufficient supply of PPE. These findings are consistent with those from studies on the outbreaks of MERS-CoV and Ebola [13,22].

In the current study, junior nurses expressed worries about their family members, corroborating a previous study by Lee et al. [23]. These emotions were prevalent among nurses who had elderly individuals or children in their families. The nurses interviewed during this research described how they had experienced strong negative emotions, such as anxiety, fear, and helplessness. Such emotions have been described in several previous studies and can be attributed to a lack of knowledge and experience, a sense of psychological helplessness, health and safety concerns, and fatigue [11,24].

The findings of this study revealed that the negative emotions encountered by the junior nurses were stronger in the first week of their clinical practice in isolation wards. Junior nurses may be provided with opportunities to undergo voluntary stress assessments as soon as they undertake pandemic prevention tasks in the initial few weeks or after a certain number of months. Healthcare management may consider supporting junior nurses throughout their adaptation process with specialised, adaptable, and continued interventions to encourage emotional release and to safeguard their mental health [13,23,25]. Solid support systems, such as sufficient PPE, training, and team support, may also be made available to help junior nurses adapt to the demands of providing holistic care to patients during a pandemic.

The participants in the current study revealed that they used several psychological strategies, such as distraction, awareness of the importance of self-care, and rationalisation, to deal with the challenges they encountered. Previous studies have reported that the application of coping strategies can assist clinicians in dealing with stress and in maintaining positive mental health when encountering an epidemic [26]. This study also found that junior nurses deal with stress through processes such as employing self-care coping strategies and seeking social support. Our results support Mak, Law, Woo, Cheung, and Lee's [27] finding that nurses' ability to adapt on a psychological level and their access to social support play important roles in their ability to undergo psychological adaptation and self-transformation when encountering outbreak stress. When acting under stress and pressure, nurses may adopt psychological self-modifications to gain confidence and build courage and resilience for emerging challenges in their clinical practice.

The interviewees in this study described how they used various methods to reduce stress, including listening to music, diary-writing, and engaging in breathing exercises. This finding corroborates previous studies on how nurses attending to patients in SARS wards employed various approaches to manage stress and pressure [23,28]. Furthermore, we found that the nurses involved in our study exhibited a strong sense of team solidarity that enabled them to cope with the hurdles at the early stage of their work in isolation wards, echoing the findings of Kim [11] and Shih, Liao, Chan, Duh, and Gau [29]. On a holistic level, junior nurses tended to modify their cognitive rationality to adjust to the demands presented by the pandemic. This could be attributed to the fact that healthcare practitioners possess strong healthcare knowledge and understanding and have a more logical and optimistic mindset [30]. Per the stress and coping model presented by the American psychologist Richard Lazarus, the extent to which stressors are effective is directly correlated with the process by which one engages in cognitive appraisal and the coping strategies involved. When operating in high-pressure situations, junior nurses continually modify their cognitive appraisal by applying their professional knowledge to seek support from members of their team, to encourage self-psychological harmony, to perform altruistic acts, and to take active steps to decrease stress and modify their nutrition, exercise, and sleep to respond to changes in the internal and external context and avoid stress-related impacts on their health and ability to perform their nursing duties [10,25].

Previous research has found that epidemics may cause significant psychological trauma to healthcare workers [16,17]. However, the outcomes of this study revealed that junior nurses developed on a psychological level when under stress. Through self-transformation, junior nurses engaged in a process of self-evaluation and ultimately responded positively—for example, by voicing their appreciation for their families and social support networks. The perception of accountability associated with professional ethics during an epidemic inspired nurses to enthusiastically contribute to anti-epidemic tasks and enhanced their sense of professional pride and identity [7,27]. These findings agree with those of a previous study [15]. Proactively supporting junior nurses to achieve psychological development during a pandemic could facilitate their psychological adjustment.

In the current study, we found that junior nurses experienced many positive emotions, such as confidence, courage, and gratitude, when providing care to patients during the pandemic. These positive emotions characterise the process of self-transformation. This finding contrasts sharply with previous research that was limited to discussing the negative emotions nurses encounter due to outbreak stress [16,17]. However, some studies have described comparable findings to ours [10,15,16]. Researchers have found that positive emotions can play a significant role in people's ability to adjust or respond to psychological trauma [31]. Positivity can have protective implications in terms of psychological trauma during tragedies and can stimulate psychological recovery from posttraumatic stress [32]. Thus, psychological support services that could be provided to junior nurses during a pandemic may include offering strong social support, encouraging positive coping styles, and promoting positive emotions.

During an outbreak, early training and confidence in skills and safety represent fundamental attributes that support nurses' willingness to engage in anti-epidemic work [33]. Mental and physical rewards also represent significant supportive elements [24]. The junior nurses who participated in the current study typically believed that their positive emotions were attributable to the multi-faceted support they received from family, friends, patients, social groups, team members, and the organisations in which they worked. Similar studies that support our findings can be identified in the literature [14–16].

4.1. Strengths

In this study, the data related to the experiences of junior nurses who provided direct care to patients with confirmed COVID-19 were compiled over nearly 6 months via a series of interviews. This helped us gain insights into the lived experiences of junior nurses, who remained an under-researched group at the time this research was undertaken. The methodology of this study enabled us to collate in-depth and reliable information that can allow other researchers to interpret the findings within a clearly described context. Unlike previous studies, our study revealed the process of self-transformation through which junior nurses developed self-care coping strategies in the face of pressure and ways to maintain positivity, confidence, and the ability to appreciate the wider support system in society. These attributes helped junior nurses to become resilient.

4.2. Limitations

First, as this study took the form of qualitative research, it involved a limited sample size. The sample in this study may be biased towards participants who had strong family and/or social support, and as reflected in the results, these participants were able to overcome some of the stress in their nursing work. This limitation could be addressed in future studies by enrolling junior nurses who may not have strong family or social support. For example, participants' perceived social support could be measured using an established and validated instrument before their interviews. Based on the measurements, researchers could further analyse and interpret the collected data, providing new perspectives on how varying levels of perceived family and/or social support may alter the coping processes of junior nurses in times of stress in their caregiving work during the COVID-19 pandemic. Caution should therefore be exercised in interpreting the results of this study, since junior nurses who do not have strong family and/or social support may have unique emotional and psychosocial needs arising from their practice in the pandemic as well as their difficulties in coping with the stress originating from their caring responsibilities at work. Second, the participants were limited to Hong Kong-based junior nurses who had recently completed their pre-licensure training. Practicing nurses who had undergone pre-licensure training abroad before returning to work in Hong Kong were not included in this study due to their much smaller proportion in public hospitals in Hong Kong. Third, because of the risks associated with a pandemic and the need to avoid infection, we could not perform focus-group interviews or collect data from on-site observations. Fourth, this study was performed over a relatively short period. Future research could examine the psychological experiences of junior nurses over a longer period.

5. Conclusions

This research employed a phenomenological approach to generate detailed insights into the transformational experiences of junior nurses who provided direct care to patients with confirmed COVID-19 in an acute care setting. In this study, the hurdles experienced by junior nurses included fear and anxiety, which may be accompanied by somatic symptoms (such as sleep disturbance). A reciprocal pattern of concern (both from the family to the participants and vice versa) was identified in our study. Social media that conveyed negative messages (for example, the death of patients with confirmed COVID-19) may have contributed to the development of negative emotions (such as anxiety) among junior nurses. Our findings also revealed that junior nurses maintained positivity through appreciation

of the important relationships in their lives and reflection upon professionalism. The process of self-transformation began when junior nurses were able to confront the hurdles in the early stage of their work in isolation wards with self-care coping strategies. Self-transformation prepared junior nurses to be resilient for future stressful events in the battle against this global pandemic. The confidence of junior nurses built up gradually during self-transformation. Ultimately, junior nurses were more capable of understanding both the negativity and positivity of their experiences. The self-transformation process also enabled junior nurses to recognise and appreciate the wider support system from various parties in society.

Author Contributions: Y.-C.Y.: Conceptualisation, methodology, formal analysis, investigation, writing the original draft, supervision, project administration. K.-H.Y.: Methodology, formal analysis, investigation, writing, reviewing, and editing. W.-K.T.: Investigation. All authors have read and agreed to the published version of the manuscript.

Funding: This research did not receive any funding.

Institutional Review Board Statement: This study was approved by the Caritas Institute of Higher Education, Research and Ethics Committee (Ref. no. HRE200133).

Informed Consent Statement: All participants provided written consent for their participation in this study. In addition, all participants were assured that their shared experience and interview content would be reported in international journals anonymously.

Data Availability Statement: The interview guide is provided in a table in the manuscript. To protect participants' privacy, the transcripts containing private and confidential data, such as the wards and the sites of practice of the participants, will not be made publicly available.

Conflicts of Interest: All authors declare that there is no conflict of interest.

References

1. Hui, D.S.; Azhar, E.I.; Madani, T.A.; Ntoumi, F.; Kock, R.; Dar, O.; Giuseppe, I.; Mchugh, T.D.; Memish, Z.A.; Drosten, C.; et al. The continuing 2019-nCoV epidemic threat of novel coronaviruses to global health—The latest 2019 novel coronavirus outbreak in Wuhan, China. *Int. J. Infect. Dis.* **2020**, *91*, 264. [CrossRef]
2. WHO Announces COVID-19 Outbreak a Pandemic. Available online: https://www.euro.who.int/en/health-topics/health-emergencies/coronavirus-covid-19/news/news/2020/3/who-announces-covid-19-outbreak-a-pandemic (accessed on 24 May 2021).
3. Wu, Z.; McGoogan, J.M. Characteristics of and important lessons from the coronavirus disease 2019 (COVID-19) outbreak in China: Summary of a report of 72 314 cases from the Chinese Center for Disease Control and Prevention. *JAMA* **2020**, *323*, 1239–1242. [CrossRef]
4. Maunder, R.; Hunter, J.; Vincent, L.; Bennett, J.; Peladeau, N.; Leszcz, M.; Sadavoy, J.; Verhaeghe, L.M.; Steinberg, R.; Mazzuli, T. The immediate psychological and occupational impact of the 2003 SARS outbreak in a teaching hospital. *Can. Med. Assoc. J.* **2003**, *168*, 1245–1251.
5. Amin, S. The psychology of coronavirus fear: Are healthcare professionals suffering from corona-phobia? *Int. J. Healthc. Manag.* **2020**, *13*, 249–256. [CrossRef]
6. Du, J.; Dong, L.; Wang, T.; Yuan, C.; Fu, R.; Zhang, L.; Liu, B.; Zhang, M.; Yin, Y.; Qin, J.; et al. Psychological symptoms among frontline healthcare workers during COVID-19 outbreak in Wuhan. *Gen. Hosp. Psychiatry* **2020**, *67*, 144–145. [CrossRef] [PubMed]
7. Aliakbari, F.; Hammad, K.; Bahrami, M.; Aein, F. Ethical and legal challenges associated with disaster nursing. *Nurs. Ethics* **2015**, *22*, 493–503. [CrossRef]
8. O'Boyle, C.; Robertson, C.; Secor-Turner, M. Nurses' beliefs about public health emergencies: Fear of abandonment. *Am. J. Infect. Control* **2006**, *34*, 351–357. [CrossRef] [PubMed]
9. Chung, B.P.M.; Wong, T.K.S.; Suen, E.S.B.; Chung, J.W.Y. SARS: Caring for patients in Hong Kong. *J. Clin. Nurs.* **2005**, *14*, 510–517. [CrossRef]
10. Honey, M.; Wang, W.Y. New Zealand nurses' perceptions of caring for patients with influenza A (H1N1). *Nurs. Crit. Care* **2013**, *18*, 63–69. [CrossRef] [PubMed]
11. Kim, Y. Nurses' experiences of care for patients with Middle East respiratory syndrome- coronavirus in South Korea. *Am. J. Infect. Control* **2018**, *46*, 781–787. [CrossRef]
12. Liu, C.; Wang, H.; Zhou, L.; Xie, H.; Yang, H.; Yu, Y.; Sha, H.; Yang, Y.; Zhang, X. Sources and symptoms of stress among nurses in the first Chinese anti-Ebola medical team during the Sierra Leone aid mission: A qualitative study. *Int. J. Nurs. Sci.* **2019**, *6*, 187–191. [CrossRef]

13. Smith, M.W.; Smith, P.W.; Kratochvil, C.J.; Schwedhelm, S. The psychosocial challenges of caring for patients with Ebola virus disease. *Health Secur.* **2017**, *15*, 104–109. [CrossRef]
14. Su, T.P.; Lien, T.C.; Yang, C.Y.; Su, Y.L.; Wang, J.H.; Tsai, S.L.; Yin, J.C. Prevalence of psychiatric morbidity and psychological adaptation of the nurses in a structured SARS caring unit during outbreak: A prospective and periodic assessment study in Taiwan. *J. Psychiatr. Res.* **2007**, *41*, 119–130. [CrossRef] [PubMed]
15. Liu, H.; Liehr, P. Instructive messages from Chinese nurses' stories of caring for SARS patients. *J. Clin. Nurs.* **2009**, *18*, 2880–2887. [CrossRef]
16. Kang, L.; Li, Y.; Hu, S.; Chen, M.; Yang, C.; Yang, B.X.; Wang, Y.; Hu, J.; Lai, J.; Ma, X.; et al. The mental health of medical workers in Wuhan, China dealing with the 2019 novel coronavirus. *Lancet Psychiatry* **2020**, *7*, e14. [CrossRef]
17. Xiang, Y.T.; Yang, Y.; Li, W.; Zhang, L.; Zhang, Q.; Cheung, T.; Ng, C.H. Timely mental health care for the 2019 novel coronavirus outbreak is urgently needed. *Lancet Psychiatry* **2020**, *7*, 228–229. [CrossRef]
18. Colaizzi, P.F. Psychological Research as the Phenomenologist Views It. In *Existential Phenomenological Alternatives for Psychology*; Valle, R.S., King, M., Eds.; Open University Press: New York, NY, USA, 1978; pp. 48–71.
19. Hu, D.; Kong, Y.; Li, W.; Han, Q.; Zhang, X.; Zhu, L.X.; Wan, S.W.; Liu, Z.; Shen, Q.; Yang, J.; et al. Frontline nurses' burnout, anxiety, depression, and fear statuses and their associated factors during the COVID-19 outbreak in Wuhan, China: A large-scale cross-sectional study. *EClinicalMedicine* **2020**, *24*, 100424. [CrossRef] [PubMed]
20. Lai, J.; Ma, S.; Wang, Y.; Cai, Z.; Hu, J.; Wei, N.; Wu, J.; Du, H.; Chen, T.; Li, R.; et al. Factors associated with mental health outcomes among health care workers exposed to coronavirus disease 2019. *JAMA Netw. Open* **2020**, *3*, e203976. [CrossRef] [PubMed]
21. Lincoln, Y.S.; Guba, E.G. But is it rigorous? Trustworthiness and authenticity in naturalistic evaluation. *New Dir. Eval.* **1986**, *1986*, 73–84. [CrossRef]
22. Kang, H.S.; Son, Y.D.; Chae, S.M.; Corte, C. Working experiences of nurses during the Middle East respiratory syndrome outbreak. *Int. J. Nurs. Pract.* **2018**, *24*, e12664. [CrossRef]
23. Lee, S.H.; Juang, Y.Y.; Su, Y.J.; Lee, H.L.; Lin, Y.H.; Chao, C.C. Facing SARS: Psychological impacts on SARS team nurses and psychiatric services in a Taiwan general hospital. *Gen. Hosp. Psychiatry* **2005**, *27*, 352–358. [CrossRef]
24. Khalid, I.; Khalid, T.J.; Qabajah, M.R.; Barnard, A.G.; Qushmaq, I.A. Healthcare workers' emotions, perceived stressors and coping strategies during MERS-CoV outbreak. *Clin. Med. Res.* **2016**, *14*, 7–14. [CrossRef]
25. The Guideline of Psychological Crisis Intervention for 2019-Ncov Pneumonia. Available online: http://www.nhc.gov.cn/jkj/s3577/202001/6adc08b966594253b2b791be5c3b9467.shtml (accessed on 24 May 2021).
26. Main, A.; Zhou, Q.; Ma, Y.; Luecken, L.J.; Liu, X. Relations of SARS-related stressors and coping to Chinese college students' psychological adjustment during the 2003 Beijing SARS epidemic. *J. Couns. Psychol.* **2011**, *58*, 410. [CrossRef]
27. Mak, W.W.; Law, R.W.; Woo, J.; Cheung, F.M.; Lee, D. Social support and psychological adjustment to SARS: The mediating role of self-care self-efficacy. *Psychol. Health* **2009**, *24*, 161–174. [CrossRef] [PubMed]
28. Wong, T.W.; Yau, J.K.; Chan, C.L.; Kwong, R.S.; Ho, S.M.; Lau, C.C.; Lau, F.L.; Lit, C.H. The psychological impact of severe acute respiratory syndrome outbreak on healthcare workers in emergency departments and how they cope. *Eur. J. Emerg. Med.* **2005**, *12*, 13–18. [CrossRef] [PubMed]
29. Shih, F.J.; Liao, Y.C.; Chan, S.M.; Duh, B.R.; Gau, M.L. The impact of the 9−21 earthquake experiences of Taiwanese nurses as rescuers. *Soc. Sci. Med.* **2002**, *55*, 659–672. [CrossRef]
30. Mishra, P.; Bhadauria, U.S.; Dasar, P.L.; Kumar, S.; Lalani, A.; Sarkar, P.; Chauhan, A.; Godha, S.; Vyas, S. Knowledge, attitude and anxiety towards pandemic flu a potential bio weapon among health professionals in Indore City. *Prz. Epidemiol.* **2016**, *70*, 41–45.
31. Waugh, C.E. The regulatory power of positive emotions in stress: A temporal-functional approach. In *The Resilience Handbook: Approaches to Stress and Trauma*; Kent, M., Davis, M.C., Reich, J.W., Eds.; Routledge/Taylor & Francis Group: New York, NY, USA, 2014; pp. 73–85.
32. Carbone, E.G.; Echols, E.T. Effects of optimism on recovery and mental health after a tornado outbreak. *Psychol. Health* **2017**, *32*, 530–548. [CrossRef] [PubMed]
33. Aoyagi, Y.; Beck, C.R.; Dingwall, R.; Nguyen-Van-Tam, J.S. Healthcare workers' willingness to work during an influenza pandemic: A systematic review and meta-analysis. *Influenza Other Respir. Viruses* **2015**, *9*, 120–130. [CrossRef]

International Journal of
Environmental Research and Public Health

MDPI

Article

Relational Capital and Post-Traumatic Growth: The Role of Work Meaning

Ting Nie [1], Mi Tian [1,*] and Hengrui Liang [2]

[1] School of Business, Macau University of Science and Technology, Macau 999078, China; tnie@must.edu.mo
[2] Independent Researcher, Xining 810016, China; henryliangt@gmail.com
* Correspondence: mtian@must.edu.mo

Abstract: Through a statistical survey of 760 front-line medical staff during the COVID-19 epidemic, this study attempts to explore the relationships between relational capital, psychological security, post-traumatic growth and the meaning of work. Data analysis verifies that trust, reciprocity, and identification can promote post-traumatic growth by enhancing the individual's psychological security. A high level of work meaning can enhance the role of trust, reciprocity and identification in promoting psychological security. Work meaning has a moderated mediating effect when trust and reciprocity affect post-traumatic growth through psychological security, but no moderated mediating effect is found when identification affects post-traumatic growth through psychological security.

Keywords: relational capital; post-traumatic growth; psychological security; work meaning

Citation: Nie, T.; Tian, M.; Liang, H. Relational Capital and Post-Traumatic Growth: The Role of Work Meaning. *Int. J. Environ. Res. Public Health* **2021**, *18*, 7362. https://doi.org/10.3390/ijerph18147362

Academic Editors: Richard Gray and Sonia Udod

Received: 11 June 2021
Accepted: 6 July 2021
Published: 9 July 2021

1. Introduction

The epidemic in 2020 has caused the entire human world to face a challenge that has not been met for a century. As of July 2021, 205 countries around the world have been affected, with more than 186 million confirmed cases and more than 4.02 million deaths (Refer online real time data from https://www.outbreak.my/zh/world accessed on 8 July 2021). People all over the world are working hard to prevent and control the epidemic. With the spread of multiple shocks of COVID-19, the world economy is in recession, industrial development and business operations have been hit hard, and everyone's lives have been affected. This has been and will be a challenge for the entire human race as well as for each individual.

In the fight against the epidemic, front-line medical staff have made tremendous contributions. However, as witnesses of the epidemic, they have been harmed both physically and mentally in the high-pressure environment of this disaster. The COVID-19 pandemic has led to a large increase in the incidence and prevalence of mental health problems, such as anxiety and depression [1], and is placing enormous stress on healthcare workers, whose mental health may have been damaged, caused by these events [2]. If medical staff are in a state of emotional exhaustion, they will naturally enter the resource preservation mode, and they are more likely to have work withdrawal behaviors the next day [3]. In particular, when the meaning of work is low, the COVID-19 crisis perceived by the health care workers increases, and their work engagement and responsibility decrease; therefore, the organization should carry out training and effective intervention to avoid deterioration of the situation [4]. The trauma brings not only harm, but many people also have re-considered their values, interpersonal relationships, and self-understanding. Because of the epidemic, some positive changes have taken place. In a sense, some have grown after trauma, due to disaster or adversity. Post-traumatic growth is exactly what contemporary positive psychology pays attention to today. Negative effects and positive effects after trauma coexist; various positive effects can promote the development of individuals and enhance their perception of happiness [5]. Previous studies have confirmed that when individuals have enough support, they can stimulate post-traumatic growth [6], but there are still some differences in the influence mechanisms of different types of support. Under the Chinese cultural background, we pay more attention to interpersonal relationships. The formation of trust, reciprocity, and identification within the organization create a special kind of capital, that is, relational capital [7]. Since COVID-related stressors can frustrate employees' sense of belonging, increase their sense of insecurity, and have a negative impact on their behaviors [8], it is meaningful for us to explore whether mutual trust and cooperation within the organization and a high degree of identification can help medical staff have a positive sense of belonging so as to better engage in work and obtain growth opportunities during the COVID-19 crisis; namely, can relationship capital promote the occurrence of post-traumatic growth by improving the individual's psychological security? In particular, when the individual has a high sense of work meaning, will this promotion effect be strengthened? This study selected medical staff that were on the front line during the outbreak of COVID-19 as the sample to explore the mediating role of psychological security between relational capital and post-traumatic growth, and to verify whether work meaning has a moderating effect.

2. Theoretical Basis and Research Hypothesis

2.1. The Impact of Relational Capital on Employee's Psychological Security

Regarding relational capital, academics generally recognize that individuals establish relational asset through mutual communication, interaction, and cooperation, including the three dimensions of trust, reciprocity and identification [7]. The enhancement of relational capital can promote mutual cooperation within the organization and gain the support of other stakeholders in the network. Krishna [9] pointed that relational capital refers to the capital rooted in the relationship, emphasizing factors such as attitudes, norms, beliefs, and values. Most scholars believe that relational capital is an important part of social capital, which has a certain influence on the perception and behavior of individuals in the organization [10,11]. Research has verified the role of relational capital in promoting individual performance. When individuals perceive higher trust and identification, they show higher work commitment [12]. The research of Chen et al. [13] found that relational capital could stimulate team creativity, which in turn helped promote team innovation. The research of Ortiz [14] examined the correlation between relational capital and the individual's knowledge recognition ability and knowledge acquisition ability. Relational capital contributes to knowledge sharing within the organization. Empirical research has verified the positive influence of relational capital on innovation vitality and innovation efficiency [15]. Relational capital can also promote knowledge transfer and value realization within the organization, which in turn has a certain stimulating effect on the overall performance of the organization [16]. Most of the research on relational capital is currently concentrated in the field of knowledge management.

Psychological security is regarded as a feeling of confidence, security and freedom that is separated from fear and anxiety, and it is the feeling of satisfying a person's various needs, now and in the future [17]. Kahn [18] believes that psychological security is the perception that individuals can fully express their true self without worrying that such behavior will negatively affect their image, status, and career. The higher an employee's perception of psychological safety, the more obvious it is that they have a positive perception of their environment, the more comfortable their behavior, and the easier it is to stimulate off-role behaviors [19]. Cong and An [20] believe that psychological security is a subjective feeling at the individual level. It is the subjective perception of dangers or risks that may appear around and threaten the body and mind, and it is the perception of whether they have the ability to deal with dangers or risks. This is mainly reflected in the sense of certainty and control. Therefore, psychological security has two main sources: the perception of whether the environment is safe and the judgment of whether one has the ability to cope with change [21]. Enterprises need to pay attention to employees' psychological safety perception, which is of great significance to the healthy development of the organization [22]. Interpersonal trust and support in an organization can help improve psychological security [18]. High-quality interpersonal relationships can promote learning within the organization through the role of psychological security [23]. If colleagues maintain a relationship of mutual trust and support and communicate frequently at work, employees' psychological security will also be enhanced [24]. The employee's perceived relationship capital can promote psychological security. Therefore, we propose Hypothesis 1:

Hypothesis 1. *Relational capital has a significant positive impact on psychological safety.*

2.2. The Mediating Role of Psychological Security

Post-traumatic growth is the positive aspect that an individual exhibits in the face of a traumatic event. It is the positive and positive psychological change experienced by the individual in the process of fighting a traumatic event [25]. The research pointed out that the post-trauma growth of an individual can be found in the improvement of interpersonal relationships, the possibility of obtaining new opportunities, the change of life philosophy, self-growth (confidence, self-efficacy, and acquisition of new coping styles) and spiritual development. Trauma is an unavoidable event in an individual's life. The individual's reaction after experiencing a traumatic event is reflected in multiple levels and multiple aspects. It is not only limited to negative health reactions, but also manifested in a series of positive cognitive modes, such as self-awareness and value change [26]. The positive and negative effects of trauma can coexist. Therefore, post-trauma growth is a very normal phenomenon. There have been a large number of studies that have confirmed the existence and influencing factors of post-traumatic growth. From an individual perspective, when their parents are disabled at an early age, individuals become more independent and more responsible for the family [27]. Women are more likely to develop post-traumatic growth than men, and as they grow older, post-traumatic growth is more pronounced [28]. Personality traits are an effective predictor of post-traumatic growth. Individuals with high extroversion, optimistic personality, self-control, and self-efficacy can effectively predict the occurrence of post-traumatic growth [29]. From the view of the trauma source, trauma related to natural disasters is more likely to stimulate the post-traumatic growth of individuals than trauma by human causes [30]. The study of Milam et al. [31] found that when individuals had religious beliefs, they were more likely to have a higher level of post-traumatic growth in the face of trauma. Social support can promote post-traumatic growth. The support of family, friends, teachers and other social forces can make individuals have a higher sense of psychological security, and are more likely to develop post-traumatic growth [32]. Brown [33] pointed out that psychological security can positively predict employees' work behavior and increase work involvement. Relational capital itself is a kind of social support. Organization members trust each other, adhere to the principle of mutual benefit, help and support each other, and have a sense of belonging to the organization, which will enhance their confidence in coping with difficulties and trauma, and strengthen their individual resistance to pressure. Individuals will have positive growth after trauma, recognize themselves and accept themselves. Therefore, we propose research Hypothesis 2:

Hypothesis 2. *Relational capital affects post-traumatic growth through psychological security. Psychological security plays a mediating role between relational capital and post-traumatic growth.*

2.3. The Moderating Effect of Work Meaning

Work meaning is the value judgment that an individual makes on the purpose of their work, according to his own values and value standards, which reflects the matching level between the individual's values, beliefs and job role [34]. Employees evaluate organizational goals according to their personal judgment standards. Employees who believe that their work is meaningful and valuable are more willing to work hard and use the autonomy granted by the organization to complete organizational goals [35]. The study of Mok and Au-Yeung [36] showed that teamwork spirit can positively affect employees' perceived work meaning. Information sharing within the organization helps employees realize the meaning of work, strive to make their own work goals consistent with the organization's development goals, and put forward valuable suggestions or opinions for the organization. Studies have found that a high-quality leader–member exchange relationship can help enhance employees' perception of job meaning [37]. The research of Zhang and Bartol [38] pointed out that when employees think that their work is meaningful and have high autonomy, their innovative behaviors are more frequent. The employee's work meaning perception will increase the employee's identification and loyalty to the organization [39]. Li Chaoping [40] verified through empirical research that job meaning has a significant positive impact on employees' organizational commitment and job satisfaction, and negatively impacts job burnout. When employees' sense of work meaning is higher, it means that employees' recognition of their work and their sense of satisfaction at work is stronger. If, at the same time, employees can perceive trust from their colleagues and experience reciprocity and a strong sense of belonging at work, meaningful work can further enhance their psychological security. When experiencing high-pressure work challenges, an individual's perception of the meaning of work and the recognition of work goals can enhance their courage and enthusiasm to cope with difficulties, and it is easier to form self-growth in this process. Therefore, we propose research Hypothesis 3 and research Hypothesis 4:

Hypothesis 3. *Work meaning has a moderating effect on the relationship between relational capital and psychological security, and high work meaning can enhance the positive effect of relational capital on psychological security.*

Hypothesis 4. *Work meaning has a moderated mediating effect on the relationship between relational capital, psychological security and post-traumatic growth.*

3. Research Design

3.1. Procedure

To verify the inner relationship between relational capital, psychological security, post-traumatic growth, and work meaning, as shown in the research model (Figure 1) we collected data in public hospitals of 19 provinces and autonomous regions, including Jiangsu, Sichuan, Ningxia, Guizhou, Yunnan, Beijing, Tianjin and Shanghai from June 2020 to August 2020. A total of 900 questionnaires were distributed and 835 were recovered, with a recovery rate of 92.8%. Of these, 760 questionnaires were valid, and the effective recovery rate was 84.4%.

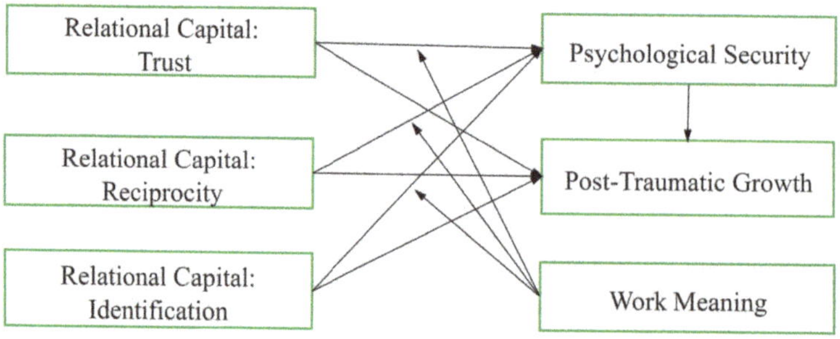

Figure 1. Research Model.

There were 124 males, accounting for 16.3% of the total sample, and 636 females, accounting for 83.7% of the total sample. The female sample was much higher than the male sample, which is consistent with the gender differences in the medical industry. The respondents were mostly young, with 471 respondents under the age of 30, accounting for

62% of the sample. There were 279 respondents at the age of 30–50, representing 36.7% of the total sample. The majority of the respondents were highly educated. There were 677 people with a bachelor's degree or above, accounting for 89% of the total sample. There were 182 doctors, representing 23.9% of the total sample, and 578 nurses, representing 76.1% of the sample. A total of 516 were medical staff working in designated hospitals for COVID-19, accounting for 67.9% of the total sample. Another 315 were medical staff directly involved in the treatment of confirmed or suspected patients with COVID-19, accounting for 41.4% of the total sample. During the outbreak of COVID-19, most medical staff carried out intensive work; 419 medical personnel worked more than 10 hours a day, representing 55% of the total sample.

3.2. Measurement

This study used mature scales, which was measured by Likert's five-point scale from 1 completely disagree to 5 completely agree. The questionnaire included demographic variables, relational capital, psychological security, post-traumatic growth, and work meaning. The data were analyzed by SPSS 22, Amos24 and Process V3.4 statistical software, mainly related to descriptive statistics, confirmatory factor analysis, correlation analysis, hierarchical regression analysis, and bootstrap analysis to validate research hypotheses. Relational capital focuses on the particular relations people have, such as respect and friendship, that influence their behaviors. It is through these ongoing personal relationships that people fulfill such social motives as sociability, approval and prestige [7]. Relational capital has three dimensions: trust, reciprocity and identification. Trust refers to an individual's expectation that members in a virtual community will follow a generally accepted set of values, norms, and principles. Reciprocity refers to the actions that are contingent on rewarding reactions from others and that cease when these expected reactions are not forthcoming. Identification is the process whereby individuals see themselves as one with another person or a group of people (Chiu et al., 2006). The measurement of relational capital is based on the research of Chiu et al. [41], which contains nine items in three dimensions; the internal consistency coefficients of trust, reciprocity and identification are 0.894, 0.801 and 0.821, respectively. Psychological security focuses on a feeling of confidence, security and freedom that is separated from fear and anxiety, and it is the feeling of satisfying a person's various needs, now and in the future (Authur S. Reber, 1996) [17]. The measurement of psychological security is based on the study of Cong Zhong and An Lijuan [20]; the scale contains fifteen items and the internal consistency coefficient is 0.834. Post-traumatic growth focuses on the positive and positive psychological change experienced by the individual in the process of fighting a traumatic event [25]. The measurement of post-traumatic growth is based on the research of Tedeschi et al. [25], which has 20 items and an internal consistency coefficient of 0.943. Work meaning focuses on the value judgment that an individual makes on the purpose of their work, according to his/her own values and value standards, which reflects the matching level between the individual's values, beliefs and the job role [34]. Measurement of work meaning is based on the research of Spreitzer [34]. The scale contains three items with an internal consistency coefficient of 0.936.

4. Results

4.1. Confirmatory Factor Analysis

First of all, we use confirmatory factor analysis to test the validity of the data obtained from this survey and verify whether there is a serious homologous bias problem. Based on the six-factor model (trust, reciprocity, identification, psychological security, post-traumatic growth, and work meaning), we compare the model fit of six factors with that of five-factor, four-factor, three-factor, and one-factor models. As shown in Table 1, the overall model fit of the six-factor model is the best ($\chi^2/df = 1.846$, TLI = 0.987, CFI = 0.992, RMSEA = 0.018). The model fit of the single-factor model ($\chi^2/df = 20.513$, TLI = 0.722, CFI = 0.790, RMSEA = 0.076) is not within the acceptable range, so the homologous deviation of this study is not serious and further statistical analysis can be carried out.

Table 1. Confirmatory factor analysis.

Model	χ^2	*df*	χ^2/df	TLI	CFI	RMSEA
Six-Factor Model	230.722	125	1.846	0.987	0.992	0.018
Five-Factor Model	347.659	131	2.654	0.975	0.983	0.020
Four-Factor Model	450.671	135	3.338	0.965	0.975	0.036
Three-Factor Model	731.929	136	5.382	0.934	0.953	0.057
Single-Factor Model	2646.192	129	20.513	0.722	0.790	0.076

4.2. Correlation Analysis

Through descriptive statistical analysis, we can understand the perceived level of relational capital, psychological security, post-traumatic growth, and work meaning in this survey with the results shown in Table 2. The medical staff surveyed have a moderate level of perceived trust (3.859), reciprocity (4.084), and identification (3.852). Reciprocal perception is the most evident in the work nature of doctors and nurses because the treatment of any patient requires a team effort, which is a process of communicating and learning from each other.

Table 2. Means, standard deviations and correlations (N = 760).

	Mean	SD	1	2	3	4	5	6	7	8	9	10
Gender	1.84	0.370										
Age	1.51	0.740	−0.262 **									
Education	2.07	0.575	−0.297 **	0.360 **								
Position	1.76	0.427	0.512 **	−0.465 **	−0.585 **							
Tenure	1.95	1.009	−0.183 **	0.831 **	0.290 **	−0.324 **						
TRU	3.86	0.858	0.010	−0.170 **	−0.100 **	0.168 **	−0.146 **					
REC	4.08	0.747	0.013	−0.159 **	−0.091 *	0.157 **	−0.130 **	0.713 **				
IDE	3.85	0.789	−0.039	−0.047	−0.099 **	0.142 **	−0.045	0.616 **	0.533 **			
PS	4.02	0.726	−0.070	−0.031	−0.030	0.068	−0.028	0.518 **	0.565 **	0.493 **		
PTG	3.98	0.723	−0.023	−0.127 **	−0.085 *	0.147 **	−0.103 **	0.539 **	0.555 **	0.494 **	0.719 **	
WM	3.93	0.813	−0.035	−0.178 **	−0.135 **	0.164 **	−0.181 **	0.590 **	0.531 **	0.607 **	0.674 **	0.641 **

Note: N = 760; ** $p < 0.01$, * $p < 0.05$; TRU, trust; REC, reciprocity; IDE, identification; PS, psychological security; PTG, post-traumatic growth; WM, work meaning.

Respondents have a stronger sense of psychological security (4.022) and a sense of meaning at work (3.926). Doctors and nurses have a high reputation in society, especially in the face of an outbreak, and their work is highly valued, which helps to stimulate professional well-being and satisfaction. In a high-pressure work environment, doctors and nurses have a moderate degree of post-traumatic growth (3.980); many respondents in this survey said that because of COVID-19, they have rethought the value of life. Despite the unprecedented challenges, they have experienced a degree of positive change in their relationships and personal development that has made them more value what they have now.

The results of the correlation analysis show that trust, reciprocity, identification, psychological security, post-traumatic growth and work meaning are significantly related with each other after gender, age, education, position, and seniority have been controlled. Trust (0.518 **), reciprocity (0.565 **) and identification (0.493 **) all have a significant positive effect on psychological security, indicating that when individuals can trust each other and help each other, and have a higher sense of identification, psychological security is also stronger; therefore, relational capital can promote the formation of individual psychological security. Trust (0.539 **), reciprocity (0.555 **), and identification (0.494 **) all have significant positive effects on post-traumatic growth. There is a significant positive correlation between psychological security and post-traumatic growth (0.719 **), which indicates that the formation of psychological security is essential for the emergence of individual post-traumatic growth, and that the stronger the psychological security, the more likely it is for the individual to experience post-traumatic growth.

4.3. Mediating Effect

The mediating effect of psychological security in the relations between relational capital and post-traumatic growth is verified by the hierarchical regression. Taking gender, age, education, position, seniority as the control variables, we discuss the mediating effect of trust, reciprocity and identification respectively in relational capital. The hierarchical regression results are shown in Table 3: Models 1–3 examine the mediating effect of psychological security between trust and post-traumatic growth. After confirming the significant influence of trust on post-traumatic growth (0.440 ***) and psychological security (0.442 ***), when psychological security as a mediating variable enters the regression equation, the effect of the mediating variable is significant (0.601 ***). Although the relationship between trust and post-traumatic growth is still significant, the effect is weaker (0.176 ***); therefore, psychological security has a partial mediating effect between trust and post-traumatic growth. Models 4–6 examine the mediating effect of psychological security between reciprocity and post-traumatic growth. After confirming the significant influence of reciprocity on post-traumatic growth (0.521 ***) and psychological security (0.552 ***), when psychological security as a mediating variable enters the regression equation, the effect of the mediating variable is significant (0.596 ***). Although the relationship between reciprocity and post-traumatic growth is still significant, the effect is weaker (0.192 ***). Therefore, psychological security has a partial mediating effect between reciprocity and post-traumatic growth. Models 7–9 examine the mediating effect of psychological security between identification and post-traumatic growth. After confirming the significant influence of identifications to post-traumatic growth (0.438 ***) and psychological security (0.447 ***), when the psychological security as a mediating variable enters the regression equation, the effect of the mediating variable is significant (0.624 ***). Although the relationship between identification and post-traumatic growth is still significant, the effect is weaker (−0.160 ***). Therefore, psychological security has a partial mediating effect between identification and post-traumatic growth. Through hierarchical regression, Hypothesis 1 and Hypothesis 2 are validated.

Table 3. Mediating effect.

	Model 1 PTG	Model 2 PS	Model 3 PTG	Model 4 PTG	Model 5 PS	Mdoel 6 PTG	Model 7 PTG	Model 8 PS	Model 9 PTG
Gender	−0.156 *	−0.171 *	−0.053	−0.165	−0.174 *	−0.061	−0.123	−0.136	−0.039
Age	−0.020	0.057	−0.054	−0.012	0.068	−0.052	−0.094	−0.018	−0.083
Education	0.006	0.010	0.000	0.004	0.008	−0.001	0.031	0.035	0.009
Position	0.160 *	0.097	0.102	0.168	0.096	0.111	0.140	0.072	0.095
Tenure	0.003	0.013	0.003	−0.005	−0.008	0.000	0.005	0.002	0.004
TRU	0.440 ***	0.442 ***	0.176 ***						
REC				0.521 ***	0.552 ***	0.192 ***			
IDE							0.438 ***	0.447 ***	0.160 ***
PS			0.601 ***			0.596 ***			0.624 ***
ΔR^2	0.229 ***	0.277 ***	0.562 ***	0.317 ***	0.328 ***	0.558 **	0.259 ***	0.247 ***	0.554 ***
F	53.487	48.030	138.079	58.312	61.331	135.575	43.294	41.113	133.626

Note: N = 760; *** $p < 0.001$, ** $p < 0.01$, * $p < 0.05$; TRU, trust; REC, reciprocity; IDE, identification; PS, psychological security; PTG, post-traumatic growth; WM, work meaning.

4.4. Moderating Effect

The process procedure is used to verify the moderating effect of work meaning between relational capital and psychological security, and the moderated mediating effect of work meaning between relational capital, psychological security and post-traumatic growth. The results are shown in Table 4.

First of all, we discuss the moderating effect of work meaning between trust and psychological security. At a high standard of work meaning, the 95% confidence interval of the moderating effect between trust and psychological security (b = 0.2386, SE = 0.0394) is [0.1612, 0.3159], and the interval does not pass zero, which means that work meaning at a high level has a moderating effect between trust and psychological security, namely, a high level of work meaning can enhance the role of trust in the promotion of psychological security. At a low level of work meaning, the 95% confidence interval of the moderating effect between trust and psychological security (b = 0.1052, SE = 0.0324) is [0.0416, 0.1678], and the interval does not pass zero, which means that work meaning at a low level has a moderating effect between trust and psychological security, namely, low level of work meaning inhibits the role of trust in promoting psychological security. When work meaning is taken into account in the mediating effects of trust between psychological security and post-traumatic growth (b = 0.0456, SE = 0.0192), the interval under the 95% confidence level is [0.0084, 0.0839] and the interval does not pass zero, so work meaning plays a moderated mediating effect on the relationship between trust, psychological security and post-traumatic growth.

Table 4. Moderating effect and moderated mediating effect.

	Moderating Effect				Moderated Mediating Effect			
Variable	Effect	SE	95% Confidence Interval		Effect	SE	95% Confidence Interval	
			Upper	Lower			Upper	Lower
TEU	0.1052	0.0324	0.0416	0.1678	0.0456	0.0192	0.0084	0.0839
	0.2386	0.0394	0.1612	0.3159				
REC	0.0706	0.0375	−0.0030	0.1442	0.0434	0.0218	0.0005	0.0867
	0.1919	0.0425	0.1086	0.2763				
IDE	0.0521	0.0317	−0.0101	0.1143	0.0309	0.0228	−0.0162	0.0738
	0.0762	0.0260	0.0253	0.1272				

Note: TRU, trust; REC, reciprocity; IDE, identification; PS, psychological security; PTG, post-traumatic growth; WM, work meaning.

Secondly, we discuss the moderating effect of work meaning between reciprocity and psychological security. At a high standard of work meaning, the 95% confidence interval of the moderating effect between reciprocity and psychological security (b = 0.1919, SE = 0.0425) is [0.1086, 0.2763], and the interval does not pass zero, which means that work meaning at a high level has a moderating effect between reciprocity and psychological security, namely, a high level of work meaning can enhance the role of reciprocity in the promotion of psychological security. At a low level of work meaning, the 95% confidence interval of the moderating effect between reciprocity and psychological security (b = 0.0706, SE = 0.0375) is [−0.0030, 0.1442], and the interval does pass zero, which means that work meaning at a low level has not a moderating effect between reciprocity and psychological security, namely, the effect of low working meaning on the intrinsic relationship between reciprocity and psychological security does not exist. When work meaning is taken into account in the mediating effects of reciprocity between psychological security and post-traumatic growth (b = 0.0434, SE = 0.0218), the interval under the 95% confidence level is [0.0005, 0.0867] and the interval does not pass zero, so work meaning plays a moderated mediating effect on the relationship between reciprocity, psychological security and post-traumatic growth.

Finally, we discuss the moderating effect of work meaning between identification and psychological security. At a high standard of work meaning, the 95% confidence interval of the moderating effect between identification and psychological security (b = 0.0762, SE = 0.0260) is [0.0253, 0.1272], and the interval does not pass zero, which means that work meaning at a high level has a moderating effect between identification and psychological security, namely, a high level of work meaning can enhance the role of identification in the promotion of psychological security. At a low level of work meaning, the 95% confidence interval of the moderating effect between identification and psychological security (b = 0.0521, SE = 0.0317) is [−0.0101, 0.1143], and the interval does pass zero, which means that work meaning at a low level does not have a moderating effect between identification and psychological security, namely, the effect of low working meaning on the intrinsic relationship between identification and psychological security does not exist. When work meaning is taken into account in the mediating effects of identification between psychological security and post-traumatic growth (b = 0.0309, SE = 0.0228), the interval under the 95% confidence level is [−0.0162, 0.0738] and the interval does pass zero, so work meaning does not play a moderated mediating effect on the relationship between identification, psychological security and post-traumatic growth. Hypothesis 3 and Hypothesis 4 are partially validated.

5. Conclusions and Discussions

The war against the epidemic has not been declared a final victory, and countless medical staff and society are continuing to fight with COVID-19. Extensive research has shown that traumatic experiences might influence physical and mental state, even resulting in post-traumatic stress disorder. At the same time, positive psychology points out that many individuals have the opportunity to grow in the process of crisis response and treatment. Our study explains a possible cause of individual post-traumatic growth from the perspective of relational capital.

Based on statistical analysis, it is proved that relational capital can promote the realization of individual post-traumatic growth through psychological security, that is, when the individual perceives mutual trust within the organization, stays in a reciprocal environment, and has a strong sense of belonging, they have higher psychological security; this also can help the individual to rebuild values, enhance the individual's response ability to the crisis and find new development opportunities, which will lead to individual growth. Work meaning plays a regulating role between relational capital and psychological security. When the individual perceives a higher level of work meaning, the promoting effect of trust, reciprocity and identification on psychological security is enhanced. However, when at the low level of work meaning, only the effect of trust on the promotion of psychological security is enhanced, while the influence of reciprocity and identification on psychological security are not affected.

The results of the study may reflect some characteristics of doctors and nurses. Compared with other social occupational groups, their overall work value perception is high, especially in an outbreak environment. From the analysis of their work characteristics, we can see that most medical staff are working in teams. Reciprocity is a basic requirement at work, and their sense of belonging is relatively high. At the same time, due to the continuous progress of medical technology, the competency requirements of doctors and nurses are increasing and the internal competition is also fiercer, which may lead to a challenge in the trust between each other. This study only confirms the existence of the moderated mediating effects of work meaning on the relationship between trust reciprocity, psychological security and post-traumatic growth.

Whether it is natural or man-made, adversity and trauma are inevitable for human beings. How to recover from trauma and make life more active is the most important issue in trauma research. Relational capital as a social support is essential for psychological rehabilitation; in particular, in Chinese culture, people pay more attention to maintaining good relations. Therefore, when encountering major setbacks or crises, relational capital is especially important so that individuals can respond and recover more quickly after the crisis. Organizations should strive to promote the formation of an internal trust mechanism and atmosphere through cultural construction and value management; they should also help members form mutually beneficial working relations through interactive learning, management by objective, knowledge sharing, etc., and enhance their sense of belonging through organizational compensation, special ceremonies, etc. Relational capital gives employees more confidence to cope with high pressure and uncertainty, and can boost their future growth. In the recruitment process, selecting employees who are more recognized for their work, and strengthening the individual's sense of work value through various publicity and training activities will also help the occurrence of post-traumatic growth. It is not an accidental phenomenon that individuals have positive feedback and growth after experiencing major crises and traumas. This study only explores the role of relational capital, but there are many individual traits, group interaction factors, organizational supportive factors that may affect the occurrence of post-traumatic growth, which also need to be further studied in future research.

Author Contributions: Conceptualization, T.N. and M.T.; methodology, T.N.; software, T.N.; validation, T.N.; formal analysis, T.N.; investigation, T.N.; resources, T.N.; data curation, T.N.; writing—original draft preparation, T.N. and M.T.; writing—review and editing, M.T. and H.L.; visualization, T.N. and M.T.; supervision, T.N.; project administration, M.T.; funding acquisition, T.N. All authors have read and agreed to the published version of the manuscript.

Funding: This research was funded by the Higher Education Fund of Macau, grant number: HSS-MUST-2020-08.

Institutional Review Board Statement: Not applicable.

Informed Consent Statement: Not applicable.

Data Availability Statement: The data presented in this study are available on request from the corresponding author.

Acknowledgments: We are thankful to the editors and anonymous reviewers for their helpful comments. They helped to improve the presentation and discussion of our topic immensely. During this pandemic season, we would like to give our thanks to the medical workers over the world who have been sacrificing themselves both physically and mentally, especially the 760 medical staff who worked at the front lines at the first outbreak of COVID-19. They contributed not only their energy and love, but also knowledge. This was not only new medical knowledge, as they also made it possible for us to achieve new knowledge through the questionnaire.

Conflicts of Interest: The authors declare no conflict of interest. The funders had no role in the design of the study; in the collection, analyses, or interpretation of data; in the writing of the manuscript, or in the decision to publish the results.

Abbreviations

The following abbreviations are used in this manuscript:

TRU	Trust
REC	Reciprocity
IDE	Identification
PS	Psychological Security
PTG	Post-Traumatic Growth
WM	Work Meaning

References

1. Dozois, D.J. Anxiety and depression in Canada during the COVID-19 pandemic: A national survey. *Can. Psychol. Psychol. Can.* **2021**, *62*, 136–142. [CrossRef]
2. Alonzi, S.; La Torre, A.; Silverstein, M.W. The psychological impact of preexisting mental and physical health conditions during the COVID-19 pandemic. *Psychol. Trauma Theory Res. Pract. Policy* **2020**, *12*, S236. [CrossRef] [PubMed]
3. Chong, S.; Huang, Y.; Chang, C.H.D. Supporting interdependent telework employees: A moderated-mediation model linking daily COVID-19 task setbacks to next-day work withdrawal. *J. Appl. Psychol.* **2020**, *105*, 1408. [CrossRef] [PubMed]
4. Liu, D.; Chen, Y.; Li, N. Tackling the negative impact of COVID-19 on work engagement and taking charge: A multi-study investigation of frontline health workers. *J. Appl. Psychol.* **2021**, *106*, 185–198. [CrossRef]
5. Joseph, S. *What Doesn't Kill Us: The New Psychology of Posttraumatic Growth*; Basic Books: New York, NY, USA, 2011.
6. Karanci, A.N.; Erkam, A. Variables related to stress-related growth among Turkish breast cancer patients. *Stress Health J. Int. Soc. Investig. Stress* **2007**, *23*, 315–322. [CrossRef]
7. Nahapiet, J.; Ghoshal, S. Social capital, intellectual capital, and the organizational advantage. *Acad. Manag. Rev.* **1998**, *23*, 242–266. [CrossRef]
8. Andel, S.A.; Shen, W.; Arvan, M.L. Depending on your own kindness: The moderating role of self-compassion on the within-person consequences of work loneliness during the COVID-19 pandemic. *J. Occup. Health Psychol.* **2021**. [CrossRef]
9. Krishna, A. *Active Social Capital: Tracing the Roots of Development and Democracy*; Columbia University Press: New York, NY, USA, 2002.

10. van Dijk, A.; Hendriks, P.; Romo-Leroux, I. Knowledge sharing and social capital in globally distributed execution. *J. Knowl. Manag.* **2016**, *20*, 327–343. [CrossRef]
11. Wiersema, M.F.; Nishimura, Y.; Suzuki, K. Executive succession: The importance of social capital in CEO appointments. *Strateg. Manag. J.* **2018**, *39*, 1473–1495. [CrossRef]
12. Batjargal, B. Internet entrepreneurship: Social capital, human capital, and performance of Internet ventures in China. *Res. Policy* **2007**, *36*, 605–618. [CrossRef]
13. Chen, J.E.; Ouyang, T.H.; Pan, S.L. The role of feedback in changing organizational routine: A case study of Haier, China. *Int. J. Inf. Manag.* **2013**, *33*, 971–974. [CrossRef]
14. Ortiz, B.; Donate, M.J.; Guadamillas, F. Inter-organizational social capital as an antecedent of a firm's knowledge identification capability and external knowledge acquisition. *J. Knowl. Manag.* **2018**, *22*, 1332–1357. [CrossRef]
15. Huang Yu-Hong, J.M.Y. Relationship, social capital and innovations of small- and micro-enterprises. *Sci. Res. Manag.* **2018**, *39*, 27–39.
16. Inkpen, A.C.; Tsang, E.W. Social capital, networks, and knowledge transfer. *Acad. Manag. Rev.* **2005**, *30*, 146–165. [CrossRef]
17. Reber, A.S. *The Penguin Dictionary of Psychology*; Penguin Press: London, UK, 1995.
18. Kahn, W.A. Psychological conditions of personal engagement and disengagement at work. *Acad. Manag. J.* **1990**, *33*, 692–724.
19. Edmondson, A. Psychological safety and learning behavior in work teams. *Adm. Sci. Q.* **1999**, *44*, 350–383. [CrossRef]
20. Zhong, C.; Lijuan, A. Developing of security questionnaire and its reliability and validity. *Chin. Ment. Health J.* **2004**, *18*, 97–99.
21. Aranzamendez, G.; James, D.; Toms, R. Finding antecedents of psychological safety: A step toward quality improvement. In *Nursing Forum*; Wiley Online Library: New York, NY, USA, 2015; Volume 50, pp. 171–178.
22. Harris, B.; Leather, P. Levels and consequences of exposure to service user violence: Evidence from a sample of UK social care staff. *Br. J. Soc. Work.* **2012**, *42*, 851–869. [CrossRef]
23. Carmeli, A.; Gittell, J.H. High-quality relationships, psychological safety, and learning from failures in work organizations. *J. Organ. Behav. Int. J. Ind. Occup. Organ. Psychol. Behav.* **2009**, *30*, 709–729. [CrossRef]
24. Siemsen, E.; Roth, A.V.; Balasubramanian, S.; Anand, G. The influence of psychological safety and confidence in knowledge on employee knowledge sharing. *Manuf. Serv. Oper. Manag.* **2009**, *11*, 429–447. [CrossRef]
25. Tedeschi, R.G.; Calhoun, L.G. The Posttraumatic Growth Inventory: Measuring the positive legacy of trauma. *J. Trauma. Stress* **1996**, *9*, 455–471. [CrossRef]
26. Janoff-Bulman, R. Assumptive worlds and the stress of traumatic events: Applications of the schema construct. *Soc. Cogn.* **1989**, *7*, 113–136. [CrossRef]
27. Morin, S.; Nelson, K.; Corbo-Cruz, N. Adolescent perceptions on the impact of growing up with a parent with a disability. *Psychology* **2015**, *5*, 311–316.
28. Vishnevsky, T.; Cann, A.; Calhoun, L.G.; Tedeschi, R.G.; Demakis, G.J. Gender differences in self-reported posttraumatic growth: A meta-analysis. *Psychol. Women Q.* **2010**, *34*, 110–120. [CrossRef]
29. Schroevers, M.J.; Teo, I. The report of posttraumatic growth in Malaysian cancer patients: Relationships with psychological distress and coping strategies. *Psycho-Oncology* **2008**, *17*, 1239–1246. [CrossRef] [PubMed]
30. Shakespeare-Finch, J.; Armstrong, D. Trauma type and posttrauma outcomes: Differences between survivors of motor vehicle accidents, sexual assault, and bereavement. *J. Loss Trauma* **2010**, *15*, 69–82. [CrossRef]
31. Milam, J.E.; Ritt-Olson, A.; Unger, J.B. Posttraumatic growth among adolescents. *J. Adolesc. Res.* **2004**, *19*, 192–204. [CrossRef]
32. Kimhi, S.; Eshel, Y.; Zysberg, L.; Hantman, S.; Enosh, G. Sense of coherence and socio-demographic characteristics predicting posttraumatic stress symptoms and recovery in the aftermath of the Second Lebanon War. *Anxiety Stress Coping* **2010**, *23*, 139–152. [CrossRef]
33. Brown, S.P.; Leigh, T.W. A new look at psychological climate and its relationship to job involvement, effort, and performance. *J. Appl. Psychol.* **1996**, *81*, 358. [CrossRef]
34. Spreitzer, G.M. Psychological empowerment in the workplace: Dimensions, measurement, and validation. *Acad. Manag. J.* **1995**, *38*, 1442–1465.
35. Thomas, K.W.; Velthouse, B.A. Cognitive elements of empowerment: An "interpretive" model of intrinsic task motivation. *Acad. Manag. Rev.* **1990**, *15*, 666–681.
36. Mok, E.; Au-Yeung, B. Relationship between organizational climate and empowerment of nurses in Hong Kong. *J. Nurs. Manag.* **2002**, *10*, 129–137. [CrossRef]
37. Aryee, S.; Chen, Z.X. Leader–member exchange in a Chinese context: Antecedents, the mediating role of psychological empowerment and outcomes. *J. Bus. Res.* **2006**, *59*, 793–801. [CrossRef]
38. Zhang, X.; Bartol, K.M. Linking empowering leadership and employee creativity: The influence of psychological empowerment, intrinsic motivation, and creative process engagement. *Acad. Manag. J.* **2010**, *53*, 107–128. [CrossRef]
39. Henderson, D.J.; Liden, R.C.; Glibkowski, B.C.; Chaudhry, A. LMX differentiation: A multilevel review and examination of its antecedents and outcomes. *Leadersh. Q.* **2009**, *20*, 517–534. [CrossRef]
40. Li, C.; Tian, B.; Shi, K. Transformational Leadership and Employee Work Attitudes: The Mediating Effects of Multidimensional Psychological Empowerment. *Acta Psychol. Sin.* **2006**, *38*, 297–307.
41. Chiu, C.M.; Hsu, M.H.; Wang, E.T. Understanding knowledge sharing in virtual communities: An integration of social capital and social cognitive theories. *Decis. Support Syst.* **2006**, *42*, 1872–1888. [CrossRef]

International Journal of
Environmental Research and Public Health

MDPI

Article

Nurses Who Are More Willing to Participate in the Fight against COVID-19: Evidence from China

Lai-Kun Tong [1], Ming-Xia Zhu [2], Si-Chen Wang [2], Pak-Leng Cheong [2] and Iat-Kio Van [2,*]

[1] Research Management and Development Department, Kiang Wu Nursing College of Macau, Macau 999078, China; chingco@kwnc.edu.mo

[2] Education Department, Kiang Wu Nursing College of Macau, Macau 999078, China; zmx@kwnc.edu.mo (M.-X.Z.); sichen@kwnc.edu.mo (S.-C.W.); joecheong@kwnc.edu.mo (P.-L.C.)

* Correspondence: van@kwnc.edu.mo; Tel.: +853-8295-6202

Abstract: When facing an infectious disease disaster, nurses' willingness to work is critical. Nurses' lack of willingness to work during a pandemic may worsen the shortage of health care personnel. The purpose of this study is to assess the willingness of nurses to participate in the fight against COVID-19 in China and to identify factors associated therewith. This cross-sectional study examines nurses working in 11 Chinese cities including Macau, Hong Kong, Shenzhen, Dongguan, Huizhou, Guangzhou, Zhaoqing, Foshan, Jiangmen, Zhongshan, and Zhuhai. Questionnaires were collected from 19 May to 7 August 2020. A total of 8065 questionnaires were received, of which 8030 valid questionnaires were included for analysis. A total of 53.4% of participants reported that they had signed up to support the COVID-19 pandemic response. Multivariate logistic regression analysis revealed that being single (OR = 0.72, 95% CI: 0.60–0.87), having no children (OR = 0.81, 95% CI: 0.68–0.97), possessing higher professional qualifications (OR = 1.25, 95% CI: 1.14–1.37), having a more prestigious professional title (OR = 1.68, 95%CI: 1.50–1.90), being an administrative supervisor (OR = 0.53, 95% CI: 0.45–0.63), having a higher caring dimensions inventory score (OR = 1.01, 95% CI: 1.01–1.01), working in a hospital (OR = 0.53, 95% CI: 0.39–0.72), and receiving employer-provided care training (OR = 0.77, 95% CI: 0.68–0.87) were predictive of nurses' willingness to participate in the fight against COVID-19. We suggest that unmarried nurses should be given priority when recruiting to fight an epidemic and, for married nurses with children who are recruited to fight an epidemic, supporting measures should be provided for childcare. We suggest strengthening workplace training of caring for nurses in order to better retain and recruit qualified support for an epidemic outbreak of infectious diseases.

Keywords: COVID-19; nurse; willingness

Citation: Tong, L.-K.; Zhu, M.-X.; Wang, S.-C.; Cheong, P.-L.; Van, I.-K. Nurses Who Are More Willing to Participate in the Fight against COVID-19: Evidence from China. *Int. J. Environ. Res. Public Health* **2021**, *18*, 7357. https://doi.org/10.3390/ijerph18147357

Academic Editors: Richard Gray and Sonia Udod

Received: 4 June 2021
Accepted: 6 July 2021
Published: 9 July 2021

1. Introduction

The coronavirus disease 2019 (COVID-19) pandemic, caused by the severe acute respiratory syndrome coronavirus 2 (SARS-CoV-2) [1], has caused more than 1.1 billion infections and nearly 2.7 million deaths worldwide, as of 15 March 2021 [2]. The prevalence of SARS-CoV-2 infection among health care workers (HCW) in different regions ranged from 0.4% to 57.06% and the estimated pooled prevalence was 11% [3]. Nurses may be more affected by the COVID-19 outbreak than other HCW, with higher rates of SARS-CoV-2 infection and psychological distress [3,4].

Nurses are the largest cadre of the HCW in all countries and play an important role in the response to a global pandemic [5]. Before the outbreak of COVID-19, there had been an extant, global shortage of nurses, and the World Health Organization had recommended that health care providers develop plans to cope with this shortage [6]. Nursing managers during the COVID-19 crisis mitigated for this shortfall by recruiting volunteers and temporary nurses [7]. When facing an infectious disease disaster, nurses' willingness to work is critical, yet the percentage of nurses willing to work during the last influenza pandemic ranged from 23.1% to 90.1%, depending on their social and professional contexts [8].

Nurses' lack of willingness to work during a pandemic may worsen the shortage of this profession. Effective preparation for the next pandemic requires assessing the willingness of nurses to have participated in the fight against COVID-19 and understanding the factors that influenced such willingness. Several studies conducted during the COVID-19 pandemic have shown that age, marital status, area of work, level of knowledge, positive professional perception, communication from managers, and risk category may be predictors of willingness [9–12].

All nurses, including general, specialist, hospital, and community nurses are the backbone of the fight against COVID-19 [13]. However, the small sample size of our studies, or the fact that participants were selected from the same institutions or from within specific groups of nurses (e.g., nurse practitioner) limited the generalizability of our results. However, Chinese nurses' participation in the fight against COVID-19 was not restricted by region. For example, more than 42,000 medical workers from across China travelled to Hubei Province to combat the epidemic [14]. Samples in this study were collected from various cities and institutions, including hospitals and community institutions, and the sample size was increased to improve sample representativeness. Existing studies have only asked participants about their willingness to work during COVID-19; however, these studies did not further explore whether their participants had indeed participated. During the COVID-19 pandemic, governments and medical institutions around the world recruited nurses to fight the disease. Therefore the willingness of nurses to participate in an epidemic is of global significance, and can be better understood by investigating whether reported willingness to work was congruent with behavior during COVID-19.

The purpose of this study is to assess the willingness of nurses to participate in the fight against COVID-19 and to identify its associated factors.

2. Materials and Methods

2.1. Ethic

This study obtained ethical approval from the Research Management and Development Department of Kiang Wu Nursing College of Macau (reference no: 2019APR01). Participants were required to give informed consent before filling completing our questionnaire. The survey was conducted anonymously. Participants could withdraw from the research or exit the survey at any time. The collected data were stored on encrypted computers and online platforms.

2.2. Study Design and Sample

Ours is a cross-sectional study conducted from 11 Chinese cities including Macau, Hong Kong, Shenzhen, Dongguan, Huizhou, Guangzhou, Zhaoqing, Foshan, Jiangmen, Zhongshan, and Zhuhai. There were 258,364 nurses in these cities. To increase the survey representativeness, the sample size was set at 3% of the nursing population, producing a required sample size of 7751.

The inclusion criteria were employment as a nurse, (accredited by the local government) in hospitals, clinics, schools, services for the elderly, etc. in the above cities, and having obtained qualification as a nurse practitioner. The exclusion criteria for this study were employment as trainees or probationary nurses, and nurses who were unwilling to participate.

2.3. Measures

The online questionnaire included four parts: (1) socio-demographic, professional information, and workplace information of the participants; (2) the caring dimensions inventory; (3) the nurse's career identity scale; and (4) willingness to participate in the fight against COVID-19.

Part 1: General information. Part 1 included questions about socio-demographic data (such as gender, age, marital status, number of children, etc.), profession and workplace-related characteristics (such as professional qualifications, professional title, professional experience, being an administrative supervisor, having received care training in college, having worked at least one year in the nursing profession and/or their present organization, type of health facility, adequacy of their regional workforce, and having received employer-provided care training, etc.) of the participants.

Part 2: The caring dimensions inventory. The caring dimensions inventory (CDI) consists of 25 items, each assessed on a 5-point Likert scale (1 = strongly disagree, 5 = strongly agree) developed by Watson and Lea to measure perceptions of caring [15], with scores ranging from 25 to 125. It is cross-culturally applicable [16,17]; the original English inventory was translated into Chinese using a systematic translation process which included a forward-backward translation, consensus meeting, pilot testing, and a psychometric analysis [18]. The Cronbach's α coefficient and the content validity index (CVI) of the Chinese version inventory were 0.97 and 0.98 respectively [19].

Part 3: The nurse's career identity scale. The nurse's career identity scale (NCI) consists of 13-item, each assessed on a 7-point Likert scale, with scores ranging from 1 to 7, where higher scores indicate a higher level of professional identity. The Chinese version of the NCI was modified by Zhao et al. [20]. Good reliability (Cronbach's α = 0.84) and validity (CVI = 0.92) of NCI in the Chinese version were demonstrated [20].

Part 4: Intention to participate in the fight against COVID-19. Willingness to participate in the fight against COVID-19 was assessed with a single question: "Have you registered to support COVID-19 pandemic response?"

2.4. Data Collection Procedure

The research team set up a liaison system in 11 cities, with a volunteer from hospitals, universities or nursing professional societies in each city to promote the survey in their respective cities. Participants could enter the electronic questionnaire platform with the QR code or URL on our recruitment poster to be presented with an informed consent procedure and, thereafter, complete the questionnaire. The electronic questionnaire was designed to be completed only once per device to avoid duplicate data. The questionnaires were collected from 19 May to 7 August 2020.

2.5. Data Analysis

Continuous variables were reported as mean $\pm$ standard deviation and a *t*-test was used for comparison between groups. Frequencies and proportions were used for categorical variables and comparison between groups was performed using chi-squared tests or Fisher's exact test. Multivariable binary logistic regression (forward stepwise likelihood ratio method) was employed to identify the predictors for nurses' willingness to participate in the fight against COVID-19. Statistical analyses were performed using SPSS 22.0 software (SPSS Inc., Chicago, IL, USA). The threshold for statistical significance was set to 0.05.

3. Results

3.1. Characteristics of Participants

A total of 8065 questionnaires were received, of which 8030 valid questionnaires were included in the analysis. The mean age of the participants was 31.9 years (SD = 8.7). The majority were female (96.6%), married (63.9%), and held a bachelor's degree (52.8%). More than 97% of participants were working in hospitals. Among the participants analyzed, approximately 70% had junior professional titles, with a mean professional experience of 11.5 years (refer to Table 1 for details).

Table 1. Characteristics of participants and their willingness to participate in the fight against COVID-19 (n = 8030).

Demographics	Categories	Oversll, n (%)/Mean (SD)	Not Registered, n (%)	Registered, n (%)	χ^2/t	p-Value
Socio-demographic characteristics						
gender					3.244	0.072
	male	274 (3.4)	113 (41.2)	161 (58.8)		
	female	7756 (96.6)	3627 (46.8)	4129 (53.2)		
age *		31.9 (8.7)	31.4 ± 8.7	32.3 ± 8.6	−0.063	0.000
marital status					14.320	0.001
	single	2741 (34.1)	1213 (44.3)	1528 (55.7)		
	married	5127 (63.9)	2464 (48.1)	2663 (51.9)		
	other	162 (2.0)	63 (38.9)	99 (61.1)		
had one or more children					4.693	0.030
	yes	4748 (59.1)	2259 (47.6)	2489 (52.4)		
	no	3282 (40.9)	1481 (45.1)	1801 (54.9)		
Profession-related characteristics						
professional qualifications					50.463	0.000
	diploma	3654 (45.5)	1859 (50.9)	1795 (49.1)		
	graduate	4240 (52.8)	1818 (42.9)	2422 (57.1)		
	postgraduate	136 (1.7)	63 (46.3)	73 (53.7)		
professional title					113.067	0.000
	junior	5542 (69.0)	2801 (50.5)	2741 (49.5)		
intermediate and senior		2488 (31.0)	939 (37.7)	1549 (62.3)		
administrative supervisor					122.711	0.000
	yes	918 (11.4)	270 (29.4)	648 (70.6)		
	no	7112 (88.6)	3470 (48.8)	3643 (51.2)		
received caring training in college					9.688	0.008
	yes	6748 (84.0)	3119 (46.2)	3629 (53.8)		
	no	869 (10.8)	398 (45.8)	471 (54.2)		
	not sure	413 (5.2)	223 (54.0)	190 (46.0)		
years in nursing profession		11.1 (8.5)	10.6 ± 8.4	11.6 ± 8.5	−5.258	0
years in present organization		9.1 (7.5)	8.6 ± 7.3	9.6 ± 7.7	−5.889	0
CDI *		107.5 (14.7)	106.4 ± 14.2	108.5 ± 15.0	−6.555	0
NCI *		6.0 (0.86)	5.9 ± 0.8	6.0 ± 0.9	−6.371	0
Workplace-related characteristics						
type of health facility					21.137	0.000
	hospital	7834 (97.6)	3617 (46.2)	4217 (53.8)		
	community	196 (2.4)	123 (62.8)	73 (37.2)		
workforce					0.159	0.924
	enough	2021 (25.0)	930 (46.2)	1082 (53.8)		
	barely enough	3146 (39.2)	1472 (46.8)	1674 (53.2)		
	not enough	2872 (35.8)	1338 (46.6)	1534 (53.4)		
provided caring training					39.031	0.000
	yes	5981 (74.5)	2664 (44.5)	3317 (55.5)		
	no	1298 (16.2)	684 (52.7)	614 (47.3)		
	not sure	751 (9.3)	392 (52.2)	359 (47.8)		

CDI, the caring dimensions inventory; NCI, the nurse's career identity scale. * Result from mean (SD) and t-test.

3.2. Nurses' Willingness to Participate in the Fight against COVID-19

A total of 53.4% of participants reported that they had registered to support the COVID-19 pandemic response. The results of the individual factors associated with nurses' willingness to participate in the fight against COVID-19 are shown in Table 1. The results show that no statistically significant difference in participatory willingness was found by gender composition within the workforce. Those who did not show willingness to participate in the fight against COVID-19 were more likely to be younger, married, have children, have lower professional qualifications or title, be in a role other than administrative supervisor, have less profession experience, have lower CDI and/or NCI scores, work in community health facilities, and not have received care training from their employer than those who were willing to participate in the fight against COVID-19.

3.3. Predictors of Nurses' Willingness

The Hosmer–Lemeshow test showed that there was no significant difference between the observed and predicted probabilities of the binary logistic regression model ($\chi2 = 10.667$, $p = 0.221$), indicating good model fit. Regarding socio-demographic factors, only marital status and parenthood were predictors of the willingness to participant in the fight against COVID-19. Unmarried nurses (OR = 0.72, 95% CI: 0.60–0.87) and those having no children (OR = 0.81, 95% CI: 0.68–0.97) were more willing to participate than those in marriages or with children. Regarding professionally related factors, nurses with higher professional qualifications (OR = 1.25, 95% CI: 1.14–1.37), a higher professional title (OR = 1.68, 95% CI: 1.50–1.90), and a higher CDI score (OR = 1.01, 95% CI: 1.01–1.01) were associated with higher willingness to participate in the fight against COVID-19. Nurses who were administrative supervisors (OR = 0.53, 95% CI: 0.45–0.63) were also more willing to participate in the pandemic response than those who were not. Regarding the influence of workplace-related factors on willingness, multivariate logistic regression analysis revealed that nurses who worked in hospitals (OR = 0.53, 95% CI: 0.39–0.72) and whose employers provided care training (OR = 0.77, 95% CI: 0.68–0.87) were more likely to participate in the fight against COVID-19 than those who worked in the community and/or whose employers did not provide such training. (Table 2).

Table 2. Predictors of willingness to participate in the fight against COVID-19 (multivariable logistic regression).

Variables	β	OR (95% CI)	p-Value
Socio-demographic characteristics			
gender		/	0.101
age		/	0.596
marital status			0.000
married vs. single [R]	−0.33	0.72 (0.60–0.87)	0.000
other vs. single [R]	0.03	1.03 (0.72–1.48)	0.878
had one or more children		0.016	
no vs. yes [R]	−0.22	0.81 (0.68–0.97)	0.016
Profession-related characteristics			
professional qualifications	0.22	1.25 (1.14–1.37)	0.000
professional title	0.52	1.68 (1.50–1.90)	0.000
administrative supervisor			0.000
no vs. yes [R]	−0.63	0.53 (0.45–0.63)	0.000
received caring training in college		0.153	
no vs. yes [R]		/	0.285
not sure vs. yes [R]		/	0.132
years in nursing profession		/	0.991
years in present organization		/	0.542
CDI	0.01	1.01 (1.01–1.01)	0.000
NCI		/	0.062
Workplace-related characteristics			
type of health facility			0.000
community vs. hospital [R]	−0.64	0.53 (0.39–0.72)	0.000
human resource		/	0.496
provided caring training			0.000
no vs. yes [R]	−0.26	0.77 (0.68–0.87)	0.000
not sure vs. yes [R]	−0.21	0.81 (0.70–0.95)	0.009
Hosmer and Lemeshow test	chi-square value = 10.667		p-value = 0.221

CDI, the caring dimensions inventory; NCI, the nurse's career identity scale. [R] = reference case; / = variable was excluded from the logistic regression model.

4. Discussion

Previous surveys have shown that 61–97% of some nursing populations are willing to participate in the fight against COVID-19 [9–11,21,22], while the results of this study show that less than 55% of Chinese nurses have signed up to support the COVID-19 pandemic response. More than 3% of nurses sent by the Chinese government to Wuhan (where the first COVID-19 case was reported) to join the battle against COVID-19 expressed their unwillingness to participate in frontline work during the COVID-19 outbreak [22]. Meta-analysis found that the pooled prevalence of anxiety, depression, and sleep disorders among nurses during the COVID-19 pandemic was 37%, 53%, and 43%, respectively [23]. Nearly 25% of nurses in one hospital reported they intended to leave the field of nursing after the COVID-19 pandemic [24]. As the COVID-19 pandemic continues to develop, the shortage of nurses has worsened. Managers must involve nurses in the response to the epidemic to alleviate workforce shortages. An Australian study has suggested that strategies to improve knowledge of the COVID-19 pandemic, preparedness of the intensive care unit, and personal concern are ineffective in promoting nurses' active participation in fighting the epidemic, and that communication from managers is most effective [9].

This survey found that gender and age were not associated with nurses' willingness to participate in the fight against COVID-19, which was consistent with the findings in other studies [9,10]. In addition, some studies showed that male and young HCW were more willing to participate in epidemic work [25,26]. This finding was not replicated, and may be explained by the proportion of male nurses in China, which is approximately 2% of the nursing workforce [27], while this proportion is much higher in other countries. Univariate analysis showed that younger nurses had a higher willingness to be participatory, but multivariate analysis showed that age was not a predictor after controlling for other factors. As in previous research, this study found that married nurses were less likely than nurses who were single to participate in the COVID-19 pandemic response, especially those who were married with children [26,28,29]. One possible reason may be that women were the main family caregivers in the observed populations, and they bore more responsibility at home in addition to their professional responsibilities. Surveys conducted by Mattingly et al. [30] and Craig [31] showed that, in some populations, compared with fathers, mothers were expected to spend more time with their children and have more overall responsibility for managing care. It is suggested that unmarried personnel should be given priority when recruiting during an epidemic, and that, to recruit married nurses who are also parents, supporting measures should be provided for childcare.

Previous studies have been inconsistent regarding the association of professional experience with nurses' willingness to participate in fighting the epidemic [12,32]. The results of multiple logistic regression analysis showed that a predictor was not professional experience, but rather professional title. It was predictive of Chinese nurses' attitudes towards dying patients, while clinical experience was not [33]. Nurses with more highly-regarded professional titles had a more positive attitude towards dying patients [33]. The incidence of case fatality rates for COVID-19 in China was 3.8% compared with 14.6% between January and April 2020 [34]. This means that nurses participating in the COVID-19 pandemic response are more likely to face caring for dying patients. However, Chinese nurses lack hospice care education and training [35]. The lack of knowledgeability surrounding hospice care was seen to put pressure on nurses caring for COVID-19 patients [36] and reduce their willingness to participate in the fight against COVID-19. As a result, we suggest medical institutions seeking to retain qualified personnel during a pandemic should strengthen nurses' training in hospice care.

Although professional esteem for nurses increased during the COVID-19 epidemic [37], the results of multiple regression in this study showed that the more significantly influencing factor of nurses' willingness to participate in the fight against the epidemic was not professional identity but perceptions of caring. Care is an important part of nursing; training in caring can improve nurses' mentality surrounding care. Additionally, the results of this study showed that the factor affecting nurses' willingness to participate in the fight against COVID-19 was not whether they had received relevant training at all during their educations, but whether their working institutions provided relevant training afterward. Nurses with no care training were 77.0% less likely to participate in the epidemic response than those with training provided by their workplaces. It is suggested that at-work institutional training is more important than academic training for improving the caring mentality of nurses. One explanation may be that, while schools do seek to develop nursing students' caring abilities, the academic process may undermine the students' valuation of care [38]. Thus, the development of caring abilities may depend upon in-service training. Less than three quarters of the nurses surveyed had received workplace training in care. We therefore suggest strengthening workplace training of caring for nurses to decrease professional reluctance during an outbreak of infectious diseases.

This present study had limitations. First, although the sample size was 3% of the total nursing population and the backgrounds of participants were matched to the population as much as possible, the sample was not randomly selected, so the representativeness of the sample was correspondingly limited. A second limitation was the cross-sectional nature of this study; it is not possible to draw causal inferences between our identified factors and nurses' willingness to participate in a pandemic response. Third, the use of the Student's t-test for between-group comparison in such a large sample was not optimal because it is sensitive to population size.

5. Conclusions

More than half of the respondents in this survey were willing to participate in the fight against COVID-19. The nurses who were married, had children, worked in the community, or were not administrative supervisors reported less willingness to participate in the fight against COVID-19, while those with higher education, professional titles, and CDI scores, or workplace training in caring, had a greater willingness to participate. It is suggested that unmarried nurses should be given priority when recruiting to fight an epidemic. When married nurses with children are recruited, supporting measures should be provided for childcare. Finally, we suggest strengthened workplace training of caring for nurses to better retain and recruit qualified support during the outbreak of infectious diseases.

Author Contributions: Conceptualization, L.-K.T. and I.-K.V.; methodology, L.-K.T. and M.-X.Z.; software, L.-K.T., S.-C.W. and P.-L.C.; validation, L.-K.T., I.-K.V. and M.-X.Z.; formal analysis, L.-K.T., S.-C.W. and P.-L.C.; investigation, L.-K.T., S.-C.W. and I.-K.V.; resources, M.-X.Z.; data curation, L.-K.T., S.-C.W. and P.-L.C.; writing—original draft preparation, L.-K.T. and I.-K.V.; writing—review and editing, M.-X.Z., S.-C.W. and P.-L.C.; visualization, M.-X.Z. and I.-K.V.; supervision, I.-K.V.; project administration, I.-K.V.; funding acquisition, I.-K.V. All authors have read and agreed to the published version of the manuscript.

Funding: This research was funded by Macao Foundation, grant number 2964/DS/2019.

Institutional Review Board Statement: The study protocol was approved by the Research Management and Development Department of Kiang Wu Nursing College of Macau (protocol code 2019APR01, dated April 2019).

Informed Consent Statement: Informed consent was obtained from all subjects involved in the study.

Data Availability Statement: All data that support the findings of this study are available from the corresponding author upon reasonable request.

Acknowledgments: Funding from Macao Foundation is gratefully acknowledged. We thank College of Nursing Hong Kong, Dongguan Nursing Society, Jiangmen Third People's Hospital, Nethersole Institute of Continuing Holistic Health Education, The Fifth Affiliated Hospital of Sun Yat-sen University, Zhaoqing Medical College, Guisu Jiang, Jun Lin, Li Zhang, Lijing Hu, and Qun Wang for help with data collection. We acknowledge Andrew Leung Luk for the linguistic editing and proofreading during the preparation of this manuscript.

Conflicts of Interest: The funders had no role in the design of the study; in the collection, analyses, or interpretation of data; in the writing of the manuscript, or in the decision to publish the results.

References

1. Coronaviridae Study Group of the International Committee on Taxonomy of Viruses. The species Severe acute respiratory syndrome-related coronavirus: Classifying 2019-nCoV and naming it SARS-CoV-2. *Nat. Microbiol.* **2020**, *5*, 536. [CrossRef]
2. World Health Organization. WHO Coronavirus (COVID-19) Dashboard. Available online: https://covid19.who.int/ (accessed on 15 March 2021).
3. Gómez-Ochoa, S.A.; Franco, O.H.; Rojas, L.Z.; Raguindin, P.F.; Roa-Díaz, Z.M.; Wyssmann, B.M.; Guevara, S.L.R.; Echeverría, L.E.; Glisic, M.; Muka, T. COVID-19 in health-care workers: A living systematic review and meta-analysis of prevalence, risk factors, clinical characteristics, and outcomes. *Am. J. Epidemiol.* **2021**, *190*, 161–175. [CrossRef] [PubMed]
4. de Pablo, G.S.; Serrano, J.V.; Catalan, A.; Arango, C.; Moreno, C.; Ferre, F.; Shin, J.I.; Sullivan, S.; Brondino, N.; Solmi, M. Impact of coronavirus syndromes on physical and mental health of health care workers: Systematic review and meta-analysis. *J. Affect. Disord.* **2020**, *275*, 48–57. [CrossRef] [PubMed]
5. Corless, I.B.; Nardi, D.; Milstead, J.A.; Larson, E.; Nokes, K.M.; Orsega, S.; Kurth, A.E.; Kirksey, K.M.; Woith, W. Expanding nursing's role in responding to global pandemics 5/14/2018. *Nurs. Outlook* **2018**, *66*, 412–415. [CrossRef] [PubMed]
6. World Health Organization. *Hospital Preparedness for Epidemics*; World Health Organization: Geneva, Switzerland, 2014.
7. Poortaghi, S.; Shahmari, M.; Ghobadi, A. Exploring nursing managers' perceptions of nursing workforce management during the outbreak of COVID-19: A content analysis study. *BMC Nurs.* **2021**, *20*, 27. [CrossRef] [PubMed]
8. Aoyagi, Y.; Beck, C.R.; Dingwall, R.; Nguyen-Van-Tam, J.S. Healthcare workers' willingness to work during an influenza pandemic: A systematic review and meta-analysis. *Influenza Other Respir. Viruses* **2015**, *9*, 120–130. [CrossRef] [PubMed]
9. Lord, H.; Loveday, C.; Moxham, L.; Fernandez, R. Effective communication is key to intensive care nurses' willingness to provide nursing care amidst the COVID-19 pandemic. *Intensive Crit. Care Nurs.* **2021**, *62*, 102946. [CrossRef] [PubMed]
10. Nashwan, A.J.; Abujaber, A.A.; Mohamed, A.S.; Villar, R.C.; Al-Jabry, M.M. Nurses' willingness to work with COVID-19 patients: The role of knowledge and attitude. *Nurs. Open* **2021**, *8*, 695–701. [CrossRef]
11. Wu, B.; Zhao, Y.; Xu, D.; Wang, Y.; Niu, N.; Zhang, M.; Zhi, X.; Zhu, P.; Meng, A. Factors associated with nurses' willingness to participate in care of patients with COVID–19: A survey in China. *J. Nurs. Manag.* **2020**, *28*, 1704–1712. [CrossRef]
12. Gan, X.; Shi, Z.; Chair, S.Y.; Cao, X.; Wang, Q. Willingness of Chinese nurses to practice in Hubei combating the coronavirus disease 2019 epidemic: A cross-sectional study. *J. Adv. Nurs.* **2020**, *76*, 2137–2150. [CrossRef]
13. Nayna Schwerdtle, P.; Connell, C.J.; Lee, S.; Plummer, V.; Russo, P.L.; Endacott, R.; Kuhn, L. Nurse Expertise: A Critical Resource in the COVID-19 Pandemic Response. *Ann. Glob. Health* **2020**, *86*, 49. [CrossRef]
14. The State Council of the People's Republic of China. Last Medical Assistance Team Leaves Hard-Hit Hubei as Epidemic Subsides. Available online: http://english.www.gov.cn/news/photos/202004/16/content_WS5e97b2c5c6d0c201c2cc104e.html (accessed on 4 June 2021).
15. Watson, R.; Lea, A. The caring dimensions inventory (CDI): Content validity, reliability and scaling. *J. Adv. Nurs.* **1997**, *25*, 87–94. [CrossRef]
16. Akansel, N.; Watson, R.; Aydin, N.; Özdemir, A. Mokken scaling of the Caring Dimensions Inventory (CDI-25). *J. Clin. Nurs.* **2013**, *22*, 1818–1826. [CrossRef]
17. Watson, R.; Hoogbruin, A.L.; Rumeu, C.; Beunza, M.; Barbarin, B.; Macdonald, J.; McCready, T. Differences and similarities in the perception of caring between Spanish and UK nurses. *J. Clin. Nurs.* **2003**, *12*, 85–92. [CrossRef]
18. Jones, P.S.; Lee, J.W.; Phillips, L.R.; Zhang, X.E.; Jaceldo, K.B. An adaptation of Brislin's translation model for cross-cultural research. *Nurs. Res.* **2001**, *50*, 300–304. [CrossRef]
19. Tong, L.-K.; Zhu, M.-X.; Wang, S.-C.; Cheong, P.-L.; Van, I.-K. A Chinese Version of the Caring Dimensions Inventory: Reliability and Validity Assessment. *Int. J. Environ. Res. Public Health* **2021**, *18*, 6834. [CrossRef]
20. Zhao, H.; Lu, T.T.; Zhang, C.Y. Testing for reliability and validity of Chinese version of the Nurse's career identity scale. *Chin. Nurs. Manag.* **2010**, *11*, 49–51.
21. Upadhyaya, D.P.; Paudel, R.; Bromberg, D.J.; Acharya, D.; Khoshnood, K.; Lee, K.; Park, J.-H.; Yoo, S.-J.; Shrestha, A.; BC, B. Frontline healthcare workers' knowledge and perception of COVID-19, and willingness to work during the pandemic in Nepal. *Healthcare* **2020**, *8*, 554. [CrossRef] [PubMed]
22. Hu, D.; Kong, Y.; Li, W.; Han, Q.; Zhang, X.; Zhu, L.X.; Wan, S.W.; Liu, Z.; Shen, Q.; Yang, J.; et al. Frontline nurses' burnout, anxiety, depression, and fear statuses and their associated factors during the COVID-19 outbreak in Wuhan, China: A large-scale cross-sectional study. *EClinicalMedicine* **2020**, *24*, 100424. [CrossRef]
23. Al Maqbali, M.; Al Sinani, M.; Al-Lenjawi, B. Prevalence of stress, depression, anxiety and sleep disturbance among nurses during the COVID-19 pandemic: A systematic review and meta-analysis. *J. Psychosom. Res.* **2021**, *141*, 110343. [CrossRef] [PubMed]
24. Said, R.M.; El-Shafei, D.A. Occupational stress, job satisfaction, and intent to leave: Nurses working on front lines during COVID-19 pandemic in Zagazig City, Egypt. *Environ. Sci. Pollut. Res.* **2021**, *28*, 8791–8801. [CrossRef]
25. Al-Hunaishi, W.; Hoe, V.C.W.; Chinna, K. Factors associated with healthcare workers willingness to participate in disasters: A cross-sectional study in Sana'a, Yemen. *BMJ Open* **2019**, *9*, e030547. [CrossRef]
26. Charney, R.L.; Rebmann, T.; Flood, R.G. Hospital Employee Willingness to Work during Earthquakes Versus Pandemics. *J. Emerg. Med.* **2015**, *49*, 665–674. [CrossRef]
27. National Health Commission of China. *China Health Yearly Statistics 2020*; Peking Union Medical College Press: Beijing, China, 2020.

28. Seale, H.; Leask, J.; Po, K.; MacIntyre, C.R. "Will they just pack up and leave?"—attitudes and intended behaviour of hospital health care workers during an influenza pandemic. *BMC Health Serv. Res.* **2009**, *9*, 30. [CrossRef]
29. Damery, S.; Draper, H.; Wilson, S.; Greenfield, S.; Ives, J.; Parry, J.; Petts, J.; Sorell, T. Healthcare workers' perceptions of the duty to work during an influenza pandemic. *J. Med. Ethics* **2010**, *36*, 12–18. [CrossRef]
30. Mattingly, M.J.; Blanchi, S.M. Gender differences in the quantity and quality of free time: The US experience. *Soc. Forces* **2003**, *81*, 999–1030. [CrossRef]
31. Craig, L. Does Father Care Mean Fathers Share?: A Comparison of How Mothers and Fathers in Intact Families Spend Time with Children. *Gend. Soc.* **2006**, *20*, 259–281. [CrossRef]
32. Luo, Y.; Feng, X.; Zheng, M.; Zhang, D.; Xiao, H.; Li, N. Willingness to participate in front-line work during the COVID-19 pandemic: A cross-sectional study of nurses from a province in South-West China. *J. Nurs. Manag.* **2021**. [CrossRef]
33. Wang, L.; Li, C.; Zhang, Q.; Li, Y. Clinical nurses' attitudes towards death and caring for dying patients in China. *Int. J. Palliat. Nurs.* **2018**, *24*, 33–39. [CrossRef]
34. Mi, Y.-N.; Huang, T.-T.; Zhang, J.-X.; Qin, Q.; Gong, Y.-X.; Liu, S.-Y.; Xue, H.-M.; Ning, C.-H.; Cao, L.; Cao, Y.-X. Estimating the instant case fatality rate of COVID-19 in China. *Int. J. Infect. Dis.* **2020**, *97*, 1–6. [CrossRef] [PubMed]
35. Ling, M.; Wang, X.; Ma, Y.; Long, Y. A Review of the Current State of Hospice Care in China. *Curr. Oncol. Rep.* **2020**, *22*, 99. [CrossRef]
36. Liu, Q.; Tao, J.; Gao, L.; He, X.; Wang, Y.; Xia, W.; Huang, L. Attitudes of Front-Line Nurses Toward Hospice Care During the COVID-19 Pandemic. *Am. J. Hosp. Palliat. Med.* ® **2020**, *38*, 204–210. [CrossRef] [PubMed]
37. Li, Z.; Zuo, Q.; Cheng, J.; Zhou, Y.; Li, Y.; Zhu, L.; Jiang, X. Coronavirus disease 2019 pandemic promotes the sense of professional identity among nurses. *Nurs. Outlook.* [CrossRef] [PubMed]
38. Murphy, F.; Jones, S.; Edwards, M.; James, J.; Mayer, A. The impact of nurse education on the caring behaviours of nursing students. *Nurse Educ. Today* **2009**, *29*, 254–264. [CrossRef]

International Journal of *Environmental Research and Public Health*

MDPI

Article

To Volunteer or Not? Perspectives towards Pre-Registered Nursing Students Volunteering Frontline during COVID-19 Pandemic to Ease Healthcare Workforce: A Qualitative Study

Betsy Seah *, Ben Ho, Sok Ying Liaw, Emily Neo Kim Ang and Siew Tiang Lau

Alice Lee Centre for Nursing Studies, Yong Loo Lin School of Medicine, National University of Singapore, Clinical Research Centre, Block MD11, Level 2, 10 Medical Drive, Singapore 117597, Singapore; benho@u.nus.edu (B.H.); nurliaw@nus.edu.sg (S.Y.L.); nuranke@nus.edu.sg (E.N.K.A.); nurlst@nus.edu.sg (S.T.L.)
* Correspondence: nurseah@nus.edu.sg; Tel.: +65-6601-3213

Abstract: COVID-19 has caused a shortage of healthcare workers and has strained healthcare systems globally. Pre-registered healthcare students with training have a duty of care and can support the healthcare workforce. This study explored factors influencing the willingness of final-year nursing students to volunteer during the COVID-19 pandemic, the role of professional identity in volunteering as healthcare workers, and strategies to improve future volunteering uptakes and processes. A qualitative study using focus-group discussions was conducted. Final-year nursing students who volunteered, students who did not volunteer, and lecturers who supervised student volunteers were recruited. Interviews were conducted online, video-recorded, and transcribed verbatim. A thematic analysis was used. The themes were "wavering thoughts on volunteering", "bringing out 'the nurse' in students through volunteering" and "gearing up to volunteer". Findings suggested the need to look beyond the simplicity of altruism to the role of professional identity, operational, and motivational factors to explain nursing students' decision to volunteer and their volunteer behavior. Providing accommodation, monetary and academic-related incentives, supporting the transitionary phase from students to "professional volunteers", promoting cohesive and positive staff–student volunteer relationships, and establishing a volunteer management team are strategies identified to improve volunteering uptake and operational processes. Our findings advocate strategic partnerships between hospitals/communities and academic institutions in providing various healthcare services during pandemics.

Keywords: COVID-19; health workforce; nursing students; professional identity; qualitative study; volunteers

Citation: Seah, B.; Ho, B.; Liaw, S.Y.; Ang, E.N.K.; Lau, S.T. To Volunteer or Not? Perspectives towards Pre-Registered Nursing Students Volunteering Frontline during COVID-19 Pandemic to Ease Healthcare Workforce: A Qualitative Study. *Int. J. Environ. Res. Public Health* **2021**, *18*, 6668. https://doi.org/10.3390/ijerph18126668

Academic Editors: Richard Gray and Sonia Udod

Received: 14 May 2021
Accepted: 20 June 2021
Published: 21 June 2021

1. Introduction

The 2019 novel coronavirus (COVID-19) pandemic has become a major health crisis affecting millions of people across the globe [1]. To manage the surge of COVID-19 patients, there was a sudden shortage of healthcare workers, and this strained healthcare systems globally. Additional roles, such as screening for potential cases, implementing quarantine and contact tracing contributed further pressures on the healthcare workforce.

In times of crisis, healthcare professionals, government agencies and volunteers from official agencies would form the formal emergency and disaster management system. However, the willingness of healthcare workers to work during a respiratory disease pandemic ranged between 23.1% and 95.8%, and was influenced by various factors such as gender, profession, perceived personal safety, awareness of pandemic risk, role-specific knowledge, pandemic response training and confidence in personal skills [2]. On the other hand, individuals volunteering their time, knowledge, skills, and resources will obtain legitimacy and become part of the formal system through agencies' volunteer recruitment [3]. Factors influencing the willingness of healthcare professionals to serve on the front line have an impact on manpower supply. Older ages, psychological stress, previous volunteering experience, perceived knowledge of disease prevention, safety concerns, and social support were associated with a willingness to serve on the front line [4–6].

Due to the healthcare workforce shortage, healthcare students are perceived to have a moral and professional obligation to volunteer, and are strongly encouraged to do so during pandemics [5]. Pre-registered healthcare students, when equipped with the right skills and knowledge, can render great support to the formal healthcare workforce. During the COVID-19 pandemic, medical students in Demark and the United Kingdom were mobilized as temporary residents, ventilator therapy assistants, or nursing assistants [7]. Similarly, final-year nursing students in Spain were deployed to work in hospitals to reinforce staffing levels, often remunerated similarly to nursing care assistants [8]. These students felt highly committed to volunteer and worked as nurses despite the uncertainty and non-completion of their nursing course [8]. However, the willingness of students to join the workforce was dependent on factors such as a sense of duty, perceived risk of infection, personal health, lack of protocol and knowledge, and perceived preparedness and skill competency required to execute volunteer duties [8–10].

In Singapore, the COVID-19 crisis evolved from multiple community cluster outbreaks in February 2020 to large endemic spreads in migrant worker dormitories, beginning in April 2020. These dormitories were high-density communal residences, with unhygienic living conditions for low-waged migrant workers who lacked equal access to healthcare and social safety-nets, and these factors elevated the risk of large outbreaks of respiratory diseases [11]. Hundreds of new migrant worker cases were detected daily, with numbers soaring to a peak of 1397 on 20 April 2020 [12]. A national task force was established to coordinate Singapore's outbreak response. As part of the public health strategy, mass testing facilitated the quick identification of cases, immediate isolation of cases, contact tracing and precautionary self-isolation of close contacts. This required trained personnel to conduct nasal swabs and serology tests on both infected and non-infected individuals, and placed manpower strains on Singapore's healthcare system. Apart from hiring short-term nasopharyngeal swabbers and swabbing assistants, Singapore's Ministry of Health sought volunteers from current and former healthcare professionals, as well as healthcare students, to support these testing efforts.

Eighty-five pre-registered final-year nursing students from a university in Singapore were approached in May 2020 to volunteer and perform venipuncture for migrant workers. Among them, only 27 (31%) volunteered. As competency in venipuncture was not part of the pre-registration undergraduate nursing curriculum in the university, these students underwent a phlebotomy course conducted by the university's nursing faculty, where they practiced venipuncture using simulated intravenous arms. Personal protective equipment (PPE) training and mask refitting were also conducted. These students were then deployed to the dormitories and received on-the-job training, with close supervision by a team of doctors, nurses, and phlebotomists from a hospital cluster. The student volunteers had to perform 20 successful venipunctures to certify their competency in phlebotomy. Thereafter, they would volunteer their phlebotomy services for six weeks. Additionally, three nursing faculty members, who also volunteered to be frontline phlebotomists, supervised or worked alongside these student volunteers.

Although the uptake of volunteering was similarly reported in Saudi Arabia [9], the authors expected the numbers to be higher, and wanted to understand how to improve future volunteering uptake and processes. By understanding the factors influencing pre-registered healthcare students' willingness to volunteer and their volunteer experience, healthcare leaders and volunteer managers can better facilitate manpower planning and volunteer recruitment for future crisis management. From an educational perspective, learning about students' decision-making on volunteering and their volunteering experiences in relation to professional identity may help to shape curriculum planning and enhance learning experiences. This study was thus undertaken to (a) explore factors influencing final-year nursing students' willingness to volunteer during the COVID-19 pandemic, (b) explore the role of professional identity in volunteering as a frontline healthcare worker among final-year nursing students, and (c) identify strategies to improve future volunteering uptakes and processes.

2. Methods

2.1. Design and Procedure

We performed a qualitative study and collected data via focus-group discussions (FGDs). Using a semi-structured interview guide, seven FGDs were conducted online via Microsoft Teams at the nursing institute of a Singapore university between September 2020 and November 2020. Prior to the start of data collection, the study protocol was approved by the University's Institutional Review Board ethics committee (IRB-2020-176). Invitation emails to participate in this study were sent to all fourth-year undergraduate nursing students, and to three lecturers who provided supervision to the student volunteers. Recruitment calls were also broadcasted by the researchers during the students' e-lecture. Interested participants contacted the research team and provided their personal contact details to arrange for the conduct of FGDs. Written informed consent was obtained from all study participants.

2.2. Participants

A total of 33 participants were recruited via purposive sampling and were grouped as follows: students who volunteered as frontline phlebotomists (3 FGDs, n = 15), students who did not volunteer (3 FGDs, n = 15), and lecturers who provided supervision to the student volunteers (1 FGD, n = 3). All 85 final-year undergraduate nursing students who were invited to volunteer as frontline phlebotomists between June and July 2020 were eligible to participate in this study. The three nursing faculty members who supervised or worked alongside the student volunteers also participated in this study. Individuals who refused to be video-recorded on Microsoft Teams were excluded. The demographic characteristics of the participants are presented in Table 1. None of the participants dropped out of the study.

Table 1. Characteristics of study participants (n = 33).

Characteristic	Nursing Students		Lecturers (n = 3)
	Volunteers (n = 15)	Non-Volunteers (n = 15)	
Gender			
Female	9	13	2
Male	6	2	1
Age (Mean ± SD)	23.5 ± 2.0	22.6 ± 0.9	-
Ethnicity			
Chinese	15	12	1
Malay	0	1	1
Indian	0	2	0
Other	0	0	1
Previous volunteering experience			
Yes	14	9	-
No	1	5	-
Prefer not to say	0	1	-

2.3. Data Collection

The research team developed an interview guide to explore the following topics: (a) the willingness of final-year nursing students to volunteer as frontline healthcare workers during the COVID-19 pandemic, (b) nursing students' consideration factors for volunteering or not volunteering as frontline healthcare workers, (c) the role of professional identity in influencing the decision and experience of volunteering as frontline healthcare workers, and (d) areas of improvement to increase voluntary participation as frontline healthcare workers and to enhance the volunteering experience. A pilot FGD involving five nursing students was conducted to test the questions and determine if they addressed the identified research aims. Data shared during the pilot FGD was not used for the analysis of this study. As the concept of professional identity was found to be abstract during the pilot FGD, several questions were rephrased to contextualize or personalize the act of volunteering, to elicit responses that addressed the study's aims. Examples of revised questions included: "Do you think nursing students are professionally obligated to volunteer in times of pandemic, and why?", and "Does your volunteering experience change the way you view yourself as a nurse?". The interview guide is presented in Table 2.

Table 2. Semi-structured interview guide.

- Willingness of final-year nursing students to volunteer as frontline healthcare personnel during the COVID-19 pandemic (volunteers/non-volunteers/lecturers)
    - Do you think healthcare students should be deployed to be frontline healthcare personnel during pandemic crises or national emergencies? Why?
    - Do you think final-year nursing students are equipped to volunteer as frontline healthcare personnel? Why?
    - Do you think if we give training to nursing students, they would be expected to volunteer? Why?
    - What are some of the volunteering activities that healthcare students can contribute?
- Nursing students' consideration factors for volunteering or not volunteering as frontline healthcare personnel (volunteers and non-volunteers)
    - What are some of the considerations to determine if you will volunteer?
    - How did you come to a decision to volunteer/not to volunteer as a frontline phlebotomist?
    - What are the top three key factors that led you to make that decision to volunteer/not volunteer?
    - Was it an easy or difficult decision to come to? Why?
- Role of professional identity in influencing the decision and experience of volunteering as frontline healthcare personnel
    - Do you think nursing students are professionally obligated/have a duty of care to volunteer in times of pandemic crisis? Why? (volunteers/non-volunteers/lecturers)
    - Do you think the students' professional identity was demonstrated during the course of their volunteering? Why? (lecturers)
    - Has your volunteering experience (volunteers)/the pandemic experience (non-volunteers) changed the way you view yourself as a nurse? In what way?
    - How was your experience of volunteering? (volunteers)
    - If you were asked to volunteer again, will you do it again? Why? (volunteers)
    - Do you feel part of the healthcare community? (volunteers/non-volunteers)
- Areas of improvement to increase voluntary participation as frontline healthcare personnel and to enhance the volunteering experience
    - What do you hope to change if you were to volunteer again? (volunteers)
    - What would discourage you to volunteer again? (volunteers)
    - What will make you change your mind to volunteer? (non-volunteers)
    - What would encourage nursing students to volunteer during a pandemic (lecturers)

All FGDs were moderated by the same researcher (B.S.); B.S. was accompanied by either colleague S.T.L. or S.Y.L., who co-moderated the sessions, took down field notes during the FGDs, and summarized content shared by participants at the end of each FGD. All the moderators (B.S., S.T.L. and S.Y.L.) were females, had completed a Ph.D., and had experience in conducting qualitative research. They were known to the participants as faculty members of the undergraduate nursing program. Where existing dependent and/or explicit relationships were involved, the researcher would not be involved in the FGD. No other persons were present except for the participants and the identified researchers. All interviews were video-recorded. The average duration of each online FGD was 92 min. No repeat focus-group interviews were conducted. Prior to the FGDs, participants completed a brief socio-demographic questionnaire. Memos were written by B.S. after the conduct of each FGD; they were shared with the two co-moderators and were used to assess data saturation.

2.4. Data Analysis

All the FGDs were transcribed verbatim. None of the transcripts were returned to participants for checking. Qualitative data were analyzed inductively using thematic analysis [13]. Coding was conducted independently by two researchers, B.S. and B.H. Two coders (B.S. and B.H.) first familiarized themselves with the data by reading and re-reading all transcripts and listened to all interview recordings. This was followed by independent coding of all transcripts with the aid of N-Vivo version 12 software and a Microsoft Excel spreadsheet, by B.S. and B.H., respectively. The two coders discussed their initial semantic codes with each other to resolve differences before they reduced these initial codes to latent codes, and to preliminary sub-themes and themes together. The entire process of data reduction was iterative. Subsequently, a consensus meeting with S.T.L. was held to reach an agreement on data interpretation and refine the sub-themes and themes.

3. Results

We identified three themes. They include (1) wavering thoughts on volunteering, (2) bringing out "the nurse" in students through volunteering, and (3) gearing up to volunteer. Table 3 depicts an overview of themes, sub-themes, and reduced codes.

Table 3. Process of data analysis.

Theme	Sub-Theme	Reduced Codes
Wavering thoughts on volunteering	Propelling intrinsic motivators	• To help • Concern for migrant workers • Personality • Apply knowledge and learn skills • Seek experiences • Have something to do • Not joining healthcare post-graduation
	Accounting for extrinsic concerns	• Pandemic uncertainty • Confidence in the healthcare system • Protecting family members • Peer influence • Academic concerns • Attractive incentives • Accountable to scholarship/sponsorship providers
Bringing out "the nurse" in students through volunteering	Displaying personal growth as a nurse	• Gaining confidence and proficiency in phlebotomy management • Appreciating pandemic management and workflow • Growing as a person • Demonstrating the attributes of a nurse
	Ascertaining the identity as a nurse	• Being part of the nursing community through volunteering • Strengthening the perceived identity of a nurse • Affirming the decision to be a nurse
	Entangled in the student role: "we are not full nurses yet"	• Duty of care as healthcare professionals • Student status • Student nurse versus employed nurse
Gearing up to volunteer	Healthcare and non-healthcare volunteering opportunities	• Healthcare students are equipped to volunteer • Ways and processes of signing up as a volunteer • Types of volunteering opportunities
	Operational workflow in managing student volunteers	• Organizing and providing details of the volunteering task • Providing venipuncture training for the volunteering task • Help is available when needed • Strategies to promote the uptake of volunteering • Strategies to promote the sustainability of volunteering

3.1. Wavering Thoughts on Volunteering

The first theme revealed the wavering thought processes of final-year nursing students making the decision to volunteer as frontline phlebotomists during the COVID-19 pandemic. Student participants found themselves in a dilemma, weighing their intrinsic motivations and the extrinsic concerns of volunteering. Although many were intrinsically motivated to volunteer and help, they wanted to *"know what I'm getting into before I make a responsible accountable decision"* as they had to consider *"the stakeholders involved and whether we would actually be helping when we offer our services to volunteer"*. Only a few of the student volunteers were not constrained by environmental considerations and stepped forward without hesitation.

> *"(It) was a very, very difficult decision ... like how difficult I would say is the email has a deadline for us to submit, right? I submitted like only 10 min before the deadline because I was deciding right up till that point."*
>
> (FGD1, P2, volunteer)

3.1.1. Propelling Intrinsic Motivators

Participants expressed that they volunteered because they wanted to contribute and help others; some were motivated by altruism, interest, and passion. A few mentioned that it was a calling, and they felt a responsibility to step up as future healthcare personnel. Three participants mentioned that they were looking for volunteering opportunities, even before the school approached them. Some participants were concerned about the mental health and welfare of migrant workers and wanted to help them. Two lecturers commented that personality played a great role; they observed that students who volunteered were more outspoken, outgoing, adventurous, and willing to learn.

As venipuncture was considered a new clinical skill, student participants had to appraise their confidence and skill competence. They recognized that confidence and clinical competence varied across peers. Some were afraid their inexperience and inabilities would burden the strained healthcare workforce. Some participants had the courage to volunteer, while others did not.

> *"There's a lot of expectations for us to be competent ... the nurses, physicians and all ... they are already very stressed, so we don't want to burden the rest also..."*
>
> (FGD1, P1, volunteer)

> *"I feel uncertain ... because ... we just completed our (clinical) attachment (placement) and personally, I feel I'm not competent enough to enter a pandemic situation when my competency in a clinical setting isn't stable."*
>
> (FGD6, P1, non-volunteer)

Student volunteers identified volunteering as a great opportunity to apply nursing knowledge and skills in *"real-life scenarios"*. They looked forward to seeking new, interesting, and meaningful learning experiences. A few mentioned that the opportunity to experience *"first-hand on the ground" "how a hot zone area works"* during pandemics was *"once in a lifetime"*. While some non-volunteers wanted a break from their clinical placement, others viewed volunteering as a purposeful activity to pass the time and avoid boredom at home. A few participants commented that some of their peers did not volunteer because they were uninterested in pursuing a career in nursing upon graduation.

3.1.2. Accounting for Extrinsic Concerns

Participants commented that the lack of information on disease transmission and management during the early phases of the pandemic brought about uncertainty, anxiety, and fear in them. A few were concerned whether they could withstand the hot, uncomfortable working environment, wearing their PPE. Only one participant expressed concern about PPE sufficiency. Most student volunteers, including lecturers, spoke of the confidence they had in their local healthcare system in ensuring safety measures were in place (e.g., decontamination procedures, protocols). Thus, concerns relating to volunteer training were afterthoughts.

> *"The last factor would be my trust in the system, knowing that your PPE is ALL there..."*
> (FGD2, P1, volunteer)

> *"Everyone was just going in the dark, and we were very much confident in the higher authority, like they will guide us."*
> (FGD3, P2, lecturer)

> *"Maybe because of our status as students we are not very clear on the decon procedures that hospital staff might be familiar with. So that kind of affects the confidence if I were to volunteer . . . what are the decontamination procedures afterward that (would) prevent me (from) bringing the virus out."*
> (FGD6, P3, non-volunteer)

Protecting their family was one of the primary factors driving students' decisions not to volunteer. Many revealed that ensuring their family members' safety outweighed their professional duties of volunteering. Volunteering at the front line meant that they would be exposed to COVID-19 and compromise the safety of their loved ones, particularly the very young and old family members who were deemed more vulnerable. As family held an important place, obtaining parental approval and encouragement contributed to their decision-making. Participants who volunteered said that their parents were supportive, and they would take additional precautionary measures (e.g., showering before going home, and minimizing mingling with family and friends). Students who did not volunteer shared about their parents' disapproval, and many would not *"go against their wishes"*.

> *"I did think of if I insisted on volunteering even though my family wasn't really keen. Then, what (are the) consequences if I end up contracting the virus? And what kind of burden will (I) put onto the family, like financially and emotionally? So in the end, I just say 'oh okay, maybe there will be other opportunities in the future to learn . . . I shouldn't be risking everything else just for my own learning."*
> (FGD6, P5, non-volunteer)

Peer influence also contributed to some participants' decision to volunteer. A few sought advice from classmates and seniors; others shared that volunteering with friends *"made the experience more fun"*. Being academically motivated, they contemplated their abilities to manage time. They wanted to fulfill their student role by performing well and completing their studies. While many participants acknowledged that the monetary incentive was highly attractive, it was not *"the biggest pushing factor although it was a key factor"* to account for the health risks involved. A few participants wanted to be accountable to their scholarship/sponsorship providers and were initially unsure whether they could both volunteer and receive monetary incentives.

3.2. Bringing Out "the Nurse" in Students through Volunteering

The second theme highlighted nursing students' enriched volunteering experiences and how the pandemic brought out the "nurse" identity among student volunteers and non-volunteers. Compared with employed registered nurses (RNs), these participants felt entangled and constrained by their "student status" in contributing as a nurse.

3.2.1. Displaying Personal Growth as a Nurse

Student participants who volunteered shared that they gained confidence and proficiency in phlebotomy management. This included technical skill competency, overcoming communication barriers with migrant workers, and observing clinical safety (e.g., patient identification, handling of sharps). Likewise, the lecturers witnessed their clinical progression and were impressed that *"by the end of the sessions, they have already mastered"* phlebotomy care management.

Student volunteers said they gained experiential knowledge about pandemic management and workflow processes. By observing the operation and organization of different zone areas in the dormitories, participants appreciated public health measures and how the local healthcare system functioned during a crisis. They recognized the importance of smooth workflow processes, workspace knowledge, protocol adherence and having buddy systems. Some were more cognizant and appreciative of the roles which laboratory technicians and hospital administrators played. Many participants spoke about the teamwork, camaraderie, and solidarity experienced within the healthcare team.

> *" . . . they (the students) saw how people from the lab... work in a pair . . . they (the students) saw this kind of coordinated movements and tried to mimic . . . because every time if you want to prepare to do the things, it takes time. So, one person does passes (of requisites), the second person (does) the withdrawal (to) collect blood. Then you swap the job or roles. So that was also a very good thing they observed and learned."*
>
> (FGD3, P2, lecturer)

> *"It was really very encouraging to see how everyone put aside their roles and positions to come and work together . . . they didn't care like how many doctors they have, how many nurses . . . senior nurses, how many students we have, as long as they meet the manpower needed . . . everyone just chip in and it doesn't matter where you come from or your experience. It just matters you contribute."*
>
> (FGD 4, P4, volunteer)

Student volunteers shared how they grew as a person through frontline volunteering. They were proud that they *"took the leap of faith"*, *"stepped out of their comfort zone"*, and proved to themselves that they could do the job; others learned to troubleshoot problems, built confidence in functioning independently and managing high risks. One participant added, and others agreed, that he learned an important skill—to *"say sorry"*.

> *'I learned . . . to say sorry. It is truly a vital skill to be very frank and to say that I am new, and I accidentally screwed up or I didn't manage to take blood. Would you allow me another try?"*
>
> (FGD 4, P2, volunteer)

Student participants mentioned how they learned and displayed the professional attributes of nurses. Through the pandemic, they saw how adaptable nurses are in performing *"multiple roles in multiple situations"*, beyond the clinical environment. Participants learned about the expanded scope of nurses and realized that *"nurses do even more"*. While student participants developed such insights, lecturers observed their spontaneity, passion, and caring demeanor. One student volunteer said, *"Caring is at the heart of what we do"*, and many learned to be *"unafraid to approach the situation"* and *"make the best decisions at that point in time"*. Others shared how they developed resilience, grit, and empathy.

3.2.2. Ascertaining an Identity as a Nurse

Student participants felt a greater sense of belonging to the nursing community after volunteering. They expressed positive feelings toward being able to contribute and enjoy meaningful interactions with migrant workers. Using nursing skills during the pandemic situation made *"us feel like we're different from the rest"*. They felt recognized for their efforts and were proud to be *"on par in terms of contribution like what the healthcare community was doing for Singapore"*. One participant shared that the staff *"valued me as part of the team though I am a novice to them"*. Those who volunteered unanimously said they would volunteer again. Conversely, those who did not volunteer felt left out, guilty, or regretted not being *"part of the whole team in fighting against COVID-19"*.

> *"I would volunteer again. Because I felt like I played my part and I want to play my part in the situation."*
>
> (FGD4, P1, volunteer)

"... they had a lack of manpower and that affected their burden at work, so I felt that if I had volunteered, ... my conscience (would have) felt a bit better."

(FGD6, P3, non-volunteer)

Regardless of their "volunteer status", the pandemic drew attention to student participants' sense of professional identity. It not only raised participants' awareness toward the public's mixed perception about nurses but also highlighted the societal value that the country placed on nurses. One participant shared how the pandemic strengthened her beliefs on what a nurse does and can do, solidifying her identity as a nurse. Some agreed that the volunteering opportunity broadened their perceptions toward the roles and responsibilities of nurses. Others mentioned that there was no change in how they view nursing, as they already knew what they *"signed up for"*.

"(The) pandemic wasn't really in the picture when I was considering to be a nurse... but now the pandemic becomes one of the things I have to overcome as a nurse ... I will be willing to learn more about emergency preparedness."

(FGD6, P2, non-volunteer)

"We should have also considered and known that with this kind of education comes a certain responsibility."

(FGF4, P2, volunteer)

Most participants affirmed that the pandemic cemented their decision of becoming a nurse and validated their choice of study in the university.

"It makes me feel like this is ... what I can, what I like to do, and what I can foresee myself to do in the future... Like (if) you can go through these very bad times, you can go through more in the future."

(FGD2, P5, volunteer)

3.2.3. Entangled in the Student Role: "We Are Not Full Nurses Yet"

Most student participants felt that full-fledged RNs have a duty of care during health crises, as nurses are equipped with specialized healthcare skills to step up. A few were conflicted that nurses had a personal choice to step up, as each had their own concerns. They shared that nurses who did not join the front line should not be viewed as *"wrong"*, *"not courageous enough"* or *"not worthy to be one"*.

"The public and nation trust us, nurses and healthcare professionals to step up and use their specialized knowledge to help out. And, to add on, they are getting paid. But then, as humans we have every right to our lives ... If patients have autonomy, I think nurses and doctors should have autonomy too... basically, knowledge is power. Power is like you can use it or you don't. It is not an obligation."

(FGD 1, P1, volunteer)

Student participants perceived that the professional obligation for RNs to step up is more prominent compared to that of nursing students. As students, they felt they should be given a choice to volunteer. Their priority was to fulfill academic requirements and learn as much as possible so that they could be competent in the future. Many wanted to contribute to the healthcare workforce but were limited by their *"student status"*; they knew they lacked clinical experience and could only perform basic tasks. One participant broached the topic that *"even in (the) clinical attachment, we were highly discouraged from going into isolation rooms... how can we be confident to attend to a pandemic crisis, to such an infectious virus?"* Compared to formal hospital staff, they were not familiar with hospital protocols and workflow. Thus, one participant said it was harder to volunteer as students.

Student participants looked up to and looked forward to being RNs. They highlighted that *"we are not really full nurses yet"* and were *"not fully part of the healthcare family"*. They lacked the RN license and were not employed. A few were concerned about their professional accountability as student volunteers. This added complexity, as they recognized that the schools would have to be accountable for them. Some participants shared that they would be more confident clinically if they were RNs. While they had the choice of volunteering as students, healthcare staff have work responsibilities. Thus, some mentioned it would be easier to convince their parents to allow them to volunteer as it would be *"part of their job"*. A number of participants hoped that they had the financial capability of employed nurses to find alternative accommodation, so that they could go ahead and volunteer, and not worry about infecting their family members.

3.3. *Gearing Up to Volunteer*

The third theme revealed the types and avenues of volunteering opportunities that nursing students could take. It also shed light on how operational workflows can be better managed for future volunteering roles during pandemics.

3.3.1. Healthcare and Non-Healthcare Volunteering Opportunities

Most participants felt that nursing students were equipped with fundamental PPE and infection control competencies to volunteer at the front line, and they *"have the potential to help a lot"*. A few participants expressed strongly that the deployment of healthcare students should precede lay individuals when outsourcing manpower during health crises. Depending on the care demands and clinical expertise needed, participants felt they could be trained and *"learned on the job"*. One student participant highlighted that *"even frontline workers might not be very prepared for this"*, and what was important was to quickly adapt and train individuals for the needed roles. Volunteer training instilled confidence and gave reassurance, by revising the required essential skills.

Alternative avenues of volunteering opportunities were shared. Prior to the university's invitation, some students expressed interest in contributing in COVID-19 related operations via the Singapore Healthcare Corps, an initiative coordinated by the Singapore Ministry of Health to provide support to healthcare and community care professionals by referring additional healthcare professionals and lay extenders to areas of need in COVID-19 operations and in community care. However, responses were slow, and participants who registered received no updates once the vacancies for volunteering opportunities were taken up. One participant joined a private home nursing agency and conducted health assessments for migrant workers living in dormitories.

Participants also shared alternative volunteering roles in which nursing students could participate. Most of them preferred to volunteer for familiar clinical-related roles that enabled them to apply their nursing knowledge. These included COVID-19 swab tests, basic ADL care and basic clinical assessment, so that hospital nurses could take on advanced responsibilities. A few suggested extending their clinical placement hours in hospitals to increase manpower. Some participants were less enthusiastic in volunteering for administrative and operational support roles. They perceived these roles as less meaningful or lacking interaction with people. On the contrary, a few highlighted that the job scope of such roles could be specified with greater clarity, as they included critical and meaningful work such as patient registration, transporting equipment, and ensuring colleagues gown and de-gown PPE properly. Options could be offered to volunteer in areas having no contact with potential or infected patients. This could ease students' concerns regarding the risks of infecting themselves and their family members.

> *"If there was an option of the logistics one, I might have gone. Because it's really the direct contact that I was worried about, especially with parents who are quite elderly and vulnerable."*
>
> (FGD5, P1, non-volunteer)

Others suggested community-based volunteering opportunities to assist vulnerable populations. They included delivering food to the elderly living alone, befriending the elderly, distributing masks, befriending migrant workers via hotlines, and translating health education materials for migrant workers.

3.3.2. Operational Workflow in Managing Student Volunteers

Participants highlighted the inadequate details of the volunteer program in the disseminated recruitment email. They were unsure about the commitment duration, on-site working conditions, decontamination process, presence of clinical supervision on-site, and whether their participation would affect their studies and graduation. Such information was only shared by lecturers during the venipuncture training. Some felt that they were kept *"in suspense"* for too long; the lack of such vital information made them feel less reassured. Some of their peers who registered were put off by the stipulated long volunteering hours, early reporting time and inconvenient volunteering sites. As such, a few withdrew. One participant suggested having a platform or point of contact for interested students to raise inquiries and assist them in making informed decisions. Information delivery could have been more organized and laid out more clearly.

> *"Initially when they send out the email, . . . the commitment is 5 days a week, 7 h a day . . . it seemed more daunting. But when I hear from my friend's experiences, it's not that frequent..."*
>
> (FGD 7, P3, non-volunteer)

Some participants felt the volunteering experiences were brief and wanted to be contacted earlier or allocated more slots so that they could contribute more. The recruitment and training of volunteers could be expedited. Some missed other volunteering opportunities. One participant attributed these negative experiences to the lack of a human resources coordinator to manage volunteers and coordinate volunteering activities.

Nonetheless, a few participants appreciated the opportunity provided by the university; they did not have to manage the administrative procedures of volunteering or worry about getting back to classes on time. Others mentioned that the university *"has done as much as they could"* to transition them to frontline phlebotomists. This included venipuncture training, certification of skill competency, coordinating volunteer schedules, lecturers overseeing the on-site safety of student volunteers, providing psychosocial assurance and advice on risk management and self-care. Having lecturers on-site gave student volunteers a sense of familiarity. They were figures of authority whom students could approach for assistance. Participants gave feedback that apart from having preceptors on-site, help was also constantly available from the ground staff.

> *"They were also very kind. If we had any difficulties locating the vein or taking the blood, we could approach any of the experienced people and they would do it for us very willingly."*
>
> (FGD 2, P4, volunteer)

Participants shared strategies to improve the uptake of future volunteering programs. A few suggested extending the program to first- and second-year nursing students, as well as students from other nursing schools, to increase volunteers. To motivate future student cohorts to volunteer, lecturers suggested producing a video montage to showcase students' volunteering experiences and inform prospective students about such volunteering opportunities. One lecturer suggested appointing student volunteers as pandemic ambassadors, to give talks and share their experiences with their peers. A few students recommended including pandemic management in the nursing curriculum, using COVID-19 as a case study. While such knowledge could prepare prospective students to be pandemic-ready, some non-volunteers cautioned that such knowledge would not change their decision to volunteer. Most non-volunteers would only change their mind if alternative accommodation were provided, as the risk of infecting family members was their key concern. A few participants suggested counting volunteering time as clinical placement hours to incentivize students to join.

> P3 (FGD 4): *"Moving forward, . . . instead of having the clinical (placement), (as) in like the clean cases, like maybe in the wards, why don't we give another option for students to clock in clinical hours . . . during the pandemic . . . ?"*

Moderator: " ... *That means the volunteer(ing) to be counted as clinical hours?"*

P3 (FGD 4): *"Yes. Because at least we have the best I would say, best of both worlds (of) being in the clean zone."*

Participants shared strategies to facilitate the smooth operation of this volunteer program and improve volunteering experiences. Some suggested providing orientation at the dormitories so that they could navigate the operational workflow processes to fit in better. Some participants wished they could have venipuncture practice on one another instead of using manikins. One participant suggested combining low-fidelity skills training with simulation to better manage patients. A few wanted to have more training sessions and an assessment on skill competency to boost their confidence. Others hoped to have more direct and closer on-site supervision for their initial venipuncture attempts.

When asked about what sustained volunteering efforts, participants identified interest, monetary incentives, peer support, camaraderie, assurance, and ease of getting help from approachable faculty members and healthcare staff. Two participants shared that following up with patients' serological results would allow them to see the impact they were making and sustain their motivation.

4. Discussion

The current study revealed the perceptions of final-year pre-registered nursing students volunteering as frontline healthcare workers during the COVID-19 pandemic, focusing on the factors influencing their decision to volunteer, the role of their professional identity as nurses to volunteer, and strategies to improve future volunteering uptake and processes. While the exploration of healthcare students' perceptions and experiences of volunteering during the COVID-19 pandemic is not new [8,9,14,15], this study contributes to the current literature by demonstrating what worked well, and the efforts to improve future operational processes when recruiting students as frontline healthcare workers to ease manpower constraints.

Our findings suggested that final-year nursing students' decisions to volunteer as frontline healthcare workers were multifaceted. We observed the interplay of intrinsic and extrinsic factors, as many faced a quandary in their decision-making. As is similar to past studies in COVID-19 and other pandemic situations [10,16,17], most of our student participants were willing and motivated to volunteer. Their motivation was accounted for by Clary and Snyder [18] as six personal and social functions that can be applied to other volunteering contexts in various crisis situations: (1) increasing expression of values such as altruism, (2) seeking learning opportunities and experiences to understand world-views during health crises, (3) enhancing personal growth and psychological development, such as through the fulfillment of their calling and passion pursuit, (4) gaining career-related clinical skills and experiences, (5) fortifying social relationships with peers and beneficiaries (e.g., migrant workers), and (6) protecting oneself from feeling bored, purposeless and guilty for not helping. As is consistent with observations made by our lecturers, Bazan et al. [19] reported that Polish medical students characterized by curious, sensitive, calm, and sociable personalities were more likely to volunteer. Individuals with such traits, linked to extraversion, agreeableness, and openness, have more salient helping identities, and are associated with a greater propensity to volunteer [20].

Protecting family safety emerged as a priority among student participants in this study and was a key determinant of the participants' decision to not volunteer. Although the fear of transmitting COVID-19 to susceptible significant others was reported among medical and nursing students in Spain, it did not stop them from volunteering [14]. Our findings highlighted the strong collectivist Asian family values and culture that Singapore students hold, regarding placing their family first. Similar findings on the fears for their family's health were reported among medical students in Indonesia [10]. Family interests are expected to overrule those of the individual [21]. As such, the provision of alternative accommodation for these non-volunteers would change their minds in stepping forward and increase the volunteering uptake. Offering concessionary prices for accommodation within the university campus could be a possible approach to support these students [15]. During the COVID-19 pandemic, non-volunteer nursing students in our study displayed the citizenship responsibilities of protecting family members, instead of assuming the professional duties of a nurse [8].

Despite this uncertainty, it was encouraging to learn that our participants had confidence in Singapore's healthcare system to enforce safety and operational measures for healthcare workers and volunteers. Some students were thus reassured enough to volunteer without worrying about training in PPE and venipuncture. This takes into consideration that our nursing students were approached in May 2020, when hundreds of new COVID-19 cases were reported daily in migrant-worker dormitories. Their confidence in Singapore's healthcare system could be attributed to the establishment of existing pandemic workflows and mitigation processes. Subsequently, when the participants were interviewed between September 2020 and November 2020, the spread of COVID-19 was under control and there were no migrant-worker cases detected. Our findings identified the importance of student volunteers having confidence in the healthcare system. During the earlier phases of the COVID-19 pandemic, healthcare student volunteers in other countries reported safety concerns related to insufficiency and limited access to PPE, and the lack of knowledge towards equipment usage [14,19].

Our study participants acknowledged that the monetary remuneration enticed them to volunteer and sustained their volunteering efforts. This differed from Lazarus et al.'s study [10], which reported a lack of association between monetary incentives and increased willingness to volunteer among undergraduate medical students in Indonesia. Additionally, our student participants suggested including volunteering as part of their clinical placement hours to incentivize peers to volunteer. Such academic-related incentives, which some healthcare education institutes in the United States and Europe employed as part of service-learning, internship programs, or curricular activities, require a prompt responsive curriculum redesign and strong hospital/community–campus partnerships [15,22,23]. While such formal or even mandatory academic incentives can encourage volunteer participation, they might reduce students' internal motivation and satisfaction regarding volunteer work [15]. To mitigate the negative effects and sustain volunteering efforts, as revealed in our findings, autonomy to choose the type and location of volunteer work could be given to students, as well as increasing students' perception of intrinsic motivation by demonstrating how volunteer work fits various goals [24,25].

The pandemic reminded student participants of the professional function of the healthcare knowledge and capabilities they were developing, which highlighted and strengthened their professional identity as nurses. While student volunteers had experiential learning, non-volunteers gained such perspectives through observations and peer-sharing. Nursing students generally related the "nurse" identity with their clinical abilities and gained new insights on the application of nursing skills [26]. At the personal level, our study participants displayed their "nurse" identity through acts of assertiveness, compassion, competence, confidence, conscience, commitment, and courage during the pandemic [27]. At the interpersonal level, they experienced continual personal growth, maturity and affirmation through professional socialization, as they cultivated their sense of belonging to the nursing community [27]. At the societal level, pandemics such as COVID-19 provided students with an opportunity to develop the psyche for forming an evolved professional identity of being "system citizens" who contribute to the needs of the healthcare system [22].

However, our findings showed that student participants' professional identity as nurses was still solidifying, which likely accounted for their wavering thoughts on volunteering. Toggling with their student role status, some participants expressed fear and uncertainty regarding their academic progress. This was also evident among final-year nursing students in Spain who were forced to work before they completed their studies [8]. Nonetheless, we observed a presenting range of professional maturity as nurses among the student volunteers. While some volunteers were in the "learner" mode of wanting to gain more skills and training, others transcended to the "professional" realm of volunteering dutifully, with the intention of serving as a nurse. As such, our study participants felt that they were "not full nurses yet" when volunteering as phlebotomists. This contrasted with Gomez-Ibanez et al.'s study [8], where final-year nursing students perceived themselves as nurses when they were pushed to mature faster professionally and function as nurses in the workforce. Volunteer administrators and educators thus need to be mindful and support such a transitionary phase of professional development among healthcare student volunteers. Examples of approaches identified were validating and addressing their academic concerns, providing adequate competency volunteer training and assessment, and empowering students to perform related clinical volunteer work independently and safely, to bridge the gap between being students and "professional" volunteers.

Student volunteers' sense of belonging to the profession was cemented as they accumulated clinical experiences through volunteering, and received consistent support and recognition from healthcare staff and the general public. Our findings supported past studies that feeling welcomed by healthcare staff, amicable staff interactions and behaviors, team comradeship and receiving appreciation are components instrumental in positive staff-student relationships, and cultivate a sense of belonging to sustain volunteering efforts [26,28]; these approaches made students feel valued and closer to being a member of the profession [26]. Thus, promoting cohesive and positive staff–student volunteer relationships, facilitating clinical guidance by allocating preceptors, providing psychosocial support, and close follow-up with students' interactions with healthcare staff are crucial in sustaining students' volunteering commitment and efforts.

Our student participants shared a wealth of alternative volunteering roles which they can contribute as part of their participatory service learning. Other studies also articulated roles in promoting pandemic safety awareness and mitigating the consequences of pandemic safety measures (e.g., social isolation) in the community, addressing pandemic-specific and non-COVID-19 healthcare and hospital operational processes, supporting daily living concerns outside the work responsibilities (e.g., childcare) of healthcare staff, and assisting in COVID-19-related research work [22,23,29]. In Singapore, we have a relatively large pool of more than 6000 nursing students, with various years of study, across different educational institutions. Identifying these potential areas of volunteering allows healthcare educational institutions, hospitals, and community agencies to tap students' capabilities and capacities for future pandemics.

Our findings highlighted the need to establish a tight volunteer management team from the university to ensure collaboration, coordination and regularly updated communication with our hospital/community partners and students. Such a team serves as a bridge between the university and hospital/community partners, attends to the details of operational processes, and facilitates smoother volunteer recruitment, training, placement, and coordination. In addition to articulating well-defined roles and clear workflows, Long et al. [22] emphasized that the first action of such a team was to ensure regulatory and safety measures were in place within the legal parameters and students' capacity. Depending on the nature of the voluntary tasks, contact proximity, and duration of contact with at-risk or infected COVID-19 patients, students may incur physical or psychological harm to themselves or others, and subject involved stakeholders to liability risks arising from their participation in spontaneous volunteering [3]. Fortunately, no needlestick injury was reported and our student volunteers were swabbed as negative for COVID-19 at the end of the program.

For healthcare students to function effectively in clinical-related volunteering roles, they need to be equipped with core competencies and well-prepared for pandemic or emergency situations [10]. Our findings revealed that students were not familiar with how healthcare systems respond during health emergencies. The lack of such knowledge was reported to be a barrier to volunteering during the COVID-19 pandemic among undergraduate healthcare students in Saudi Arabia [9]. Despite previous historical encounters with SARS, MERS and swine flu, not many universities, including our own, embed pandemic preparedness and education on the logistical challenges specific to pandemics in the undergraduate curriculum to ensure prospective healthcare workers are adequately prepared for future public health emergencies [30]. While our findings revealed that knowledge on pandemic preparedness might not increase the volunteering uptake, it could increase prospective healthcare professionals' reception, willingness, readiness, and confidence in managing future health emergencies. Our findings also shared strategies for healthcare educational institutions to showcase and encourage volunteerism among students during health emergencies.

Strengths and Limitations

One key strength of this study is the participation of nursing student volunteers and non-volunteers, as well as all the faculty involved in supervising the student volunteers on-site. The inclusion of different stakeholders for data source triangulation captured wide-ranging perspectives and allowed data validation [31]. Additionally, investigator triangulation via independent coding was performed by two researchers, followed by extensive discussion of results with other team members to enhance trustworthiness [31].

One limitation of this study is that considering the impact of the COVID-19 outbreak, e.g., incidence and mortality rate, and how Singapore's response to the virus differed from other countries, the findings of this study might be context-specific and might not be generalizable to other nursing student populations. The second limitation of this study was the small sample size of faculty members included, as there were only three faculty members who supervised or worked alongside the student volunteers. Another study limitation that might affect the generalizability of this study is the lack of ethnic representation among the nursing student volunteers sampled.

5. Conclusions

Our study affirmed that pre-registered nursing students are uniquely positioned to contribute gainfully during pandemics. These nursing students brought their health knowledge, awareness of the delivery of healthcare, understanding of COVID-19 as a societal challenge, professional maturity, and commitment to serve healthcare needs [22]. They should be considered as contingent resources in times of healthcare emergency crises, and they have the capacity and capability to take on both frontline and supportive roles to ease the burden on the healthcare workforce and the cost on society. Thus, our findings advocate strategic partnerships between the hospital/communities and academic institutions in providing various healthcare services during pandemic crises.

Our findings highlighted the importance of addressing pre-registered nursing students' extrinsic concerns to improve the volunteering uptake. Strategies identified included providing accommodation, as well as monetary and academic-related incentives. From the education and clinical perspectives, emergency preparedness and the scope of professional responsibilities during a pandemic should be introduced to the curriculum of pre-registered nursing students, to cultivate the "readiness to serve" attitude and aptitude in times of healthcare emergencies. Additionally, supporting the transitionary phase from students to "professional volunteers", promoting cohesive and positive staff-student volunteer relationships, and establishing volunteer management teams were strategies that were identified to improve operational processes when engaging pre-registered nursing students as frontline workers.

In summary, our findings suggested that we must look beyond the simplicity of altruism to the role of professional identity, operational, and motivational factors to explain final-year nursing students' intentions to volunteer and their volunteer behavior.

Author Contributions: Conceptualization, B.S., E.N.K.A. and S.T.L.; methodology, B.S., S.Y.L. and S.T.L.; formal analysis, B.S., B.H. and S.T.L.; writing—original draft preparation, B.S. and S.T.L.; writing—review and editing, B.S., S.Y.L. and S.T.L.; supervision E.N.K.A.; project administration, E.N.K.A. and S.T.L.; funding acquisition, S.T.L. All authors have read and agreed to the published version of the manuscript.

Funding: This research was funded by the Alice Lee Centre for Nursing Studies, Yong Loo Lin School of Medicine, National University of Singapore.

Institutional Review Board Statement: The study was conducted according to the guidelines of the Declaration of Helsinki, and approved by the Institutional Review Board of National University of Singapore (IRB-2020-176 and approved on 7 August 2020).

Informed Consent Statement: Informed consent was obtained from all subjects involved in the study.

Data Availability Statement: Raw data on the focus group discussion transcripts could be made available upon request. The data are not publicly available due to privacy.

Acknowledgments: We would like to thank all study participants who were involved in this study.

Conflicts of Interest: The authors declare no conflict of interest.

References

1. The World Health Organization Coronavirus Disease (COVID-19) Outbreak. Available online: https://www.who.int/emergencies/diseases/novel-coronavirus-2019 (accessed on 21 March 2021).
2. Aoyagi, Y.; Beck, C.R.; Dingwall, R.; Nguyen-Van-Tam, J.S. Healthcare workers' willingness to work during an influenza pandemic: A systematic review and meta-analysis. *Influenza Other Respir Viruses* **2015**, *9*, 120–130. [CrossRef] [PubMed]
3. Whittaker, J.; McLennan, B.; Handmer, J. A review of informal volunteerism in emergencies and disasters: Definition, opportunities and challenges. *Int. J. Disaster Risk Reduct.* **2015**, *13*, 358–368. [CrossRef]
4. Oh, N.; Hong, N.; Ryu, D.H.; Bae, S.G.; Kam, S.; Kim, K.Y. Exploring Nursing Intention, Stress, and Professionalism in Response to Infectious Disease Emergencies: The Experience of Local Public Hospital Nurses During the 2015 MERS Outbreak in South Korea. *Asian Nurs. Res.* **2017**, *11*, 230–236. [CrossRef] [PubMed]
5. Rosychuk, R.J.; Bailey, T.; Haines, C.; Lake, R.; Herman, B.; Yonge, O.; Marrie, T.J. Willingness to volunteer during an influenza pandemic: Perspectives from students and staff at a large Canadian university. *Influenza Other Respir Viruses* **2008**, *2*, 71–79. [CrossRef]
6. Turtle, L.; McGill, F.; Bettridge, J.; Matata, C.; Christley, R.; Solomon, T. A survey of UK healthcare workers' attitudes on volunteering to help with the Ebola outbreak in West Africa. *PLoS ONE* **2015**, *10*, e0120013. [CrossRef]
7. Rasmussen, S.; Sperling, P.; Poulsen, M.S.; Emmersen, J.; Andersen, S. Medical students for health-care staff shortages during the COVID-19 pandemic. *Lancet* **2020**, *395*, e79–e80. [CrossRef]
8. Gomez-Ibanez, R.; Watson, C.; Leyva-Moral, J.M.; Aguayo-Gonzalez, M.; Granel, N. Final-year nursing students called to work: Experiences of a rushed labour insertion during the COVID-19 pandemic. *Nurse Educ. Pr.* **2020**, *49*, 102920. [CrossRef] [PubMed]
9. AlOmar, R.S.; AlShamlan, N.A.; AlAmer, N.A.; Aldulijan, F.; AlMuhaidib, S.; Almukhadhib, O.; Algarni, S.A.; Alshaibani, A.; Darwish, M.; Al Shammari, M. What are the barriers and facilitators of volunteering among healthcare students during the COVID-19 pandemic? A Saudi-based cross-sectional study. *BMJ Open* **2021**, *11*, e042910. [CrossRef]
10. Lazarus, G.; Findyartini, A.; Putera, A.M.; Gamalliel, N.; Nugraha, D.; Adli, I.; Phowira, J.; Azzahra, L.; Ariffandi, B.; Widyahening, I.S. Willingness to volunteer and readiness to practice of undergraduate medical students during the COVID-19 pandemic: A cross-sectional survey in Indonesia. *BMC Med. Educ.* **2021**, *21*, 138. [CrossRef]
11. Yi, H.; Ng, S.T.; Farwin, A.; Pei Ting Low, A.; Chang, C.M.; Lim, J. Health equity considerations in COVID-19: Geospatial network analysis of the COVID-19 outbreak in the migrant population in Singapore. *J. Travel Med.* **2020**, *28*, taaa159. [CrossRef]
12. Ministry of Health COVID-19 Situation Report. Available online: https://covidsitrep.moh.gov.sg/ (accessed on 31 May 2021).
13. Braun, V.; Clarke, V. Using thematic analysis in psychology. *Qual. Res. Psychol.* **2006**, *3*, 77–101. [CrossRef]
14. Collado-Boira, E.J.; Ruiz-Palomino, E.; Salas-Media, P.; Folch-Ayora, A.; Muriach, M.; Balino, P. "The COVID-19 outbreak"-An empirical phenomenological study on perceptions and psychosocial considerations surrounding the immediate incorporation of final-year Spanish nursing and medical students into the health system. *Nurse Educ. Today* **2020**, *92*, 104504. [CrossRef]
15. Chawlowska, E.; Staszewski, R.; Lipiak, A.; Giernas, B.; Karasiewicz, M.; Bazan, D.; Nowosadko, M.; Cofta, M.; Wysocki, J. Student Volunteering as a Solution for Undergraduate Health Professions Education: Lessons From the COVID-19 Pandemic. *Front Public Health* **2020**, *8*, 633888. [CrossRef]
16. Cervera-Gasch, Á.; González-Chordá, V.M.; Mena-Tudela, D. COVID-19: Are Spanish medicine and nursing students prepared? *Nurse Educ. Today* **2020**, *92*, 104473. [CrossRef]
17. Yonge, O.; Rosychuk, R.J.; Bailey, T.M.; Lake, R.; Marrie, T.J. Willingness of university nursing students to volunteer during a pandemic. *Public Health Nurs.* **2010**, *27*, 174–180. [CrossRef]
18. Clary, E.G.; Snyder, M. The Motivations to Volunteer: Theoretical and Practical Considerations. *Curr. Dir. Psychol. Sci.* **1999**, *8*, 156–159. [CrossRef]
19. Bazan, D.; Nowicki, M.; Rzymski, P. Medical students as the volunteer workforce during the COVID-19 pandemic: Polish experience. *Int. J. Disaster Risk Reduct.* **2021**, *55*, 102109. [CrossRef] [PubMed]
20. Matsuba, M.K.; Hart, D.; Atkins, R. Psychological and social-structural influences on commitment to volunteering. *J. Res. Personal.* **2007**, *41*, 889–907. [CrossRef]

21. Tan, C. "Our shared values" in Singapore: A Confucian perspective. *Educ. Theory* **2012**, *62*, 449–463. [CrossRef]
22. Long, N.; Wolpaw, D.R.; Boothe, D.; Caldwell, C.; Dillon, P.; Gottshall, L.; Koetter, P.; Pooshpas, P.; Wolpaw, T.; Gonzalo, J.D. Contributions of Health Professions Students to Health System Needs During the COVID-19 Pandemic: Potential Strategies and Process for U.S. Medical Schools. *Acad. Med.* **2020**, *95*, 1679–1686. [CrossRef]
23. Bahethi, R.R.; Liu, B.Y.; Asriel, B.; Blum, J.R.; Huxley-Reicher, Z.; Agathis, A.Z.; Pathak, S.; Sainte Willis, M.; Muller, D. The COVID-19 Student WorkForce at the Icahn School of Medicine at Mount Sinai: A Model for Rapid Response in Emergency Preparedness. *Acad. Med.* **2021**, *96*, 859. [CrossRef]
24. Stukas, A.A.; Snyder, M.; Clary, E.G. Understanding and encouraging volunteerism and community involvement. *J. Soc. Psychol.* **2016**, *156*, 243–255. [CrossRef]
25. Henney, S.M.; Hackett, J.; Porreca, M.R. Involuntary Volunteerism: What Happens When You Require People to "Do Good? *J. Serv. Learn. High.* **2017**, *6*, 13.
26. Clements, A.J.; Kinman, G.; Leggetter, S.; Teoh, K.; Guppy, A. Exploring commitment, professional identity, and support for student nurses. *Nurse Educ. Pr.* **2016**, *16*, 20–26. [CrossRef] [PubMed]
27. Ohlén, J.; Segesten, K. The professional identity of the nurse: Concept analysis and development. *J. Adv. Nurs.* **1998**, *28*, 720–727. [CrossRef] [PubMed]
28. Levett-Jones, T.; Lathlean, J.; Higgins, I.; McMillan, M. Staff-student relationships and their impact on nursing students' belongingness and learning. *J. Adv. Nurs.* **2009**, *65*, 316–324. [CrossRef] [PubMed]
29. Gresh, A.; LaFave, S.; Thamilselvan, V.; Batchelder, A.; Mermer, J.; Jacques, K.; Greensfelder, A.; Buckley, M.; Cohen, Z.; Coy, A.; et al. Service learning in public health nursing education: How COVID-19 accelerated community-academic partnership. *Public Health Nurs.* **2021**, *38*, 248–257. [CrossRef] [PubMed]
30. O'Byrne, L.; Gavin, B.; McNicholas, F. Medical students and COVID-19: The need for pandemic preparedness. *J. Med. Ethics* **2020**, *46*, 623–626. [CrossRef]
31. Carter, N.; Bryant-Lukosius, D.; DiCenso, A.; Blythe, J.; Neville, A.J. The use of triangulation in qualitative research. *Oncol. Nurs. Forum.* **2014**, *41*, 545–547. [CrossRef]

International Journal of
Environmental Research and Public Health

MDPI

Article

Evaluation of the Risk of Anxiety and/or Depression during Confinement Due to COVID-19 in Central Spain

Rosa M Cárdaba-García [1,2,3], Lucia Pérez Pérez [1,2,4], Virtudes Niño Martín [1,2,5], Inés Cárdaba-García [6], Carlos Durantez-Fernández [7,*] and Elena Olea [1,2,8]

1 Nursing Department, Faculty of Nursing, University of Valladolid, 47005 Valladolid, Spain; rosacardaba@yahoo.es (R.M.C.-G.); lperezp@saludcastillayleon.es (L.P.P.); vninoger@gmail.com (V.N.M.); olea@ibgm.uva.es (E.O.)
2 Nursing Care Research (GICE), Faculty of Nursing, University of Valladolid, 47005 Valladolid, Spain
3 Emergencies Management (SACYL), 40002 Segovia, Spain
4 Primary Care Management Valladolid West (SACYL), 47012 Valladolid, Spain
5 Primary Care Management Valladolid East (SACYL), 47010 Valladolid, Spain
6 General Hospital of Segovia (SACYL), 40002 Segovia, Spain; inescardaba@gmail.com
7 Faculty of Health Sciences, University of Castilla-La Mancha, 45600 Talavera de la Reina, Spain
8 Department of Biochemistry and Molecular Biology and Physiology, University of Valladolid, 47005 Valladolid, Spain
* Correspondence: carlos.durantez@uclm.es; Tel.: +34-925-72-1010 (ext. 5678)

Abstract: (1) Background: The confinement of the population in response to the COVID-19 pandemic was related to an increased risk of suffering from anxiety and/or depression in previous studies with other populations. (2) Methods: descriptive study using surveys (Goldberg Anxiety and Depression Scale) with 808 participants over 18 years of age between 14 and 20 of May 2020 during the confinement due to the SARS-CoV-2 virus in Spain. (3) Results: 63% of the participants were at risk of suffering from anxiety and 64.9% were at risk of depression. Variables reaching statistical significance were: age (t anxiety = −0.139 and t depression = −0.153), gender (t anxiety = −4.152 and t depression = −4.178), marital status (anxiety F = 2.893 and depression F = 3.011), symptoms compatible with COVID-19 (t anxiety = −4.177 and t depression = −3.791), previous need for psychological help (t anxiety = −5.385 and t depression = −7.136) and need for such help at the time of the study (t anxiety = −9.144 and depression = −10.995). In addition, we generated two regression models that estimate the risk of anxiety and depression. (4) Conclusions: more than half of the participants were at risk of suffering from anxiety and/or depression, confirming the negative effect of confinement on the population.

Keywords: SARS-CoV-2; pandemic; confinement; Spain; depression; anxiety

Citation: Cárdaba-García, R.M.; Pérez Pérez, L.; Niño Martín, V.; Cárdaba-García, I.; Durantez-Fernández, C.; Olea, E. Evaluation of the Risk of Anxiety and/or Depression during Confinement Due to COVID-19 in Central Spain. *Int. J. Environ. Res. Public Health* **2021**, *18*, 5732. https://doi.org/10.3390/ijerph18115732

Academic Editors: Richard Gray and Sonia Udod

Received: 20 April 2021
Accepted: 25 May 2021
Published: 27 May 2021

1. Introduction

The pandemic produced by the SARS-CoV-2 virus has generated a global emergency, which has led to a series of measures that have included the confinement of the population in Spain and other countries [1,2].

On 31 December 2019, the WHO received a statement from the Chinese authorities of several cases of atypical pneumonia in the city of Wuhan [2,3]. A week later, this disease was termed COVID-19 (coronavirus disease 2019) after it was discovered that it was caused by a new coronavirus [4]. Months later, the virus spread rapidly throughout the world, with Spain being one of the most affected countries [5]. For this reason, the Spanish Government published a Royal Decree 463/2020 [6] on March 14 in the Official State Gazette, declaring a state of alarm for the management of the health crisis caused by COVID-19. Among other measures, the decree obliged the population to confine themselves to their homes from 15 March to 3 May 2020 [7]. This restriction of freedom of movement with the aim of controlling viral transmission was maintained at the time of the study, despite the relaxation of some of these restrictions. It was not until the publication of Order SND/380/2020, of 30 April, that the confinement measures were somewhat relaxed for the population over 14 years of age to allow outdoor sports [8]. Therefore, the Spanish population had remained strictly isolated in their homes for a little less than two consecutive months.

Although containment measures were necessary to control the outbreak, the possible consequences that confinement may have on the mental health of the population are still worrying [9–11]. Even the WHO recommended that the impact of confinement on people be quickly assessed to implement timely health measures that mitigate its harmful effects [12]. No similar situation has existed in Europe in recent years, but preliminary studies provide evidence of the deterioration of mental health in the population due to confinement. In China, two studies show higher rates of anxiety, depression, alcohol consumption and a lower proportion of mental well-being than usual in the population during the pandemic [13,14]. A study in India, with 1000 respondents with the Depression Anxiety Stress Scales (DASS21) questionnaire, presents significant differences between depression, anxiety and stress according to age, gender and employment [15]. In addition, in Italy, the mental health of the population has been affected and yet there have been fewer hospital admissions for psychological causes [16,17]. In the United Kingdom, research has been conducted that predicts anxiety and depression as a function of the presence of low income or loss of income and pre-existing health conditions in self and others [18]. Similarly in Denmark, higher rates of anxiety and depression due to confinement have also been found [19]. In Spain, the geographical area most affected by COVID-19 disease has been the center of the country [20], however, there is not previous research specifically investigating the mental health of the confined population in this region.

According to the prevalence of anxiety and depression in the aforementioned studies, we propose as working hypothesis that the confinement of the population of Spain was related to a greater risk of anxiety and/or depression. Hence, the objective of this study was to determine the risk of suffering from anxiety and/or depression in the Spanish population confined to regions of central Spain due to COVID-19.

2. Materials and Methods

2.1. Study Design

This is a descriptive study with a survey methodology carried out on a confined population. The data were collected from 14 to 20 May 2020. At that moment, the population had been confined to their homes for two months and de-escalation in Phase 0 had begun throughout Spain.

The study included persons residing in the central region of Spain during confinement, over 18 years of age, Spanish-speaking, with sufficient technical skills to answer an online survey and who voluntarily consented to participate in the study. We excluded Spaniards residing in other geographic areas than the central part of the country, those under 18 years of age, individuals who do not speak Spanish, those who don´t have the ability to handle online questionnaires and those who checked the refusal box in the study participation, even though they had completed the questionnaire.

2.2. Population and Ethical Aspects

We included the entire population over 18 years of age residing in central regions of Spain during the state of alarm due to SARS-CoV-2, who voluntarily accepted participation in the study on the indicated dates. A sample of 808 people who met the inclusion criteria was obtained.

The study was approved by the Ethics Committee for Drug Research of the Valladolid East health area, with registration code PI 20-1803 NO HCUV on 14 May 2020. This study conforms to the STROBE Initiative (Strengthening the Reporting of Observational Studies in Epidemiology) for observational studies of the EQUATOR Initiative [21].

2.3. Outcome Measures

The study variables we aimed to describe and correlate were: age, gender, marital status, being a health worker, place of confinement, number of confined people in the home, having been dismissed from work, suffering from COVID-19 symptoms (fever, headache, dry cough, sore throat, dyspnea, nausea and vomiting, diarrhea, fatigue, ageusia, and anosmia) [16], undergoing COVID-19 diagnostic tests (rapid antigen detection test or viral RNA detection by RT-PCR), a family member or friend who suffered from COVID-19, previous need for mental healthcare, current need for mental healthcare, being at risk of suffering from anxiety and/or depression.

2.4. Data Collection

Due to the conditions at the time of study, sampling was non-probabilistic through volunteering and secondarily by chain referral to obtain the largest possible sample. Recruitment was carried out through social networks (WhatsApp®, Facebook® and Twitter®), in which the link to the questionnaire was disseminated through Google Forms® on Google Drive®.

For data collection, we used a self-administered and anonymous questionnaire in which all the aforementioned variables were collected, using the Goldberg Anxiety and Depression Scale (GADS) [22,23] (Appendix A; Table A1). This screening tool measures the possibility of suffering from anxiety and/or depression. It consists of two subscales with nine items each, whose answers are dichotomous in a Yes/No format, and in which one point is assigned to an affirmative answer and 0 to a negative answer. The first four items of each of the subscales determine the risk of suffering from anxiety (in 4 points) and/or depression (in $\geq$2 points). Higher scores in each subscale are related to a higher risk, but the total score of the instrument (anxiety score and depression score) is not meaningful and generally not used, unless the first items show alteration. The anxiety scale has a sensitivity of 82% and the depression scale with 85%. The positive predictive value for anxiety is 0.56 and for depression 0.85 [22].

2.5. Data Analysis

We used descriptive analysis with measures of sample distribution (frequencies and percentages), centrality (mean) and dispersion (standard deviation [SD]) of the variables. Quantitative variables were analyzed using a normality test (Kolmogorov–Smirnov), using parametric tests (ANOVA, Student's t-test and Pearson's correlation coefficient) for the inferential analysis of the results and the total scores of the anxiety and depression subscales.

In an attempt to search for predictive models of factors related to anxiety and depression, we decided to use a Bayesian probability model. A multiple regression analysis was done in successive steps, from which predictive models with significant variables ($p \leq 0.01$) and model equations were obtained, both for anxiety and depression. For data analysis, we used IBM SPSS Statistics, version 24.0 (SPSS Inc., Chicago, IL, USA). In all tests, a confidence level of 95% and a p-value below 0.05 were considered significant.

3. Results

3.1. Descriptive Data

In total, 808 participants were included, who were between 18 and 80 years old, with a mean of 43.4 years (95% CI: 42.7–44.0, SD 19.0). The vast majority resided in the Autonomous Community of Castilla y León (76.6%); only 85 (10.5%) participants lived alone. The average number of cohabitants in a household was 2.35 (95% CI: 1.9–2.8, SD 1.3). Most participants had kept their jobs, had not been infected with COVID-19, had not presented compatible symptoms or required diagnostic tests. Regarding the need for psychological and psychiatric help, 244 people (30.2%) had needed it at some point in their life, while at the time of study, 10.8% were in need. 31.4% believed that confinement was negatively affecting cohabitation in their homes (Table 1).

Table 1. Frequency distribution and percentages of general variables (* N = 808), Spain, 2020.

Variables	Values: Frequency (N)/Percentage (%)
Gender	
Male	158 (19.6)
Female	650 (80.4)
Age (years)	
<40	325 (40.2)
40–49	221 (27.4)
50–59	151 (18.7)
>60	111 (13.7)
Marital status	
Married	354 (43.8)
Partnered	73 (9.0)
Separated or divorced	63 (7.8)
Single	306 (37.9)
Widowed	12 (1.5)
Healthcare worker	
Yes	172 (21.3)
Autonomous community	
Castilla y León	619 (76.6)
Madrid	85 (10.5)
Other	104 (12.9)
Number of cohabitants	
2	270 (33.4)
3	202 (25.0)
4	203 (25.1)
More than 4	48 (5.9)
Lived alone	85 (10.5)
Dismissal from work	
Yes	60 (7.4)
COVID-19 diagnostic	
Yes	30 (3.7)
Diagnostic COVID-19 test	
Yes	109 (13.5)
COVID-19 symptoms	
Yes	151 (18.7)
Family member or friend with COVID-19	
Yes	395 (48.9)
Previous psychological help	
Yes	244 (30.2)
Current psychological help	
Yes	87 (10.8)
Confinement in the household († n = 727)	
Yes	254 (34.9)

* N—total number of participants in the sample; † n—number of participants that were evaluated.

Table 2 shows the results of the anxiety and depression subscales in the GADS. To verify the reliability of the results, Crombach's α was calculated at 0.859 for the total scale (18 items), and at 0.793 and 0.776 for the anxiety (nine items) and depression (nine items) subscales, respectively, which confers validity to the results.

Table 2. Affirmative responses in anxiety and depression subscales of the GADS * († $N = 808$), Spain, 2020.

Key Symptom	Values: Frequency (*N*)/Percentage (%)
Anxiety Subscale of the GADS *	
Anguished and nervous	402 (49.8)
Worried	586 (72.5)
Irritable	377 (46.7)
Difficulty relaxing	435 (53.6)
Bad sleep quality	472 (58.4)
Headache	417 (41.6)
Tremor and/or tingling and/or dizziness and/or sweating and/or diarrhea	201 (24.9)
Worried about health	449 (55.6)
Difficulty falling asleep	472 (58.4)
Depression Subscale of the GADS *	
Key Symptom	**Values: Frequency (*N*)/Percentage (%)**
Low energy levels	464 (57.4)
Loss of interest in things	314 (38.9)
Loss of self-confidence	163 (20.2)
Hopelessness	188 (23.3)
Difficulties concentrating	422 (42.2)
Weight loss	150 (18.6)
Wakes up earlier than usual	369 (45.7)
Slowness in carrying out activities	383 (47.4)
Feeling worse in the morning	244 (30.2)

* Goldberg Anxiety and Depression Scale; † *N*—total number of participants in the sample.

Considering the cutoff number of the first four items of each subscale, 63% (509) of the sample was at risk of suffering from anxiety (4 points in the first four items of the anxiety subscale) and 64.9% (524) were at risk of depression (≥2 in the first four items of the depression subscale) (Table 3). The mean anxiety subscale score was 4.72, (95% CI 3.78–5.66, SD 1.43); while in the depression subscale, the mean of responses was 3.34 (95% CI 2.46–4.22, SD 1.36).

Table 3. Prevalence of anxiety and depression symptoms according to GADS * ($N = 808$), Spain, 2020.

Variables	Frequency († $n = 808$)	Percentage %	CI 95%
Symptoms of anxiety			
Yes (=4)	509	63	59.6–66.4
No (<4)	299	37	33.6–40.4
Symptoms of depression			
Yes (≥2)	524	64.9	61.5–68.1
No (<2)	284	35.1	31.8–38.4

* Goldberg Anxiety and Depression Scale; † *n*—number of participants that were evaluated.

3.2. Inferential Analysis

We performed parametric tests after verifying the normal distribution of the total scores on the anxiety and depression subscales to determine the relationship between sociodemographic variables, COVID-19-related variables, and the results of the GADS questionnaire subscales (Table 4).

Table 4. Inferential analysis between variables and scale GADS † (N = 808), Spain, 2020.

Variables	Pearson Correlation Coefficient (r)	
	Anxiety	**Depression**
Age	−0.139 *	−0.153 *
Number of cohabitants	0.044	0.027
Variables	**ANOVA (F)**	
	Anxiety	**Depression**
Marital status	2.893 **	3.011 **
Cohabitation	13.636 **	10.007 **
Geographical place	0.934	1.220
Variables	**Student *t*-Test (*t*)**	
	Anxiety	**Depression**
Gender	−4.152 **	−4.178 **
COVID symptoms	−4.177 **	−3.791 **
Health profession	−1.694	1.651
Job dismissal	−1.554	−1.546
COVID diagnostic	0.104	0.010
COVID tests	−1.226	−2.324 *
COVID diagnostic of family member or friend	−2.183 *	−1.851
Psychological or psychiatric care (pre pandemic)	−5.385 *	−7.136 **
Psychological or psychiatric care (during pandemic)	−9.144 **	−10.995 **

* $p < 0.05$; ** $p < 0.01$; † Goldberg Anxiety and Depression Scale.

In relation to age, the Pearson correlation coefficient was −0.139 for anxiety and −0.153 for depression, both weakly statistically significant (p = 0.01 bilateral). It is shown that at an older age the risk of suffering from anxiety and depression decreases. Concerning gender differences, we compared means with the Student's t test, obtaining the value t = −4.152 (p = 0.000) in anxiety, and a value t = −4.178 (p = 0.000) in depression. Both anxiety and depression symptoms were much more frequent in women.

Among the variables that showed significant results in both anxiety and depression scores, we identified the marital status of the participants (ANOVA anxiety F = 2.893; p = 0.002 and ANOVA depression F = 3.011; p = 0.002), having had symptoms compatible with COVID-19 (t anxiety = −4.177; p = 0.000 and t depression = −3.791; p = 0.000) and cohabitation (ANOVA anxiety F = 13.636; p = 0.000 and ANOVA depression F = 10.007; p = 0.000). Nonetheless, the number of cohabitants did not reach statistical significance according to Pearson's correlation coefficient, 0.044 for anxiety and 0.027 for depression (p = 0.01 bilateral).

In contrast, the variables that did not show a statistically significant relationship were: the geographical place of residence (anxiety ANOVA: F = 0.934; p = 0.495 and depression ANOVA: F = 1.220; p = 0.279), health profession (anxiety t = −1.694; p = 0.091; and t depression = −1.651; p = 0.099), job dismissal (t anxiety = −1.554; p = 0.121 and t depression = −1.546; p = 0.123) and having been diagnosed with SARS-CoV-2 infection (t anxiety = 0.104; p = 0.917 and t depression = 0.010; p = 0.992).

Having undergone diagnostic tests for COVID-19 had no statistical significance for anxiety (t = −1.226; p = 0.221), but it did for depression (t = −2.324; p = 0.020). However, having a family member or friend who had suffered from SARS-CoV-2 produced statistically significant differences in anxiety (t = −2.183; p = 0.029), but not in depression (t = −1.851; p = 0.065).

Finally, subjects who previously required psychological or psychiatric care were more likely to suffer from anxiety (t = −5.385; p = 0.000) and depression (t = −7.136; p = 0.000). Similar results were obtained if such help was needed at the time of the study (t anxiety = −9.144; p = 0.000 and t depression = −10.995; p = 0.000).

3.3. Regression Analysis

We did a successive step multiple linear regression analysis to determine which variables played a more important role in producing anxiety and depression symptoms ($p < 0.01$) (Table 5).

Table 5. Models of regression analysis. Theorem 1 and Theorem 2 (N = 808), Spain, 2020.

Factor	Theorem 1					
	B	Standard Error	β	t	p	CI 95%
Constant	10.226	1.077		9497	0.000	8.102–12.35
Cohabitation	1.400	0.301	0.322	4.658	0.000	0.807–1.003
Age	−0.033	0.010	−0.225	−3.259	0.001	−0.052–−0.013
COVID symptoms	1.394	0.447	0.197	3.118	0.002	0.512–2.275
Factor	**Theorem 2**					
	B	Standard Error	β	t	p	CI 95%
Constant	11.221	0.867		12.944	0.000	9.511–12.931
Age	−0.046	0.009	−0.333	−4.968	0.000	−0.064–−0.028
Cohabitation	1.281	0.279	0.308	4.600	0.000	0.732–1.830

$$\text{Total anxiety score} = 10.226 + (1400 \times \text{cohabitation}) - (0.03 \times \text{age}) + (1.394 \times \text{COVID symptoms}) \tag{1}$$

Theorem 1. *The variables 'living with someone during confinement', 'age' and 'presenting symptoms of COVID infection' increase the score on the anxiety subscale of the GADS instrument and therefore the subjective perception of suffering from anxiety. The results determine a predictor model of anxiety ($R^2 = 0.245$).*

$$\text{Total depression score} = 11.221\ (-0.046 \times \text{age}) + (1.281 \times \text{cohabitation}) \tag{2}$$

Theorem 2. *The variables 'age' and 'living with someone during confinement' increase the score on the depression subscale of the GADS instrument and therefore the subjective perception of suffering from depression, with a predictive model of depression ($R^2 = 0.289$).*

4. Discussion

Taking into account the research findings, the working hypothesis can be partially accepted, since the factors age, gender, marital status, suffering from symptoms compatible with COVID-19 and requiring previous or current psychological care, were related to having an increased risk of anxiety and/or depression. Having undergone a diagnostic test for SARS-CoV-2 increased the risk of depression whereas having a family member or friend sick with COVID-19 increased the risk of anxiety.

Based on the results, it seems logical to say that confinement has had a negative effect on the population of central Spanish areas, which has been at risk of suffering from symptoms of anxiety and depression, results comparable with other studies carried out in Spain [3,5] and other countries [13–19].

It is surprising that unemployment was not identified as an essential factor for either depression or anxiety, since it is usually related to symptoms thereof in other studies [5,7,15,18,24]. The reason for this result is unknown, however, it may be related to participants responding more positively to a temporary dismissal that resulted from a reversible adjustment of employment levels due to the pandemic. Similarly, ample scientific literature describes the risk of suffering from anxiety and depression in the health professions [1,7,25]. In both cases, the low representation of these groups in the sample may have influenced the results. The economic influence of the pandemic should be carefully monitored by public organizations to support financially and psychologically numerous self-employed professions [26].

The low rates of positive COVID-19 diagnoses are consistent with epidemiological data published by the Ministry of Health, according to which around 5% of the population had developed antibodies to SARS-CoV-2 at the time of study [27]. The frequency of symptoms compatible with SARS-CoV-2 was higher than the percentage of positive diagnostic tests, probably, as other authors point out, because these symptoms are sometimes nonspecific as is the case with fever, dry cough, and gastrointestinal symptoms [28].

Unsurprisingly, having required psychological help previously or at the time of study was related to the presence of anxious–depressive symptoms. However, some participants had had professional help at some point in their life but not during the pandemic. The cause of this effect is unknown, and it should be studied in depth in future research, since it contradicts the existing literature [17,29,30].

That younger people are at greater risk of anxiety and depression than older people was not surprising, coinciding with Ahmeda et al. [14]. Age was the variable that most influenced the presence of anxious–depressive symptoms together with gender, as corroborated by other studies [13,15,18,19]. In China, the most affected age range is 21 to 40 years [14]. In India, 15 to 35 years of age [15]. In the United Kingdom, early ages are the most affected [18] and in Denmark the middle ages [19].

Having to undergo a diagnostic test for COVID-19 increases the risk of depression. This result agrees with that of Chinese researchers who related it to mechanisms of anticipation of suffering the disease [31]. In addition, having a close person diagnosed as COVID-19-positive was related to anxiety, as also pointed out by Inchausti et al. [7] and Alamri et al. [32].

Living with at least two people has been considered an advantage since it may provide emotional support [18], but not all the scientific literature agrees on this point. Some studies highlight the need for a space of solitude within your own home, which is more complicated if you live with someone [23,33]. Jimenez et al. agree on quality of cohabitation and age were found to be key variables in the psychological impact of confinement [34]. Our results show that, during confinement, the number of cohabitants was not relevant for the development of anxiety or depression. However, cohabitation in general was relevant, as it constituted a risk factor for suffering from anxiety and depression. Marital status was another variable that had an influence on presenting anxious–depressive symptoms, and is related to cohabitation. Some research has revealed a greater perceived social support by people who have a partner, which seems of utmost importance during confinement [18,23].

Finally, it should be noted that the study provides a reality that, in the early stages of the pandemic, when the absolute priority was the lives of people, was not taken into account. Although some authors have published studies on this subject [34], in the case of Spain there is not much research and even less in our population group belonging to the central region of the country. The findings of this research show the possibility of suffering from anxiety and depression in a situation of home confinement and justify the creation of health programs to prevent this alteration of psychological health, as well as early detection, follow-up and treatment of the problems generated by isolation in the home in the face of an illness that entails major changes in living and working habits. Certain skills such as self-efficacy and the possibility that increasing self-compassion may be used to promote better mental health in similar situations [35–37].

Limitations

We encountered difficulties during the study due to the circumstances associated with its design, which is why we might have incurred a selection bias in the participants due to a non-randomized sample. We assumed this bias due to the impossibility of accessing a large sample volume in such short period of time with other sampling methods. Due to the time required for approval by the ethics committee and the different rates of de-escalation in the different autonomous communities, most of the sample came from Castilla y León and Madrid, which impedes generalizing the results to the entire country. This sampling, however, strengthens the homogeneity of our data since both regions were still in Phase

0 of the de-escalation on the dates of study. Based on these issues, we propose to obtain a representative sample of the national population in the future. In addition, the use of a Likert scale questionnaire may generate response biases such as social desirability and acquiescence response [38,39], validation data can help quantify or mitigate this issue [40,41].

5. Conclusions

This study aimed to assess the risk of anxiety and/or depression during confinement due to the COVID-19 pandemic in the Spanish population. We found that 63% of the sample was at risk of suffering from anxiety and 64.9% at risk of depression.

The factors age, gender, marital status, suffering from symptoms compatible with COVID-19 and needing previous or current psychological help, were related to a greater risk of anxiety and/or depression. The risk of anxiety was fundamentally related to cohabitation, age and presenting symptoms compatible with COVID-19, while the risk of depression was mainly related to cohabitation and age.

In conclusion, taking care of the mental health of the population is essential in situations of confinement due to a pandemic. This requires developing action plans that allow an immediate response in the event of a further wave of SARS-CoV-2 or pandemics caused by other infectious agents.

Author Contributions: Conceptualization, R.M.C.-G. and I.C.-G.; methodology, E.O.; software, C.D.-F.; validation, L.P.P., V.N.M. and R.M.C.-G.; formal analysis, R.M.C.-G.; investigation, I.C.-G.; resources, L.P.P.; data curation, E.O.; writing—original draft preparation, R.M.C.-G.; writing—review and editing, C.D.-F.; visualization, I.C.-G.; supervision, R.M.C.-G.; project administration, R.M.C.-G.; funding acquisition, V.N.M. All authors have read and agreed to the published version of the manuscript.

Funding: This research received no external funding.

Institutional Review Board Statement: The study was conducted according to the guidelines of the Declaration of Helsinki, and approved by the Ethics Committee for Drug Research of the Valladolid East Health Area (PI 20-1803 NO HCUV on 14 May 2020).

Informed Consent Statement: Informed consent was obtained from all subjects involved in the study.

Data Availability Statement: The data presented in this study are available on request from the corresponding author.

Conflicts of Interest: The authors declare no conflict of interest. The funders had no role in the design of the study; in the collection, analyses, or interpretation of data; in the writing of the manuscript, or in the decision to publish the results.

Appendix A

Table A1. Self-administered questionnaire.

1. Age
2. Sex
- Male
- Female
- Other
3. Relationship status
- Married
- Cohabitation
- Separated/Divorced
- Widower/Widow
- Single

Table A1. *Cont.*

4. Are you a Health worker? - Yes - No 5. Where are you confined? - Castile and León - Madrid - Other 6. How many people, including you, are living confined at home? - Just me - 2 - 3 - 4 - More than 4 7. Do you have a job dismissal due to COVID-19? - Yes - No 8. Do you have been diagnosed with COVID-19? - Yes - No 10. Do you have been tested for COVID-19? - Yes - No 11. Do you have had any symptoms compatible with COVID-19? - Yes - No 12. Do you have anyone in your family or friends diagnosed with COVID-19? - Yes - No 13. Do you have ever needed psychological or psychiatric help? - Yes - No 14. Are you needing psychological or psychiatric help these days? - Yes - No 15. Do you think that confinement is negatively affecting your coexistence? - Yes - No 16. Regarding the last week of confinement (Goldberg Anxiety and Depression Scale) *

* Participants answered 18 anxiety and depression-related questions from the Goldberg Anxiety and Depression Scale (GADS), which are copyrighted and cannot be disseminated without permission from the authors who created and validated the questionnaire for this purpose.

References

1. Ibáñez-Vizosó, J.E.; Alberdi-Páaramo, I.; Díaz-Marsá, M. International Mental Health perspectives on the novel coronavirus SARS-CoV-2 pandemic. *Rev. Psiquiatr. Salud Ment.* **2020**, *13*, 111–113.
2. Fernández-Riquelme, S. Primera Historia de la crisis del Coronavirus en España. *La Razón Histórica Rev. Hispanoam. Hist. Ideas Políticas Soc.* **2020**, *46*, 12–22.
3. Ozamiz-Etxebarria, N.; Dosil-Santamaria, M.; Picaza-Gorrochategui, M.; Idoiaga-Mondragon, N. Niveles de estrés, ansiedad y depresión en la primera fase del brote del COVID-19 en una muestra recogida en el norte de España. *Cad. Saúde Pública* **2020**, *36*, e00054020. [CrossRef] [PubMed]
4. Cruz, M.P.; Santos, E.; Cervantes, M.V.; Juárez, M.L. COVID-19, una emergencia de salud pública mundial. *Rev. Clínica Española* **2021**, *221*, 55–61. [CrossRef]
5. Sandín, B.; Valiente, R.M.; García-Escalera, J.; Chorot, P. Psychological impact of the COVID-19 pandemic: Negative and positive effects in Spanish people during the mandatory national quarantine. *Rev. Psicopatología Psicol. Clínica* **2020**, *25*, 1–22. [CrossRef]
6. Real Decreto 463/2020. Boletín Oficial del Estado, n° 67, 14 de Marzo de 2020. pp. 25390–25400. Available online: https://www.boe.es/eli/es/rd/2020/03/14/463 (accessed on 20 April 2021).
7. Inchausti, F.; García-Poveda, N.V.; Prado-Abril, J.; Sánchez-Reales, S. La Psicología Clínica ante la Pandemia COVID-19 en España. *Clínica Salud* **2020**, *31*, 105–107. [CrossRef]

8. Orden SND/380/2020. Boletín Oficial del Estado, n° 121, 30 de Abril de 2020. pp. 30925–30929. Available online: https://www.boe.es/eli/es/o/2020/04/30/snd380/con (accessed on 20 April 2021).
9. Urzúa, A.; Vera-Villarroel, P.; Caqueo-Urízar, A.; Polanco-Carrasco, R. La Psicología en la prevención y manejo del COVID-19. Aportes desde la evidencia inicial. *Rev. Int. Psicol. Ter. Psicol.* **2020**, *38*, 103–118.
10. Ramírez-Ortiz, J.; Castro-Quintero, D.; Lerma-Córdoba, C.; Yela-Ceballos, F.; Escobar-Córdoba, F. Mental health consequences of the COVID-19 pandemic associated with social isolation. *Colomb. J. Anesthesiol.* **2020**, *48*, e930. [CrossRef]
11. Qiu, J.; Shen, B.; Zhao, M.; Wang, Z.; Xie, B.; Xu, Y. A nationwide survey of psychological distress among Chinese people in the COVID-19 epidemic: Implications and policy recommendations. *Gen. Psychiatry* **2020**, *33*, e100213. [CrossRef]
12. Tricco, A.C.; Langlois, E.V.; Straus, S.E. *Rapid Reviews to Strengthen Health Policy and Systems: A Practical Guide*; World Health Organization: Geneva, Switzerland, 2017; Available online: https://www.who.int/alliance-hpsr/resources/publications/rapid-review-guide/en/ (accessed on 20 April 2021).
13. Meng, H.; Xu, Y.; Dai, J.; Zhang, Y.; Liu, B.; Yang, H. Analyze the psychological impact of COVID-19 among the elderly population in China and make corresponding suggestions. *Psychiatry Res.* **2020**, *289*, 112983. [CrossRef]
14. Ahmed, M.Z.; Ahmed, O.; Zhou, A.; Sang, H.; Liu, S.; Ahmad, A. Epidemic of COVID-19 in China and associated Psychological Problems. *Asian J. Psychiatry* **2020**, *51*, 102092. [CrossRef]
15. Husain-Kazmi, S.S.; Hasan, K.; Talib, S.; Saxena, S. COVID-19 and Lockdown: A study on the Impact on Mental Health 19. *SRNN* **2020**, 1–13. [CrossRef]
16. Girardi, P. COVID-19: An Epidemiological Perspective. Ph.D. Thesis, Dipartimento di Psicologia dello Sviluppo e della Socializzazione Universita' degli Studi di Padova, Padova, Italy, 2020.
17. Clerici, M.; Durbano, F.; Spinogatti, F.; Vita, A.; De Girolamo, G.; Micciolo, R. Psychiatric hospitalization rates in Italy before and during COVID-19: Did they change? An analysis of register data. *Ir. J. Psychol. Med.* **2020**, *37*, 283–290. [CrossRef] [PubMed]
18. Shevlin, M.; McBride, O.; Murphy, J.; Miller, J.G.; Hartman, T.K.; Levita, L.; Mason, L.; Martinez, A.P.; McKay, R.; Stocks, T.V.A.; et al. Anxiety, depression, traumatic stress and COVID-19-related anxiety in the UK general population during the COVID-19 pandemic. *BJPsych Open* **2020**, *6*, e125. [CrossRef] [PubMed]
19. Sønderskov, K.M.; Dinesen, P.T.; Santini, Z.I.; Østergaard, S.D. The depressive state of Denmark during the COVID-19 pandemic. *Acta Neuropsychiatr.* **2020**, *32*, 226–228. [CrossRef]
20. Pollán, M.; Pérez-Gómez, B.; Pastor-Barriuso, R.; Oteo, J.; Hernán, M.A.; Pérez-Olmeda, M.; Sanmartín, J.L.; Fernández-García, A.; Cruz, I.; de Larrea, N.F.; et al. Prevalence of SARS-CoV-2 in Spain (ENE-COVID): A nationwide, population-based seroepidemiological study. *Lancet* **2020**, *396*, 535–544. [CrossRef]
21. Vandenbroucke, J.P.; Von Elm, E.; Altman, D.G.; Gøtzsche, P.C.; Mulrow, C.D.; Pocock, S.J.; Poole, C.; Schlesselman, J.J.; Egger, M. Strengthening the reporting of observational studies in epidemiology (STROBE): Explanation and elaboration. *Gac. Sanit.* **2009**, *23*, 158.e1–158.e28. [CrossRef]
22. Goldberg, D.; Bridges, K.; Duncan-Jones, P.; Grayson, D. Detecting anxiety and depression in general medical settings. *BMJ* **1988**, *297*, 897–899. [CrossRef]
23. Montón, C.; Pérez-Echevarría, M.J.; Campos, R. Escalas de ansiedad y depresión de Goldberg: Una guía de entrevista eficaz para la detección del malestar psíquico. *Aten. Primaria* **1993**, *12*, 345–349.
24. García-Hernández, A.M. Duelo y confinamiento. *Rev. Ene Enfermería* **2020**, *14*, 1–7.
25. Sher, L. COVID-19, anxiety, sleep disturbances and suicide. *Sleep Med.* **2020**, *70*, 124. [CrossRef]
26. Dalewski, B.; Palka, L.; Kiczmer, P.; Sobolewska, E. The Impact of SARS-CoV-2 Outbreak on the Polish Dental Community's Standards of Care—A Six-Month Retrospective Survey-Based Study. *Int. J. Environ. Res. Public Health* **2021**, *18*, 1281. [CrossRef]
27. Ministerio de Sanidad de España. Madrid. Available online: https://www.mscbs.gob.es/gabinete/notasPrensa.do?id=4950 (accessed on 20 April 2021).
28. Becerra-García, J.A.; Giménez, G.; Sánchez-Gutiérrez, T.; Barbeito Resa, S.; Calvo Calvo, A. Síntomas psicopatológicos du-rante la cuarentena por COVID-19 en población general española: Un análisis preliminar en función de variables sociodemo-gráficas y ambientales-ocupacionales. *Rev. Esp. Salud Publica* **2020**, *94*, e1–e11.
29. Vieta, E.; Pérez, V.; Arango, C. Psychiatry in the aftermath of COVID-19. *Rev. Psiquiatr. Salud Ment.* **2020**, *13*, 105–110. [CrossRef]
30. Crespo-Facorro, B. Mental health and the SARS-CoV-2 pandemic. *Rev. Psiquiatr. Salud Ment.* **2020**, *13*, 55–56. [CrossRef] [PubMed]
31. Liu, N.; Zhang, F.; Wei, C.; Jia, Y.; Shang, Z.; Sun, L.; Wu, L.; Sun, Z.; Zhou, Y.; Wang, Y.; et al. Prevalence and predictors of PTSS during COVID-19 outbreak in China hardest-hit areas: Gender differences matter. *Psychiatry Res.* **2020**, *287*, 112921. [CrossRef] [PubMed]
32. Alamri, H.S.; Algarni, A.; Shehata, S.F.; Al Bshabshe, A.; AlShehri, N.N.; AlAsiri, A.M.; Hussain, A.H.; Alalmay, A.Y.; AlShehri, E.A.; AlQarni, Y.; et al. Prevalence of Depression, Anxiety, and Stress among the General Population in Saudi Arabia during Covid-19 Pandemic. *Int. J. Environ. Res. Public Health* **2020**, *17*, 9183. [CrossRef]
33. Pérez-Martínez, J.A. Diario de un mes de confinamiento (12 de marzo de 2020–15 de abril de 2020). *La Razón Histórica* **2020**, *46*, 32–38.
34. Jiménez, Ó.; Sánchez-Sánchez, L.C.; García-Montes, J.M. Psychological Impact of COVID-19 Confinement and Its Relationship with Meditation. *Int. J. Environ. Res. Public Health* **2020**, *17*, 6642. [CrossRef] [PubMed]
35. Gutiérrez-Hernández, M.; Fanjul, L.; Díaz-Megolla, A.; Reyes-Hurtado, P.; Herrera-Rodríguez, J.; Enjuto-Castellanos, M.; Peñate, W. COVID-19 Lockdown and Mental Health in a Sample Population in Spain: The Role of Self-Compassion. *Int. J. Environ. Res. Public Health* **2021**, *18*, 2103. [CrossRef]

36. Marle, C.J.-L.; Parmentier, F.; Vinchon, F.; Storme, M.; Borteyrou, X.; Lubart, T. Evolution and impact of self-efficacy during French COVID-19 confinement: A longitudinal study. *J. Gen. Psychol.* **2021**, *148*, 360–381. [CrossRef] [PubMed]
37. Waters, L.; Algoe, S.B.; Dutton, J.; Emmons, R.; Fredrickson, B.L.; Heaphy, E.; Moskowitz, J.T.; Neff, K.; Niemiec, R.; Pury, C.; et al. Positive psychology in a pandemic: Buffering, bolstering, and building mental health. *J. Posit. Psychol.* **2021**, 1–21. [CrossRef]
38. Kreitchmann, R.S.; Abad, F.J.; Ponsoda, V.; Nieto, M.D.; Morillo, D. Controlling for Response Biases in Self-Report Scales: Forced-Choice vs. Psychometric Modeling of Likert Items. *Front. Psychol.* **2019**, *10*, 2309. [CrossRef] [PubMed]
39. Morillo, D.; Abad, F.J.; Kreitchmann, R.S.; Leenen, I.; Hontangas, P.; Ponsoda, V. The Journey from Likert to Forced-Choice Questionnaires: Evidence of the Invariance of Item Parameters. *Rev. Psicol. Trab. Organ.* **2019**, *35*, 75–83. [CrossRef]
40. Bauhoff, S. Self-Report Bias in Estimating Cross-Sectional and Treatment Effects. In *Encyclopedia of Quality of Life and Well-Being Research*; Metzler, J.B., Ed.; Springer: Dodlerk, The Netherlands, 2014; pp. 5798–5800.
41. Harpe, S.E. How to analyze Likert and other rating scale data. *Curr. Pharm. Teach. Learn.* **2015**, *7*, 836–850. [CrossRef]

MDPI
St. Alban-Anlage 66
4052 Basel
Switzerland
www.mdpi.com

International Journal of Environmental Research and Public Health Editorial Office
E-mail: ijerph@mdpi.com
www.mdpi.com/journal/ijerph